Handbook of Evidence-Based Radiation Oncology

2nd Edition

Handbook of Evidence-Based Radiation Oncology

2nd Edition

Eric K. Hansen, MD
The Oregon Clinic
Radiation Oncology
Providence St. Vincent Medical Center
Portland, Oregon, USA

Mack Roach, III, MD, FACR
Professor, Radiation Oncology and Urology
Chair, Department of Radiation Oncology
UCSF Helen Diller Family Comprehensive Cancer Center
University of California San Francisco
San Francisco, California, USA

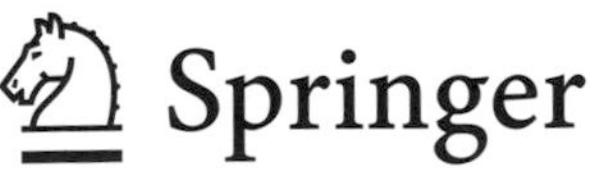

Dr. Eric K. Hansen
The Oregon Clinic,
Providence St. Vincent Medical Center,
Portland, OR, USA
e-mail: eric.hansen@providence.org

Dr. Mack Roach III
University of California,
San Francisco, CA, USA
e-mail: mroach@radonc.ucsf.edu

ISBN: 978-0-387-92987-3 e-ISBN: 978-0-387-92988-0

DOI: 10.1007/978-0-387-92988-0

Springer New York Heidelberg Dordrecht London

Library of Congress Control Number: 2009942763

Cover designer: Joe Piliero

Printed on acid-free paper

Springer is part of Springer Science+Business Media (www.springer.com)

Dedication

To Keith Hansen – Compassionate and dedicated physician; loving husband, father, and grandfather. You were larger than life!

Preface to the 2nd Edition

The first edition of *Handbook of Evidence-Based Radiation Oncology* was extremely successful and well received by the worldwide oncology community. In the second edition, we have kept the same concise format in order to remain a practical quick reference guide. Yet we have also added new content and features based on the valuable feedback from readers. All chapters have been revised and include the latest key studies and radiotherapy techniques. Color figures are included for the first time. Three new chapters have been written, including management of the neck and unknown primary of the head and neck, urethral cancer, and clinical radiobiology and physics. An appendix on use of IV contrast has been added as well.

We are particularly pleased that our second edition includes the newly published 2010 AJCC and 2008 FIGO staging systems. We recognize that there will be a transition period in which the previous staging systems will continue to be widely used. For this reason and at the AJCC's specific demand, the previous staging systems are included as well.

We have again strived to maintain a balance of including the most important information for practitioners while also limiting the size of the handbook so that it did not become a full-sized textbook. As before, we strongly encourage readers to refer to the primary literature for further details and references not included here. Although this handbook provides treatment algorithms and suggestions, it remains the professional responsibility of the practitioner, relying on experience and knowledge of the patient, to determine the best treatment for each individual.

We are grateful to all the contributing authors, including multiple new ones, for their hard work and dedication. We believe *Handbook of Evidence-Based Radiation Oncology* will continue to be an invaluable resource for students, resident physicians, fellows, and other practitioners of radiation oncology.

Last, we owe special thanks to our families for their patience during our work on this new edition.

Eric K. Hansen
Mack Roach, III

Portland, OR
San Francisco, CA

Preface to the 1st Edition

Management of patients in radiation oncology is constantly evolving as the medical literature continues to grow exponentially. Our practices have become increasingly evidence-based. In this setting, it is critical to have a practical and rapid reference. The *Handbook of Radiation Oncology* is designed with this purpose in mind.

Each clinical chapter is organized in a concise manner. First, important "pearls" of epidemiology, anatomy, pathology, and presentation are highlighted. The key facets of the work-up are then listed followed by staging and/or risk classification systems. Treatment recommendations are provided based on stage, histology, and/or risk classification. Brief summaries of key trials and studies provide the rationale for the treatment recommendations. Practical guidelines for radiation techniques are described. Finally, complications of treatment and follow-up guidelines are listed.

This handbook grew out of a practical need for a rapid reference for students, resident physicians, fellows, and other practitioners of radiation oncology. To be concise and portable, we limited the potential pages and pages of references that could have been included in the handbook (so that it did not become a textbook). Numerous sources were used to compile the information in each chapter, including the primary literature, each of the outstanding radiation oncology reference books (*Textbook of Radiation Oncology, Principles and Practice of Radiation Oncology, Radiation Oncology Rationale Technique Results, Clinical Radiation Oncology*, and *Pediatric Radiation Oncology*), the National Comprehensive Cancer Network Guidelines (at www.nccn.org), the National Cancer Institute's Physician Data Query Cancer Information Summaries (at www.cancer.gov), the American Society for Therapeutic Radiology and Oncology Annual Meeting Educational Sessions, and the notes of the radiation oncology residents at UCSF. Because a lengthy book could easily be written for many of the individual chapters, readers are encouraged to refer to the primary literature and the sources listed above for further details and references not listed in this handbook.

The handbook provides guidelines and suggestions, but it cannot replace the experience of clinicians skilled in the art of radiation oncology. It is the professional responsibility of the practitioner, relying on experience and knowledge of the patient, to determine the best treatment for each individual. Moreover, changes in care may become necessary and appropriate as new research is published, clinical experience is expanded, and/or changes occur in government regulations.

We thank all the contributors for their hours of hard work. We owe them a debt of gratitude for their excellent chapters and their promptness that made the task of editing this handbook much easier.

Eric K. Hansen — Portland, OR
Mack Roach, III — San Francisco, CA

Contents

VII. GENITOURINARY SITES

VIII. GYNECOLOGIC SITES

IX. LYMPHOMAS AND MYELOMA

X. MUSCULOSKELETAL SITES

XI. PEDIATRIC (NON-CNS)

XII. PALLIATION

Contributors

R. Scott Bermudez, MD
Radiation Oncology, University of California San Francisco,
San Francisco, CA, USA

Thomas Thanh Bui, MD
Radiation Oncology, University of California San Francisco,
San Francisco, CA, USA

Linda W. Chan, MD
Radiation Oncology, University of California San Francisco,
San Francisco, CA, USA

Chien Peter Chen, MD
Radiation Oncology, University of California San Francisco,
San Francisco, CA, USA

Hans T. Chung, MD
Radiation Oncology, Sunnybrook Odette Cancer Centre,
University of Toronto, Toronto, ON, Canada

Joy Coleman, MD
Radiation Oncology, Elmhurst Memorial Hospital, Elmhurst, IL, USA

Charlotte Dai Kubicky, MD, PhD
Radiation Medicine, Oregon Health and Science University,
Portland, OR, USA

William Foster, MD
Radiation Oncology, University of California San Francisco,
San Francisco, CA, USA

Barbara Fowble, MD
Radiation Oncology, University of California San Francisco,
San Francisco, CA, USA

Amy M. Gillis, MD
Radiation Oncology, Kaiser Permanente, San Francisco, CA, USA

Alexander R. Gottschalk, MD
Radiation Oncology, University of California San Francisco, San Francisco, CA, USA

Daphne A. Haas Kogan, MD
Radiation Oncology, University of California San Francisco, San Francisco, CA, USA

Eric K. Hansen, MD
Radiation Oncology, The Oregon Clinic,
Providence St. Vincent Medical Center, Portland, OR, US

I-Chow Hsu, MD
Radiation Oncology, University of California San Francisco, San Francisco, CA, USA

Kim Huang, MD
Radiation Oncology, University of California San Francisco, San Francisco, CA, USA

Siavash Jabbari, MD
Radiation Oncology, University of California San Francisco, San Francisco, CA, USA

Tania Kaprealian, MD
Radiation Oncology, University of California San Francisco, San Francisco, CA, USA

David A. Larson, MD, PhD
Radiation Oncology, University of California San Francisco, San Francisco, CA, USA

Brian Lee, MD, PhD
Radiation Oncology, Swedish Hospital, Seattle, WA, USA

Lawrence Margolis, MD
Radiation Oncology, University of California San Francisco, San Francisco, CA, USA

Kavita K. Mishra, MD, MPH
Radiation Oncology, University of California San Francisco, San Francisco, CA, USA

Brian Missett, MD
Radiation Oncology, Kaiser Permanente Santa Clara, Santa Clara, CA, USA

Jean L. Nakamura, MD
Radiation Oncology, University of California San Francisco, San Francisco, CA, USA

Marc B. Nash, MD
Radiation Oncology, University of California San Francisco, San Francisco, CA, USA

Catherine Park, MD
Radiation Oncology, Helen Diller Family Comprehensive Cancer Center, University of California San Francisco, San Francisco, CA, USA

Sunanda Pejavar, MD
Radiation Oncology, University of California San Francisco, San Francisco, CA, USA

Jean Pouliot, PhD
Physics Division, Radiation Oncology, University of California San Francisco, San Francisco, CA, USA

Gautam Prasad, MD, PhD
Radiation Oncology, University of California San Francisco, San Francisco, CA, USA

Jeanne Quivey, MD, FACR
Radiation Oncology, University of California San Francisco, San Francisco, CA, USA

James L. Rembert, MD
Alta Bates Summit Comprehensive Cancer Center, Berkeley, CA, USA

Mack Roach III, MD
Department of Radiation Oncology, University of California San Francisco, San Francisco, CA, USA

Naomi R. Schechter, MD
Radiation Oncology, University of California San Francisco,
San Francisco, CA, USA

Stephen L. Shiao, MD, PhD
Radiation Oncology, University of California San Francisco,
San Francisco, CA, USA

Jocelyn L. Speight, MD, PhD
Board Certified Radiation Oncologist, San Francisco, CA, USA

Stuart Y. Tsuji, MD, PhD
Radiation Oncology, University of California San Francisco,
San Francisco, CA, USA

Alice Wang-Chesebro, MD
Providence Portland Radiation Oncology, The Oregon Clinic, P.C.,
Portland, OR, USA

William M. Wara, MD
Radiation Oncology, University of California San Francisco,
San Francisco, CA, USA

Fred Y. Wu, MD, PhD
Radiation Oncology, University of California San Francisco,
San Francisco, CA, USA

Sue S. Yom, MD
Radiation Oncology, University of California San Francisco,
San Francisco, CA, USA

Jennifer S. Yu, MD, PhD
Radiation Oncology, University of California San Francisco,
San Francisco, CA, USA

PART I
Skin

1

Chapter 1
Skin Cancer

Tania Kaprealian, James Rembert, Lawrence W. Margolis, and Sue S. Yom

COMMON SKIN CARCINOMAS

PEARLS

- Basal cell carcinoma (BCC) and squamous cell carcinoma (SCC) of skin are the most common malignancies in the US.
- Greater than one million unreported cases of BCC and SCC occur annually.
- Main histologic types: BCC (65%), SCC (35%), adnexal (5%), melanoma (1.5%).
- More common in men (4:1).
- Median age: 68 (SCC and BCC).
- Most common predisposing factor: UV exposure.
- Other predisposing factors: chronic irritation, trauma, occupational exposure, genetic disorders (phenylketonuria, basal cell nevus syndrome [Gorlin's], xeroderma pigmentosum, giant congenital nevi), immunosuppression (drug-induced, leukemia/lymphoma, HIV).
- Common routes of spread: lateral and deep along path of least resistance, perineural invasion (60–70% are asymptomatic), and regional LN.
- *Basal cell carcinoma.*
  - Pathologic subtypes: nodulo-ulcerative (50%), superficial (33%), morpheaform (sclerosing), infiltrative, pigmented, fibroepithelial tumor of Pinkus, and basosquamous (rare, almost always on face, metastatic rate same as SCC).
  - Only 0.1% perineural spread (mostly with recurrent, locally advanced, after irradiation failure), and "skip areas" common.
  - Most common CN affected: V and VII.
  - Grow very slowly and <0.01% metastasize (regional LN (66%) > lung, liver, bones (20%)).

- *Squamous cell carcinoma.*
  - Pathologic subtypes: *Bowen's disease (CIS)* grows slowly as a sharply demarcated plaque, and is treated with surgery, cryotherapy, topical 5-FU, or RT (40 Gy/10 fx). *Erythroplasia of Queyrat* is Bowen's of the penis. *Marjolin's Ulcer* is SCC within a burn scar. *Verrucous* carcinoma is low grade, exophytic, and often anogenital, oral, or on the plantar surface of the foot. *Spindle cell* presents most commonly on sun-exposed areas of whites >40-year old.
  - Approximately 7% PNI (associated with nodal involvement and base of skull invasion).
  - Nodal involvement.
    - Well differentiated: 1%.
    - Poorly differentiated, recurrent, >3 cm greatest dimension, >4 mm depth, or located on lips: 10%.
    - Located on burn scars/osteomyelitic site: 10–30%.
  - Distant Mets: 2% to lung, liver, bones.
    - Factors that determine distant mets: anatomic site, duration and size of lesion, depth or dermal invasion, and degree of differentiation.
  - SCC originating from normal appearing skin vs. sun-damaged skin appears to invade more rapidly and has greater incidence of metastases.
- *Adnexal and eccrine carcinomas* of the skin are more aggressive than SCC with propensity for nodal and hematogenous spread.
- *Melanoma and Merkel cell carcinomas* will be briefly discussed after the following discussion of SCC/BCC.

WORKUP

- H&P. Palpate for nonsuperficial extent of tumor. For head/face lesions, do a detailed CN exam. Evaluate regional LN.
- Biopsy.
- CT or MRI for suspected nodal involvement. MRI if PNI suspected, and for lesions of medial/lateral canthi, to rule out orbit involvement. CT is useful to rule out suspected bone invasion.

STAGING: NONMELANOMA SKIN CARCINOMA

Editors' note: All TNM stage and stage groups referred to elsewhere in this chapter reflect the 2002 AJCC staging nomenclature unless otherwise noted as the new system below was published after this chapter was written.

(AJCC 6TH ED., 2002)

Primary tumor (T)
- TX: Primary tumor cannot be assessed
- T0: No evidence of primary tumor
- Tis: Carcinoma in situ
- T1: Tumor 2 cm or less in greatest dimension
- T2: Tumor more than 2 cm, but not more than 5 cm, in greatest dimension
- T3: Tumor more than 5 cm in greatest dimension
- T4: Tumor invades deep extradermal structures (i.e., cartilage, skeletal muscle, or bone)

Regional lymph nodes (N)
- NX: No regional lymph node metastasis can be assessed
- N0: No regional lymph node metastasis
- N1: Regional lymph node metastasis

Distant metastasis (M)
- MX: Distant metastasis cannot be assessed
- M0: No distant metastasis
- M1: Distant metastasis

Note: In case of multiple simultaneous tumors, the tumor with the highest T category will be classified and the number of separate tumors will be indicated in parentheses, e.g., T2 (5).

Stage grouping
- 0: TisN0M0
- I: T1N0M0
- II: T2–3N0M0
- III: T4N0M0, AnyTN1M0
- IV: M1

~5-Year local control

All comers: Mohs 99%, other tx ~90%

RT for SCC: T1 98%, T2 80%, T3 50%

RT for BCC: up to 5–10% better than SCC

Used with the permission from the American Joint Committee on Cancer (AJCC), Chicago, IL. The original source for this material is the AJCC Cancer Staging Manual, Sixth Edition (2002), published by Springer Science+Business Media.

(AJCC 7TH ED., 2010)

Primary tumor (T)*
- TX: Primary tumor cannot be assessed
- T0: No evidence of primary tumor
- Tis: Carcinoma in situ
- T1: Tumor 2 cm or less in greatest dimension with less than two high-risk features**
- T2: Tumor greater than 2 cm in greatest dimension or Tumor any size with two or more high-risk features*
- T3: Tumor with invasion of maxilla, mandible, orbit, or temporal bone
- T4: Tumor with invasion of skeleton (axial or appendicular) or perineural invasion of skull base

**Note*: Excludes cSCC of the eyelid

**High-risk features for the primary tumor (T) staging

Depth/invasion: >2 mm thickness, Clark level ≥IV, Perineural invasion.

Anatomic location: Primary site ear, Primary site nonhair-bearing lip.

Differentiation: Poorly differentiated or undifferentiated.

Regional lymph nodes (N)
- NX: Regional lymph nodes cannot be assessed
- N0: No regional lymph node metastases
- N1: Metastasis in a single ipsilateral lymph node, 3 cm or less in greatest dimension
- N2: Metastasis in a single ipsilateral lymph node, more than 3 cm but not more than 6 cm in greatest dimension; or in multiple ipsilateral lymph nodes, not more than 6 cm in greatest dimension; or in bilateral or contralateral lymph nodes, not more than 6 cm in greatest dimension

continued

N2a: Metastasis in a single ipsilateral lymph node, more than 3 cm but not more than 6 cm in greatest dimension
N2b: Metastasis in multiple ipsilateral lymph nodes, not more than 6 cm in greatest dimension
N2c: Metastasis in bilateral or contralateral lymph nodes, not more than 6 cm in greatest dimension
N3: Metastasis in a lymph node, more than 6 cm in greatest dimension

Distant metastasis (M)
M0: No distant metastases
M1: Distant metastases

Anatomic stage/prognostic groups
0: Tis N0 M0
I: T1 N0 M0
II: T2 N0 M0
III: T3 N0 M0
T1–T3 N1 M0
IV: T1–T3 N2 M0
T Any N3 M0
T4 N Any M0
T Any N Any M1

TREATMENT RECOMMENDATIONS

- Six major therapies: cryotherapy, curettage/electrodesiccation, chemotherapy, surgical excision, Mohs micrographic surgery, and RT
- Treatment indications
  - *Cryotherapy*: small, superficial BCC, and well-differentiated SCC with distinct margins
  - *Curettage and electrodesiccation*: same indications as cryotherapy, but typically not used for recurrences or cancers overlying scar tissue, cartilage, or bone
  - *Chemotherapy*
    - *Imiquimod or topical 5-FU*: premalignant or superficial lesions confined to epidermis, or large superficial areas of actinic keratosis
    - *Systemic:* not typically used but PR 60–70%, CR 30%
  - *Surgical excision*: reconstructive advances have made more patients surgical candidates
  - *Mohs micrographic surgery*: maximal skin sparing through staged micrographic examination of each horizontal and deep margin; if persistent positive margins or perineural invasion should be followed by post-op RT
  - *RT:* typically recommended for primary and recurrent lesions of the central face >5 mm (especially for the eyelids, tip/ala of the nose, and lips) and large lesions (>2 cm) on the ears, forehead, and scalp that would potentially have poor functional and cosmetic outcomes after Mohs
- Positive margins after excision
  - One-third BCC recur if lateral margin + and >50% if deep margin+
  - Most SCC recur at + margin and can recur loco-regionally with <50% salvage rate if LN+
  - Both types should be retreated with reexcision or radiotherapy if + margin. For SCC, retreatment should be done immediately
- *Post-op RT indications*: + margins, PNI of named nerve, >3 cm primary, extensive skeletal muscle invasion, bone/cartilage invasion, and SCC of the parotid
- *Relative RT contraindications*: age <50 (cosmetic results worsen over time), postradiation recurrences (suboptimal salvage rates with reirradiation – use Mohs), area prone to repeated trauma (dorsum of hand, bony prominence, belt line), poor blood supply (below knees/ elbows), high occupational sun exposure, impaired lymphatics, exposed cartilage/bone, Gorlin's syndrome, CD4 count <200

continued

- Approximately 5-year local control
  - All comers: Mohs 99%, other treatment(tx)~90%
  - RT for SCC: T1 98%, T2 80%, T3 50%
  - RT for BCC: up to 5–10% better than SCC

RADIATION TECHNIQUES

SIMULATION AND FIELD DESIGN

- Superficial/orthovoltage X-rays and megavoltage electrons are most commonly used to cure skin cancers.
- Orthovoltage advantages: less margin on skin surface, less expensive than electrons, D_{max} at skin surface, skin collimation with lead cutout (0.95 mm Pb for <150 kV beam; 1.9 mm Pb for >150 kV beam).
- Most common orthovoltage energies: 50, 100, 150, 200, 250, 300 kV; must specify filter/HVL.
- Select an energy so that the 90% depth dose encompasses tumor (90% IDL: 50 kV [0.7 mm Al] ~1 mm; 100 kV [4–7 mm Al] ~5 mm; 150 kV [0.52 mm Cu] 1.0 cm).
- Orthovoltage is not appropriate for >1 cm deep lesions.
- *f* factor (roentgen-rad conversion): increases dramatically below 300 kV which can lead to much higher dose to tissue with high atomic number (e.g., bone). Thus, if carcinomas invade bone, megavoltage beams give a more homogeneous distribution. There is little variation in dose delivered to cartilage, regardless of orthovoltage energy.
- Must specify filtration (HVL's) in orthovoltage beams; generally choose thickest filter providing a dose rate >50 cGy/min (Al typically for 50/100 kV and Cu for higher energy; now most machines provide only one filter per energy).
- RBE of orthovoltage X-rays is 10–15% higher than RBE of megavoltage electrons/photons, so must raise daily and total doses by 10–15% with megavoltage electrons/photons compared to suggested orthovoltage doses.
- Lead shields should be used to block the lens, cornea, nasal septum, teeth, etc. as appropriate.
- Backscattered electrons/photons can lead to conjunctival/mucosal irritation. For eyelids, thin coating of dental acrylic/wax should be used; for other areas, a thicker coating should be applied.
- General orthovoltage margins.

- Tumor size <2 cm = 0.5–1.0 cm horizontal margin; tumor size >2 cm = 1.5–2 cm horizontal margin. Deep margin should be at least 0.5 cm deeper than the suspected depth of tumor.
- Additional margin is needed in these circumstances.
  - *Electrons*: lateral constriction of isodose curves in deep portion of tumor volume increases with decreasing field sizes, so add 0.5 cm additional margin at skin surface.
  - *Recurrent and morpheaform BCC*: infiltrate more widely, so add extra 0.5–1.0 cm margin at skin surface.
  - *High-risk SCC*: 2 cm margin around tumor should be used if possible, and consider including regional LN.
  - *PNI*: if present, include named nerve retrograde to the skull base. Consider IMRT.

- Nodal treatment should be considered for recurrences after surgery and is indicated for poorly differentiated, >3 cm tumors, and/or large infiltrative-ulcerative SCC; consider IMRT depending on anatomy.
- Irradiation of a *graft* should not begin until after it is well-healed and healthy (usually 6–8 weeks), and the entire graft should be included in the target volume.

DOSE PRESCRIPTIONS (ORTHOVOLTAGE)

- Less than 2 cm: 3 Gy/fx to 45–51 Gy
- >2 cm (no cartilage involvement): 2.5 Gy/fx to 50–55 Gy
- >2 cm (cartilage involved): 2 Gy/fx to 60–66 Gy
- For electrons, add 10–15% to the daily and total dose to account for lower RBE. While treating cartilage, always keep daily dose <3 Gy/fx
- Prescription points: orthovoltage = D_{max}, electrons = D_{max} or 95%

SPECIAL RECOMMENDATIONS BY ANATOMIC SITE

- Dorsum of hand and feet
  - Generally, avoid RT at these locations due to high risk of necrosis due to repeated trauma to the region. If ≤4 mm in thickness, radioactive surface molds can be used.
  - As a rule, lesions beyond elbow and knees are at risk of poor healing and ulceration after RT due to poor vascular supply, especially for elderly.
- Eyelid
  - Surgery preferred for lesions 5 mm or less.
  - Radiation is very effective for lesions 0.5–2 cm. With lead shielding, the lens dose is negligible as is the risk of

RT-induced cataracts. Ophthalmic anesthetic drops are applied prior to insertion of shield.

- Ectropion/epiphora can occur regardless of treatment modality. Fifty percent are improved with corrective surgery.
- Mild conjunctivitis can occur due to the use of eye-shields and from RT.
- Lacri-Lube ophthalmic ointment can improve burning/pruritis.
- For tumors of 0.5–2 cm, recommended dose is 48 Gy/16 fx over 3.5 weeks with 100 kV/0.19 mmCu or equivalent.

- Lip
  - RT/Mohs/surgery are all good options.
  - Place lead shield behind lip to shield teeth/mandible.
  - For tumors <2.0 cm, recommended dose is 48 Gy/16 fx using 150 kV X-rays with 0.52 mm Cu HVL or 6–9 MeV electrons with appropriate bolus. Energy selection may vary depending on the depth of the lesion being treated, see above.
  - Include neck nodes if SCC recurrent, grade 3, >3 cm greatest dimension, or >4 mm thickness.
- Nose and ear
  - Place wax covered lead strip in nose to prevent irritation.
  - Include nasolabial fold for nasal ala lesions.
  - Use wax bolus on irregular surfaces for homogeneity.
  - For tumors 0.5–2.0 cm, recommended dose is 52.8 Gy/16 fx over 3.5 weeks with electrons or 45–51 Gy/15–17 fx using orthovoltage.
  - Selection of electron and orthovoltage energy will depend on the depth of the lesion, see above.

DOSE LIMITATIONS

- Cartilage: chondritis rare if <3 Gy/day given.
- Skin: larger volumes of tissue do not tolerate radiation as well, and thus, require smaller daily fractions; moist desquamation is expected.
- Bone: see *f* factor discussion above.

COMPLICATIONS

- Telangectasias, skin atrophy, hypopigmentation, skin necrosis (~3%), osteoradionecrosis (~1%), chondritis/cartilage necrosis (rare if fx <300 cGy/day), hair loss/ loss of sweat glands.

FOLLOW-UP (ADAPTED FROM NCCN 2009 RECOMMENDATIONS)

- BCC: H&P, complete skin exam q6–12 months for life
- SCC localized: H&P q3–6 months for 2 years, then q6–12 months for 3 years, then q1 year for life
- SCC regional: H&P q1–3 months for year 1, then q2–4 months for year 2, then q4–6 months for years 3–5, then q6–12 months for life

MERKEL CELL CARCINOMA (MCC)

- Rare, deadly (mortality rate > melanoma), neuroendocrine malignancy of the skin
- No consensus on management due to lack of randomized data to compare treatment modalities
- Prior to publication of the new AJCC 7th Ed staging (below), many institutions (including UCSF) use a simpler system: Stage I = localized (IA ≤2 cm; IB >2 cm); II = LN+; III = DM

STAGING (AJCC 7TH ED., 2010): MERKEL CELL CARCINOMA

Primary tumor (T)

TX: Primary tumor cannot be assessed
T0: No evidence of primary tumor (e.g., nodal/metastatic presentation without associated primary)
Tis: In situ primary tumor
T1: Less than or equal to 2 cm maximum tumor dimension
T2: Greater than 2 cm, but not more than 5 cm maximum tumor dimension
T3: Over 5 cm maximum tumor dimension
T4: Primary tumor invades bone, muscle, fascia, or cartilage

Regional lymph nodes (N)

NX: Regional lymph nodes cannot be assessed
N0: No regional lymph node metastasis
cN0: Nodes negative by clinical exam* (no pathologic node exam performed)
pN0: Nodes negative by pathologic exam
N1: Metastasis in regional lymph node(s)
N1a: Micrometastasis**
N1b: Macrometastasis***
N2: In-transit metastasis****

**Note*: Clinical detection of nodal disease may be via inspection, palpation, and/or imaging.
**Micrometastases are diagnosed after sentinel or elective lymphadenectomy.
***Macrometastases are defined as clinically detectable nodal metastases confirmed by therapeutic lymphadenectomy or needle biopsy.
****In-transit metastasis: a tumor distinct from the primary lesion and located either (1) between the primary lesion and the draining regional lymph nodes or (2) distal to the primary lesion.

continued

Distant metastasis (M)

M0: No distant metastasis
M1: Metastasis beyond regional lymph nodes
  M1a: Metastasis to skin, subcutaneous tissues, or distant lymph nodes
  M1b: Metastasis to lung
  M1c: Metastasis to all other visceral sites

Anatomic stage/prognostic groups

Patients with primary Merkel cell carcinoma with no evidence of regional or distant metastases (either clinically or pathologically) are divided into two stages: Stage I for primary tumors ≤2 cm in size, and Stage II for primary tumors >2 cm in size. Stages I and II are further divided into A and B substages based on the method of nodal evaluation

Patients who have pathologically proven node negative disease (by microscopic evaluation of their draining lymph nodes) have improved survival (substaged as A) compared with those who are only evaluated clinically (substaged as B). Stage II has an additional substage (IIC) for tumors with extracutaneous invasion (T4) and negative node status, regardless of whether the negative node status was established microscopically or clinically. Stage III is also divided into A and B categories for patients with microscopically positive and clinically occult nodes (IIIA) and macroscopic nodes (IIIB). There are no subgroups of Stage IV Merkel cell carcinoma

0: Tis N0 M0
IA: T1 pN0 M0
IB: T1 cN0 M0
IIA: T2/T3 pN0 M0
IIB: T2/T3 cN0 M0
IIC: T4 N0 M0
IIIA: Any T N1a M0
IIIB: Any T N1b/N2 M0
IV: Any T Any N M1

- Local recurrences common (postsurgery alone ~75%, with adjuvant RT ~15%).
- Approximately 20% have + LN at diagnosis, and sentinel LN biopsy is rapidly becoming the standard means of assessing nodal status and should be performed before resection of the primary site.
- Distant metastases develop in 50–60% of cases, usually within 10 months of diagnosis.
- Role of chemotherapy is unclear, but with the high rate of DM, it is occasionally given either concurrently or after RT. Platinum-based regimens similar to those for SCLC are commonly used (cisplatin or carboplatin with etoposide or irinotecan).
- The UCSF approach to radiotherapy for MCC is as follows:
  - Clinically N0 nodes: 45–50 Gy/1.8–2.0 Gy fx
  - Microscopic disease/–margins: 45–50 Gy/1.8–2.0 Gy fx
  - Microscopic disease/+ margins: 55–60 Gy/1.8–2.0 Gy fx
  - Macroscopic disease: 55–60 Gy/1.8–2.0 Gy fx
  - Cover primary site, in-transit lymphatics, regional LN with wide margins

1

  - May consider eliminating RT to regional LN if small primary cancer with negative SLN, or if regional LND performed for positive SLN, but patient cN0
  - Margins on primary site = 2 cm in head and neck, 3–5 cm elsewhere depending on site
- Three-year DSS for local/regional disease ~75%.
- Three-year OS: localized ~70–80%, nodal metastasis ~50–60%, distant metastasis ~30%.
- Data suggest almost no MCC-related deaths occur after 3 years from diagnosis.

FOLLOW-UP (ADAPTED FROM NCCN 2009 RECOMMENDATIONS)

- q1–3 months for year 1, q3–6 months for year 2, then annually for life.

MELANOMA

PEARLS

- Incidence increased by 1,800% from the 1930s and increasing 3.1% per year 1992–2004. Rising incidence not due to increased surveillance or changes in diagnostic criteria. 1/87 Americans will be diagnosed with melanoma.
- Mainly Caucasians. Caucasian:African American: 10:1.
- 62,480 new cases and 8,420 deaths from melanoma in 2008.
- Fifteen percent derive from preexisiting melanocytic nevi.
- Less than 10% develop in noncutaneous sites.
- Gender difference in predominant locations: M = trunk, F = extremities.
- Approximately 15% have + LN at diagnosis (~5% for T1, ~25% for >T1).
- Approximately 5% have DM at diagnosis (1/3 with no evidence of primary).
- Subtypes: superficial spreading (~65%), nodular (~25%), lentigo maligna (least common – 7%), acral lentiginous (5% in whites, but most common form in dark-skinned populations).
- Lentigo maligna has the best prognosis with LN mets in only 10% cases, and 10-year OS 85% after WLE alone. Hutchinison's freckle = lentigo maligna involving epidermis only.
- Acral lentiginous generally presents on palms, soles, or subungual.

- Most powerful prognostic factor for recurrence and survival: sentinel LN status.
- >20% chance of involved sentinel LN if melanoma is >2 mm thick.
- ≥20% risk of regional recurrence in those with involved regional LN treated with surgery alone, especially with ECE or multiple LN involvement.
- Other prognostic factors: ulceration, thickness (Breslow = measured depth, Clark = related to histologic level of dermis), anatomic site (trunk worse), gender (male worse), age (young better), number of nodes.
- ABCD rule outlining warning signs of most common type of melanoma: A – asymmetry, B – border irregularity, C – color, D – diameter > 6 mm.
- Clark levels: I = epidermis only, II = invasion of papillary dermis (localized), III = filling papillary dermis compressing reticular dermis, IV = invading reticular dermis, V = invades subcutaneous tissues.

WORKUP

- Less than 1 mm thick lesions – same as for SCC/BCC
- >1 mm thick lesions – need CBC, LFTs, CXR, evaluation of suspicious nodes, pelvic CT if inguino-femoral adenopathy

STAGING: MELANOMA

Editors' note: All TNM stage and stage groups referred to elsewhere in this chapter reflect the 2002 AJCC staging nomenclature unless otherwise noted as the new system below was published after this chapter was written.

(AJCC 6TH ED., 2002)

Primary tumor (T)

TX: Primary tumor cannot be assessed
T0: No evidence of primary tumor
Tis: Melanoma in situ
T1: Melanoma ≤1.0 mm with or without ulceration
- T1a: Melanoma ≤1.0 mm in thickness and level II or III, no ulceration
- T1b: Melanoma ≤1.0 mm in thickness and level IV or V, or with ulceration

T2: Melanoma 1.01–2.0 mm in thickness with or without ulceration
- T2a: Melanoma 1.01–2.0 mm in thickness, no ulceration
- T2b: Melanoma 1.01–2.0 mm in thickness, with ulceration

T3: Melanoma 2.01–4.0 mm in thickness with or without ulceration
- T3a: Melanoma 2.01–4.0 mm in thickness, no ulceration
- T3b: Melanoma 2.01–4.0 mm in thickness, with ulceration

T4: Melanoma greater than 4.0 mm in thickness with or without ulceration
- T4a: Melanoma >4.0 mm in thickness, no ulceration
- T4b: Melanoma >4.0 mm in thickness, with ulceration

Regional lymph nodes (N)

NX: No regional lymph node metastasis can be assessed
N0: No regional lymph node metastasis
N1: Metastasis in one lymph node
- N1a: Clinically occult (microscopic) metastasis
- N1b: Clinically apparent (macroscopic) metastasis

N2: Metastasis in 2–3 regional nodes or intralymphatic regional metastasis
- N2a: Clinically occult (microscopic) metastasis
- N2b: Clinically apparent (macroscopic) metastasis
- N2c: Satellite or in-transit metastasis without nodal metastasis

(AJCC 7TH ED., 2010)

Primary tumor (T)

TX: Primary tumor cannot be assessed (e.g., curettaged or severely regressed melanoma)
T0: No evidence of primary tumor
Tis: Melanoma in situ
T1: Melanomas 1.0 mm or less in thickness
T2: Melanomas 1.01–2.0 mm
T3: Melanomas 2.01–4.0 mm
T4: Melanomas more than 4.0 mm

Note: a and b subcategories of T are assigned based on ulceration and number of mitoses per mm^2 as shown below.

T classification	*Thickness (mm)*	*Ulceration status/mitoses*
T1	≤1.0	a) Without ulceration and mitosis <1/mm^2
		b) With ulceration or mitoses ≥1/mm^2
T2	1.01–2.0	a) Without ulceration
		b) With ulceration
T3	2.01–4.0	a) Without ulceration
		b) With ulceration
T4	>4.0	a) Without ulceration
		b) With ulceration

Regional lymph nodes (N)

NX: Patients in whom the regional nodes cannot be assessed (e.g., previously removed for another reason)
N0: No regional metastases detected

continued

N3: Metastasis in 4 or more regional nodes, or matted metastatic nodes, or in-transit metastasis or satellite(s) with metastasis in regional node(s)

Distant metastasis (M)
MX: Distant metastasis cannot be assessed
M0: No distant metastasis
M1: Distant metastasis
 M1a: Metastasis to skin, subcutaneous tissues, or distant lymph nodes
 M1b: Metastasis to lung
M1c: Metastasis to all other visceral sites or distant metastasis at any site associated with an elevated LDH

Clinical stage grouping*		**Pathologic stage grouping****		**5-Year survival**	
0:	TisN0M0	0:	TisN0M0	IA:	>95%
IA:	T1aN0M0	IA:	T1aN0M0	IB:	~90%
IB:	T1b–2aN0M0	IB:	T1b–2aN0M0	IIA:	~80%
IIA:	T2b–3aN0M0	IIA:	T2b–3aN0M0	IIB:	~65%
IIB:	T3b–4aN0M0	IIB:	T3b–4aN0M0	IIC:	~45%
IIC:	T4bN0M0	IIC:	T4bN0M0	IIIA:	~65%
III:	AnyT N1–3M0	IIIA:	T1–4aN1a/ 2aM0	IIIB:	~50%
IV:	M1	IIIB:	T1–4bN1a/ 2aM0		(30–50% if
			T1–4aN1b/2bM0		N2c)
			T1–4a/bN2cM0	IV:	~7–20%
		IIIC:	T1–4bN1b/2bM0		
			AnyTN3M1		
		IV:	M1		

N1–3: Regional metastases based upon the number of metastatic nodes and presence or absence of intralymphatic metastases (in-transit or satellite metastases)

Note: N1–3 and a–c subcategories assigned as shown below

N classification	*Number of metastatic nodes*	*Nodal metastatic mass*
N1	1 node	Micrometastasis* Macrometastasis**
N2	2–3 nodes	Micrometastasis* Macrometastasis** In-transitmet(s)/satellite(s) without metastatic nodes
N3	4 or more metastatic nodes, or matted nodes, or in-transit met(s)/ satellite(s) with metastatic node(s)	

*Micrometastases are diagnosed after sentinel lymph node biopsy and completion of lymphadenectomy (if performed).
**Macrometastases are defined as clinically detectable nodal metastases confirmed by therapeutic lymphadenectomy or when nodal metastasis exhibits gross extracapsular extension.

Distant metastasis (M)
M0: No detectable evidence of distant metastases
M1a: Metastases to skin, subcutaneous, or distant lymph nodes
M1b: Metastases to lung
M1c: Metastases to all other visceral sites or distant meta- stases to any site combined with an elevated serum LDH

Note: Serum LDH is incorporated into the M category as shown below.

continued

Notes: Clinical staging includes microstaging of the primary melanoma and clinical/radiological evaluation for metastases. By convention, it should be used after complete excision of the primary melanoma with clinical assessment for regional and distant mets.
**Pathologic staging includes microstaging of the primary melanoma and pathologic information about the regional lymph nodes after partial or complete lymphadenectomy. Pathologic Stage 0 or Stage IA patients are the exception; they do not require pathologic evaluation of their lymph nodes.

Used with the permission from the American Joint Committee on Cancer (AJCC), Chicago, IL. The original source for this material is the AJCC Cancer Staging Manual, Sixth Edition (2002), published by Springer Science+Business Media.

M classification	*Site*	*Serum LDH*
M1a	Distant skin, subcutaneous, or nodal mets	Normal
M1b	Lung metastases	Normal
M1c	All other visceral metastases	Normal
	Any distant metastasis	Elevated

Anatomic stage/prognostic groups

Clinical staging*				Pathologic staging**			
Stage 0	Tis	N0	M0	0	Tis	N0	M0
Stage IA	T1a	N0	M0	IA	T1a	N0	M0
Stage IB	T1b	N0	M0	IB	T1b	N0	N0
	T2a	N0	M0		T2a	N0	M0
Stage IIA	T2b	N0	M0	IIA	T2b	N0	M0
	T3a	N0	M0		T3a	N0	M0
Stage IIB	T3b	N0	M0	IIB	T3b	N0	M0
	T4a	N0	M0		T4a	N0	M0
Stage IIC	T4b	N0	M0	IIC	T4b	N0	M0
Stage III	Any T	≥N1	M0	IIIA	T1–4a	N1a	M0
					T1–4a	N2a	M0
				IIIB	T1–4b	N1a	M0
					T1–4b	N2a	M0
					T1–4a	N1b	M0
					T1–4a	N2b	M0
					T1–4a	N2c	M0
				IIIC	T1–4b	N1b	M0
					T1–4b	N2b	M0
					T1–4b	N2c	M0
					T1–4b	N3	M0
					Any T	N3	M0
Stage IV	Any T	Any N	M1	IV	Any T	Any N	M1

*Clinical staging includes microstaging of the primary melanoma and clinical/radiologic evaluation for metastases. By convention, it should be used after complete excision of the primary melanoma with clinical assessment for regional and distant metastases.

continued

**Pathologic staging includes microstaging of the primary melanoma and pathologic information about the regional lymph nodes after partial or complete lymphadenectomy. Pathologic Stage 0 or Stage IA patients are the exception; they do not require pathologic evaluation of their lymph nodes.

Used with the permission from the American Joint Committee on Cancer (AJCC), Chicago, IL. The original source for this material is the AJCC Cancer Staging Manual, Seventh Edition (2010), published by Springer Science+Business Media.

STAGING (AJCC 7TH ED., 2010): MUCOSAL MELANOMA OF THE HEAD AND NECK

- This is a new chapter for classification of this rare tumor

Primary tumor (T)
T3: Mucosal disease
T4a: Moderately advanced disease. Tumor involving deep soft tissue, cartilage, bone, or overlying skin
T4b: Very advanced disease. Tumor involving brain, dura, skull base, lower cranial nerves (IX, X, XI, XII), masticator space, carotid artery, prevertebral space, or mediastinal structures

Regional lymph nodes (N)
NX: Regional lymph nodes cannot be assessed
N0: No regional lymph node metastases
N1: Regional lymph node metastases present

Distant metastasis (M)
M0: No distant metastasis
M1: Distant metastasis present

Anatomic stage/prognostic groups
III: T3 N0 M0
IVA: T4a N0 M0
T3–T4a N1 M0
IVB: T4b Any N M0
IVC: Any T Any N M1

Used with the permission from the American Joint Committee on Cancer (AJCC), Chicago, IL. The original source for this material is the AJCC Cancer Staging Manual, Seventh Edition (2010), published by Springer Science+Business Media.

TREATMENT RECOMMENDATIONS

PRIMARY

- Surgery: SLN biopsy followed by WLE and completion of regional LN dissection if SLN+.
- Minimum surgical margins: Tis = 5 mm, T1 = 1 cm, T2–T4 = 2 cm; retrospective studies suggest no benefit in LC, DFS, OS with >2 cm margins.
- Primary RT rarely indicated with the exception of lentigo maligna melanomas on the face that would cause severe cosmetic/functional deficits with surgery. These can be treated with a 1.5 cm margin with 50 Gy/20fx with 100–250 kV photons. For medically inoperable patients, hyperthermia can improve response and local control, especially for tumors >4 cm [Overgaard].

ADJUVANT

- N-, 1–4 mm without ulceration, ≤1 mm with ulceration = none standard
- Less than 4 mm with ulceration/Clark IV–V = clinical trial, if available, or observation

- >4 mm or N+ = high-dose interferon alpha, clinical trial, or observation
- Consider RT to primary site: close or positive margins, recurrent disease, Breslow >4 mm with ulceration or satellitosis, desmoplastic subtype (controversial)

REGIONAL NODES

- Elective lymph node dissection (ELND) is controversial. Four phase III RCTs have not shown a benefit in survival with ELND vs. delayed therapeutic lymphadenectomy. However, benefit has been seen in overall survival in certain patient subsets, i.e., patients ≤60 years, nonulcerative melanomas, tumors located on limbs, and melanomas 1–2 mm thick.
- Sentinel lymph node biopsy, though does not have reported benefit in overall survival, has been accepted by the surgical community. Predicts survival and provides prognostic information.
- Patients who are unable to undergo completion surgery due to medical comorbidities are candidates for elective nodal irradiation which is superior to observation.
- Predictors of regional recurrence after nodal dissection alone include extracapsular extension ("matted"), ≥4 lymph nodes positive, lymph node size >3 cm in diameter, lymph nodes located in cervical basin, clinically palpable lymph nodes removed during a therapeutic resection vs. an elective dissection, and recurrent disease which increases the chance for recurrence.
    - Presence of 1 of these factors has a 30–50% rate of regional recurrence
    - Adjuvant RT reduces recurrence rate to 5–20%
- MD Anderson treatment algorithm for radiation of clinically apparent lymph nodes.
    - Cervical nodes: presence of any 1 of the following – extracapsular extension, >2 cm, >2 involved lymph nodes, recurrent disease
    - Axillary nodes: presence of any 1 of the following – extracapsular extension, >3 cm, >4 involved lymph nodes, recurrent disease
    - Groin/pelvic nodes: higher threshold due to morbidity of lymphedema
        - BMI <25 kg/m^2: presence of any 1 of the following – extracapsular extension, >3 cm, >4 involved lymph nodes, recurrent disease

- BMI >25 kg/m^2: presence of extracapsular extension and 1 of the following – >3 cm, >4 involved lymph nodes

STUDIES

- *Interferon alpha*: [ECOG 1684/1690/1694]. Three randomized trials established a role for high-dose IFN-α in T4/N+ patients. IFN-α provides ~10% absolute improvement in RFS, and possibly improves 5-year OS. Benefits not seen when high-dose IFN-α compared with low-dose [ECOG 1680] or GM2 ganglioside vaccine [ECOG 1694].
- *Chemotherapy ± Biochemotherapy*: E3695 Atkins et al. (2008): 395 patients randomized to cisplatin, vinblastine, dacarbazine (CVD) alone or concurrent with interleukin-2 and interferon alfa-2b (BCT). Median PFS was longer for BCT group, 4.8 vs. 2.9 months ($p=0.15$). No difference in median OS, 9 vs. 8.7 months. Greater grade 3 or higher toxicities with BCT than CVD, 95 vs. 73% ($p=0.001$). Temozolomide is under investigation, but in a randomized phase III trial, did not show greater efficacy in Stage IV melanoma than the current standard, dacarbazine (EORTC 18032, 33rd ESMO, 2008).
- *Monoclonal antibodies*: phase I/II trials of tremelimumab and ipilimumab showing antitumor activity in patients with metastatic melanoma.
- *Melanoma vaccines*: no randomized phase III trials demonstrate a survival benefit, but multiple trials pending.

ADJUVANT RT

- Ang et al. (1990): 83 patients with >1.5 mm thick primary or cN+ received 24–30 Gy in 4–5 fx with improved LC over historic controls treated with surgery alone.
- Ang et al. (1994). Phase II trial of adjuvant RT in H&N melanoma patients with a projected LRR rate 50%. Seventy-nine patients had WLE of a ≥1.5 mm primary or Clark's IV–V, 32 patients had WLE and elective LND, and 63 patients had LND after neck relapse. RT was 6 Gy/fx given biweekly to 30 Gy over 2.5 weeks. Results: 5-year LRC 88%, OS 47%. Five-year OS by pathologic parameters: ≤1.5 mm-100%, 1.6–4 mm 72%, >4 mm 30%, >3 LN+ 23%, 1–3LN+ 39%. Minimal acute/late toxicity.
- Chang et al. (2006): 56 patients with high-risk disease treated with hypofractionation, 30 Gy in five fractions (41 patients) or with conventional fractionation, median 60 Gy in 30 fractions

and 1 patient with b.i.d. fractionation (15 patients). No difference in LRC, OS, and CSS between two fractionation schemes. Two patients with severe late complications, osteoradionecrosis of temporal bone and xrt plexopathy, received hypofractionation.

- TROG 96.06 (Burmeister 2006): 234 N+ patients treated adjuvantly with 48 Gy in 20 fractions. If involved margins, 50 Gy in 21 fractions. Forty-seven percent were radiated to the axilla, 33% to head and neck, 20% to ilio-inguinal. One patient received adjuvant interferon. At 5 years, infield regional relapse was 6.8%. Five-year OS 36%, PFS 27%, and regional control 91%. Grade 3 lymphedema 9% in axillary RT patients and 19% in ilio-inguinal RT patients.

DEFINITIVE RT

- RTOG 8305 (Sause IJROBP 1991) showed comparable clinical response for both 32 Gy in 4 fx vs. 50 Gy in 20 fx; however, this trial contained large tumors which were loosely size-stratified <5 cm vs. ≥5 cm.

HYPERTHERMIA

- Overgaard et al. (1995): 70 patients with metastatic/recurrent melanoma randomized to 24 Gy or 27 Gy in 3 fx over 8 days alone or followed by hyperthermia (43°C for 60 min). HT improved LC (26→48%), as did 27 Gy LC (25→56%).

RADIATION TECHNIQUES

SIMULATION AND FIELD DESIGN

- Target volume for primary lesion: primary site with a 2–4-cm margin.
- Nodal target volume depends on primary site:
  - Head and neck: preauricular, postauricular lymph nodes for high facial and scalp primaries, and ipsilateral levels I through V lymph nodes, including ipsilateral supraclavicular fossa.
  - Axilla: levels I through III lymph nodes. For bulky high axillary disease, include supraclavicular fossa and low cervical lymph nodes.
  - Groin: include entire scar and regions with confirmed nodal disease. In cases with positive inguinal lymphadenopathy,

may include external iliac lymph nodes; though, this will lead to increased toxicity.

DOSE PRESCRIPTIONS

- No data to support the commonly held idea that melanoma is radioresistant
- Radiobiologic data suggest that melanoma cell lines have large shoulder on dose-response curve favoring hypofractionation
- Dose recommendations for SCC/BCC can be followed for treating melanoma, but hypofractionation approaches remain popular due to high reported LC rates
- Treatment setup and dose
  - Head and neck:
    - Cervical disease: open neck position, treat with electrons
    - Frontal, temporal, preauricular region, cheek: 2–3 fields
    - Tissue bolus is used to reduce dose to temporal lobe and larynx
    - Elective/adjuvant RT dose: 6 Gy/fraction to 30 Gy delivered twice weekly
    - If microscopic residual disease is present: an additional boost fraction is given for total dose of 36 Gy
  - Axilla: supine with treatment arm akimbo, AP/PA
    - Dose: 6 Gy/fraction to 30 Gy delivered twice weekly
  - Groin: unilateral frog-leg position
    - Dose: 6 Gy/fraction to 30 Gy delivered twice weekly
  - Consider less hypofractionated schedule if morbidity is a major concern

DOSE LIMITATIONS

- Dose to spinal cord or small bowel not to exceed 24 Gy over four fractions

COMPLICATIONS

- Site dependent:
  - Most sites: erythema, moist skin desquamation
  - Late complications: thinning of subcutaneous fat with mild to moderate fibrosis
  - Postoperative lymphedema, particularly in patients with high body-mass index or treated with adjuvant RT to groin
  - Other late effects include osteitis or fracture, joint stiffness, and neuropathy

FOLLOW-UP (ADAPTED FROM NCCN 2009 RECOMMENDATIONS)

- Stage IA – annual skin exam for life (directed H&P 3–12 months for 5 year then annually as clinically indicated)
- Stage IB–III – q3–6 months × 2 years, q3–12 months × 2 years, then annually for life

REFERENCES

Ang KK, Byers RM, Peters LJ. Regional radiotherapy as adjuvant treatment for head and neck malignant melanoma. Arch Otolaryngol Head Neck Surg. 1990;116(2):169-172.

Ang KK, Peters LJ, Weber RS. Postoperative radiotherapy for cutaneous melanoma of the head and neck region. Int J Radiat Oncol Biol Phys. 1994; 30(4):795-798.

Atkins MB, Hsu J, Lee S, et al. Phase III trial comparing concurrent biochemotherapy with cisplatin, vinblastine, dacarbazine, interleukin-2, and interferon alfa-2b with cisplatin, vinblastine, and dacarbazine alone in patients with metastatic malignant melanoma (E3695): A trial coordinated by the Eastern Cooperative Oncology Group. J Clin Oncol. 2008;26:5748-5754.

Burmeister BH, Mark Smithers B, Burmeister E, et al. A prospective phase II study of adjuvant postoperative radiation therapy following nodal surgery in malignant melanoma –Trans Tasman Radiation Oncology Group (TROG) Study 96.06. Radiother Oncol. 2006;81:136-42.

Chang DT, Amdur RJ, Morris CG, et al. Adjuvant radiotherapy for cutaneous melanoma: comparing hypofractionation to conventional fractionation. Int J Radiat Oncol Biol Phys. 2006;66(4):1051-1055.

Overgaard J, Gonzalez D, Hulshof MC. Randomised trial of hyperthermia as adjuvant to radiotherapy for recurrent or metastatic malignant melanoma. European Society for Hyperthermic Oncology. Lancet. 1995;345(8949): 540-543.

FURTHER READING

Ang KK, Weber RS. Cutaneous Carcinoma. In: Gunderson L, Tepper J, editors. Clinical Radiation Oncology, 2nd ed. Philadelphia: Churchill Livingstone; 2007. pp. 853-864.

Balch CM, Soong S, Ross MI, et al. Long-term results of a multi-institutional randomized trial comparing prognostic factors and surgical results for intermediate thickness melanomas (1.0-4.0). Ann Surg Oncol. 2000;7:87-97

Ballo MT, Ang KK. Malignant Melanoma. In: Gunderson L, Tepper J, editors. Clinical Radiation Oncology, 2nd ed. Philadelphia: Churchill Livingstone; 2007. pp. 865-877.

Ballo MT, Zagars GK, Gershenwald JE, et al. A critical assessment of adjuvant radiotherapy for inguinal lymph node metastases from melanoma. Ann Surg Oncol. 2004;11:1079-1084.

Bonnen MD, Ballo MT, Myers JN, et al. Elective radiotherapy provides regional control for patients with cutaneous melanoma of the head and neck. Cancer. 2003;100:383-389.

Camacho LH, Antonia S, Sosman J, et al. Phase I/II trial of tremelimumab in patients with metastatic melanoma. J Clin Oncol. 2009; 27:1075-1081.

Dana-Farber Cancer Institute. Merkel Cell Carcinoma: Information for Patients and Their Physicians. Available at: http://www.merkelcell.org. Accessed on January 12, 2005.

Doubrovsky A, de Wilt JH, Scolyer RA, et al. Sentinel node biopsy provides more accurate staging than elective lymph node dissection in patients with cutaneous melanoma. Ann Surg Oncol. 2004;11:829-836.

Greene FL. American Joint Committee on Cancer, American Cancer Society. AJCC Cancer Staging Manual. 6th ed. New York: Springer Verlag; 2002.

Kirkwood JM, Ibrahim JG, Sondak VK, et al. High- and low-dose alfa-2b in high-risk melanoma: First analysis of intergroup trial E1690/S9111/C9190. J Clin Oncol. 2000;18:2444-2458.

Kirkwood JM, Ibrahim JG, Sosman JA, et al. High-dose interferon alfa-2b significantly prolongs relapse-free and overall survival compared with the GM2-KLH/QS-21 vaccine in patients with resected stage IIB-III melanoma: Results of intergroup trial E1694/S9512/C509801. J Clin Oncol. 2001;19:2370-2380.

Kirkwood JM, Strawderman MH, Ernstoff MS, et al. Interferon alfa-2b adjuvant therapy of high-risk resected cutaneous melanoma: The Eastern Cooperative Oncology Group trial EST 1684. J Clin Oncol. 1996;14:7-17.

Margolin KA, Sondak VK. Melanoma and Other Skin Cancers. In: Pazdur R, Coia L, Hoskins W, Wagman L, editors. Cancer Management: A Multidisciplinary Approach. 8th ed. New York: CMP Healthcare Media; 2004. pp. 509-538.

National Comprehensive Cancer Network. Clinical Practice Guidelines in Oncology: Basal Cell and Squamous Skin Cancers. Available at: http://www.nccn.org/professionals/physician_gls/PDF/nmsc.pdf. Accessed on May 7, 2009.

National Comprehensive Cancer Network. Clinical Practice Guidelines in Oncology: Merkel Cell Carcinoma. Available at: http://www.nccn.org/professionals/physician_gls/PDF/mcc.pdf. Accessed on May 7, 2009.

National Comprehensive Cancer Network. Clinical Practice Guidelines in Oncology: Melanoma. Available at: http://www.nccn.org/professionals/physician_gls/PDF/melanoma.pdf. Accessed on May 7, 2009.

Rigel DS, Friedman RJ, Kopf AW. The incidence of malignant melanoma in the United States: issues as we approach the 21st century. J Am Acad Dermatol. 1996;34:839-847.

Sim FH, Taylor WF, Pritchard DJ, et al. Lymphadenectomy in the management of stage I malignant melanoma: a prospective randomized study. Mayo Clin Proc. 1986;61:697-705.

Solan M, Brady L. Skin Cancer. In: Perez CA, Brady LW, Halperin EC, et al., editors. Principles and Practice of Radiation Oncology. 5th ed. Philadelphia: Lippincott Williams and Wilkins; 2008. pp. 690-701.

Sause WT, Cooper JS, Rush S, et al. Fraction size in external beam radiation therapy in the treatment of melanoma. Int J Radiat Oncol Biol Phys 1991; 20(3): 429-432.

Veronesi U, Adamus J, Bandiera DC, et al. Delayed regional lymph node dissection in stage I melanoma of the skin of the lower extremities. Cancer. 1982;49:2420-2430.

Weber JS, O'Day S, Urba W, et al. Phase I/II study of ipilimumab for patients with metastatic melanoma. J Clin Oncol. 2008;26:5950-5956.

Wilder RB, Margolis LW. Cancer of the Skin. In: Leibel SA, Phiilips TL, editors. Textbook of radiation oncology. 2nd ed. Philadelphia: Saunders; 2004. pp. 1483-1501.

PART II
Central Nervous System

Chapter 2
Central Nervous System

Charlotte Dai Kubicky, Linda W. Chan, Stuart Y. Tsuji, Jean L. Nakamura, Daphne Haas-Kogan, and David A. Larson

II

INTRODUCTION

- This chapter will discuss malignant glioma, low-grade glioma, brainstem glioma, optic glioma, CNS lymphoma, ependymoma, choroid plexus tumor, meningioma, acoustic neuroma, craniopharyngioma, pituitary tumor, pineal tumor, medulloblastoma, primary spinal cord tumor, arteriovenous malformation, and trigeminal neuralgia. Brain metastases will be discussed in the palliative care chapter.

ANATOMY

- Meninges (outer to inner) = dura mater → arachnoid mater → subarachnoid space → pia mater.
- Precentral gyrus = primary motor strip; postcentral gyrus = primary somatosensory cortex. Medial = body, lower extremities, feet. Lateral = trunk, arms, head.
- Brain gray matter is peripheral and white matter is central.
- Broca's (motor) area = dominant frontal lobe just superior to lateral sulcus (Sylvian fissure) = site of expressive aphasia (comprehend but not fluent).
- Wernicke's (sensory) area = dominant temporal lobe at posterior end of lateral sulcus = site of receptive aphasia (fluent but not comprehend).
- Diencephalon = thalamaus, hypothalamus, and pineal gland.
- Telencephalon = olfactory lobes, cerebral hemispheres, basal ganglia, amygdalae.
- Mesencephalon = tectum, crus cerebri, superior and inferior colliculi, cerebral aqueduct.
- Only CN IV exits from dorsal surface of midbrain.
- CSF: choroid plexus produces → lateral ventricles → foramen of Monroe → third ventricle → cerebral aqueduct of Sylvius → fourth ventricle → foramen of Magendie and two lateral foramina of Lushka.

- Caverous sinus contains CN III, IV, V1, V2, VI and the internal carotid artery. Cavernous involvement commonly produces CN VI palsy.
- Tumors with a high propensity for CSF spread include medulloblastomas, primitive neuroectodermal tumors (PNET), and CNS lymphoma. Germ-cell tumors and ependymomas have a lower propensity for CSF spread.
- CN exits:
  - Superior orbital fissure = CN III, IV, VI, V1
  - Foramen rotundum = V2
  - Foramen ovale = V3
  - Foramen spinosum = middle meningeal artery and vein
  - Internal auditory meatus = CN VII, VIII
  - Jugular foramen = CN IX, X, XI
  - Hypoglossal canal = CN XII
- Lateral plain film.
  - Hypothalamus = 1 cm superior to sellar floor.
  - Optic canal = 1 cm superior and 1 cm anterior to the hypothalamus.
  - Pineal body (supratentorial notch) = 1 cm posterior and 3 cm superior to external acoustic meatus.
  - Lens = 1 cm posterior to anterior eyelid, 8 mm posterior to line connecting lateral canthus. Median globe size = 2.5 cm.
  - Location of cribiform plate cannot always be correctly identified with lateral plain film alone (Gripp et al. 2004).
- Spinal cord.
  - Thirty-one pairs of spinal nerves: 8 cervical, 12 thoracic, 5 lumbar, 5 sacral, 1 coccygeal.
  - Spinal cord white matter is peripheral and gray matter is central.
  - Pia mater covers cord and condenses into dentate ligaments.
  - Arachnoid contains CSF (normal pressure 70–200 mm H_2O lying down, 100–300 mm H_2O sitting or standing, ~150 mg total volume).
  - Dura ends at S2.
  - Cord ends at L1 in adults, conus ends at ~L2 in adults, cord ends ~L3–4 in newborns.

EPIDEMIOLOGY

- Twenty-one thousand eight hundred and ten new malignant primary brain tumors and 13,070 deaths in the US in 2008.

- Malignant tumors comprise ~40% of all primary brain/CNS tumors.
- Adult primary CNS tumors: 30–35% meningioma, 20% GBM, 10% pituitary, 10% nerve sheath, 5% low-grade glioma, <5% anaplastic astrocytoma, <5% primary CNS lymphoma.
- Of adult gliomas, ~80% are high-grade and ~20% are low-grade.
- Children: 20% of all pediatric tumors (second to ALL). Twenty percent JPA, 15–20% malignant glioma/GBM, 15% medulloblastoma, 5–10% pituitary, 5–10% ependymoma, <5% optic nerve glioma.
- Possible etiologic associations: rubber compounds, polyvinyl chloride, N-nitroso compounds, and polycyclic hydrocarbons.
- Prior ionizing RT has been associated with new meningiomas, gliomas, and sarcomas (~2% at 20-year).

GENETICS

- NF-1: von Recklinghausen, chromosome 17q11.2, 1/3,500 live births, *NF1* encodes neurofibromin, autosomal dominant, 50% germline, 50% new mutations, peripheral nerve sheath neurofibromas, café au lait spots, optic and intracranial gliomas, and bone abnormalities.
- NF-2: chromosome 22, 1/50,000 live births, *NF2* encodes merlin, autosomal dominant, bilateral acoustic neuromas, gliomas, ependymomas, and meningiomas.
- von Hippel-Lindau: chromosome 3, autosomal dominant, renal clear cell carcinoma, pheochromocytoma, hemangioblastoma, pancreatic tumors, and renal cysts.
- Tuberous sclerosis (Bourneville's disease): TSC1 on chromosome 9, TSC2 on chromosome 16, autosomal dominant, subependymal giant cell astrocytoma, retinal and rectal hamartomas.
- Retinoblastoma: Rb tumor suppressor gene, chromosome 13.
- Li-Fraumeni syndrome: germline p53 mutation = breast, sarcoma, and brain CA.
- Turcot's syndrome: primary brain tumors with colorectal CA.
- Neuroblastoma: N-myc amplication commonly seen and serves as a prognostic factor.

IMAGING

- MRI: T1 pre and postgadolinium, T2, and FLAIR (fluid attenuation inversion recovery, removes increased CSF signal on T2).
- Tumor Enhancement with gadolinium correlates with breakdown of the blood–brain barrier (BBB).

- Tumor: high grade – increased signal on T1 postgadolinium and T2 (T2 also shows edema). Low grade – increased signal on T2/FLAIR.
- Acute blood = increased signal on T1 pregadolinium.
- Post-op MRI should be performed within 48 h to document any residual disease after surgical intervention.
- JPA: enhancing nodule, highly vascular, 50% associated with cysts, high uptake on PET.
- Grade 2 glioma: nonenhancing, hypointense on T1, hyperintense on T2/FLAIR, well-circumscribed, solid, round, calcifications associated with oligodendroglioma.
- Grade 3 glioma: enhancing with gadolinium, infiltrative, less well-defined borders, mass effect (sulcal effacement, midline shift, ventricular dilatation, and vasogenic edema).
- GBM: rim enhancing, central necrosis, irregular borders, and mass effect.
- Dural tail sign: this could represent tumor or increased vascularity, linear meningeal thickening and enhancement associated with some tumors adjacent to meninges, reported in 60% of meningioma, also seen in chloroma, lymphoma, and sarcoidosis.
- MR spectroscopy: NAA = neuronal marker, choline = marker of cellularity and cellular integrity, creatine = marker of cellular energy, lactate = marker of anaerobic metabolism. Tumor = increased choline, decreased creatine, decreased NAA. Necrosis = increased lactate, decreased choline, creatine, and NAA.
- Dynamic MR perfusion: astrocytoma = increased relative cerebral blood volume (CBV), generally increasing with grade. Oligodendroglioma = even low-grade, may have high CBV due to hypervascularity. Radiation necrosis and tumefactive demyelinating lesions = low CBV.
- The use of gadolinium-based MR contrast has been associated with development of nephrogenic systemic fibrosis (NSF) in patients with chronic kidney disease maintained on dialysis. For patients with GFR < 30, gadolinium-based MR contrast should be avoided. For patients with GFR of 30-100, use of contrast is determined on a case by case basis, based on institutional protocols (Kuo et al. 2007)

PATHOLOGY

- World Health Organization Grading System of gliomas: WHO Grade 1 = JPA, Grade 2 = fibrillary astrocytoma, Grade 3 = anaplastic astrocytoma, Grade 4 = glioblastoma multiforme.

- Astrocytoma grading (AMEN) = nuclear *a*typia, *m*itoses, *e*ndothelial proliferation, *n*ecrosis.
- Pearls: pseudopalisading and necrosis = GBM, Rosenthal fibers = JPA, psammoma bodies = meningioma, verocay body = schwannoma, Schiller-Duval body = yolk-sac tumor, Fried-egg = oligodendroglioma, pseudorosette = ependymoma, Homer-Wright rosettes = medulloblastoma, pineoblastoma, Flexner-Wintersteiner rosettes = pineoblastoma.

RADIATION TECHNIQUE

FRACTIONATED EBRT

- Simulate patient with head mask.
- 3DCRT or IMRT for most lesions. 3DCRT provides better dose homogeneity, fewer hot spots. Inverse planning may allow greater sparing of critical structures and/or deliver hot spots in center of (hypoxic) tumor. Must be determined on a case-by-case basis.
- Fuse planning CT and MRI (pre-op vs. post-op) to help delineate target volume. Post-op MRs are better than pre-op MRs in most cases.

GENERAL GUIDELINES FOR TARGET VOLUMES

- Individualize tumor volume based on propensity to infiltrate, follow disease extension along the white matter tracts (e.g., internal capsule and corpus collosum) and use nonuniform margin.
- High-grade gliomas:
  GTV1 = T1 enhancement + T2/FLAIR. CTV1 = GTV1 + 2 cm margin.
  Boost: GTV2 = T1 enhancement. CTV2 = GTV2 + 2 cm.
  PTV = CTV + 0.3–0.5 cm.
- Low-grade gliomas.
  These tumors are often nonenhancing and tumor may be best visualized on FLAIR.
  GTV = T1 enhancement or FLAIR for oligodendrogliomas.
  CTV = GTV + 1–2 cm margin.
  PTV = CTV + 0.3–0.5 cm.

DOSE TOLERANCE GUIDELINES

EBRT using 1.8–2.0 Gy/fx	SRS Max point dose
Whole brain 50 Gy	Brainstem 12 Gy
Partial brain 60 Gy	Optic nerve and chiasm 8 Gy
Brainstem 54 Gy	Visual pathway 12 Gy
Spinal cord 45 Gy	
Chiasm 50–54 Gy	
Retina 45 Gy	
Lens 10 Gy	
Inner ear 30 Gy (increasing risk of hearing deficit with increasing dose)	
Epilation 20–30 Gy	
Lacrimal gland: 30 Gy transient, 60 Gy permanent	

- Fetal dose from cranial RT = 0.05–0.1% of total dose (<0.1 Gy).
- Individual patient dose constraints should be determined based on physicians' clinical judgment and experience.

POSSIBLE RADIATION COMPLICATIONS

- *Acute*: alopecia, radiation dermatitis, fatigue, transient worsening of symptoms due to edema, nausea, and vomiting (particularly with brainstem [area postrema] and posterior fossa [PF] radiation), and otitis externa. Mucositis, esophagitis, and myelosuppression are associated with cranio-spinal irradiation. Subside within 4–6 weeks after radiation. Dose-related.
- *Subacute* (6 weeks to 6 months after RT): somnolence, fatigue, neurologic deterioration, perhaps caused by changes in capillary permeability and transient demyelination.
- *Late* (6 months to many years after RT): radiation necrosis, diffuse leukoencephalopathy (especially with chemo, but not necessarily correlated with clinical symptoms), hearing loss, retinopathy, cataract, visual changes, endocrine abnormalities (if hypothalamic-pituitary axis is irradiated), vasculopathy, Moyamoya syndrome, decreased new learning ability, short-term memory, and problem solving skills.

FUNCTIONAL STATUS

See Appendix A.

II

MALIGNANT GLIOMAS

PEARLS

- Most common primary malignant CNS tumor in adults.
- Majority are glioblastoma.
- Multicentric tumors in <5% of cases.
- Incidence rises with age, peaks at 45–55-year (bimodal based on primary vs. transformation).
- Presentation: #1 headache (50%), #2 seizures (20%).
- Prognostic factors: age, histology, KPS, extent of surgery, duration of symptoms (see RPA below).
- Survival benefit from the addition of temozolomide to RT seen in patients with MGMT promoter methylation.

RTOG RPA CLASSES FOR MALIGNANT GLIOMA

I and II: anaplastic astrocytoma, age ≤50, normal mental status, or age >50, KPS >70, symptoms >3 month	MS: 40–60 months
III and IV: anaplastic astrocytoma, age ≤50, abnormal MS, or age >50, symptoms <3 month; Glioblastoma age <50 or age >50 and KPS ≥70	MS: 11–18 months
V and VI: glioblastoma, age >50, KPS <70 or abnormal mental status	MS: 5–9 months

- EORTC adaptation of RPA classes III-V, GBM only (based on updated Stupp data):
  - Class III (MS 17 month): age <50, WHO PS 0
  - Class IV (MS 15 month): age <50, WHO PS 1–2; age ≥50, GTR or STR, MMSE ≥27
  - Class V (MS 10 month): age ≥50, MMSE <27, biopsy only

TREATMENT RECOMMENDATIONS

General management	■ Dexamethasone before/after surgery when clinically indicated; taper gradually ■ Surgical decompression for increased ICP ■ Antiseizure medications as indicated, ensure therapeutic levels
Resectable, or partially resectable, operable	■ GTR/STR → RT (60 Gy) + concurrent temozolomide qd → temozolomide ×6c monthly (Stupp et al. 2005, 2009) ■ Or 40 Gy/15 fx for age ≥60 and KPS >50 (Roa et al. 2004)

	■ Or 30 Gy/10 fx for age ≥65 and KPS <50 (Bauman et al. 1994)
Inoperable	■ RT (60 Gy) + concurrent temozolomide qd → temozolomide ×6c monthly (Stupp et al. 2005, 2009)
Recurrence	■ Steroids if clinically indicated ■ If local and resectable and/or symptomatic: surgery → chemo ■ If local and unresectable: chemo and/or highly conformal RT or SRS ■ If diffuse: chemo + best supportive care ■ If poor KPS: best supportive care

STUDIES

RT VS. OBSERVATION

- Keime-Guibert (NEJM 2007): randomized 81 patients >70 year with GBM and KPS >70 after surgery (~50% biopsy only, ~30% GTR) to best supportive care ± RT (1.8/50.4 Gy to T1 enhancing + 2 cm). Trial stopped early because RT improved MS (4.3→7.3 month; 53% relative reduction in death) and MPFS (1.4→3.7 month) independent of the extent of surgery, with no difference in QOL and cognitive evaluations.
- Walker et al. (1979) *BTSG*: pooled three randomized trials. Compared observation vs. WBRT 45 vs. 50 vs. 55 vs. 60 Gy. MS increased with higher doses, 4→7→9→10 month.
- Walker et al. (1978) *BTSG 6901* – phase III: 222 patients (90% GBM, 10% AA) → surgery → randomized to observation vs. BCNU alone vs. WBRT 50–60 Gy alone vs. WBRT + BCNU. RT was WB to 50 Gy, then boost to 60 Gy. RT ± BCNU improved MS by 3–6 month vs. observation or BCNU alone.

DOSE AND FRACTIONATION

- Roa et al. (2004) – phase III: 100 patients with GBM age ≥60 and KPS ≥50 randomized to 60 Gy/30 fx vs. 40 Gy/15 fx. No difference in MS (5.1 vs. 5.6 month). Fewer patients in the short course RT arm required increased steroids (23 vs. 49%).
- Bauman et al. (1994): single arm prospective study. Twenty-nine patients with GBM age ≥65 and KPS ≤50 treated with WBRT (30 Gy/10 fx). RT increased MS vs. best supportive care (10 vs.1 month).

- *MRC* (Bleehen and Stenning 1991) randomized 474 patients to 45 Gy/20 fx vs. 60 Gy/30 fx. No adjuvant chemo. MS 12 month (60 Gy) vs. 9 month (45 Gy, $p = 0.007$).
- *RTOG 9305* (Souhami et al. IJROBP 2004): phase III trial of 203 patients randomized to postoperative SRS, followed by EBRT (60 Gy) plus BCNU, vs. EBRT and BCNU alone. Dose of radiosurgery dependent on tumor size (range 15–24 Gy). No difference in survival (MS 13.5 month) or patterns of failure.
- *RTOG 0023* (Cardinale et al. IJROBP 2006): phase II trial of 76 patients who were given 50 Gy and four weekly stereotactic radiotherapy boosts, to a cumulative dose of 70–78 Gy. After the RT, 6 cycles of BCNU given. MS 12.5 month, no improvement compared to historical data.

CHEMO-RT

- *EORTC/NCIC* (Stupp et al. 2005, 2009) – phase III: 573 patients with newly diagnosed glioblastoma (16% biopsy only, 40% GTR, 44% STR) randomized to RT alone vs. RT + concurrent and adjuvant temozolomide. RT was 60 Gy/30 fx. Temozolomide was concurrent daily (75 mg/m^2/day) and adjuvant (150–200 mg/m^2/day × 5 days) q4 weeks × 6 month. Concurrent and adjuvant temozolomide significantly improved MS (14.6 vs. 12.1 month) and 5-year OS (9.8 vs. 1.9%). MGMT gene promoter methylation was the strongest predictor for outcome and benefit from temozolomide.
- Walker et al. (1980) *BTSG 7201* – phase III: 476 patients (84% GBM, 11% AA) → surgery → randomized to MeCCNU alone vs. RT alone vs. RT + MeCCNU vs. RT + BCNU. RT was WB 60 Gy/30–35 fx. RT ± chemo increased MS compared to chemo alone (37–43 vs. 31 weeks). No difference between MeCCNU and BCNU.
- *RTOG 94–02* (Cairncross et al. JCO 2006) – phase III: 289 patients with pure or mixed anaplastic oligodendroglioma → surgery → randomized to PCV chemo ×4c → RT vs. RT alone. RT was 50.4 Gy → boost to 59.4 Gy. No difference in MS (4.9 vs. 4.7 year), but PCV chemo improved PFS (2.6 vs. 1.7 year). Patients with 1p/19q loss had longer PFS and OS. Benefit of PCV only observed for PFS in patients with 1p/19q loss.
- *EORTC 26951* (van den Bent et al. JCO 2006): 368 patients with anaplastic oligodendroglioma or oligoastrocytoma randomized after resection to RT → PCV × 6c, or RT alone. RT was 45 Gy → boost to 59.4 Gy. Median OS (40 vs. 31 month, $p = 0.23$), PFS (23 vs. 13 month, $p = 0.002$). 1p/19q loss was associated with better PFS and OS. In contrast to RTOG 9402, there was no differential benefit of PCV based on 1p/19q status.

DOSE

- EBRT: 1.8–2 Gy/fx to 45–46 Gy followed by boost to 59.4–60 Gy
- GTV1 = T1 enhancement + T2/FLAIR. CTV1 = GTV1 + 2 cm margin
- Boost: GTV2 = T1 enhancement. CTV2 = GTV2 + 2 cm
- PTV = CTV + 0.3–0.5 cm

FOLLOW-UP

- MRI 2–6 weeks after RT and then every 2 month.

LOW-GRADE GLIOMA

PEARLS

- Ten percent of primary intracranial tumors, 20% of gliomas.
- Oligodendrogliomas account for <5% of intracranial tumors.
- Age of onset: 30–40 year for WHO Grade II and 10–20 year for JPA.
- Presentation: seizures (60–70%, better prognosis) > headache > paresis.
- Favorable prognostic factors: age <40 year, good KPS, oligo subtype, GTR, low proliferative indices, 1p/19q deletions for oligodendroglioma.
- MS: low-grade pure oligodendroglioma (120 month) > low-grade mixed oligoastrocytoma > low-grade astrocytoma (60 month) ≥ anaplastic oligodendroglioma (60 month) > anaplastic astrocytoma (36 month) > GBM (12 month).

TREATMENT RECOMMENDATIONS

JPA, subependymal giant cell astrocytoma, subependymoma, grade 2 pleo-morphic astrocytoma, dysembryoblastic neuroepithelial tumor	GTR → observation STR → consider observation vs. reresection vs. chemo vs. RT vs. SRS, depending on the location of tumor, symptoms, age of patient
Oligodendroglioma, oligoastrocytoma, astrocytoma (adults)	Maximal safe resection (GTR or STR) → Observation if age <40 years, oligodendroglioma, GTR, good function. Serial MRIs, if progresses → RT 50–54 Gy (UCSF standard dose for low-grade gliomas is 54 Gy)

	Or, immediate post-op RT to 54 Gy. No survival benefit, but RT delays time to relapse by ~2 years (EORTC study) QOL gained by delaying recurrence must be weighted against QOL lost due to late toxicities of RT
Oligodendroglioma, oligoastrocytoma, astrocytoma (children)	Maximal safe resection (GTR or STR) → observation and serial MRIs. Adjuvant chemo may prolong DFS and delay need for RT. Adjuvant RT may improve DFS, but not recommended for children <3 years. Consider second surgery for operable progression and RT for inoperable progression (doses 45–54 Gy)

STUDIES

TIMING OF RT

- *EORTC 22845* (Karim et al. 2002; van den Bent et al. 2005) – phase III: 311 patients (WHO 1–2, 51% astro., 14% oligo., 13% mixed oligo-astro) treated with surgery (42% GTR, 19% STR, 35% biopsy) randomized to observation vs. post-op RT to 54 Gy. RT improved median progression-free survival (5.3 year vs. 3.4 year), 5-year PFS (55 vs. 35%), but not OS (68 vs. 66%). Sixty-five percent of patients in the observation arm received salvage RT. No difference in rate of malignant transformation (66–72%).

DOSE

- *EORTC 22844* (Karim et al. 1996) – phase III: 343 patients (WHO 1–2, astro., oligo. and mixed) treated with surgery (25% GTR, 30% STR, 40% biopsy) randomized to post-op RT 45 Gy vs. 59.4 Gy (shrinking fields). No difference in OS (59%) or PFS (49%). Five-year OS oligo vs. astro = 75 vs. 55%, <40 year vs. ≥40 year = 80 vs. 60%. Age <40 year, oligo histology, low T-stage, GTR, and good neurologic status are important prognostic factors.
- *INT/NCCTG* (Shaw et al. 2002) – phase III: 203 patients (WHO 1–2, astro, oligo, mixed) treated with surgery (14% GTR, 35% STR, 51% Bx) randomized to post-op RT 50.4 Gy vs. 64.8 Gy. No difference in 5-year OS (72% low dose vs. 64% high dose). Best survival in patients <40 year, tumor <5 cm, oligo histology and GTR. Increased Grade 3–5 toxicity (2.5 vs. 5%) with higher dose. Pattern of failure: 92% in field, 3% within 2 cm of RT field.

- Shaw et al. (1989) – retrospective study: 5/10-year OS surgery alone = 30/10%, surgery + <53 Gy = 50/20%, surgery + > 53Gy = 67/40%.

ROLE OF CHEMOTHERAPY

- *INT/RTOG 9802* (ASCO abstract 2008): phase III of low-grade gliomas. Low-risk (<40 year + GTR) observed until symptoms. Two hundred and fifty one high-risk (≥40 year or STR or biopsy) patients randomized to RT alone vs. RT → PCV ×6 cycles q8 weeks. RT 54 Gy to FLAIR + 2 cm margin. No boost. Five-year OS was 72 vs. 63% ($p = 0.33$), 5-year PFS was 63 vs. 46% ($p = 0.06$). For 2-year survivors, OS for 3 additional year was 84 vs. 72% ($p = 0.03$), and PFS was 74 vs. 52% ($p = 0.02$), suggesting a benefit to PCV chemo in the high-risk subgroup.
- Ongoing RTOG and EORTC trials investigating the use of temozolomide.

DOSE

- EBRT: 1.8 Gy/fx to 50.4–54 Gy.
- These tumors are often nonenhancing and tumor may be best visualized on FLAIR.
- GTV = T1 enhancement or FLAIR.
- CTV = GTV + 1–2 cm margin.
- PTV = CTV + 0.3–0.5 cm.

FOLLOW-UP

- MRI 2–6 weeks after RT, then every 6 month for 5 years, then annually.

BRAINSTEM GLIOMA

PEARLS

- Most common in young patients.
- Accounts for 5% of adult, and 15% of pediatric CNS tumors.
- Incidence peaks between age 4–6 year.
- Seventy to eighty percent are high-grade astrocytomas, remaining are low-grade astrocytomas, ependymomas, PNETs, and atypical teratoid-rhabdoid tumors.
- Biopsy can be associated with high mortality and morbidity, so sometimes not performed.
- MRI and presentation to determine grade.

- High-grade tumors > infiltrative, often originate in the Pons, extend alone white matter tracts into the cerebellum or diencephalon, diffusely expand the brainstem, younger age, rapid onset of symptoms, multiple neurological deficits.
- Low-grade tumors > focal lesions in the midbrain or thalamus, or dorsally exophytic lesions, older age, and indolent course.
- Differential diagnosis (nondiffuse): abscess, neurofibromatosis, demyelinating diseases, AVM, encephalitis.
- Two to five-year OS 45–66% in adults and 20–30% in children overall, but MS only 11 month for high-grade gliomas.

TREATMENT RECOMMENDATIONS

Steroids	■ Can help to stabilize or improve neurologic symptoms
Shunts	■ May be necessary in severe hydrocephalus
Surgery	■ Role is limited, generally not indicated in diffuse pontine lesions. Dorsally exophytic tumors and cervicomedullary tumors may be surgically resected
Radiation	■ Conventional fractionation to 54–60 Gy. Recommend 3DCRT ■ For diffuse lesions, cover the tumor with 2 cm margin or the entire brainstem (diencephalon to C2) and any cerebellar extension with margin ■ No benefit of dose escalation above 72 Gy at 1-Gy b.i.d. ■ No benefit of hyperfractionation (Pediatric Oncology Group)
Chemotherapy	■ No benefit of adjuvant CCNU, vincristine, prednisone, temozolomide vs. RT ■ No survival benefit of neoadjuvant chemotherapy ■ High-dose chemo with stem-cell rescue showed no benefit in Phase I/II trials

OPTIC GLIOMA

PEARLS

- Five percent of all CNS tumors in the pediatric age group
- Subdivided into: optic nerve gliomas, chiasmatic gliomas, and chiasmatic/hypothalamic gliomas (bulky lesions)

- Ten to fifteen percent of NF-1 patients have optic glioma; 25–40% of childhood optic pathway tumors have NF-1
- Presentation: *optic nerve tumors*: asymptomatic, long standing proptosis, impaired visual acuity, optic nerve atrophy; *chiasmal tumors*: decreased visual acuity, temporal field defects *chiasmatic/hypothalamic tumors*: nystagmus, visual field deficits, impaired visual acuity, hydrocephalus, increased intracranial pressure
- MRI: small and well circumscribed, homogenous enhancement
- Biopsy not necessary for diagnosis

TREATMENT RECOMMENDATIONS

Optic nerve and chiasmatic tumors	Chemo first for all patients and reserve RT for chemo failures
Chiasmatic/ hypothalamic tumors	CSF diversion if indicated. Maximal safe surgical resection. Chemo. Reserve RT (45–50 Gy) for patients who progress on or after chemo (~50% can avoid RT at 5-years)

SURVIVAL

- Long-term OS 90–100%.
- Long-term PFS 60–90%.
- For chiasmatic/hypothalamic gliomas: LC 70–80% and long-term OS 50–80%.

CNS LYMPHOMA

PEARLS

- Approximately 2% of intracranial tumors.
- Rapidly rising incidence (3–10×) in the last two decades in both immunocompetent and immunodeficient populations.
- EBV present in 60–70% of immunodeficient, and 15% immunocompetent patients.
- Median age: 55 year in immunocompetent, and 31 year in immunocompromised patients.
- Multifocal tumors: 25–50% of immunocompetent, and 60–80% of immunodeficient patients.
- MRI: single or multiple periventricular masses, intensely enhancing.

- In AIDS patients, smaller lesions may demonstrate ring enhancement. Differential diagnosis includes toxoplasmosis.
- Leptomeningeal involvement in 1/3 of patients.
- Retinal and vitreous seeding in 15–20% of patients.
- In primary intraocular lymphoma, 80% develop CNS involvement within 9 month.
- Histology: 90% are DLBCL.
- Presentation: focal deficits, seizures, headache, lethargy, confusion. Neck or back pain (spinal cord involvement). Blurred vision or floaters (ocular involvement, which presents in ~20% of patients).
- Workup: MRI brain and spine, biopsy, ophthalmologic exam, CXR, CSF cytology, CBC, EBV titer, HIV testing. CT chest, abdomen, and pelvis and bone marrow biopsy, consider testicular ultrasound for elderly men, consider PET scan. Hold steroids, if possible prior to diagnostic procedures
- Systemic or intrathecal methotrexate given with RT has synergistic neurotoxicity.

TREATMENT RECOMMENDATIONS

Surgery	■ Biopsy for tissue diagnosis. Extensive resection does not improve OS
Steroids	■ Should be withheld until after biopsy. Ninety percent have clinical response. Forty percent have shrinkage. Ten percent have complete resolution on imaging. Response is short-lived and tumor recurs within weeks to month after steroids are stopped
General management	■ If KPS ≥40 and acceptable renal function → high-dose methotrexate-based regimen *followed by* WBRT 24–36 Gy at 1.8–2-Gy/fx, If PR → boost gross disease to 45 Gy. If CSF positive or spinal MRI positive, consider intrathecal chemotherapy. If eye exam positive, intraocular chemotherapy or RT to globe ■ If KPS <40 or renal dysfunction → WBRT. If CSF positive or spinal MRI positive, consider intrathecal chemotherapy and focal spinal RT. If eye exam positive, RT to globe. Consider nonmethotrexate chemo alternatives ■ For patients >60, may omit WBRT if CR to chemo and reserve RT for recurrence ■ For leptomeningeal spread, use intrathecal chemo or CSI to 39.6 Gy with additional 5.4–10.8 Gy to gross disease ■ See Chap. 3 regarding ocular lymphoma

STUDIES

- *RTOG 83–15* (Nelson et al. 1992) – phase II: 41 patients with CNS lymphoma treated with 40 Gy WBRT + 20 Gy boost to tumor bed. Eighty-eight percent of recurrences were within the boost field. MS 12.2 month 2-year OS 28%. Better survival in patients with KPS >70 and Age <60.
- *RTOG 88–06* (Schultz et al. 1996) – phase I/II: 51 patients with HIV-negative CNS lymphoma treated with CHOD × 2 (cytoxan, adriamycin, vincristine, dexamethasone) → WB to 41.4 Gy and boost to 59.4 Gy. No difference in MS when compared with RTOG 83–15.
- *RTOG 93–10* (DeAngelis et al. 2002) – phase II: 102 HIV-negative CNS lymphoma patients treated with chemo ×5 (IV/IT MTX, vincristine, procarbozine) → WBRT 45 Gy → high-dose cytarabine. Fifty-eight percent CR, 36% PR, MPFS 24 month, MS 36.9 month. Fifteen percent patients with severe delayed neurotoxicity. Better survival in patients <60 year (50 vs. 22 month, $p < 0.001$).
- MSKCC experience (Gavrilovic, et al. 2006): 57 patients treated with high-dose MTX ± RT. Five-year OS 74% for patients <60 year treated with RT, but no difference in MS for patients >60 year with or without RT (29 month). 25% neurotoxicity for patients <60 year vs. 75% for >60 year with RT vs. 3% if no RT.

SURVIVAL

- RT alone MS 12 month, 2-year OS 20–30%.
- Chemo (high-dose MTX-based) + WBRT MS 30–60 month, 2-year OS 55–75%.
- Survival recursive partitioning analysis (JCO 2006 Abrey et al. 2006). From MSKCC, confirmed with RTOG data.
  - I: Age <50: MS 8 year, failure-free survival (FFS) 2 year.
  - II: Age ≥50 and KPS ≥70: MS 3 year, FFS 1.8 year.
  - III: Age ≥50 and KPS <70: MS 1 year, FFS 0.6 year.

EPENDYMOMA

PEARLS

- Ependymal cells form the lining of the ventricular system and the central spinal canal.

- Less than 5% of adult brain tumors, incidence peaks at 35 years old.
- Ten percent of pediatric brain tumors, incidence peaks at 5 years old.
  - Most intracranial lesions are located in the PF and arise from floor of the fourth ventricle.
  - Ten to thirty percent of fourth ventricular tumors extend down through the foramen magnum to the upper C-spine.
- Sixty percent of primary spinal cord tumors are ependymomas.
- Increased frequency of spinal cord ependymomas in patients with NF2.
- Less than 7% incidence of CSF spread at diagnosis, up to 15% ultimately, rare without local progression.
- CSF relapse 5–15%. More common with infratentorial and high-grade tumors.
- Complete resection of the PF tumors is difficult due to proximity to fourth ventricle, CNs, and major vessels.
- Complete resection is the single most important prognostic factor.
- Other good prognostic factors: low grade and age >2–4 year.
- CSF and MRI spine required to assess spine. Lumbar puncture and spine MRI should be delayed 2-3 weeks after surgery to avoid false positive results.
- Pediatric patients should be enrolled in clinical trials whenever possible.

TREATMENT RECOMMENDATIONS

Symptomatic hydrocephalus	**Steroids and/or CSF diversion**	**Outcomes**
Ependymoma resectable	■ Maximal safe surgical resection ■ Negative MRI spine and CSF ■ GTR → limited field RT (54–60 Gy) ■ STR → limited field RT ■ Positive MRI spine or CSF → CSI (30–36 Gy, boost gross disease, 54–60 Gy for brain lesions and 45 Gy for spine lesions)	5-year PFS Adults: GTR 50–55% STR 0–25% Peds (most infratentorial with post-op RT) GTR 60–80% STR 30–45% 5-year OS low-grade 60–90%

continued

Anaplastic ependymoma resectable	■ Maximal safe surgical resection ■ Negative MRI spine and CSF GTR or STR → limited field RT (54–60 Gy) ■ Positive MRI spine or CSF → CSI (30–36 Gy, boost gross disease 54–60 Gy for brain lesions and 45 Gy for spine lesions)	5-year OS up to 50–60% with surgery, RT, and chemo
Unresectable	■ Negative CSF → limited field RT (54–60 Gy) ■ Positive MRI spine or CSF → CSI (30–36 Gy, boost gross disease 54–60 Gy for brain lesions and 45 Gy for spine lesions)	5-year OS 20–30%
Recurrence	■ Maximal surgical resection ■ Post-op RT if no prior RT, consider SRS ■ Chemotherapy, best supportive care	
Children <4 years	■ Maximal safe surgical resection. If STR → chemo (platinum-based compounds and cyclophosphamide) and delay RT to avoid toxicities	5-year PFS/OS: 40/45%

FOLLOW-UP

- MRI brain and spine (if initially positive) every 3–4 month for the first year, every 4–6 month for the second year, then every 6–12 month.

CHOROID PLEXUS TUMORS

PEARLS

- Less than 2% of all glial tumors.
- Most common location: lateral ventricles in children, the fourth ventricle in adults.
- Benign (WHO grade I) = choroid plexus papilloma, 60–80%, papillary formation, lack of mitosis, and normal tissue invasion.

- Malignant (WHO grade III) = choroid plexus carcinoma, 20–40%, nuclear atypia, pleomorphism, frequent mitoses, and invasion of subependymal brain tissue.
- Most commonly present with hydrocephalus due to CSF overproduction and flow obstruction.
- Up to 30% of children present with metastatic disease at diagnosis.
- Workup: MRI brain and spine, CSF cytology.

TREATMENT RECOMMENDATIONS

General management	■ Maximal safe resection is first-line therapy for both choroid plexus papilloma and carcinoma
Choroid plexus papilloma	■ GTR and spine negative → observation ■ STR and spine negative → RT to post-op bed 50–54 Gy ■ STR and spine positive (rare!) → CSI 36 Gy + LF boost 54 Gy and boost to mets 45–54 Gy ■ No role for chemotherapy
Choroid plexus carcinoma	■ GTR and spine negative → observation, consider RT ■ STR and spine negative → RT to post-op bed to 54 Gy ■ STR and spine positive → CSI 36 Gy + LF boost 54 Gy and boost to mets 45–54 Gy ■ Consider chemotherapy

SURVIVAL

- Choroid plexus papilloma 5-year OS 90–100%.
- Choroid plexus carcinoma 5-year OS 20–30%.

MENINGIOMA

PEARLS

- Thirty percent of primary intracranial neoplasms
- Most common benign intracranial tumor in adults
- Eight thousand six hundred new cases in the US in 2002
- Incidence increases with age, peaks in the sixth and seventh decades
- F:M = 2:1 for all meningiomas and 1:1 for anaplastic meningiomas (rhabdoid and papillary)

- Locations: cerebral convexities, falx cerebri, tentorium cerebelli, cerebellopontine angle, sphenoid ridge, and spine
- Possible risk factors: ionizing radiation, viral infection, sex hormones, NF2, loss of chromosome 22q.

WORKUP

- H&P: historically, most common presentation was headaches > personality change/confusion > paresis. Symptoms correlate with location: cranial neuropathy (cerebellopontine angle), headaches or seizures (convexities, falx), visual loss (sphenoid ridge wing or optic nerve involvement). Increased use of CT/MRI brain scans has led to a rising incidence, particularly for asymptomatic lesions (autopsy series suggest prevalence of 2–3%).
- CT: extraaxial, well-circumscribed and smooth, with moderate to intense homogenous enhancement with contrast, often minimal edema (consistent with slow growth). Bony changes (destruction or hyperostosis, reflects disease involvement and not reactive change) in 15–20%. Malignant meningiomas may frequently invade the brain.
- MRI: isointense on T1 and T2, intensely enhance with gadolinium.
- Dural tail sign: linear meningeal thickening and enhancement adjacent to a peripherally located cranial mass, reported in 60% of meningiomas, also seen in chloroma, lymphoma, and sarcoidosis.
- Slower tumor growth has been linked to calcification, homogeneous enhancement and iso to hypointense T2 signal.

TREATMENT RECOMMENDATIONS

Resectable, operable	■ Observation, if asymptomatic and slow-growing. ■ GTR (often facilitated by pre-op angiography ± embolization) → observation and serial MRIs. ■ If recurrence → RT. Alternative, definitive RT, or SRS
Unresectable, operable	■ STR → RT. Alternative, definitive RT, or SRS
Inoperable	■ RT alone or SRS alone
Malignant meningioma	■ GTR or STR → RT to 60 Gy with 2–3 cm margin
Recurrence	■ RT or SRS or surgery as salvage therapy

STUDIES

POST-OP EBRT

- Goldsmith et al. (1994): 140 patients from USCF with STR + post-op RT for benign (84%) and malignant (16%) meningiomas. Five-year OS 85% for benign, 58% for malignant. Improved PFS in patients who received >52 Gy (95 vs. 65% benign, 65 vs. 15% malignant). No benefit of aggressive STR vs. biopsy alone if post-op RT given. Patients with benign tumors treated after 1980 (when CT and MRI were used for treatment planning) had better 5yr PFS compared to those treated before 1980 (98% vs. 77%, P=0.002).

SRS

- Kondziolka et al. (1999): 99 patients from U. Pittsburgh, 43% SRS alone, 57% surgery + SRS, median tumor margin dose 16 Gy, max dose 32 Gy, median tumor volume 4.7 cc. LC 95%, PFS 93% at 5–10-year.
- Stafford et al. (2001): 190 patients from Mayo Clinic, 59% had prior surgery, 12% with atypical or malignant histology. Median tumor margin dose was 16 Gy. Median prescription isodose volume was 8.2 cm^3. Five-year LC for patients with benign, atypical, and malignant tumors were 93, 68, and 0%, respectively. Five-year CSS for patients with benign, atypical, and malignant tumors were 100, 76, and 0%, respectively.
- EORTC 26021–22021: phase III study randomizing benign Grade I incompletely resected intracranial meningiomas to observation vs. EBRT or SRS. Trial closed in 3/2006, *Results pending.*

DOSES

- EBRT: 54 Gy for benign, 60 Gy for malignant.
- SRS or FSRT: individual dose chosen based on tumor volume, location, surgical history, and radiosensitivity of nearby structures.

SURVIVAL

- WHO I: 5-year PFS for GTR 88–98%, for STR alone 43–83%, and for STR + RT 88–98%. 5/10/15-year OS 85/75/70%.
- Malignant: surgery + RT, 40–50% 5-year PFS.

FOLLOW-UP

- MRI every 4 months for 1 year, every 6 months for 2 years, then annually.

ACOUSTIC NEUROMA

PEARLS

- Six percent of intracranial tumors.
- Arise from Schwann cells of myelin sheath of peripheral nerves.
- Sporadic (unilateral, age 40–50 year) or associated with NF 2 (bilateral).
- Slow growing, well-circumscribed, expansile, displace adjacent nerves.
- Symptoms: progressive sensorineuronal hearing loss and vestibular deficits. May affect CN VII function. Expansion into cerebellopontine angle may lead to CN V symptoms. Hydrocephalus may occur.
- Screening: pure tone and speech audiometry (selective loss of speech discrimination common).
- Thin slice, gadolinium-enhanced MRI through the cerebellopontine angle is the imaging modality of choice.
- Suspected NF should have neuraxis imaging.

TREATMENT RECOMMENDATIONS

- *Surgery*: 90% are total or near-total resection (<10% LF). STR without post-op RT (45% LF) vs. STR with post-op RT (6% LF). Preservation of CN VII function >60%. Preservation of useful hearing 30–50%, depending on lesion size and surgical technique.
- *SRS*: >90% LC. Dose 12–13 Gy single fraction, increased complications with >14 Gy. Similar outcome with fractionated and single fraction SRS. Preservation of CN VII function >90%. Preservation of useful hearing ~75%. Preservation of CN V function =90%.
- *EBRT*: dose 54 Gy/1.8 Gy fx. Preservation of CN VII function >95%. Preservation of useful hearing ~75%. Preservation of CN V function ~95%.

STUDIES

- Koh et al. (2007): 60 patients treated with FSRT (50 Gy/2 Gy fx). Five-year LC 96%, useful hearing preservation 77%. No new cranial nerve toxicity.
- Chopra et al. (2007): 216 patients treated with SRS (12–13 Gy marginal dose). Ten-year LC 98%. Preservation of serviceable hearing among hearing patients was 74%. CN V function preservation was 95%, CN VII was 100%.

CRANIOPHARYNGIOMA

PEARLS

- Benign, partially cystic, epithelial tumors.
- Arise from Rathke's pouch in the sellar region.
- Five to ten percent of pediatric intracranial tumors, ages 5–14 year.
- Bimodal distribution: 55% occur in children and 45% are over age 20 year with another peak between 55 and 65 year.
- Present with neuroendocrine deficits such as diabetes insipidus or growth failure, visual field cuts, decreased acuity, increased ICP, cognitive and behavioral changes.
- MRI: solid nodule (calcified and contrast enhancing) with cystic component filled lipoid, cholesterol laden fluid ("crankcase oil").
- May develop invaginations into adjacent brain, causing a glial reaction.

TREATMENT RECOMMENDATIONS

- Maximal safe resection.
- If GTR → observation (LC 85–100%).
- If STR → post-op EBRT to 54 Gy at 1.8-Gy/fx (LC 75–90%), or observation (LC 30%).
- Cyst decompression for nonresectable lesions prior to RT may ease sparing of critical structures and sometimes may be required during the course of RT.
- SRS: for small primaries or recurrent tumors.
- Intralesional bleomycin and intracavitary injection of radioactive colloid are effective in shrinking and fibrosing cysts,

although data are limited. Treatment toxicity can mimic disease progression with multiple endocrinopathies, visual loss, seizures, other cranial neuropathies, motor neuropathies, and neurocognitive deficits.

- For children <3 year, limited surgery and close follow-up, defer RT.

SURVIVAL

- Long-term event-free survival 80–100%.

PITUITARY TUMORS

PEARLS

- Ten to fifteen percent of primary brain tumors.
- 2.5: 1 incidence (female to male).
- Long natural history with insidious onset of symptoms; often slow (or no) detectable radiologic progression.
- The pituitary gland is surrounded by anterior and posterior clinoids; superiorly by anterior cerebral arteries, the optic nerves, and chiasm; laterally by cavernous sinuses (CN III, IV, V1, V2, VI, internal carotid artery); inferiorly by sphenoid sinus.
- Nearly all pituitary tumors arise from the anterior lobe, which is derived from Rathke's pouch (an evagination of ectodermal tissue from NPX).
- Anterior lobe produces GH, PRL, ACTH, TSH, FSH, LH, controlled by hypothalamic portal system hormones.
- Posterior lobe produces ADH and oxytocin.
- Seventy-five percent functional, 25% nonfunctional.
- Tumors secreting prolactin are the most common secreting tumors (30%), followed by GH (25%) → ACTH → TSH (rare).
- Macroadenomas: ≥1 cm; microadenomas: <1 cm.
- MEN-1: autosomal dominant, pituitary, parathyroid, pancreatic island cell tumors.
- Mass effect on stalk (infundibulum) causes increased PRL because of the loss of inhibition from hypothalamus. A similar effect after radiation of the stalk can be observed with persistent PRL elevation.
- Immunohistochemistry to identify subtype.
- After radiation therapy, prolactin and growth hormone levels normalize over several year. ACTH usually normalizes within 1 year.

WORKUP

- H&P: headache, visual field testing (bitemporal hemianopsia, superior temporal deficits, homonymous hemianopsia, central scotoma, etc), CN deficits (involvement of cavernous sinus), sleep/appetite/behavior changes (compression of hypothalamus), growth abnormalities, cold or heat intolerance.
- Imaging: MRI (thin cuts with contrast) or CT (look for bone destruction), skeletal survey when indicated.
- Complete endocrine evaluation.
  - Prolactin
  - Basal GH, IGF-1, glucose suppression, insulin tolerance, TRH stimulation
  - Serum ACTH, 24-h urine 17-hydroxycorticosteroids and free cortisol, dexamethasone suppression
  - Gonadal: LH, FSH, plasma estrodial, testosterone
  - Thyroid: TSH, T3, T4
  - Basal plasma or urinary steroids; cortisol response to insulin-induced hypoglycemia and plasma ACTH response to metyrapone
- Acromegaly = headache, changes in facial/skull/hand bones, heat intolerance, wt gain. Dx = GH >10 ng/mL, not suppressed by glucose, or elevated IGF-1.
- Prolactinoma = amenorrhea, infertility, decreased libido, impotence galactorrhea, PRL >20 ng/mL.
- Cushing's disease = bilateral adrenal hyperplasia, central obesity, HTN, glucose intolerance, hirsutism, easy bruising, osteoporosis. Diagnosis = elevated cortisol, not suppressed with low-dose dexamethasone, partially suppressed with high-dose dexamethasone, normal or moderately elevated plasma ACTH. In adrenal tumors, ACTH is depressed.

TREATMENT RECOMMENDATIONS

TREATMENT MODALITIES

Medical management	■ Bromocriptine for prolactinomas, somatostatin analogs and pegvisomant (GH receptor antagonist) for GH-secreting tumors, and ketoconazole, metapyone, mitotane for ACTH-secreting tumors may be used ■ Frequent relapse when discontinued ■ Provide temporary control of remission while awaiting response to RT

continued

Surgery	■ Immediate decompression ■ Microadenomas ■ Maximal safe resection even for unresectable tumors, which may result in better normal tissue sparing by making SRS feasible
Radiation	■ Indications: medically inoperable (especially with hypopituitarism), STR with persistent post-op hypersecretion, or large tumor with extrasellar extension. Consider SRS or fractionated stereotactic radiotherapy

TREATMENT AND OUTCOME BY TUMOR TYPE

Nonfunctioning pituitary tumors	■ Surgery → observation or RT vs. definitive RT alone ■ 10-year DFS 90% (S+RT) vs. 80% (RT alone)
GH-secreting	■ Surgery → observation → RT 45–50 Gy for recurrent GH elevation. Or, RT alone 45–50 Gy for inoperable patients ■ 10-year DFS 70–80% (S+RT) vs. 60–70% (RT alone)
Prolactin-secreting	■ Observation vs. medical management vs. surgery vs. RT, individualize treatment based on symptoms, side effect profile, and patient preferences. Ten-year DFS 80–90%
ACTH-secreting	■ Surgery → observation → RT 45–50 Gy for recurrent ACTH elevation. RT alone 45–50 Gy for inoperable patients. Surgery results in more rapid normalization of hormones than RT alone. Ten-year remission rate 50–60%
TSH-secreting	■ Aggressive, always treat with post-op RT
Histiocytosis X	■ 5–15 Gy in 3–8 fx

DOSE

- 1.8 Gy/fx to 45–50 Gy for nonfunctioning, or 50.4–54 Gy for functioning.
- No more than 5% of dose inhomogeneity in tumor volume.
- 1.8–54 Gy for TSH and to 50.4 Gy for ACTH-secreting tumors.
- Radiosurgery: dose prescribed to the tumor margin: 12–20 Gy for nonfunctioning tumors, 15–30 Gy for functioning adenomas. Keep optic chiasm dose <8 Gy.

SURVIVAL

- No difference in OS between surgery, surgery + RT, or RT alone; best therapy based on minimizing side effects.

FOLLOW-UP

- Post-RT contrast-enhanced MRI every 6 month ×1 year, then annually.
- Endocrine testing every 6 month – 1 year. Assess hormonal response and monitor gonadal, thyroid and adrenal function for hypopituitarism.
- Formal visual field testing before RT for baseline and annually.

PINEAL TUMORS

PEARLS

- Adults: 1% of adult brain CA. Thirty to fourty percent are germinomas and 10–20% NGGCTs.
- Children: 5% of pediatric brain CA. Fifty percent are germ-cell tumors and 25–33% pineal parenchymal tumors. Incidence peaks at age 10–12 year. M:F 3:1.
- Nongerminomatous germ-cell tumors (NGGCTs) include embryonal carcinoma (produces both β-HCG and AFP), endodermal sinus tumor (elevated AFP), choriocarcinoma (elevated β-HCG), malignant teratoma.
- Pineoblastoma and NGGCTs more commonly have CSF dissemination.
- Presenting symptoms: sellar (visual field cut), suprasellar (endocrinopathies), and pineal (hydrocephalus, Parinaud's (see below)).
- Classic triad = diabetes insipidus, precocious or delayed sexual development, visual deficits.
- Workup = MRI brain and spine, baseline ophthalmologic exam, CSF cytology and serum markers (β-HCG and AFP).

PINEOBLASTOMA

- Highly malignant primitive embryonal tumor, variant of PNET, WHO grade IV.
- Associated with bilateral retinoblastoma = trilateral retinoblastoma.
- Presents with rapidly raised ICP and enlarged head circumference.
- MRI: multilobulated, heterogeneous enhancement, with areas of necrosis and/or hemorrhage.
- Leptomeningeal spread at diagnosis in up to 50% cases.

PINEOCYTOMA

- Slow-growing tumor. WHO grade II.
- Most common in teens. Present with raised ICP.
- Parinaud's syndrome: limited upward gaze, lid retraction, retraction nystagmus, pupils that react more poorly to light than to accommodation.
- MRI: spherical, well-circumscribed, homogeneous enhancement, hypointense on T1, hyperintense on T2.

PINEAL PARENCHYMAL TUMOR OF INTERMEDIATE DIFFERENTIATION

- Moderately high cellularity, mild nuclear atypia, occasional mitoses.
- No pineocytomatous rosettes.
- Rare tumor, optimal treatment need to be decided on an individual basis.

GERMINOMAS

- Germinoma = like seminoma in men, dysgerminoma in women
- MRI: hypodense, well-circumscribed, homogeneous enhancement
- Mildly elevated β -HCG, but not AFP

NGGCT

- Elevated serum or CSF AFP and marked elevated B-HCG
- Less radiosensitive than germinoma
- Extent of resection correlates with survival

TREATMENT RECOMMENDATIONS AND OUTCOME

Histology	Recommended treatment
Pineoblastoma	■ Treat like medulloblastoma: maximal safe resection (to determine risk category) → CSI (23.4–39 Gy) + local boost to 54–55.8 Gy + chemo (5-year OS 50–70%). Radiosurgery boost possible for gross residual. If no CSI, poor outcome. MPFS 11–14 month. Five-year OS 50–70%

continued

Pineocytoma	■ Treat like low-grade glioma: surgery when possible. ■ If GTR, observe. If STR → post-op RT (residual + 1–1.5 cm margin; 50–55 Gy). Five-year OS 60–90%
Germinoma	■ MRI of neuraxis. RT alone or chemo followed by RT. Prophylactic neuraxis RT is controversial, not done at UCSF. Consider partial cranial field: whole ventricular irradiation to 24–30 Gy, boost to primary to 45–50 Gy. If there is neuraxis or subependymal spread, or multiple midline tumors → CSI 24–36 Gy + primary disease to 45–50 Gy. Five-year OS 80–90%, spinal relapse 10–20%
NGGCT	■ Maximal safe resection → platinum-based chemo. MRI and lumbar puncture. If negative neuraxis, consolidative local RT. If positive neuraxis, CSI 30–36 Gy + primary disease 50–54 Gy. Five-year OS 20–40%

MEDULLOBLASTOMA

PEARLS

- Twenty percent of pediatric CNS tumors, 40% of all PF tumors.
- The second most common pediatric CNS tumor: low-grade glioma 35–50%, medulloblastoma 20%, brainstem glioma 10–15%, high-grade glioma 10%.
- M:F = 2:1.
- Median age 5–6 year in children and 25 year in adults.
- Thirty to forty percent of patients have CSF spread at the time of diagnosis.
- Bad prognostic factors: male, age <5 year, M1 disease.
- At diagnosis, 2/3 of patients are standard risk and 1/3 are high risk.
- Common presentation: vomiting, nausea, ataxia, headaches, papilledema, CN palsy, and motor weakness.
- Differential diagnosis of Posterior Fossa (PF) mass: medulloblastoma, ependymoma, astrocytoma, brainstem glioma, JPA, and metastasis.
- PF syndrome = difficulty swallowing, truncal ataxia, mutism, respiratory failure in 10–15% of children after PF craniotomy for medulloblastoma.
- PCV chemo = cisplatin, CCNU, vincristine.

WORKUP

- H&P
- MRI of the brain (pre-op and post-op within 24–48 h after surgery)
- MRI of the spine to rule-out leptomeningeal spread
- CSF cytology
- Bilateral bone marrow biopsy
- Consider bone scan and CXR
- Baseline audiometry, IQ, TSH, CBC, and growth measurements

STAGING

Chang system (Chang et al. 1969)

T1:	≤3 cm
T2:	>3 cm
T3a:	> 3cm with extension into the aqueduct of Sylvius and/or the foramen of Luschka
T3b:	> 3cm with unequivocal extension into the brainstem
T4:	> 3cm with extension up past the aqueduct of Sylvius and/or down past the foramen magnum
M0	No metastases
M1	Microscopic cells in CSF
M2	Gross Nodular seeding in cerebellar, cerebral subarachnoid space, third or lateral ventricles
M3	Gross Nodular seeding in spinal subarachnoid space
M4	Extraneuraxial metastasis

Risk categories

Standard risk: age >3 years and GTR/STR with <1.5 cm^2 residual and M0

High risk: age <3 years or >1.5 cm^2 residual, or M+

Survival

Standard-risk DFS 60–90%

High-risk DFS 20–40%, increased to 50–85% with adjuvant chemo

TREATMENT RECOMMENDATIONS

General management	■ Hydrocephalus and increased ICP: steroids and VP shunt before attempting resection
Standard risk	■ Surgical resection → CSI 23.4 Gy at 1.8-Gy/fx with PF boost to 54 Gy with concurrent vincristine → PCV chemo. DFS ~80%
High risk Residual >1.5 cm^2 M+	■ Surgical resection → post-op CSI 36–39 Gy at 1.8-Gy/fx, with entire PF and mets >1 cm boosted to 54 Gy with concurrent vincristine → PCV chemo. DFS ~60%
Infants <3-year old	■ Surgery → intensive chemo. Reserve RT for salvage (Duffner et al. 1993; Rutkowski et al. 2005). DFS ~30–40%

STUDIES

ROLE OF CHEMOTHERAPY

- Evans et al. (1990) *CCSG/RTOG* – phase III: 233 patients with medulloblastoma → surgery → randomized to post-op RT vs. post-op chemo-RT followed by chemo × 1 year. RT was CSI 35–40 Gy with PF boost to 50–55 Gy + spinal mets to 50 Gy. Chemo was concurrent vincristine, adjuvant vincristine, CCNU, and prednisone ×1 year. Five-year OS 65% in both arms. Chemo improved EFS in T3–4, M1–3 (46% for chemo-RT vs. 0% for RT alone).
- Tait et al. (1990) *SIOP I* – phase III: 286 patients with medulloblastoma → surgery → randomized to post-op RT vs. post-op chemo-RT followed by chemo × 1 year. RT was CSI 30–35 Gy/PF boost to 50–55 Gy. Five-year/10-year OS 53/45%. Initial DFS and OS benefit of chemo disappeared with longer F/U secondary to late failures in chemo arm. Subgroups T3–4 and gross residual disease still benefited from chemo.
- *PNET 3* (Taylor et al. 2003) – phase III: 217 patients with M0–1 medulloblastoma → surgery → randomized to post-op RT vs. post-op chemo-RT. Chemo was vincristine/etoposide/carboplatin/cyclophosphomide. Patients 3–16-year old received CSI 35 Gy + 20 Gy PF boost. Trial closed early due to low accrual in RT-alone arm. Five-year OS 71%. Five-year EFS significantly better for chemo-RT arm (74 vs. 60%, $p = 0.04$). Follow-up QOL paper reported poorer outcomes in behavior and quality of life for chemo-RT arm (Bull et al. 2007).

TIMING OF CHEMOTHERAPY

- Bailey et al. (1995) *SIOP II*: 364 patients with low-risk (GTR/STR, no brainstem involvement, M0) and high-risk (gross residual, brainstem invasion, or M+) medulloblastoma. All low-risk patients randomized to surgery + chemo → RT vs. surgery → RT. Chemo was vincristine, procarbazine, and methotrexate. RT was randomized to either standard dose 35 Gy CSI + 20 Gy PF boost vs. low-dose 25 Gy CSI + 30 Gy PF boost. All high-risk patients received 35 Gy CSI + adjuvant vincristine and CCNU. Results: pre-RT chemo did not improve 5-year EFS (58% with chemo and 60% without chemo). For low-risk, no difference with RT alone for 35 vs. 25 Gy (5-year EFS 75 vs. 69%).

STANDARD/AVERAGE/LOW RISK

- Thomas et al. (2000) *POG8631/CCG923:* 88 low-risk (age 3–21, Chang T1–3a, residual <1.5 cm, M0) medulloblastoma → randomized to CSI 23.4 Gy/PF 54 Gy vs. CSI 36 Gy/PF 54 Gy. No chemo. A trend toward improved outcome with 36 Gy. However, overall EFS is suboptimal in the absence of chemo.
- *POG A9961* (JCO 2006): 379 average-risk medulloblastoma patients (age 3–21, no disseminated disease, residual <1.5 cm) → CSI 23.4 Gy/PF 55.8 Gy randomized one of two adjuvant chemotherapy regimens (CCNU, cisplatin, vincristine vs. CPM, cisplatin, vincristine). Five-year EFS 82 vs. 80%, 5-year OS 87 vs. 85%, respectively.
- Merchant et al. (2008): 86 newly diagnosed, average-risk medulloblastoma. RT began within 28 days of definitive surgery, and consisted of CSI (23.4 Gy), conformal RT to PF (36 Gy), and primary site RT (55.8 Gy). Five-year EFS 83%, comparable to historical CSI + PF RT.

HIGH-RISK

- Zeltzer et al. (1999) *CCG 921*: high-risk patients (age 1.5–21, or M1–4, or T3–4, or residual >1.5 cm^2) randomized to CSI 36 Gy/PF 54 Gy/spinal mets 50.4–54 Gy (age <3 received CSI 23.4 Gy/PF 45 Gy) + vincristine → VCP ×8 vs. "8 in 1" chemo × 2 → RT → "8 in 1" chemo × 8. "8 in 1" chemo was vincristine, prednisone, lomustine, hydroxyurea, procarbazine, cisplatin, cyclophosphamide, and cytarabine. Better 5-year PFS with VCP (63 vs. 45%, $p = 0.006$). Seventy-eight percent 5-year PFS for M0, >3-year old, ≤1.5 cm^2 residual.
- Tarbell et al. (2000) *POG 9031*: 226 high-risk patients. randomized to chemo1 → RT → chemo2 vs. RT → chemo1 → chemo2. Chemo1 was cisplatin/etoposide × 7 weeks. Chemo2 was vincristine/cyclophosphamide. RT was CSI 35.2–44 Gy/PF 53.2–56.8 Gy. Results: no difference in 5-year EFS (70% RT first vs. 66% chemo first).
- (Gajjar et al. 2006) St. Jude *Medullo-96*: 134 patients (age 3–21). Low-risk patients received CSI (23.4 Gy)/PF (36 Gy)/primary bed (55.8). High-risk patients received CSI 39.6 Gy/boost to 55.8 Gy. All patients received dose-intensive chemo × 4 cycles. Low-risk 5-year EFS 83%; high risk 70%.

INFANTS

- Duffner et al. (1993): this study addressed whether RT can be delayed by giving chemo post-op and delay RT until >3 year age. Patients <3 year with malignant brain tumors (including medulloblastoma, malignant glioma, brainstem glioma, ependymoma, PNET, etc.) underwent surgery → age <2 years, 24 month of chemo; age >2 year, 12 month of chemo → if disease progression → reresect or RT. Chemo was cyclophosphamide + vincristine × 2 → cisplatin + etoposide × 1. RT was CSI 35.2 Gy/PF 54 Gy (reduced to 24 Gy/50 Gy if complete response after surgery/chemo). Thirty-nine percent CR after the first 2 cycles of chemo. No difference in 2-year PFS (39 vs. 33%) and OS (53 vs. 55%) between two groups (<2 vs. >2 years). Thirty-four percent PFS and 46% OS for medulloblastoma at 2 year. These results suggest that it is safe to delay RT until age >3 year.

- Rutkowski et al. (2005) *German BTSG* – phase II: 43 patients (age <3) with medulloblastoma → surgery (40% GTR, 32% STR, 28% macro mets) → intensive chemo ×3c (cyclophosphamide, vincristine, methotrexate, carboplatin, and etoposide) and intrathecal methotrexate. Five-year PFS was 82 vs. 50 vs. 33% and 5-year OS was 93 vs. 56 vs. 38% for GTR vs. STR vs. macro mets. For M0 patients, 5-year PFS and OS were 68% and 77%, respectively. Sixty-two percent chemo response rate in patients with measurable disease after surgery. Age >2, desmoplastic histology and M0 were good prognostic factors. Mean IQ after treatment was lower than healthy controls, but higher than those who received RT. This study shows that lengthy remission can be obtained with intensive post-op chemo in children <3 year, reserving RT for salvage.
- Geyer (JCO 2005) *CCG 9921*: 284 patients <3-year-old w malignant brain tumors → surgery (167 <1.5 cm residual, 117 >1.5 cm residual) → randomized to two induction chemo regimens (no difference in response rate or EFS). Patients with residual dz after induction chemo or w mets at presentation received RT (tumor + 1.5 cm margin or CSI, respectively) at age 3 year (18 month for medullo or supra PNET) or after 8 cycles chemo. Five-year EFS 27%, OS 43%. Fifty-eight percent of patients alive at 5-year did not receive RT. For medullo, 5-year EFS 32%. For supra PNET, 5-year EFS 17%.

ONGOING TRIALS

- *P9934*: A phase I/II study evaluating the safety and efficacy of systemic chemo, second look surgery and IFRT for children ≥8 month and ≤36 month with nonmetastatic (M0) medulloblastoma.

- *ACNS0331*: A phase III randomized study comparing limited target volume boost irradiation and reduced dose CSI to18 Gy to standard dose RT in children with newly diagnosed standard-risk medulloblastoma.
- *ACNS0334:* Phase III randomized trial for children <36 month with high-risk medulloblastoma or PNET. Trial designed to evaluate the addition of high-dose methotrexate to the four drug induction chemo regimen of vincristine, etoposide, cyclophosphamide, cisplatin. Patients then undergo second surgery, followed by consolidation and PBSC rescue. RT at discretion of individual institution.

TREATMENT PLANNING

TRADITIONAL PRONE TECHNIQUE

- Simulate patient prone, hyperextend the neck to avoid PA beam exiting through mouth. Head mask for immobilization. Use CT for treatment planning. Anesthesia may be required for patients unable to cooperate.
- Simulate the spine field first.
  - Superior border: C2 without exiting through mouth (slight neck hyperextension may help minimize exit through mouth).
  - Inferior border: bottom of S2 or lowest level of the thecal sac as seen on MRI.
  - Lateral borders: 1 cm lateral to the lateral edge of pedicles, increase by 1–2 cm in sacrum to cover spreading of neural foramen inferiorly.
  - Field length <35 cm, use 100 cm SSD; >35 cm, use 120 cm SSD.
  - In some patients, two adjacent spinal fields may be required to encompass the spine. When two spinal fields are used, match at depth of mid spinal cord.
  - Use CT or MRI to determine depth of spinal cord.
- Simulate the cranial field second. Two parallel-opposed lateral fields.
  - Superior border flash the skin. Inferior border 0.5–1 cm on cribiform plate, 1 cm on middle cranial fossa. One centimerer anterior to the vertebral bodies, 2–2.5 cm posterior to eye markers. May angle gantry to align eyelid markers to avoid radiation to the lens.
- *Collimator angle* (of the cranial field) to match diverging spinal fields = arctan(1/2 length superior spine field/SSD).

- *Couch angle* (of the spinal field) to match diverging cranial fields = arctan(1/2 length cranial field/SAD). The foot of couch is rotated toward the side treated. Alternative to couch angle is to beam split lower border of the cranial field to avoid any overlaps at any depth with upper border of the spinal field.
- Various beamsplit techniques may be utilized to avoid overlaps at depth (see Fig. 2.1).
- *Gap shift* = For every 9 Gy, extend the cranial field inferiorly by 1 cm, shift the upper spine field inferiorly by 1 cm, and shorten the lower spine field by 1 cm. Need to recalculate couch angle each time.
- *PF boost*: use 3DCRT and CT/MRI for planning.

SUPINE TECHNIQUE (SOUTH ET AL. 2008)

- Patient simulated supine on CT with thermoplastic mask immobilization. Isocenter set at level of C2 vertebral body and marked on mask. Two CT scans then obtained, both covering the isocenter: one of head with 3 mm spacing, one of spine with 5 mm spacing.
- Brain, spinal cord, and OARs outlined on planning CT.
- Brain lateral fields are half-beam blocked and set with Y2 = 20 cm, Y1 = 0 cm.
- An 11° collimator rotation is used to match the beam divergence of the superior border of the spinal field because the spine field isocenter is always located 20 cm inferior to the C2 brain field isocenter. If an inferior spinal field is required, its iso is always located 30 cm inferior to the superior spine field iso The length of the superior portion of the inferior spine field is adjusted with asymmetric jaws in order to match the inferior limit of the superior spine field at the depth of the posterior surface of the vertebral body at that level. The length of the inferior portion of the inferior spine field is adjusted with asymmetric jaws to cover the caudal extent of the thecal sac.
- All fields use a common 100 cm SAD, so only the couch need be moved longitudinally to treat each field.
- Surface gaps are confirmed with the spine fields in the anterior position as measured from the reconstructed sagittal CT images obtained from the treatment planning system.
- Feathering is accomplished with the use of asymmetric jaws. The inferior jaw of the brain fields is opened by 1 cm every 9 Gy, while the superior border of the superior spinal field is

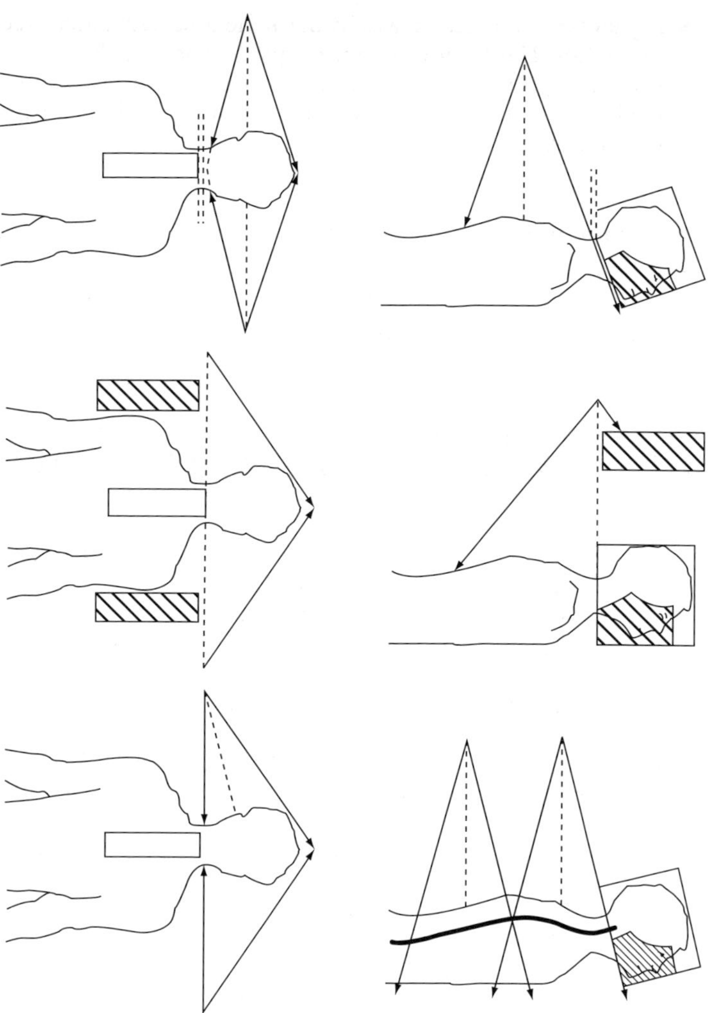

Fig. 2.1 Various techniques of cranio-spinal irradiation

decreased by 1 cm. The small change in FS is a negligible difference in divergence, so 11° collimation can still be used. With an inferior spine field, the inferior border of the superior spine field is decreased by 1 cm every 9 Gy and the superior border of the inferior field is increased by 1 cm.

- All fields are imaged on a daily basis the first week, then weekly thereafter. The anterior surface gaps are checked daily.
- If the cranial field length exceeds 20 cm, the half-beam blocked fields may be treated at extended SAD with a fixed lateral couch translation.

ALTERNATIVE DELIVERY METHODS

- Protons may be employed to reduce exit dose.
- Tomotherapy may avoid the need to match fields, but greater whole body dose exposure.

PRIMARY SPINAL CORD TUMORS

PEARLS

- Primary spinal cord tumors account for 4% of all CNS tumors overall, and 6% of CNS tumors in children.
- 2/3 extramedullary, 1/3 intramedullary.
- Intramedullary = astrocytoma (most common), ependymoma, and oligodendroglioma.
- Intradural-extramedullary = meningioma, ependymoma, nerve sheath tumors.
- Extradural = metastasis, bone osteogenic sarcoma, chondrosarcoma, chordoma, myeloma, epidural hemangiomas, lipomas, extradural meningiomas, and lymphomas.
- Astrocytomas are more common in C/T spine and frequently associated with cysts.
- Ependymomas are more common in L/S spine.
- Presentation: focal pain, segmental or nerve root weakness, sensory deficit in dermatomal distribution, incontinence.
- Brown-Séquard Syndrome = ipsilateral loss of motor function and fine touch sensation, and contralateral loss of pain and temperature sensation.
- Workup: MRI spine, CSF cytology, MRI brain for ependymoma, lymphoma, AA, metastases and GBM, CT chest for sarcomas, no LP before MRI.
- MRI: nearly all spinal cord tumors enhance with gadolinium, including low-grade gliomas.
- CSF: increased protein, possible xanthochromia (with extradural compression).

TREATMENT RECOMMENDATIONS

All tumors resectable, operable	Maximal safe surgical resection	Outcomes
Low-grade glioma, GTR	Observation	5-year OS 60–90% 5-year DFS 40%
Low-grade glioma, STR	RT to 50–54 Gy	5-year OS 60–90% 5-year DFS 40%
High-grade glioma	RT to 54 Gy. Consider adjuvant chemo	5-year OS 0–30% MS 6–24 month
Ependymoma	RT to 50–54 Gy ± CSI (for documented neuraxis dissemination)	5-year OS 60–100% 5-year DFS 60–90% Low-grade OS: 85–100% High-grade OS: 25–70%
Meningioma, GTR	Observation	
Meningioma, STR	Observation, or RT to 50–54 Gy or SBRT	
Spinal cord sarcomas, vertebral body chondro sarcomas, chordomas, osteogenic sarcomas	SBRT or charged particle beams	
Recurrent tumor	Surgical resection or reirradiation	

ARTERIOVENOUS MALFORMATION

PEARLS

- Average age 30 year.
- Annual rate of spontaneous hemorrhage ~2–4% with morbidity 20–30% per bleed and mortality 1%/year or 10–15% per bleed.
- There is a period of decreased risk of hemorrhage during latent interval after SRS treatment before complete angiographic resolution.
- After angiographic obliteration, lifetime risk of hemorrhage is ≤1%.
- SRS produces progressive thickening of the vascular wall and luminal thrombosis.

- Obliteration takes several years.
- Treatment.
  - Microsurgical resection or SRS are both options.
  - Treat entire nidus, but not feeding arteries or draining veins.
  - Tailor dose according to volume and location.
- Maruyama et al. (2005) reviewed 500 patients treated with SRS who were followed with serial exams, MRI and/or angiography. Mean dose 21 Gy. Cumulative 4-year obliteration rate 81%, 5 year 91%. Hemorrhage risk reduced by 54% during latency period and by 88% after obliteration compared to before SRS.
- Obliteration rate at 2-year for lesions <2 cm is 90–100% and for >2 cm is 50–70%.
- F/U: MRI every 6 month × 1–3 year, then annually. Once MRI shows obliteration, obtain angiogram to confirm (gold standard).

TRIGEMINAL NEURALGIA

PEARLS

- Disorder of the sensory nucleus of CN V causing episodic, paroxysmal, severe pain lasting seconds to minutes, followed by a pain free period in the distribution of one or more of its divisions.
- Peak age 60 year. F:M 2:1.
- Often precipitated by stimulation (e.g., shaving, brushing teeth, wind).
- Obtain MRI to rule-out neoplasm in cerebellopontine angle.
- Medical management is standard treatment (carbamazepine, gabapentin, antidepressants, etc.).
- Surgical options include nerve blocks, partial sensory rhizotomy, balloon decompression of the Gasserian ganglion, microvascular decompression, and peripheral nerve ablation (radiofrequency, neurectomy, cryotherapy).
- SRS may also be used with dose of ~80 Gy to 100% isodose line.
- Median time to pain relief with SRS is ~1 month. Approximately 50–60% become pain free, ~10–20% have decreased severity or frequency of pain, and ~5–10% have slight improvement only. Less than 10% developed facial numbness.

REFERENCES

Abrey LE, Ben-Porat L, Panageas KS et al. Primary Central Nervous System Lymphoma: The Memorial Sloan-Kettering Cancer Center Prognostic Model. J Clin Oncol 2006; 36: 5711-5715.

Bailey CC, Gnekow A, Wellek S, et al. Prospective randomised trial of chemotherapy given before radiotherapy in childhood medulloblastoma. International Society of Paediatric Oncology (SIOP) and the (German) Society of Paediatric Oncology (GPO): SIOP II. Med Pediatr Oncol 1995;25:166-178.

Bull KS, Spoudeas HA, Yadegarfar G, et al. Reduction of health status 7 yrs after addition of chemotherapy to craniospinal irradiation for medulloblastoma: a follow-up study in PNET3 trial survivors on behalf of the CCLG (formerly UKCCSF). J Clin Oncol 2007;25: 4239-4245.

Bauman GS, Gaspar LE, Fisher BJ, et al. A prospective study of short-course radiotherapy in poor prognosis glioblastoma multiforme. Int J Radiat Oncol Biol Phys 1994;29:835-839.

Bleehen NM, Stenning SP. A Medical Research Council trial of two radiotherapy doses in the treatment of grades 3 and 4 astrocytoma. The Medical Research Council Brain Tumour Working Party. Br J Cancer 1991;64:769-774.

Cairncross G, Berkey B, Shaw E, et al. Phase III trial of chemotherapy plus radiotherapy compared with radiotherapy alone for pure and mixed anaplastic oligodendroglioma: intergroup radiation therapy oncology group trial 9402. J Clin Oncol 2006;24:2707-2714.

Cardinale R, Won M, Choucair A, et al. A phase II trial of accelerated radiotherapy using weekly stereotactic conformal boost for supratentorial glioblastoma multiforme: RTOG 0023. Int J Radiat Oncol Biol Phys 2006;65:1422-1428.

Chang CH, Housepian EM, Herbert C Jr. An operative staging system and a megavoltage radiotherapeutic technic for cerebellar medulloblastomas. Radiology 1969; 93(6): 1351-1359.

Chopra R, Kondziolka D, Niranjan A, et al. Long-term follow-up of acoustic schwannoma radiosurgery with marginal tumor doses of 12 to 13 Gy. Int J Radiat Biol Phys 2007;63:845-851.

DeAngelis LM, Seiferheld W, Schold SC, et al. Combination chemotherapy and radiotherapy for primary central nervous system lymphoma: Radiation Therapy Oncology Group Study 93-10. J Clin Oncol 2002;20:4643-4648.

Duffner PK, Horowitz ME, Krischer JP, et al. Postoperative chemotherapy and delayed radiation in children less than three years of age with malignant brain tumors. N Engl J Med 1993;328:1725-1731.

Evans AE, Jenkin RD, Sposto R, et al. The treatment of medulloblastoma. Results of a prospective randomized trial of radiation therapy with and without CCNU, vincristine, and prednisone. J Neurosurg 1990;72:572-582.

Gajjar A, Chintagumpala M, Ashley D, et al. Risk-adapted craniospinal radiotherapy followed by high-dose chemotherapy and stem-cell rescue in children with newly diagnosed medulloblastoma (St Jude Medulloblastoma-96): long-term results from a prospective, multicentre trial. Lancet Oncol 2006;7:813-820.

Gavrilovic IT, Hormigo A, Yahalom J, et al. Long-term follow-up of high-dose methotrexate-based therapy with and without whole brain irradiation for newly diagnosed primary CNS lymphoma. J Clin Oncol. 2006;24:4570-4574.

Geyer JR, Sposto R, Jennings M, et al. Multiagent chemotherapy and deferred radiotherapy in infants with malignant brain tumors: a report from the Children's Cancer Group. J Clin Oncol 2005;23:7621-7631.

Goldsmith BJ, Wara WM, Wilson CB, et al. Postoperative irradiation for subtotally resected meningiomas. A retrospective analysis of 140 patients treated from 1967 to 1990. J Neurosurg 1994;80:195-201.

Gripp S, Kambergs J, Wittkamp M, et al. Coverage of anterior fossa in whole-brain irradiation. Int J Radiat Oncol Biol Phys 2004;59:515-520.

Karim AB, Maat B, Hatlevoll R, et al. A randomized trial on dose-response in radiation therapy of low-grade cerebral glioma: European Organization for Research and Treatment of Cancer (EORTC) Study 22844. Int J Radiat Oncol Biol Phys 1996;36:549-556.

Karim AB, Afra D, Cornu P, et al. Randomized trial on the efficacy of radiotherapy for cerebral low-grade glioma in the adult: European Organization for Research and Treatment of Cancer Study 22845 with the Medical Research Council study BRO4: an interim analysis. Int J Radiat Oncol Biol Phys 2002;52:316-324.

Keime-Guibert F, Chinot O, Taillandier L, et al. Radiotherapy for Glioblastoma in the Elderly. NEJM 2007; 356:1527-1535.

Koh E, Millar B, Menard C, et al. Fractionated stereotactic radiotherapy for acoustic neuroma. Single-institution experience at the Princess Margaret Hospital. Cancer 2007;109:1203-1210.

Kondziolka D, Levy EI, Niranjan A, et al. Long-term outcomes after meningioma radiosurgery: physician and patient perspectives. J Neurosurg 1999;91:44-50.

Kuo PH, Kanak E, Abu-Alfa AK, et al. Gadolinium-based MR contrast agents and nephrogenic systemic fibrosis. Radiology 242; 647-649.

Maruyama K, Kawahara N, Shin M, et al. The risk of hemorrhage after radiosurgery for cerebral arteriovenous malformations. N Engl J Med 2005;352:146-153.

Merchant TE, Kun LE, Krasin MJ, et al. Multi-institutional prospective trial of reduced-dose craniospinal irradiation (23.4 Gy) followed by conformal posterior fossa (36 Gy) and primary site irradiation (55.8 Gy) and dose-intensive chemotherapy for average-risk medulloblastoma. Int J Radiat Oncol Biol Phys 2008;70:782-787.

Nelson DF, Martz KL, Bonner H, et al. Non-Hodgkin's lymphoma of the brain: can high dose, large volume radiation therapy improve survival? Report on a prospective trial by the Radiation Therapy Oncology Group (RTOG): RTOG 8315. Int J Radiat Oncol Biol Phys 1992;23:9-17.

Pomeroy SL. Treatment and prognosis of medulloblastoma. Uptodate Online 17.3. www.uptodate.com. Assessed Feb. 21, 2010.

Roa W, Brasher PM, Bauman G, et al. Abbreviated course of radiation therapy in older patients with glioblastoma multiforme: a prospective randomized clinical trial. J Clin Oncol 2004;22:1583-1588.

Rutkowski S, Bode U, Deinlein F, et al. Treatment of early childhood medulloblastoma by postoperative chemotherapy alone. N Engl J Med 2005;352:978-986.

Schultz C, Scott C, Sherman W, et al. Preirradiation chemotherapy with cyclophosphamide, doxorubicin, vincristine, and dexamethasone for primary CNS lymphomas: initial report of radiation therapy oncology group protocol 88-06. J Clin Oncol 1996;14:556-564.

Shaw EG, Daumas-Duport C, Scheithauer BW, et al. Radiation therapy in the management of low-grade supratentorial astrocytomas. J Neurosurg 1989; 70:853-861.

Shaw E, Arusell R, Scheithauer B, et al. Prospective randomized trial of low- versus high-dose radiation therapy in adults with supratentorial low-grade glioma: initial report of a North Central Cancer Treatment Group/Radiation Therapy Oncology Group/Eastern Cooperative Oncology Group study. J Clin Oncol 2002;20:2267-2276.

Souhami L, Seiferheld W, Brachman D, et al. Randomized comparison of stereotactic radiosurgery followed by conventional radiotherapy with carmustine for patients with glioblastoma multiforme: Report of Radiation Therapy Oncology Group 93-05 protocol. Int J Radiat Oncol Biol Phys 2004;60:853-860.

South M, Chiu JK, The BS, et al. Supine craniospinal irradiation using intrafractional junction shifts and field-in-field dose shaping: early experience at Methodist hospital. Int J Radiat Oncol Biol Phys 2008;71(2):477-483.

Stafford SL, Pollock BE, Foote RL, et al. Meningioma radiosurgery: tumor control, outcomes, and complications among 190 consecutive patients. Neurosurgery 2001;49(5):1029-1037.

Stupp R, Hegi ME, Mason WP, et al. Effects of radiotherapy with concomitant and adjuvant temozolomide versus radiotherapy alone on survival in glioblastoma in a randomised phase III study: 5-year analysis of the EORTC/NCIC trial. Lancet Oncol 2009;10:459-466.

Stupp R, Mason WP, van den Bent MJ, et al. Radiotherapy plus concomitant and adjuvant temozolomide for glioblastoma. New Engl J Med 2005;352:987-996.

Tait DM, Thornton-Jones H, Bloom HJ, et al. Adjuvant chemotherapy for medulloblastoma: the first multi-centre control trial of the International Society of Paediatric Oncology (SIOP I). Eur J Cancer 1990;26:464-469.

Tarbell NJ, Smith AR, Adams J, et al. The challenge of conformal radiotherapy in the curative treatment of medulloblastoma. Int J Radiat Oncol Biol Phys 2000;46:265-266.

Taylor RE, Bailey CC, Robinson K, et al. Results of a randomized study of preradiation chemotherapy versus radiotherapy alone for nonmetastatic medulloblastoma: The International Society of Paediatric Oncology/United Kingdom Children's Cancer Study Group PNET-3 study. J Clin Oncol 2003;21:1581-1591.

Thomas PR, Deutsch M, Kepner JL, et al. Low-stage medulloblastoma: final analysis of trial comparing standard-dose with reduced-dose neuraxis irradiation. J Clin Oncol 2000;18:3004-3011.

Van den Bent MJ, de Witte O, Hassel MB, et al. Long-term efficacy of early versus delayed radiotherapy for low-grade astrocytoma and oligodendroglioma in adults: the EORTC 22845 randomized trial. Lancet 2005;366:985-990.

Van den Bent MJ, Carpentier AF, Brandes AA, et al. Adjuvant procarbazine, lomustine, and vincristine improves progression-free survival but not overall survival in newly diagnosed anaplastic oligodendrogliomas and oligoastrocytomas : a randomized European organisation for research and treatment of cancer phase III trial. J Clin Oncol 2006;24:2715-2722.

Walker MD, Alexander E, Jr., Hunt WE, et al. Evaluation of BCNU and/or radiotherapy in the treatment of anaplastic gliomas. A cooperative clinical trial. J Neurosurg 1978;49:333-343.
Walker MD, Strike TA, Sheline GE. An analysis of dose-effect relationship in the radiotherapy of malignant gliomas. Int J Radiat Oncol Biol Phys 1979;5:1725-1731.
Walker MD, Green SB, Byar DP, et al. Randomized comparisons of radiotherapy and nitrosoureas for the treatment of malignant glioma after surgery. N Engl J Med 1980;303:1323-1329.
Zeltzer PM, Boyett JM, Finlay JL, et al. Metastasis stage, adjuvant treatment, and residual tumor are prognostic factors for medulloblastoma in children: conclusions from the Children's Cancer Group 921 randomized phase III study. J Clin Oncol 1999;17:832-845.

FURTHER READING

Batchelor T, Loeffler S. Primary CNS lymphoma. J Clin Oncol 2006;24:1281-1288.
Bauman GS, Fisher B, Schild S, et al. Meningioma, ependymoma, and other adult brain tumors. In: Gunderson LL, Tepper JE, editors. Clinical radiation oncology. 2nd ed: Elsevier; 2007. pp 539-566.
Berger C, Thiesse P, Lellouch-Tubiana A, et al. Choroid plexus carcinomas in childhood: clinical features and prognostic factors. Neurosurgery 1998;42:470-475.
Broniscer A, Iacono L, Chintagumpala M, et al. Role of temozolomide after radiotherapy for newly diagnosed diffuse brainstem glioma in children: results of a multiinstitutional study (SJHG-98). Cancer 2005;103:133-139.
Brown PD, Shaw EG. Low-grade gliomas. In: Gunderson LL, Tepper JE, editors. Clinical radiation oncology. 2nd ed: Elsevier; 2007. pp 493-514.
Carter M, Nicholson J, Ross F, et al. Genetic abnormalities detected in ependymomas by comparative genomic hybridisation. Br J Cancer 2002; 86:929-939.
Central Brain Tumor Registry of the United States. 2009 CBTRUS Statistical Report: Primary Brain and Central Nervous System Tumors Diagnosed in the United States in 2004-2005. Available at: http://www.cbtrus.org/reports/reports.html Accessed on June 15, 2009.
Cha S. Perfusion MR imaging of brain tumors. Top Magn Reson Imaging 2004;15:279-289.
Cheuk AV, Chin LS, Petit JH, et al. Gamma knife surgery for trigeminal neuralgia: Outcome, imaging, and brainstem correlates. Int J Radiat Oncol Biol Phys 2004;60:537-541.
Chung HT, Ma R, Toyota B, et al. Audiologic and treatment outcomes after linear accelerator-based stereotactic irradiation for acoustic neuroma. Int J Radiat Oncol Biol Phys 2004;59:1116-1121.
Cowper SE. Nephrogenic systemic fibrosis: an overview. J Am Coll Radiol 2008;5:23-28.
Fiveash JB, Nordal RA, Markert JM, et al. High-grade gliomas. In: Gunderson LL, Tepper JE, editors. Clinical radiation oncology. 2nd ed: Elsevier; 2007. pp 515-537.
Freeman CR, Farmer J, Taylor RE. Central nervous system tumors in children. In: Perez CA, Brady LW, Halperin EC, et al., editors. Principles and practice of radiation oncology. 5th ed: Lippincott Williams and Wilkins; 2008. pp 1822-1849.
Freire JE, Brady LW, Shields JA, et al. Eye and orbit. In: Perez CA, Brady LW, Halperin EC, et al., editors. Principles and practice of radiation oncology. 4th ed: Lippincott Williams and Wilkins; 2004. pp 876-896.
Fulton DS, Urtasun RC, Scott-Brown I, et al. Increasing radiation dose intensity using hyperfractionation in patients with malignant glioma. Final report of a prospective phase I-II dose response study. J Neurooncol 1992; 14:63-72.
Gilbertson RJ, Bentley L, Hernan R, et al. ERBB receptor signaling promotes ependymoma cell proliferation and represents a potential novel therapeutic target for this disease. Clin Cancer Res 2002;8:3054-3064.
Goldsmith BJ. Meningeal tumors. In: Leibel SA, Phillips TL, editors. Textbook of radiation oncology. 2nd ed: Saunders; 2004. pp 497-514.
Gupta N. Choroid plexus tumors in children. Neurosurg Clin N Am 2003;14:621-631.
Gururangan S, Friedman HS. Recent advances in the treatment of pediatric brain tumors. Oncology (Huntingt) 2004;18:1649-1661; discussion 1662, 1665-1646, 1668.
Huang D, Halberg FE. Pituitary tumors. In: Leibel SA, Phillips TL, editors. Textbook of radiation oncology. 2nd ed: Saunders; 2004. pp 533-548.
Hukin J, Steinbok P, Lafay-Cousin L, et al. Intracystic bleomycin therapy for craniopharyngioma in children. Cancer 2007;109:2124-2131.
Jemal A, Siegel R, Ward E, et al. Cancer statistics, 2008. CA Cancer J Clin 2008;58:71-96.
Kondziolka D, Lunsford LD, Flickinger JC. Stereotactic radiosurgery for the treatment of trigeminal neuralgia. Clin J Pain 2002;18:42-47.

Lunsford LD, Niranjan A, Flickinger JC, et al. Radiosurgery of vestibular schwannomas: summary of experience in 829 cases. J Neurosurg 2005;102 Suppl:195-199.

Maire JP, Caudry M, Darrouzet V, et al. Fractionated radiation therapy in the treatment of stage III and IV cerebello-pontine angle neurinomas: long-term results in 24 cases. Int J Radiat Oncol Biol Phys 1995;32:1137-1143.

Maire JP, Caudry M, Guerin J, et al. Fractionated radiation therapy in the treatment of intracranial meningiomas: local control, functional efficacy, and tolerance in 91 patients. Int J Radiat Oncol Biol Phys 1995;33:315-321.

Merchant TE. Central nervous system tumors in children. In: Gunderson LL, Tepper JE, editors. Clinical radiation oncology. 2nd ed: Elsevier; 2007. pp 1575-1591.

Michalski JM. Spinal canal. In: Perez CA, Brady LW, Halperin EC, et al., editors. Principles and practice of radiation oncology. 5th ed: Lippincott Williams and Wilkins; 2008. pp 765-777.

Mirimanoff R, Gorlia T, Mason W, et al. Radiotherapy and temozolomide for newly diagnosed glioblastoma: recursive partitioning analysis of the EORTC 26981/22981- NCIC CE3 Phase III randomized trial. J Clin Oncol 2006;24:2563-2569.

Nakamura M, Roser F, Michel J, et al. The natural history of incidental meningiomas. Neurosurgery 2003;52:62-71.

Narayana A, Leibel SA. Primary and metastatic brain tumors in adults. In: Leibel SA, Phillips TL, editors. Textbook of radiation oncology. 2nd ed: Saunders; 2004. pp 463-497.

National Comprehensive Cancer Network. Clinical Practice Guidelines in Oncology: Central Nervous System Tumors. Available at: http://www.nccn.org/professionals/physician_gls/PDF/cns.pdf. Accessed on June 25, 2009.

Packer RJ, Gajjar A, Vezina G, et al. Phase III study of craniospinal radiation therapy followed by adjuvant chemotherapy for newly diagnosed average-risk medulloblastoma. J Clin Oncol 2006;24:4202-4208.

Roberge D, Shenouda G, Souhami L. Pituitary. In: Halperin EC, Perez CA, Brady LW, editors. Principles and practice of radiation oncology. 5th ed: Lippincott Williams & Wilkins; 2008. pp 751-764.

Shaw EG, Debinski W, Robbins ME. Central nervous system tumors overview. In: Gunderson LL, Tepper JE, editors. Clinical radiation oncology. 2nd ed: Elsevier; 2007. pp 459-491.

Sheehan J, Pan HC, Stroila M, et al. Gamma knife surgery for trigeminal neuralgia: outcomes and prognostic factors. J Neurosurg 2005;102:434-441.

Shrieve DC, Larson DA, Loeffler JS. Radiosurgery. In: Leibel SA, Phillips TL, editors. Textbook of radiation oncology. 2nd ed: Saunders; 2004. pp 549-564.

Siker ML, Donahue BR, Vogelbaum MA, et al. Primary intracranial neoplasms. In: Halperin EC, Perez CA, Brady LW, editors. Principles and practice of radiation oncology. 5th ed: Lippincott Williams & Wilkins; 2008. pp 717-750.

Silvani A, Eoli M, Salmaggi A, et al. Combined chemotherapy and radiotherapy for intracranial germinomas in adult patients: a single-institution study. J Neurooncol 2005;71:271-276.

Varia MA, Ewend MG, Sharpless J, et al. Pituitary tumors. In: Gunderson LL, Tepper JE, editors. Clinical radiation oncology. 2nd ed: Elsevier; 2007. pp 567-589.

Weil MD, Hass-Kogan DA, Wara WM. Pediatric central nervous system tumors. In: Leibel SA, Phillips TL, editors. Textbook of radiation oncology. 2nd ed: Saunders; 2004. pp 1199-1214.

Wolff JE, Sajedi M, Coppes MJ, et al. Radiation therapy and survival in choroid plexus carcinoma. Lancet 1999;353:2126.

III

PART III
Head and Neck

Chapter 3

Malignant and Benign Diseases of the Eye and Orbit

III

Tania Kaprealian, Kavita K. Mishra, Alice Wang-Chesebro, and Jeanne Marie Quivey

GENERAL PEARLS

- All eye/orbit malignancies are uncommon: per ACS, approximately 2,390 new cases/year.
- Percentage of malignant tumors increases with age, due to increases in primary orbital lymphoma (OL) and metastatic lesions in the elderly (both in choroid and in the orbit).
- Most common intraocular malignancy in adults: choroidal metastasis, usually adenocarcinoma, especially from lung, breast, and prostate.
- Most common primary eye malignancy in adults: uveal melanoma.
- Most common primary eye malignancy in children: retinoblastoma.
- Most common primary orbital malignancy in adults: lymphoma.
- Most common primary orbital malignancy in children: rhabdomyosarcoma.
- This chapter will discuss uveal melanoma, OL, intraocular lymphoma (IOL), thyroid ophthalmopathy, and orbital lymphoid hyperplasia (for Retinoblastoma and Rhabdomyosarcoma, see Part XI).

UVEAL MELANOMA

PEARLS

- Most common primary intraocular malignancy in adults.
- Ocular melanomas represent ~3–5% of all melanomas, of which 85% are uveal, 5% conjunctival, and 10% other.
- In the US, ~1,500–2,000 cases/year.
- Thought to arise from melanocytes of the uveal tract (pigmented layer of the eye that includes the iris, ciliary body, and choroid).
- Average age at diagnosis is 60 years (peak incidence 60–79).
- Male-to-female ratio is 1.3:1.
- Risk factors: light eyes, melanocytosis in affected eye, arc welding, history of sun/snow burn.
- Xeroderma pigmentosum, oculodermal melanocytosis, and dysplastic nevus syndrome may predispose to melanoma.
- Histologic subtypes: spindle cell (grade 1), mixed cell (grade 2), epithelioid cell (grade 3).
- Presentation: ~1/3 asymptomatic, found on exam; patient reports visual distortion, field loss, floaters, scotomas, flashing lights, unilateral cataract, pain.
- Patterns of spread: (1) intraocular spread, including vitreous seeding; (2) extrascleral extension (15% of patients); (3) metastasis may occur after a prolonged disease-free interval; typically liver (~90%), also skin and lung; brain mets are rare.
- Poor prognostic factors include larger tumor diameter, greater thickness, ciliary body invasion, near fovea/macula, scleral penetration, optic nerve invasion, mixed/epithelioid cell type, high mitotic rate, Ki-67+, pleomorphic nucleoli, lymphocytic infiltration, monosomy of chromosome 3, gene expression profiling, and older age.
- Collaborative Ocular Melanoma Study (COMS) size classification: small melanomas (1–3 mm thick and 5–16 mm in largest dimension), medium-sized melanomas (2.5–10 mm thick, and ≤16 mm in largest dimension), and large melanomas (>10 mm thick and/or >16 mm in largest dimension).

WORKUP

- H&P includes measurement of tumor diameter/thickness, location, geometry, and tumor coloration.
- Labs: CBC, LFTs, LDH.
- Imaging: fundus photography, fluorescein angiography, ocular ultrasound (Kretz A&B), and MRI. CT of chest/abdomen if LFTs are elevated.

STAGING: UVEAL MELANOMA

Editors' note: All TNM stage and stage groups referred to elsewhere in this chapter reflect the 2002 AJCC staging nomenclature unless otherwise noted as the new system below was published after this chapter was written.

(AJCC 6TH ED., 2002)

Primary tumor (T)

All uveal melanomas

TX: Primary tumor cannot be assessed
T0: No evidence of primary tumor
Tis: Carcinoma *in situ*

Iris

T1: Tumor limited to iris
- T1a: Tumor limited to iris not more than 3 clock hours in size
- T1b: Tumor limited to iris more than 3 clock hours in size
- T1c: Tumor limited to iris with melanomalytic glaucoma

T2: Tumor confluent with or extending into the ciliary body and/or choroid
- T2a: Tumor confluent with or extending into the ciliary body and/or choroids with melanomalytic glaucoma

T3: Tumor confluent with or extending into the ciliary body and/or choroid with scleral extension
- T3a: Tumor confluent with or extending into the ciliary body with scleral extension and melanomalytic glaucoma

T4: Tumor with extraocular extension

Ciliary body and choroid

T1: Tumor 10 mm or less in greatest diameter and 2.5 mm or less in greatest height (thickness)
- T1a: Tumor 10 mm or less in greatest diameter and 2.5 mm or less in greatest height (thickness) without microscopic extraocular extension
- T1b: Tumor 10 mm or less in greatest diameter and 2.5 mm or less in greatest height (thickness) with microscopic extraocular extension
- T1c: Tumor 10 mm or less in greatest diameter and 2.5 mm or less in greatest height (thickness) with macroscopic extraocular extension

(AJCC 7TH ED., 2010)

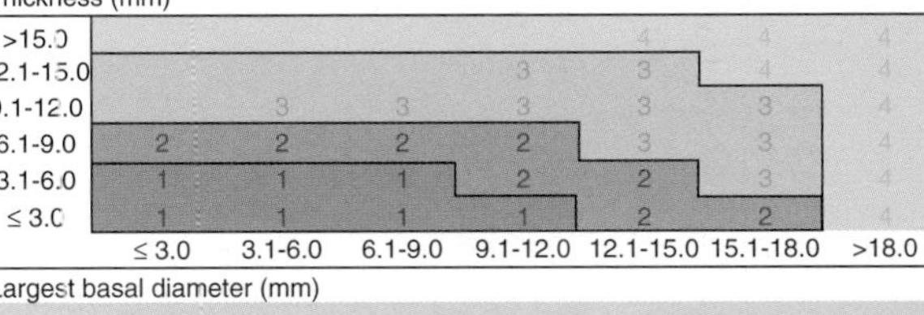

Classification for ciliary body and choroid uveal melanoma based on thickness and diameter

Primary tumor (T)

All uveal melanomas

TX Primary tumor cannot be assessed
T0: No evidence of primary tumor

*Iris****

T1: Tumor limited to the iris
- T1a: Tumor limited to the iris not more than 3 clock hours in size
- T1b: Tumor limited to the iris more than 3 clock hours in size
- T1c: Tumor limited to the iris with secondary glaucoma

T2: Tumor confluent with or extending into the ciliary body, choroid, or both
- T2a: Tumor confluent with or extending into the ciliary body, choroid, or both, with secondary glaucoma

T3: Tumor confluent with or extending into the ciliary body, choroid, or both, with scleral extension

continued

T2*: Tumor greater than 10 mm, but not more than 16 mm in greatest basal diameter and between 2.5 and 10 mm in maximum height (thickness)

- T2a: Tumor greater than 10 mm, but not more than 16 mm in greatest basal diameter and between 2.5 and 10 mm in maximum height (thickness) without microscopic extraocular extension
- T2b: Tumor 10–16 mm in greatest basal diameter and between 2.5 and 10 mm in maximum height (thickness) with microscopic extraocular extension
- T2c: Tumor 10–16 mm in greatest basal diameter and between 2.5 and 10 mm in maximum height (thickness) with macroscopic extraocular extension

T3*: Tumor more than 16 mm in greatest diameter and/or greater than 10 mm in maximum height (thickness) without extraocular extension

T4: Tumor more than 16 mm in greatest diameter and/or greater than 10 mm in maximum height (thickness) with extraocular extension

**Note*: When basal dimension and apical height do not fit this classification, the largest tumor diameter should be used for classification.

Regional lymph nodes (N)

- NX: No regional lymph node metastasis cannot be assessed
- N0: No regional lymph node metastasis
- N1: Regional lymph node metastasis

Distant metastasis (M)

- MX: Distant metastasis cannot be assessed
- M0: No distant metastasis
- M1: Distant metastasis

Stage grouping

- I: T1N0M0, T1a-1cN0M0
- II: T2N0M0, T2a-2cN0M0
- III: T3N0M0, T4N0M0
- IV: Any T N1 M0; Any T Any N M1

10-Year CSS/OS by stage

- I: ~95/80%
- II: ~80/60%
- III: ~60/40%
- IV: MS ~6 months

- T3a: Tumor confluent with or extending into the ciliary body, choroid, or both, with scleral extension and secondary glaucoma

T4: Tumor with extrascleral extension

- T4a: Tumor with extrascleral extension less than or equal to 5 mm in diameter
- T4b: Tumor with extrascleral extension more than 5 mm in diameter

Ciliary body and choroid

Primary ciliary body and choroidal melanomas are classified according to the four tumor size categories below:

T1: Tumor size category 1

- T1a: Tumor size category 1 without ciliary body involvement and extraocular extension
- T1b: Tumor size category 1 with ciliary body involvement
- T1c: Tumor size category 1 without ciliary body involvement, but with extraocular extension less than or equal to 5 mm in diameter
- T1d: Tumor size caategory 1 with ciliary body involvement and extraocular extension less than or equal to 5 mm in diameter

T2: Tumor size category 2

- T2a: Tumor size category 2 without ciliary body involvement and extraocular extension
- T2b: Tumor size category 2 with ciliary body involvement
- T2c: Tumor size category 2 without ciliary body involvement but with extraocular extension less than or equal to 5 mm in diameter
- T2d: Tumor size category 2 with ciliary body involvement and extraocular extension less than or equal to 5 mm in diameter

T3: Tumor size category 3

- T3a: Tumor size category 3 without ciliary body involvement and extraocular extension
- T3b: Tumor size category 3 with ciliary body involvement

continued

T3c: Tumor size category 3 without ciliary body involvement, but with extraocular extension less than or equal to 5 mm in diameter
T3d: Tumor size category 3 with ciliary body involvement and extraocular extension less than or equal to 5 mm in diameter

T4: Tumor size category 4
- T4a: Tumor size category 4 without ciliary body involvement and extraocular extension
- T4b: Tumor size category 4 with ciliary body involvement
- T4c: Tumor size category 4 without ciliary body involvement, but with extraocular extension less than or equal to 5 mm in diameter
- T4d: Tumor size category 4 with ciliary body involvement and extraocular extension less than or equal to 5 in diameter
- T4e: Any tumor size category with extraocular extension more than 5 mm in diameter

Regional lymph nodes (N)
NX: Regional lymph nodes cannot be assessed
N0: No regional lymph node metastasis
N1: Regional lymph node metastasis

Distant metastasis (M)
M0: No distant metastasis
M1: Distant metastasis
- M1a: Largest diameter of the largest metastasis 3 cm or less
- M1b: Largest diameter of the largest metastasis 3.1–8.0 cm
- M1c: Largest diameter of the largest metastasis 8 cm or more

Anatomic stage/prognostic groups
I: T1a N0 M0
IIA: T1b-d N0 M0
T2a N0 M0

continued

III

IIB:	T2b N0 M0
	T3a N0 M0
IIIA:	T2c-d N0 M0
	T3b-c N0 M0
	T4a N0 M0
IIIB:	T3d N0 M0
	T4b-c N0 M0
IIIC:	T4d-e N0 M0
IV:	Any T N1 M0
	Any T Any N M1a-c

TREATMENT RECOMMENDATIONS

2002 Stage	Recommended treatment
Small, indeterminate pigmented lesions	■ Serial observation (COMS showed no difference in survival with early treatment, and vision preserved longer with observation). ~2/3 do not grow ■ If growth, then consider surgery, laser, protons/charged particles, plaque, or SRS
Medium-sized lesions (T2)	■ Options: ■ Surgery: enucleation, orbital exenteration, local resection ± adjuvant RT ■ Proton radiotherapy, helium, or SRS ■ I-125 brachytherapy (other isotopes also used)
Large-sized lesions (T3+)	■ Enucleation standard. Select large tumors, may consider eye-conserving options above
Recurrent lesion without metastases	■ Options: ■ Surgical salvage: enucleation ■ Re-irradiation (Marucci et al. 2006)

STUDIES

- Only randomized study of plaques vs. particles: *UCSF/Berkeley* (Char et al. 1993): 184 patients with T2/T3 lesions randomized to 70 GyE with helium (5 fx in 5–7 days, <2 min fx) vs. I-125 plaque (0.7–0.75 Gy/h at apex). LC was 100% He vs. 83% I-125; subsequent enucleation He 9.3% vs. I-125 17.3%. No survival differences. Different toxicities: more dry eye, epiphora, neovascular glaucoma with He vs. temporary strabismus unique to brachytherapy.
- UCSF (Quivey et al. 1993): 449 patients treated with I-125; ~13% recurred locally; increased local failure with smaller tumor height, closer proximity to fovea/disk and optic nerve, larger diameter, lower radiation dose.
- COMS (1997, 2006, 2004): three part multicenter randomized study.
  - Small tumors: 204 patients with small/T1 nonprogressive tumors enrolled for observational study with treatment only if progression documented. Five-year OS 94%, 8-year OS 85%; 5-year DSS 99%; 8-year DSS 96%. No apparent loss of survival and good preservation of vision with close follow-up of small lesions.
  - Medium tumors/T2: 1,317 patients with selected T2 tumors (not abutting optic disk) randomized to brachytherapy ($n = 657$) vs. enucleation ($n = 660$). No difference in 5-year OS (81–82%).

Approximately 60% patients who died had DM at death. Visual acuity declined over time with brachytherapy plaque patients 5-year LF ~10%, 5-year eye retention ~85%. Twelve-year update: OS 57–59%, 12-year CSS 79–83%.

- Large tumors: 1,003 patients with large-sized tumors randomized to enucleation vs. pre-op 20 Gy EBRT + enucleation. No OS difference (5-year OS ~60%, 5-year DSS 73%). Ten-year update: OS 39%, CSS 55–60%.

- Egger et al. (2001): 2,435 patients treated with protons 54.5 Gy in four fractions. Five-year LC 96%, 10-year 95%. Near fovea increased LF 5 years ~30%. LC correlated with CSS. Approximately 990 patients treated after 1993 with contemporary practice, 5-year LC 99%, 5-year CSS 88%.
- Gragoudas et al. (2000, 2006) 188 patients randomized to proton therapy 50 cobalt GyE and 70 CGE in five fractions. No difference in ocular toxicity or 5-year LC. Overall, >2,000 patients treated at Harvard cyclotron with protons for uveal melanoma, 5-year LC 97% and 15-year LC 95%, 5-year OS 78.5%.
- *Metastatic progression – COMS 26* (Diener-West et al. 2005): COMS medium and large trial patients were followed prospectively for metastatic progression. Metastatic melanoma rate at 5 years 25%, 10 years 34%, with increased tumor size as poor prognostic factor. MS (median survival) ~6 months. Most common sites included: ~90% liver, 30% lung, 20% bone.

RADIATION TECHNIQUES

PROTON/CHARGED PARTICLE THERAPY

- Surgical placement of tantalum rings for tumor localization purpose: perilimbal incision made and rectus muscles isolated with suture slings; melanoma localized with transillumination and 3–5 marker rings sutured in position around the tumor base.
- Treatment planning: use EYEPLAN software with around the tumor base tantalum ring coordinates, ultrasound measurements, surgeon's mapping, fundus photo, MRI to build model of patient eye, tumor, and normal structures.
- Field design: 2–2.5 mm margin on tumor. Optimize gaze angle, field collimation, and beam depth and width of Bragg peak to ensure tumor coverage and minimize dose to critical structures (ON, disk, macula, lens, ciliary body, etc.)
- Dose prescription: 56 GyE in five fractions (GyE = Gray equivalent = dose in Gy × RBE of protons 1.1). Typical treatment duration 1–2 min/fx.

EPISCLERAL PLAQUE

- Field design: tumor + margin to include scleral thickness (1 mm) + 1–2 mm around tumor.
- One millimeter spacer (or contact lens) used to minimize hot spots over individual seeds.
- Surgical placement with general or local anesthesia, and as above, localize melanoma with transillumination. Suture dummy plaque into place, and verify position. Then suture radioactive plaque, irrigate eye with antibiotic solution, close conjunctiva, and place lead eye shield.
- Patient usually discharged in 24 h, return for plaque removal in 4–7 days.
- Dose prescription: minimum tumor I-125 dose 85 Gy; dose rate 0.60–1.05 Gy/h.
- ABS guidelines: plaques not advised for large tumors: peripapillary or macular tumors due to lower LC and poorer visual outcome. Also not suitable for gross extrascleral extension, ring melanoma, and tumor involving more than half of the ciliary body (Nag et al. 2003).

III

STEREOTACTIC RADIOSURGERY (SRS)

- Treatment planning, dose prescription/homogeneity, and method of eye fixation/monitoring vary for typical duration of each treatment fraction of up to 1 h (concerns of corneal dryness and fatigue). Doses include 25–40 Gy single fx to 50% isodose line; 48–70 Gy multifraction.
- SRS/SRT generally deliver higher doses to normal structures (i.e., ipsilateral lacrimal gland, contralateral eye, thyroid, and peripheral organs) and has greater tumor inhomogeneity compared with either proton therapy or plaque (Weber et al. 2005; Zytkovicz et al. 2007).

OUTCOMES

- LC higher for charged particles/protons vs. plaques in prospective randomized and retrospective data. Five-year LC particles ~92–99%. Five-year LC plaque ~81–96%.
- Need RCT and longer follow-up to evaluate relative outcomes and toxicity for SRS.
- Overall survival rates are comparable between surgery and radiation techniques of plaque and charged particles.

COMPLICATIONS

- Episcleral plaque: RT retinopathy up to 43% (depends on the length of follow-up), optic atrophy, cystoid macular edema, cataracts, vitreous hemorrhage, neovascular glaucoma, central retinal vein occlusion, scleral necrosis, secondary strabismus (5%).
- Proton/helium: increased anterior complications from entrance beam including epiphora, dry eye, lash loss, neovascular glaucoma, cataract, telangectasias, hemorrhage, maculopathy, retinopathy, and optic neuropathy.
- Need for enucleation for complications or tumor recurrence.
- Vision loss variable; depends on initial visual acuity, tumor location/size, distance/dose to macula, disk, and nerve.

FOLLOW-UP

- H&P including ocular ultrasound and fundus photo every 3–6 months initially, then annually. LFTs or abdominal imaging ± CXR annually.

ORBITAL LYMPHOMA

PEARLS

- Includes lymphoid malignancies of the conjunctiva, lacrimal apparatus, eyelids, uvea, and intraconal and extraconal retrobulbar areas.
- In contrast to IOL, OL is generally an indolent disease.
- Most lesions are low-grade B-cell lymphomas.
- Most common histology: extranodal marginal zone B-cell lymphoma or mucosa-associated lymphoid tissue (MALT).
- Common presentations: orbital mass, proptosis, eye swelling, diplopia, salmon colored conjunctival mass, and increased tearing.
- Most patients present in seventh decade of life.

WORKUP

- H&P includes fundoscopy and measurement of tumor including exophthalmometer if proptosis.
- Labs: CBC, LFTs.
- Imaging: fine cut orbit CT and MRI. Brain MRI. Rule out systemic lymphoma with CT chest, abdomen, and pelvis.

- Tissue diagnosis: biopsy of lesion with immunohistochemistry and flow cytometry analysis; also bone marrow biopsy for systemic work-up.

STAGING (AJCC 7TH ED., 2010): ORBITAL LYMPHOMA

Primary tumor (T)

TX: Lymphoma extent not specified
T0: No evidence of lymphoma
T1: Lymphoma involving the conjunctiva alone without orbital involvement
  T1a: Bulbar conjunctiva only
  T1b: Palpebral conjunctiva ± fornix ± caruncle
  T1c: Extensive conjunctival involvement
T2: Lymphoma with orbital involvement ± any conjunctival involvement
  T2a: Anterior orbital involvement (± conjunctival involvement)
  T2b: Anterior orbital involvement (± conjunctival involvement + lacrimal involvement)
  T2c: Posterior orbital involvement (± conjunctival involvement ± anterior involvement and ± any extraocular muscle involvement)
  T2d: Nasolacrimal drainage system involvement (± conjunctival involvement but not including nasopharynx)
T3: Lymphoma with preseptal eyelid involvement (defined above)16 ± orbital involvement ± any conjunctival involvement
T4: Orbital adnexal lymphoma extending beyond orbit to adjacent structures such as bone and brain
  T4a: Involvement of nasopharynx
  T4b: Osseous involvement (including periosteum)
  T4c: Involvement of maxillofacial, ethmoidal, and/or frontal sinuses
  T4d: Intracranial spread

Regional lymph node (N)

NX: Involvement of lymph nodes not assessed
N0: No evidence of lymph node involvement
N1: Involvement of ipsilateral regional lymph nodes*
N2: Involvement of contralateral or bilateral regional lymph nodes*
N3: Involvement of peripheral lymph nodes not draining ocular adnexal region
N4: Involvement of central lymph nodes

**Note*: The regional lymph nodes include preauricular(parotid), submandibular, and cervical.

Distant metastasis (M)

M0: No evidence of involvement of other extranodal sites
M1a: Noncontiguous involvement of tissues or organs external to the ocular adnexa (e.g., parotid glands, submandibular gland, lung, liver, spleen, kidney, breast, etc.)
M1b: Lymphomatous involvement of the bone marrow
M1c: Both M1a and M1b involvement

- Ann Arbor staging system often used as for other lymphomas (see Chap. 35).
- Working Formulation and REAL classifications of NHL used to characterize low-grade vs. intermediate/high-grade lesions for management decisions.

TREATMENT RECOMMENDATIONS

Extent of disease	Treatment options
Low grade, limited disease	Best results seen with RT alone, dose 30–30.6 Gy, in 1.5–1.8 Gy fractions
Intermediate/high grade, or systemic disease with orbital involvement	Combined systemic chemo (e.g., CHOP) and RT to orbit (40 Gy). For CD20+, add rituximab

STUDIES

- Esik et al. (1996): review of 37 patients with OL treated with RT after biopsy (17 patients), surgery alone (13 patients), or chemo (7 patients). Median RT dose 34.8 Gy. Ten-year local RFS was 100% with RT, 0% with surgery alone, and 42% with chemo. Twenty-year CSS was 100% with RT, 67% with surgery alone, and 0% with chemo.
- Stanford (Le et al. 2002): series of 31 patients with MALT lymphoma treated with 30–40 Gy (mean 34 Gy) using 9–20 MeV electrons for conjunctival lesions, 6 MV photons for retrobulbar; lens shielded. Ten-year OS 73%, LC 100%. Ten-year freedom from relapse 71% with most failures extranodal mucosa. No difference with dose ≤34 vs. >34 Gy. Two patients had retinal damage >34 Gy.
- Bolek et al. (1999): series of 38 patients, 20 with limited disease treated with curative intent, 18 with extensive disease. Median dose 25 Gy. LC achieved in 37/38 patients. For patients treated curatively, 5-year CSS was 89% for low grade, and 33% for intermediate/high grade. Cataracts: 7/21 patients without shielding, 0/17 with shielding.
- Pfeffer et al. (2004): 23 patients with OL were retrospectively reviewed. Twelve patients with limited disease were treated to partial orbital volumes and 11 patients with more extensive disease received whole orbit RT. Dose was 20–30 Gy for low-grade lymphoma and 24–40 Gy for intermediate- to high-grade lymphoma. All patients had complete response to RT. Four patients treated with partial orbital RT had intraorbital recurrence in previously uninvolved regions not covered in the initial target volume. These patients were salvaged with RT or surgery. No intraorbital recurrences seen in patients treated with whole orbit RT.

RADIATION TECHNIQUES

EBRT

- Set up patient supine, immobilize head with thermoplastic mask.
- Place radio-opaque markers at lateral canthus or radio-opaque contact lens to help define fields.
- For anterior lesions involving eyelid or bulbar conjunctiva, use electron beam 6–9 MeV with 0.5–1.0 cm bolus.
- Lens shield used if tumor coverage is not compromised. Lens block can be placed directly on the cornea after topical anesthetic if mounted on a Lucite conformer. Daily placement of block should carefully place it within limbus. Hanging blocks provide less reliable shielding when using electron beams.
- Lacrimal lesions as well as those involving intra- or extraconal spread benefit from more sophisticated planning techniques: obtain CT for 3D CRT/IMRT planning.
- Dose prescription: 30 Gy in 1.8–2 Gy fractions with CT/MRI planning.

COMPLICATIONS

- Acute: mild skin erythema.
- Late: depends on technique and shielding; includes cataracts, vitreous hemorrhage, retinopathy, second tumors in field of irradiation, dry eye, and glaucoma.

FOLLOW-UP

- H&P every 3 months for 1 year, every 4 months for second year, every 6 months for third and fourth year, then annually.

INTRAOCULAR LYMPHOMA

PEARLS

- Very rare: a subset of primary CNS lymphomas, which account for 1–2% extranodal lymphomas.
- Confined to neural structures; distinguished from OLs, which involve the uvea and ocular adnexa of the orbit, lacrimal gland, and conjunctiva.
- Histology: usually diffuse large B-cell non-Hodgkin's lymphoma.

- Median age of onset in immunocompetent patients is late 50s–60s.
- More common in men.
- Of the patients who develop primary intraocular lymphoma (PIOL), 60–80% will go on to develop CNS disease within 3 years.
- Conversely, 25% of patients with primary CNS lymphoma without initial eye involvement will develop IOL.
- Common presentations: blurred vision, floaters; less common: red eye, photophobia, ocular pain, uveitis; ocular disease is bilateral in ~80% cases.
- Recurs in 50% of cases.
- No universal staging system.
- Optimum treatment remains unclear.

WORKUP

- H&P includes fundoscopy, slit lamp examination, measurement of tumor; thorough CNS evaluation.
- Labs: CBC, LFTs, ESR, lumbar puncture – CSF for cytology, chemistry, cytokine analysis; immunohistochemistry and flow cytometry of lymphoma cells from CSF/vitrectomy/biopsy.
- Brain/orbit MRI. Consider stereotactic brain biopsy for suspicious brain lesions, fluorescein angiography, and ocular ultrasound.
- Systemic workup (CT chest, abdomen, pelvis, and bone marrow biopsy).
- Tissue diagnosis: diagnostic vitrectomy, vitreous aspiration needle tap. Patients suspected of having IOL with no lesion on imaging should have diagnostic vitrectomy on eye with more severe vitreitis/worse visual acuity.
- If vitrectomy is nondiagnostic, consider chorioretinal biopsy or enucleation.

TREATMENT RECOMMENDATIONS

Extent of disease	Treatment options
Limited to eye	Combined chemo-RT: use high-dose systemic chemo ± intrathecal chemo + RT (ocular + brain) or chemo alone
Eye disease with primary CNS lymphoma	Combined chemo-RT. Ocular RT ± whole brain RT, from 20 to 45 Gy at 1.8–2 Gy/fx
Refractory/recurrent	Chemo alone or high-dose chemo and stem cell rescue

STUDIES

- Hoffman et al. (2003): series of 14 HIV negative patients with IOL. Most had lymphoma elsewhere; 64% had bilateral disease; 29% had prior systemic lymphoma; 57% had PCNSL; 29% non-B cell. Ten out of 14 (71%) received combined chemo-RT (most common 40 Gy in 20–25 fx). Four out of fourteen received chemo alone. Seventy-nine percent of patients died of lymphoma with 16-month median survival. Patients without CNS involvement had improved survival (50 vs. 10%). RT complications included cataracts (50%), dry eye (40%), punctuate keratopathy (20%), retinopathy (20%), and optic atrophy (10%).
- Berenbom et al. (2007): 12 patients with 21 eyes diagnosed with PIOL retrospectively reviewed. Six patients were treated with RT and chemotherapy, 4 patients chemotherapy alone, 1 patient RT alone, and 1 patient no treatment. No relapses seen in patients treated with RT compared with two relapses in patients who did not receive RT. Complications of RT include dry eye, cataract, and mild retinopathy. RT is effective and has acceptable complications.

THYROID OPHTHALMOPATHY

PEARLS

- Usually in association with Graves' disease but can arise in association with Hashimoto's thyroiditis.
- Histopathology: T-cell predominant lymphocytic infiltration of orbital tissues; also glycosaminoglycans in periorbital fat and extraocular muscles.
- Present with exophthalmos, impaired extraocular muscle involvement, diplopia, blurred vision, periorbital edema, chemosis (conjunctival edema), lid retraction, and compressive optic neuropathy.

WORKUP

- H&P includes measurement of proptosis with Hertel exophthalmometer.
- Labs: CBC, chemistries, thyroid function tests.
- Imaging: orbit CT, MRI.

TREATMENT RECOMMENDATIONS

- If stable, no threat of impending visual loss, begin with treatment of underlying thyroid disorder.
- If moderate symptomatic/progressive/refractory to thyroid treatment, options include orbital RT ± systemic immunosuppressive agents, especially IV corticosteroids, oral steroids, cyclosporine, others.
- For visual loss unresponsive to corticosteroids (loss of color vision, a key symptom of optic nerve compression), decompressive surgery.
- EBRT: 20 Gy in 10 fx, see 50–80% response rate.

STUDIES

- Upenn Study (Prummel et al. 1993): 56 patients with moderately severe Graves' ophthalmopathy (no corneal involvement or loss of visual acuity) euthyroid for at least 2 months, randomized to 3 months oral prednisone + sham RT vs. retrobulbar RT to 20 Gy + placebo capsules. Results: same rate of responders/no change/failures (RT 46/40/14%, prednisone 50/36/14%), but steroid therapy had much higher minor, moderate, and major complications rates. Note that 75% of all patients (71% RT, 79% prednisone) ultimately needed decompressive/squint/rehabilitation surgery, regardless of treatment.
- *Stanford series* (Lanciano et al. 1990): 311 patients treated from 1968 to 1988, most with 20 Gy. Some patients treated from 1979 to 1983 received 30 Gy, but no benefit was noted from increased dose. Results: improved or complete resolution of soft tissue changes 80%, proptosis 51%, eye muscle impairment 61%, visual acuity 61%. Of 1/3 patients who were on steroids when starting RT, 76% were able to discontinue use. Treatment well-tolerated with 10% acute toxicity.
- Prummel et al. (2004): double-blind RCT. Forty-four patients received orbital RT and 44 patients received sham RT. RT-treated patients had significant improvement in eye motility and diplopia. RT may not be associated with improvement in quality of life.
- Bradley et al. (2008): literature review of five observational studies and nine RCTs regarding orbital RT for Graves opthalmopathy. Three of the RCTs were sham controlled and none showed that RT was better than sham for improving proptosis, lid fissure, or soft tissue changes (i.e., eyelid swelling). Two of the 3 RCTs had improved vertical range of motion in

RT-treated subjects compared to controls. Risk of radiation retinopathy is 1–2% within 10 years of RT.

RADIATION TECHNIQUES

SIMULATION AND FIELD DESIGN

- Set up patient supine; immobilize head with thermoplastic mask. Highly recommend cutting out around eyes to allow verification of clinical set-up.
- Place radio-opaque markers at lateral canthus or radio-opaque contact lens to define fields.
- Place the beam split anterior field border 11–12 mm behind cornea to spare lens (Fig. 3.1).
- Fields: usually lateral opposed, although angled opposed beams needed for marked asymmetry of proptosis, extending from just behind the lens of the globe to the anterior clinoids with superior and inferior margins defined by the bony orbit; general range of 4 × 4 to 5.5 × 5.5 cm with appropriate shielding.

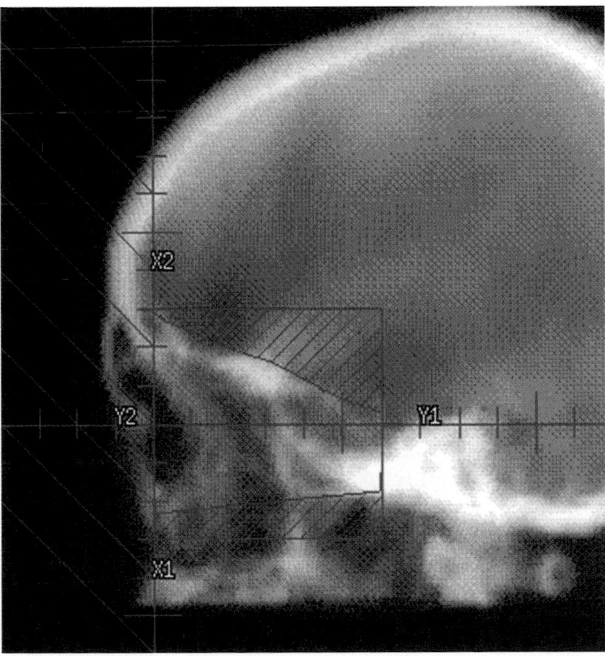

Fig. 3.1 Lateral DRR of a field used to treat thyroid ophthalmopathy

- Techniques to minimize divergence into contralateral lens.
  - Half beam block anterior edge of field (preferred).
  - Alternatively, angle lateral fields 5° posteriorly (can use CT scan to ensure the optimal beam angle is selected).
- Dose prescription: 20 Gy in 2 Gy fx.
- Dose limitation: lens<10 Gy.

ORBITAL PSEUDOTUMOR/ LYMPHOID HYPERPLASIA/ PSEUDOLYMPHOMA

PEARLS

- Very rare benign orbital mass lesions in which mature lymphocytes (polyclonal) are noted.
- Usually present with soft tissue swelling, orbital pain, proptosis, extraocular muscle involvement, and less common decreased visual acuity.

WORKUP

- A diagnosis of exclusion: need to rule out lymphoma, metastatic carcinoma, sarcoma, and infectious causes of orbital inflammation.
- H&P exam includes measurement of tumor diameter, location, and geometry.
- Labs: CBC, LFTs, ESR, lumbar puncture – CSF for cytology, chemistry, and cytokine analysis.
- Imaging: brain/orbit CT, MRI.
- Tissue diagnosis: biopsy to rule out malignancy; may analyze with flow cytometry for clonality and immunohistochemistry.

TREATMENT RECOMMENDATIONS

- First line: corticosteroids; ~50% patients have durable complete response.
- If contraindications to steroid therapy, unacceptable toxicities with steroids, or refractory/recurrent: EBRT most commonly 20 Gy in 10 fx.
- Local control rates with radiation, 74–100% for doses 380–3,600 cGy.

TRIALS/STUDIES

- Lanciano et al. (1990): series of 26 orbits in 23 patients with orbital pseudotumor, of whom 87% had a trial of corticosteroids before RT treated with 20 Gy in 10 fx. Results: 66% durable complete response; 11% had local relapse and went on to achieve CR with more treatment or spontaneously. Eleven percent had PR; only 11% had no response.

III

RADIATION TECHNIQUES

- Simulation and field design: as per thyroid ophthalmopathy.
- Dose prescription: 20 Gy in 2 Gy fxs.

COMPLICATIONS

- Acute: mild skin erythema.
- Late: depends on technique and shielding; includes cataracts, vitreous hemorrhage, retinopathy, hypopituitarism, and second tumors in the field of irradiation, especially with >60 Gy.

FOLLOW-UP

- H&P every 3 months for 1 year, every 4 months for second year, every 6 months for third and fourth years, then annually.

REFERENCES

Berenbom A, Davila RM, Lin H-S, et al. Treatment outcomes for primary intraocular lymphoma: implications for external beam radiotherapy. Eye 2007;21:1198-1201.

Bhatia S, et al. Curative radiotherapy for primary orbital lymphoma. IJROBP 2002;54:818-821.

Bolek T, et al. Radiotherapy in the management of orbital lymphoma. IJROBP 1999;44:31-36.

Bradley EA, Gower EW, Bradley DJ, et al. Orbital radiation for graves ophthalmopathy. Ophthalmology 2008;115:398-409.

Char D, Quivey J, et al. Helium ions versus I-125 brachytherapy in management of uveal melanoma. A prospective, dynamically balanced trial. Ophthalmology 1993;100:1547-1554.

COMS. Mortality in patients with small choroidal melanoma. COMS report no. 4. Arch Ophthalmol 1997;115:886.

COMS. The COMS randomized trial of iodine 125 brachytherapy for choroidal melanoma: V. Twelve-year mortality rates and prognostic factors: COMS report no. 28. Arch Ophthalmol 2006;124:1684.

COMS. The COMS randomized trial of pre-enucleation radiation of large choroidal melanoma: IV. Ten-year mortality findings and prognostic factors. COMS report no 24. Am J Ophthalmol 2004;138(6):936.

Diener-West M, et al. Development of metastatic disease after enrollment in the COMS trials for treatment of choroidal melanoma: COMS report no. 26. Arch Ophthalmol 2005; 123(12):1639.

Egger E, et al. Maximizing local tumor control and survival after proton beam radiotherapy of uveal melanoma. Int J Radiat Oncol Biol Phys 2001;51:138.

Esik O, et al. Retrospective analysis of different modalities for treatment of primary orbital non-Hodgkin's lymphomas. Radiother Oncol 1996;38:13-18.

Gragoudas ES, et al. A randomized controlled trial of varying radiation doses in the treatment of choroidal melanoma. Arch Ophthalmol 2000;118:773.

Gragoudas ES. Proton beam irradiation of uveal melanomas: the first 30 years. Invest Ophthalmol Vis Sci 2006;47:4666-4673.

Hoffman PM, et al. Intraocular lymphoma: a series of 14 patients with clinicopathological features and treatment outcomes. Eye 2003;17:513-521.

Lanciano R, et al. The results of radiotherapy for orbital pseudotumor. IJROBP 1990;18:407

Le Q, et al. Primary radiotherapy for localized orbital malt lymphoma. IJROBP 2002;52:657-663.

Marucci L, Lane AM, Li W, et al. Conservation treatment of the eye: conformal proton reirradiation for recurrent uveal melanoma. IJROBP 2006;64:1018-1022.

Nag S, et al. The American Brachytherapy Society recommendations for brachytherapy of uveal melanomas. IJROBP 2003;56:544.

Pfeffer MR, Rabin T, Tsvang L, et al. Orbital lymphoma: is it necessary to treat the entire orbit? IJROBP 2004;60:527-530.

Prummel M, et al. Randomized double-blind trial of prednisone versus radiotherapy in Graves' ophthalmopathy. Lancet 1993;342:949-954.

Prummel MF, Terwee CB, Gerding MN, et al. A randomized controlled trial of orbital radiotherapy versus sham irradiation in patients with mild Graves' ophthalmopathy. J Clin Endocrinol Metab 2004;89:15-20.

Quivey J, Char D, et al. High intensity 125-iodine (125I) plaque treatment of uveal melanoma. IJROBP 1993;26(4):613-618.

Shields J, et al. Survey of 1264 patients with orbital tumors and simulating lesions. Ophthalmology 2004;111:997-1008.

Weber DC, Bogner J, Verwey J, et al. Proton beam radiotherapy versus fractionated stereotactic radiotherapy for uveal melanomas: a comparative study. IJROBP 2005;63:373-384.

Zytkovicz A, et al: Peripheral dose in ocular treatments with Cyberknife and Gamma Knife radiosurgery compared to proton radiotherapy. Phys Med Biol 2007;52(19):5957.

FURTHER READING

Akpek E, et al. Intraocular-central nervous system lymphoma: clinical features, diagnosis, and outcomes. Ophthalmology 1999;106:1805-1810.

Bell D, et al. Choroidal melanoma: natural history and management options. Cancer Control 2004;11(5):296-303.

Chan C, Wallace D. Intraocular lymphoma: update on diagnosis and management. Cancer Control 2004;11(5):285-295.

Char D, et al. Primary intraocular lymphoma (ocular reticulum cell sarcoma) diagnosis and management. Ophthalmology 1988;95:625 630.

COMS. The COMS randomized trial of pre-enucleation radiation of large choroidal melanoma II: initial mortality findings: COMS report no. 10. Am J Ophthamol 1998;124:779-796.

COMS. The COMS randomized trial of iodine 125 brachytherapy for choroidal melanoma III: initial mortality findings: COMS report no. 18. Arch Ophthalmol 2001;119:969-982.

Daftari I, et al. Newer radiation modalities for choroidal tumors. Int Ophthal Clin 2006;46:69.

Diener-West M, et al. Screening for metastasis from choroidal melanoma: the COMS Group report 23. JCO 2004;22:2438-2444.

Kath R, et al. Prognosis and treatment of disseminated uveal melanoma. Cancer 1993;72(7): 2219-2223.

Kujala E, et al. Very long term prognosis of patients with malignant uveal melanoma. Invest Ophthalmol Vis Sci 2003;44:4651-4659.

Mishra KK, Quivey J, Char D. Uveal melanoma. In: Leibel S, Phillips T, editors. Textbook of Radiation Oncology, 3rd ed. Chapter 64 In press.

Nguyen LN, Ang K. The orbit. In: Cox J, Ang K, editors. Radiation Oncology. 8th ed. St. Louis: Mosby; 2003. pp 282-292.

Pelloski CE, et al. Clinical stage IEA-IIEA orbital lymphomas: outcomes in the era of modern staging and treatment. Radiother Oncol 2001;59:145-151.

Peterson IA, et al. Prognostic factors in the radiotherapy of Graves' ophthalmopathy. IJROBP 1990;19:259-264.

Peterson K, et al. The clinical spectrum of ocular lymphoma. Cancer 1993;72:843-849.

Rosenthal S. Benign disease. In: Leibel SA, Phillips TL, editors. Textbook of Radiation Oncology. 2nd ed. Philadelphia: Saunders; 2004. pp 1525-1543.

Shields C, Shields J. Diagnosis and management of retinoblastoma. Cancer Control 2004;11(5): 317-327.

Stafford SL, et al. Orbital lymphoma: radiotherapy outcome and complications. Radiother Oncol 2001;59:139-144.

Chapter 4
Cancer of the Ear

Fred Y. Wu, Eric K. Hansen, and Sue S. Yom

III

PEARLS

- The ear consists of pinna (auricle), external auditory canal (EAC), tympanic membrane, middle ear (containing the auditory ossicles), and inner ear in the petrous portion of the temporal bone (consisting of the bony and membranous labyrinth).
- Primary middle ear and temporal bone tumors are rare, but external ear cutaneous malignancies may involve these structures.
- BCC >> SCC for malignancies of the external ear, but SCC accounts for 85% of EAC, middle ear, and mastoid tumors.
- Nodal metastases occur in <15% with lymphatic drainage to parotid, cervical, and postauricular nodes.

WORKUP

- H&P with otoscopy and careful LN exam. CBC, chemistries, BUN/Cr. CT, MRI. Biopsy. Audiologic testing.

STAGING

- No site-specific AJCC/UICC staging system exists; may use histology appropriate staging (e.g., skin).
- Several proposed staging systems for EAC and middle ear; modified University of Pittsburgh system often cited (Hirsch 2002).

TREATMENT RECOMMENDATIONS

- Tumors of the external ear may be treated with surgery or RT (either EBRT or IS brachytherapy). Surgery is used if the lesion has invaded the cartilage or extends medially into the auditory canal. Advanced lesions or close/+ margins require post-op RT. Treatment of the lymphatics may be indicated for tumors >4 cm or for cartilage invasion.

- Tumors of the middle ear or temporal bone may be treated with surgery or RT. Surgery may require mastoidectomy or subtotal or total temporal bone resection. Post-op RT is generally required to increase LRC.
- LC depends on the extent of disease, and ranges from 40 to 100%.
- Preoperative RT and chemo-RT remain under investigation (Nakagawa et al. 2006).

STUDIES

- Clark and Soutar (2008): Metaanalysis of LN metastases from auricular SCC. Metastatic rate is 11.2%, commonly to parotid and upper cervical chain. Usually develops within 12 months and half will die.
- Osborne et al. (2008): For locally advanced auricular malignancies, found no pathologic evidence of occult parotid metastasis in 19 patients with clinical N0 stage. Recommended parotidectomy only for clinically positive parotid disease.
- Gal et al. (1999): 21 patients with auricular cutaneous carcinoma invading temporal bone; this carries poor prognosis, as does SCC histology. OS is 63%. Trend toward increased survival with post-op radiation.
- Pfreundner et al. (1999): 27 primary carcinomas of EAC and middle ear. Five years OS 61%. Five years LC 50%. Five years OS by stage: T1-T2 86%, T3 50%, T4 41%. Complete resection and clear margins were prognostic. All patients with dural invasion died.
- Madsen et al. (2008): 68 primary cancers of EAC and middle ear in Denmark. Five years LRC rates for surgery, RT, or surgery + RT were 55.6, 47.4, and 45.3%, respectively. Of 28 recurrences, 24 were purely local.

RADIATION TECHNIQUES

SIMULATION AND FIELD DESIGN

- Superficial tumors of the pinna may be treated with electrons or orthovoltage photons. For small tumors, 1 cm margins are adequate, but for larger lesions, 2–3 cm margins are required (see Chap. 1).
- Treatment volumes for advanced tumors of the EAC or middle ear include the entire ear canal and temporal bone with 2–3 cm margin, and the ipsilateral preauricular, postauricular, and upper level II nodes.

- Advanced or unresectable tumors may be treated definitively with high energy electrons (energy appropriate for tumor depth) alone or mixed with photons, or with 3DCRT/IMRT if coverage of nodal volumes is desired.
- Immobilization with a thermoplastic mask will be necessary.
- Use water or wax bolus to fill EAC and surrounding concha for pinna tumors to decrease complications and improve homogeneity and superficial dose delivery.

DOSE PRESCRIPTIONS

- Tumors of the pinna may be treated with 1.8–2 Gy per fraction to 50 Gy for small, thin lesions <1.5 cm, 55 Gy for larger tumors, 60 Gy for minimal or suspected cartilage or bone invasion, or 65 Gy for large lesions with bone or cartilage invasion.
- Tumors of the auditory canal or temporal bone: postoperative, 54–60 Gy; definitive, 66–70 Gy, and may consider chemo-RT.

DOSE LIMITATIONS

- Limit temporal bone to ≤70 Gy to minimize risk of osteoradionecrosis (~10% for doses >65 Gy).

COMPLICATIONS

- Cartilage necrosis of the pinna and/or temporal bone necrosis is possible if careful planning is not used.
- Neurosensory: hearing compromise or loss.
- Chronic otitis media.
- Xerostomia.

FOLLOW-UP

- Frequent H&P with otoscopy every 3–4 months for 1–2 years, then every 6 months for 1–2 years, then annually.

Acknowledgment We thank Dr. M. Kara Bucci for her contribution to this chapter in the first edition.

REFERENCES

Chao KSC, Devineni VR. Ear. In: Perez CA, Brady LW, Halperin EC, et al., editors. Principles and Practice of Radiation Oncology. 5th ed. Philadelphia: Lippincott Williams & Wilkins; 2005. pp. 800–806.

Clark R, Soutar D. Lymph node metastases from auricular squamous cell carcinoma. A systematic review and meta-analysis. J Plast Reconstr Aesthet Surg 2008;61:1140–1147.

Gal T, Futran N, Bartels L, et al. Auricular carcinoma with temporal bone invasion: outcome analysis. Otolaryngol Head Neck Surg 1999;121: 62–65.
Hirsch BE. Staging system revision. Arch Otolaryngol Head Neck Surg 2002;128:93–94.
Madsen A, Gundgaard M, Hoff C, et al. Cancer of the external auditory canal and middle ear in Denmark from 1992 to 2001. Head Neck 2008;1332–1338.
Nakagawa T, Kumamoto Y, Natori Y, et al. Squamous cell carcinoma of the external auditory canal and middle ear: an operation combined with preoperative chemoradiotherapy and a free surgical margin. Otol Neurotol 2006;27:242–248.
Osborne R, Shaw T, Zandifar H, et al. Elective parotidectomy in the management of advanced auricular malignancies. Laryngoscope 2008;118: 2139–2145.
Pfreundner L, Schwager K, Willner J, et al. Carcinoma of the external auditory canal and middle ear. Int J Radiat Oncol Biol Phys 1999;44: 777–788.

FURTHER READING

Chao and Devineni 2005, Hussey and Wen 2003, Jereczek-Fossa et al. 2003, Lin et al. 2000"
Hussey DH, Wen B-C. The Temporal Bone, Ear, and Paraganglia. In: Cox JD, Ang KK, editors. Radiation Oncology: Rationale, Technique, Results. 8th ed. St. Louis: Mosby; 2003. pp. 293–309.
Jereczek-Fossa B, Zarowski A, Milani F, et al. Radiotherapy-induced ear toxicity. Cancer Treat Rev 2003;29:417–430.
Lin R, Hug E, Schaefer R, et al. Conformal proton radiation therapy of the posterior fossa: a study comparing protons with three-dimensional planned photons in limiting dose to auditory structures. IJROBP 2000;48:1219–1226.

Chapter 5

Nasopharyngeal Cancer

Gautam Prasad, James Rembert, Eric K. Hansen, and Sue S. Yom

III

PEARLS

- Uncommon in the US, but WHO III (undifferentiated) common in Southern China and Hong Kong (e.g., third most common cancer among men in Hong Kong).
- Strongly associated with EBV (70% of patients have + titers).
- Two peak ages: 15–25 years and 50–60 years. More common among men (2:1).
- Alcohol and tobacco are associated with WHO type I (keratinizing SCC).
- Borders of the nasopharynx: anterior = posterior end of nasal septum and choanae; posterior = clivus and C1-2 vertebral bodies; superior = sphenoid bone/sinus; inferior = roof of soft palate.
- The parapharyngeal and masticator spaces are lateral to the nasopharynx. Villaret/jugular foramen syndrome = extension to the parapharyngeal space causing symptoms related to involvement of CN IX–XII and cervical sympathetics. Involvement of the masticator space causes trismus.
- The Eustachian tubes enter the lateral nasopharynx, and the posterior aspect of the orifice creates a protuberance (torus tubarius). Rosenmueller's fossa is posterior to the torus tubarius and is the number 1 location for nasopharyngeal cancer.
- Tumors spread along the walls of nasopharynx, and can occlude the Eustachian tube, erode into bone, and involve CN V2 (foramen rotundum) or CN V3 (foramen ovale). Jacod/petrosphenoidal syndrome = extension through foramen lacerum to cavernous sinus (containing CN III, IV, V1, V2, VI) may extend into middle cranial fossa.

- Undifferentiated carcinoma is the most common; WHO type 1 (keratinizing SCC, 25% of cases in the US), WHO type 2 (nonskeratinizing SCC, 12% of the US cases), and WHO type 3 (undifferentiated carcinoma, 99% of cases where endemic).
- Lymphoepithelioma = WHO III with high lymphoid component. It has higher LRC, but the same OS due to an increased rate of DM.
- Other tumors include lymphoma, minor salivary gland tumors, plasmacytomas, melanomas, chordomas, and rhabdomyosarcomas.
- Less than 10% of tumors have intracranial extension.
- Seventy percent of patients have clinically involved lymph nodes, 90% have subclinical nodes, and 40–50% have bilateral nodes.
- Metastases correlate with N stage (but not T stage): N0–N1 = 10–20% DM, N2 = 30–40% DM, and N3 = 40–70% DM.
- Before IMRT, recurrence was predominantly local, but with IMRT, distant recurrence is more common than LR.

WORKUP

- *H&P*. Common signs/symptoms include hearing loss, otitis media, neck mass, nasal obstruction, epistaxis, headache, diplopia, trismus. Perform fiberoptic nasopharyngolaryngoscopy and thorough oropharyngeal and neck exam. Also perform otoscopy. Thorough CN exam is critical.
- Labs: CBC, LFTs, BUN/Cr, baseline TSH, EBV IgA/DNA titer.
- MRI head/neck with contrast; ±CT head/neck with contrast. CT optimally demonstrates cortical bone, and MRI, medullary bone. A normal-appearing basisphenoid (clivus) on CT may demonstrate marked tumor infiltration on MRI.
- CXR. For Stage III/IV, consider CT of chest and abdomen + bone scan, or PET/CT scan.
- All patients should have a pre-RT dental evaluation and audiology testing.

STAGING: NASOPHARYNGEAL CANCER

Editors' note: All TNM stage and stage groups referred to elsewhere in this chapter reflect the 2002 AJCC staging nomenclature unless otherwise noted as the new system below was published after this chapter was written.

(AJCC 6TH ED., 2002)

Primary tumor (T)

TX: Primary tumor cannot be assessed
T0: No evidence of primary tumor
Tis: Carcinoma in situ
T1: Tumor confined to the nasopharynx
T2: Tumor extends to soft tissues
T2a: Tumor extends to the oropharynx and/or nasal cavity without parapharyngeal extension*
T2b: Any tumor with parapharyngeal extension*
T3: Tumor involves bony structures and/or paranasal sinuses
T4: Tumor with intracranial extension, and/or involvement of cranial nerves, infratemporal fossa, hypopharynx, orbit, or masticator space

**Note*: Parapharyngeal extension denotes posterolateral infiltration of tumor beyond the pharyngobasilar fascia.

Regional lymph nodes (N)

NX: No regional lymph node metastasis can be assessed
N0: No regional lymph node metastasis
N1: Unilateral metastasis in lymph node(s), 6 cm or less in greatest dimension, above the supraclavicular fossa
N2: Bilateral metastasis in lymph node(s), 6 cm or less in greatest dimension, above the supraclavicular fossa
N3: Metastasis in lymph node(s) >6 cm and/or to supraclavicular fossa
N3a: Greater than 6 cm in dimension
N3b: Extension to the supraclavicular fossa

Distant metastasis (M)

MX: Distant metastasis cannot be assessed
M0: No distant metastasis
M1: Distant metastasis

(AJCC 7TH ED., 2010)

Primary tumor (T)

TX: Primary tumor cannot be assessed
T0: No evidence of primary tumor
Tis: Carcinoma in situ
T1: Tumor confined to the nasopharynx, or tumor extends to oropharynx and/or nasal cavity without parapharyngeal extension
T2: Tumor with parapharyngeal extension*
T3: Tumor involves bony structures of skull base and/or paranasal sinuses
T4: Tumor with intrac ranial extension and/or involvement of cranial nerves, hypopharynx, orbit, or with extension to the infratemporal fossa/masticator space

**Note*: Parapharyngeal extension denotes posterolateral infiltration of tumor.

Regional lymph nodes (N)

NX: No regional lymph node metastasis can be assessed
N0: No regional lymph node metastasis
N1: Unilateral metastasis in cervical lymph node(s), 6 cm or less in greatest dimension, above the supraclavicular fossa, and/or unilateral or bilateral, retropharyngeal lymph nodes, 6 cm or less, in greatest dimension*
N2: Bilateral metastasis in cervical lymph node(s), 6 cm or less in greatest dimension, above the supraclavicular fossa*
N3: Metastasis in a lymph node(s)* >6 cm and/or to supraclavicular fossa*
N3a: Greater than 6 cm in dimension
N3b: Extension to the supraclavicular fossa**

**Note*: Midline nodes are considered ipsilateral nodes.

continued

Stage grouping

0: TisN0M0
I: T1N0M0
IIA: T2aN0M0
IIB: T2bN0M0, T1-2N1M0
III: T3N0M0, T3N1M0, T1-3N2M0
IVA: T4N0-2M0
IVB: Any T, N3, M0
IVC: Any T, any N, M1

~3-Year OS by stage

I: 70–100%
II: 65–100%
III: 60–90%
IV: 50–70%

Used with the permission from the American Joint Committee on Cancer (AJCC), Chicago, IL. The original source for this material is the AJCC Cancer Staging Manual, Sixth Edition (2002), published by Springer Science + Business Media.

***Note*: Supraclavicular zone or fossa is relevant to the staging of nasopharyngeal carcinoma and is the triangular region originally described by Ho. It is defined by three points: (1) the superior margin of the sternal end of the clavicle, (2) the superior margin of the lateral end of the clavicle, (3) the point where the neck meets the shoulder (Fig. 4.2). Note that this would include caudal portions of levels IV and VB. All cases with lymph nodes (whole or part) in the fossa are considered N3b.

Distant metastasis (M)

MX: Distant metastasis cannot be assessed
M0: No distant metastasis

Stage grouping

0: TisN0M0
I : T1N0M0
II: T1N0M0, T2N0-1M0
III: T1-2N2M0, T3N0-2M0
IVA: T4N0-2M0
IVB: Any T, N3, M0
IVC: Any T, any N, M1

Used with the permission from the American Joint Committee on Cancer (AJCC), Chicago, IL. The original source for this material is the AJCC Cancer Staging Manual, Seventh Edition (2010), published by Springer Science + Business Media.

TREATMENT RECOMMENDATIONS

2002 AJCC stage	Recommended treatment
Stage I–IIA	■ RT alone (2/70 Gy)
Stage IIB–IVB	■ Concurrent chemo-RT followed by adjuvant chemo ■ 2/70 Gy + cisplatin 100 mg/m^2 on days 1, 21, 42 → cisplatin/5-FU × 3c ■ Neck dissection for persistent/recurrent neck nodes ■ IMRT may improve LRC and reduces severe xerostomia 80% →35–40% ■ Neoadjuvant chemo (e.g., using taxanes) is under investigation
Stage IVC	■ Platinum-based combination chemo; if CR, definitive RT, otherwise palliative RT dose to metastatic sites
Local Recurrence	■ Reirradiation with IMRT, SRS, or brachytherapy. Cumulative dose is limited with respect to surrounding normal tissue tolerance. Alternative, surgery
Pediatric	■ COG ARAR 0331 protocol Stage I–IIA: RT alone (1.8/61.2 Gy for Stage I; 1.8/66.6 Gy for Stage IIa) with daily amifostine Stage ≥ IIB: Cisplatin/5-FU ×3c → RT (CR/PR to chemo 1.8/61.2 Gy, SD to chemo 1.8/70.2 Gy) with daily amifostine and concurrent cisplatin ×3c 2–3/36–46 Gy to unresectable metastases

STUDIES

RT ± CHEMOTHERAPY

- Al Sarraf et al. (1998), *Int 0099*: 147 patients with Stage III–IV disease randomized to RT (2/70 Gy) vs. chemo-RT (2/70 Gy + concurrent cisplatin (100 mg/m^2) × 3 → adjuvant cisplatin/5-FU × 3 cycles). Used old staging, so many Stage II would now be included. Chemo-RT improved 3-year OS (47→78%) and PFS (24→69%). Trial stopped early due to OS benefit. Criticized because poor LRC and OS for RT alone group, and high % of WHO I tumors (rare outside the US).
- Wee et al. (2005). Confirmed Int 0099 results with 221 patients from Singapore with Stage III–IV disease and same randomization. Chemo-RT improved 2-year OS (78→85%), DFS (57→75%), and DM (30→13%).

- Chan et al. (2005) (IJROBP). Phase III study showing benefit of weekly, low-dose (40 mg/m^2) cisplatin with RT vs. RT alone in 350 patients. Cisplatin-RT improved 5-year OS (59→70%) with main benefit seen in T3/T4. Relative low toxicity compared to Int 0099 chemo.
- Baujat et al. (2006). Pooled meta-analysis of 1,753 patients in eight published clinical trials comparing RT alone to Chemo-RT. OS benefit only observed with concomitant chemo (HR 0.60). Maximum EFS benefit seen with concomitant chemo (HR 0.63).
- RTOG 0615 (closed to accrual). Phase II for Stage IIB–IVB using IMRT/3DCRT (2.12/70 Gy + concurrent cisplatin/bevacizumab → 5-FU/cisplatin/bevacizumab ×3c; planned expansion to Phase III).

Neoadjuvant chemotherapy

- There have been numerous studies which demonstrated no OS advantage with neoadjuvant chemo + RT vs. RT alone including using cisplatin-5-FU (Chan IJROBP 1995), cisplatin-epirubicin-bleomycin (INCSG IJROBP 1996), cisplatin-epirubicin (Chua et al. 1998), and cisplatin-bleomycin-5-FU (Ma et al. 2001).
- Hui et al. (2009): 65 patients with Stage III–IV disease randomized to cisplatin/docetaxel × 2c → chemo-RT (2/66 Gy + concurrent cisplatin) versus chemo-RT alone. Neoadjuvant chemo improved 3-year OS (68→94%), but 3-year EFS (60→88%) not statistically significant. Most patients had non-IMRT plans.
- GORTEC-NPC2006 (open to accrual). Phase III for Stage IIB–IVB comparing neoadjuvant TPF chemo (docetaxel/cisplatin/5-FU ×3c) + RT (2/70 Gy) with weekly cisplatin (40 mg/m^2) vs. upfront chemo-RT alone.

EBV TITERS

- Lin et al. (2004): 99 patients with III–IV disease. EBV titer <1,500 copies/mL had increased OS and RFS. Persistently elevated EBV titer 1 week after completion of sequential chemo-RT had worse OS, RFS.
- Leung et al. (2008): 376 patients. On multivariate analysis, high EBV DNA (>4,000 copies/mL) and low EBV DNA (≤4,000 copies/mL) were predictive of OS ($p = 0.005$). EBV DNA load was better prognostic than UICC staging especially for Stage II.

IMRT

- Lee, UCSF (Lee et al. 2002, 2003): 67 patients treated with IMRT to 70 Gy. Excellent 4-year OS (88%) and LRC (97%).
- RTOG 0225 (closed to accrual). Phase II for Stage I-IVB using IMRT (2.12/70 Gy) and (for T2b or N+) concurrent cisplatin → cisplatin/5-FU ×3c. Two-year locoregional control 90.5%, PFS 73%, OS 79%.
- Kam et al. (2007): 60 patients with T1-2bN0-1 NPC randomized to 2D vs. IMRT. IMRT reduced 1 year observer-rated severe xerostomia (82 > 39%) and improved salivary flow rate. Subjective feeling of recovery not significantly different between arms.
- Pow et al. (2006): 51 patients with Stage II disease randomized to IMRT vs. 2DRT. The mean parotid dose was 68 Gy for 2DRT and 42 for IMRT. At 1 year, IMRT patients had improved salivary flow and surveys indicated improved physical/emotional health.

III

RADIATION TECHNIQUES

SIMULATION AND FIELD DESIGN

- Patient set-up supine, and immobilized with head and neck thermoplastic mask or equivalent device.
- Planning CT scan obtained with IV contrast if available. A pre-chemo MRI is critical for definition of GTV. Use CT-MRI fusion if available.
- In every case, the entire GTV must be treated to the entire prescription dose. Except in the case of very early T1-T2N0 tumors, it is not possible to accomplish this without exceeding normal tissue tolerances with conventional 2D planning. 3DCRT or IMRT is necessary for the final conedown.
- *IMRT volumes*: CTV70 = gross disease (GTV = primary and LN ≥ 1 cm) plus microscopic disease margin. CTV63 for involved nodes near critical structures. CTV56-59.4 includes the entire nasopharynx, sphenoid sinus, cavernous sinus, base of skull, posterior 1/2 of nasal cavity (~2 cm), posterior 1/3 of maxillary sinuses, posterior ethmoid sinus, pterygoid fossa, lateral and posterior pharyngeal walls to the level of the midtonsillar fossa, the retropharyngeal nodes, and bilateral cervical nodes including level V and supraclavicular nodes. CTV54 includes low-risk nodal regions as determined by the clinician per case. PTV = CTV plus planning margin.

- IMRT plan can be matched isocentrically to a conventional low neck field.
- *Conventional set-up* = three fields (lateral opposed fields covering primary and upper neck, with isocentric match to a low neck field). Use a central larynx block on low neck field, then full cord block after 42 Gy.
- *Conventional borders*: superior = generously cover sphenoid sinus and base of skull. Inferior = match at plane above true vocal cords (to block larynx in AP field). Posterior = spinous processes. Anterior = 2–3 cm anterior to GTV (and include pterygoid plates and posterior 1/3 of maxillary sinuses).
- If supraclavicular nodes involved historically used a mediastinal 8 cm wide T field with inferior border 5 cm below the head of the clavicle.
- Use wedges and compensators as needed.

DOSE PRESCRIPTIONS

- *Conventional*: 2/42 Gy → off cord boost to 50 Gy with a posterior neck electron field → conedown to GTV + 2 cm margin to 70 Gy. For the neck, N0 = 50 Gy, nodes <3 cm = 66 Gy, and nodes ≥3 cm = 70 Gy.
- *IMRT per RTOG 0615*: CTV70 (GTV + 5 mm) = 2.12/70 Gy, CTV56-59.4 = 1.8/56–59.4 Gy, CTV54 1.64/54 Gy in 33 fractions.
- *Rotterdam NPX applicator*: optional boost after 66–70 Gy to gross disease. Use 1 week after EBRT (T1–T3 60 Gy EBRT → HDR 3 Gy ×6; T4 70 Gy EBRT → HDR 3 Gy ×4).

DOSE LIMITATIONS

- *EBRT*: partial brain 60 Gy, brainstem 54 Gy (60 Gy point dose), cord 45 Gy, optic chiasm 54 Gy, retina 45 Gy, lens 10 Gy, lacrimal gland 30 Gy, ear (sensorineuronal hearing loss) 45 Gy, parotid mean dose 26 Gy, TMJ max dose 70 Gy.
- *SRS*: brainstem 12 Gy, optic nerves or chiasm 8 Gy

COMPLICATIONS

- Acute: mucositis, dermatitis, xerostomia.
- Late: soft tissue fibrosis, trismus, xerostomia, hearing loss, vasculopathy, osteoradionecrosis, temporal lobe necrosis, hypothyroidism, hypopituitarism (if included)

FOLLOW-UP

- H&P every 1–3 months first year, every 2–4 months second year, every 4–6 months years 3–5, then every 6–12 months
- MRI at 2 and 4 months post-RT, then every 6 months or as clinically indicated
- TSH every 6–12 months
- Dental cleaning every 3 months for lifetime

III

Acknowledgment We thank Dr. M. Kara Bucci for her contribution to this chapter in the first edition.

REFERENCES

Al-Sarraf M, LeBlanc M, Giri PG, et al. Chemoradiotherapy versus radiotherapy in patients with advanced nasopharyngeal cancer: phase III randomized Intergroup study 0099. J Clin Oncol 1998;16:1310-1317.

Baujat, B, Audry H, Bourhis J, et al. Chemotherapy in locally advanced nasopharyngeal carcinoma: an individualized patient data meta-analysis of eight randomized trials and 1753 patients. Int J Radiat Oncol Phys 2006;64:47-56.

Chan AT, Teo PM, Leung TW, et al. A prospective randomized study of chemotherapy adjunctive to definitive radiotherapy in advanced nasopharyngeal carcinoma. Int J Radiat Oncol Phys 2005a;33:569-77.

Chan AT, Leung SF, Ngan RK, et al. Overall survival after concurrent cisplatin-radiotherapy compared with radiotherapy alone in locoregionally advanced nasopharyngeal carcinoma. J Natl Cancer Inst 2005b;97:536-539.

Children's Oncology Group. Protocols: ARA 0331. Available at: https://members.childrensoncologygroup.org/prot/default.asp (password required). Accessed on February 10, 2009.

Chua DT, Sham JS, Choy D, et al. Preliminary report of the Asian-Oceanian Clinical Oncology Association randomized trial comparing cisplatin and epirubicin followed by radiotherapy versus radiotherapy alone in the treatment of patients with locoregionally advanced nasopharyngeal carcinoma. Cancer 1998;83:2270-2283.

ClinicalTrials.gov. Induction chemotherapy and chemoradiotherapy in nasopharyngeal cancers (GORTEC-NPC2006). Available at: http://clinicaltrials.gov/ct2/show/NCT00828386. Accessed on March 10, 2009.

Garden AS. The Nasopharynx. In: Cox JD, Ang KK, editors. Radiation oncology: rationale, technique, results. 8th ed. St. Louis: Mosby; 2003. pp. 178-195.

Greene FL, American Joint Committee on Cancer, American Cancer Society. AJCC cancer staging manual. 6th ed. New York: Springer; 2002.

Hui, EP, Ma BB, Leung SF, et al. Randomized phase II trial of concurrent cisplatin-radiotherapy with or without neoadjuvant docetaxel and cisplatin in advanced nasopharyngeal carcinoma. J Clin Oncol 2009;27:242-249.

International Nasopharynx Cancer Study Group. Preliminary results of a randomized trial comparing neoadjuvant chemotherapy (cisplatin, epirubicin, bleomycin) plus radiotherapy vs. radiotherapy alone in stage IV (≥ N2, M0) undifferentiated nasopharyngeal carcinoma: a positive effect on progression-free survival. Int J Radiat Oncol Phys 1996;35: 463-469.

Kam MK, Leung SF, Zee B, et al. Prospective randomized study of intensity-modulated radiotherapy on salivary gland function in early-stage nasopharyngeal carcinoma patients. J Clin Oncol 2007;25:4873-4879.

Lee N, Xia P, Quivey JM, et al. Intensity-modulated radiotherapy in the treatment of nasopharyngeal carcinoma: an update of the UCSF experience. Int J Radiat Oncol Biol Phys 2002;53: 12-22.

Lee N, Xia P, Fischbein NJ, et al. Intensity-modulated radiation therapy for head-and-neck cancer: the UCSF experience focusing on target volume delineation. Int J Radiat Oncol Biol Phys 2003;57:49-60.

Lee N, Fu K. Cancer of the Nasopharynx. In: Leibel SA, Phillips TL, editors. Textbook of radiation oncology. 2nd ed. Philadelphia: Saunders; 2004. pp. 579-600.

Lee AW, Perez CA, Law SC, et al. Nasopharynx. In: Halperin EC, Perez CA, Brady LW, editors. Principles and practice of radiation oncology. 5th ed. Philadelphia: Lippincott Williams & Wilkins; 2008. pp. 820-857.

Leung SF, Zee B, Ma BB, et al. Plasma Epstein-Barr viral deoxyribonucleic acid quantitation complements tumor-node-metastasis staging prognostication in nasopharyngeal carcinoma. J Clin Oncol 2008;24:5414-5418.

Lin JC, Wang WY, Chen KY, et al. Quantification of plasma Epstein-Barr virus DNA in patients with advanced nasopharyngeal carcinoma. N Engl J Med 2004;350(24):2461-2470.

Ma J, Mai HQ, Hong MH, et al. Results of a prospective randomized trial comparing neoadjuvant chemotherapy plus radiotherapy with radiotherapy alone in patients with locoregionally advanced nasopharyngeal carcinoma. J Clin Oncol 2001;19:1350-1357.

National Comprehensive Cancer Network. Clinical Practice Guidelines in Oncology: Head and Neck Cancers. Available at: http://www.nccn.org/professionals/physician_gls/PDF/head-and-neck.pdf. Accessed on February 10, 2009.

National Cancer Institute. Nasopharyngeal Cancer (PDQ): Treatment. Available at: http://cancer.gov/cancertopics/pdq/treatment/nasopharyngeal/healthprofessional/. Accessed on February 10, 2009.

Pow EH, Kwong DL, McMillan AS, et al. Xerostomia and quality of life after intensity-modulated radiotherapy vs. conventional radiotherapy for early-stage nasopharyngeal carcinoma: initial report on a randomized controlled clinical trial. Int J Radiat Onc Biol Phys 2006;66:981-991.

Radiation Therapy Oncology Group. RTOG Head & Neck Cancer Protocols. Available at: http://www.rtog.org/members/active.html#headneck. Accessed on February 10, 2009.

Wee J, Tan EH, Tai BC, et al. Randomized trial of radiotherapy versus concurrent chemo-radiotherapy followed by adjuvant chemotherapy in patients with American Joint Committee on Cancer/International Union Against Cancer Stage III and IV nasopharyngeal cancer of the endemic variety. J Clin Oncol 2005;23:6730-6738.

Chapter 6

Nasal Cavity and Paranasal Sinus Cancer

III

Chien Peter Chen, Brian Missett, and Sue S. Yom

PEARLS

- Maxillary cancers are most common (70%).
- Incidence higher in Japan and South Africa.
- More common in males (4:1).
- Ohngren's line runs from the medial canthus to the angle of the mandible.
- Tumors superior-posterior to Ohngren's line have a poorer prognosis.
- Histology: most common is SCC. Adenoid cystic, esthesioneuroblastoma, plasmacytoma, lymphoma, melanoma, and sarcoma also seen.
- Lymphatic drainage of maxillary antrum to submandibular, parotid, jugulodigastric, retropharyngeal, and jugular nodes.
- See Chap. 12 for more information on esthesioneuroblastoma.

WORKUP

- H&P, nasal endoscopy, CT/MRI, biopsy, CXR
- Consider serum blood tests including IGF-1, free thyroxin, cortisol, prolactin to get baseline pretreatment levels

STAGING: NASAL CAVITY AND PARANASAL SINUS CANCER

Editors' note: All TNM stage and stage groups referred to elsewhere in this chapter reflect the 2002 AJCC staging nomenclature unless otherwise noted as the new system below was published after this chapter was written.

(AJCC 6TH ED., 2002)

Primary tumor (T)

Maxillary sinus

Tis: Carcinoma in situ

T1: Tumor limited to maxillary sinus mucosa with no erosion or destruction of bone

T2: Tumor causing bone erosion or destruction including extension into the hard palate and/or middle nasal meatus, except extension to posterior wall of the maxillary sinus and pterygoid plates

T3: Tumor invades any of the following: posterior wall of maxillary sinus, subcutaneous tissues, floor or medial wall of orbit, pterygoid fossa, and/or ethmoid sinuses

T4a: Tumor invades anterior orbital contents, skin of cheek, pterygoid plates, infratemporal fossa, cribriform plate, sphenoid or frontal sinuses

T4b: Tumor invades any of the following: orbital apex, dura, brain, middle cranial fossa, cranial nerves other than maxillary division of trigerminal verve (V2), nasopharynx, or clivus

Primary tumor – ethmoid sinus and nasal cavity

Ethmoid sinus subsites: Right, left

Nasal cavity subsites: Septum, wall, floor, vestibule

Tis: Carcinoma in situ

T1: Tumor restricted to any one subsite, with or without bony invasion

T2: Tumor invading two subsites in single region or extending to involve an adjacent region within the nasothemoidal complex, with or without bony invasion

T3: Tumor extends to invade the medial wall or floor of orbit, maxillary sinus, palate, or cribriform plate

T4a: Tumor invades any of the following: anterior orbital contents, skin of nose or cheek, minimal extension to anterior cranial fossa, pterygoid plates, sphenoid or frontal sinuses

(AJCC 7TH ED., 2010)

Primary tumor (T)

TX: Primary tumor cannot be assessed

T0: No evidence of primary tumor

Tis: Carcinoma in situ

Maxillary sinus

T1: Tumor limited to maxillary sinus mucosa with no erosion or destruction of bone

T2: Tumor causing bone erosion or destruction including extension into the hard palate and/or middle nasal meatus, except extension to posterior wall of maxillary sinus and pterygoid plates

T3: Tumor invades any of the following: bone of the posterior wall of maxillary sinus, subcutaneous tissues, floor or medial wall of orbit, pterygoid fossa, ethmoid sinuses

T4a: Moderately advanced local disease. Tumor invades anterior orbital contents, skin of cheek, pterygoid plates, infratemporal fossa, cribriform plate, sphenoid or frontal sinuses

T4b: Very advanced local disease. Tumor invades any of the following: orbital apex, dura, brain, middle cranial fossa, cranial nerves other than maxillary division of trigeminal nerve (V2), nasopharynx, or clivus

Nasal cavity and ethmoid sinus

T1: Tumor restricted to any one subsite, with or without bony invasion

T2: Tumor invading two subsites in a single region or extending to involve an adjacent region within the nasoethmoidal complex, with or without bony invasion

T3: Tumor extends to invade the medial wall or floor of the orbit, maxillary sinus, palate, or cribriform plate

T4a: Moderately advanced local disease. Tumor invades any of the following: anterior orbital contents, skin of nose or cheek, minimal extension to anterior cranial fossa, pterygoid plates, sphenoid or frontal sinuses

continued

T4b: Tumor invades any of the following: orbital apex, dura, brain, middle cranial fossa, cranial nerves other than V2, nasopharynx or clivus

Regional lymph nodes (N)

Nx: Regional lymph nodes cannot be assessed
N1: Metastasis in a single ipsilateral lymph node, 3 cm or less in greatest dimension
N2a: Metastasis in a single ipsilateral lymph node more than 3 cm, but not more than 6 cm in greatest dimension
N2b: Metastasis in multiple ipsilateral lymph nodes, not more than 6 cm in greatest dimension
N2c: Metastasis in bilateral or contralateral lymph nodes, not more than 6 cm in greatest dimension
N3: Metastasis in a lymph node, more than 6 cm in greatest dimension

Metastases (M)

Mx: Distant metastasis cannot be assessed
M0: No distant metastasis
M1: Distant metastasis

Stage grouping		**~2/5-Years OS (maxillary sinus) (%)**	
0:	TisN0M0		
I:	T1N0M0	I:	80/55
II:	T2N0M0	II:	67/44
III:	T3N0, T1-3N1M0	III:	60/40
IVA:	T4aN0-1, T1-4aN2M0	IV:	51/27
IVB:	T4b any N, Any T N3M0		
IVC:	Any M1		

Used with the permission from the American Joint Committee on Cancer (AJCC), Chicago, IL. The original source for this material is the AJCC Cancer Staging Manual, Sixth Edition (2002), published by Springer Science+Business Media.

T4b: Very advanced local disease. Tumor invades any of the following: orbital apex, dura, brain, middle cranial fossa, cranial nerves other than (V2), nasopharynx, or clivus

Regional lymph nodes (N)

NX: Regional lymph nodes cannot be assessed
N0: No regional lymph node metastasis
N1: Metastasis in a single ipsilateral lymph node, 3 cm or less in greatest dimension
N2: Metastasis in a single ipsilateral lymph node, more than 3 cm, but not more than 6 cm in greatest dimension, or in multiple ipsilateral lymph nodes, not more than 6 cm in greatest dimension, or in bilateral or contralateral lymph nodes, not more than 6 cm in greatest dimension
- N2a: Metastasis in a single ipsilateral lymph node, more than 3 cm, but not more than 6 cm in greatest dimension
- N2b: Metastasis in multiple ipsilateral lymph nodes, not more than 6 cm in greatest dimension
- N2c: Metastasis in bilateral or contralateral lymph nodes, not more than 6 cm in greatest dimension

N3: Metastasis in a lymph node, more than 6 cm in greatest dimension

Distant metastasis (M)

M0: No distant metastasis
M1: Distant metastasis

Anatomic stage/prognostic groups	
Stage 0	Tis N0 M0
Stage I	T1 N0 M0
Stage II	T2 N0 M0
Stage III	T3 N0 M0
	T1-T3 N1 M0
Stage IVA	T4a N0 M0
	T4a N1 M0
	T1-T3 N2 M0
	T4a N2 M0

continued

Stage IVB	T4b Any N M0 Any T N3 M0
Stage IVC	Any T Any N M1

Used with the permission from the American Joint Committee on Cancer (AJCC), Chicago, IL. The original source for this material is the AJCC Cancer Staging Manual, Seventh Edition (2010), published by Springer Science+Business Media.

TREATMENT RECOMMENDATIONS

2002 Stage	Recommended treatment
Nasal cavity and ethmoid sinus	■ T1-2N0: Resection → post-op RT for close/+ margins or PNI. Alternatively, definitive RT. ■ Choice depends on size, location and expected cosmetic outcome ■ T3-4N0: Resectable: resection → post-op RT Unresectable or inoperable: Definitive RT or chemo-RT ■ N+: Resection + neck dissection → post-op ■ RT or chemo-RT. Alternatively, definitive chemo-RT
Maxillary sinus	■ T1-2N0: Resection → post-op RT for close margin, PNI, adenoid cystic. For + margin, re-resect (if possible) → post-op RT ■ T3-4N0 resectable: Resection → post-op RT or chemo-RT ■ Unresectable or inoperable: Definitive RT or chemo-RT ■ N+: Resection + neck dissection → post-op RT or chemo-RT. Alternatively, definitive chemo-RT

STUDIES

- Allen et al. (2008): 68 patients with nasal cavity or nasal septum cancer. Forty-seven percent received definitive RT. Nineteen percent received neck RT. Five years and 10 years LC 86 and 76%, DFS 86 and 78%, OS 82 and 62%.
- Le et al. (2000): 97 patients with maxillary sinus tumors. Fifty-six had surgery first and 41 had pre-op or definitive RT. Twelve percent LN relapse at 5 years. T3-4 SCC were associated with a high incidence of initial nodal involvement and nodal relapse. None of the patients presenting with SCC histology and N0 necks had nodal recurrence after elective neck radiation. Recommended elective ipsilateral neck RT for T3-4 SCC.
- Bristol et al. (2007): 146 patients with maxillary sinus tumors treated with post-op radiotherapy. Group 1 included 90 patients treated before 1991. Group 2 included 56 patients treated after 1991, when radiotherapy technique incorporated coverage of the base of skull for patients with perineural invasion, elective neck RT in SCC or undifferentiated histology, and techniques to improve dose homogeneity to target. No difference in 5 years OS (51 vs. 62%), RFS, LRC, DM between the two groups, but base of skull and nodal failures reduced in at-risk patients.

Advanced age, need for enucleation, and positive margins were independent predictors of worse OS. Need for enucleation predicted worse LRC.

- Dulguerov et al. (2001): 220 patients with nasal cavity and paranasal sinus cancer. Five years OS 40%, local control rate 59%. Prognostic factors: histology, T stage, primary site, and treatment type. Local extension factors associated with worse survival: extension to pterygomaxillary fossa, extension to frontal and sphenoid sinuses, erosion of cribriform plate, and invasion of the dura. In the presence of an intraorbital invasion, enucleation was associated with better survival.
- Chen et al. (2007): 127 patients with sinonasal carcinoma. Five years OS, LRC, DFS were 52, 62, and 54%, respectively. No significant difference in 5-year OS rates for patients treated in 1960s, 1970s, 1980s, 1990s, and 2000s. Significantly reduced incidence of severe (Grade 3 and 4) toxicity over the decades.
- Some physicians extrapolate from the Bernier and Cooper studies (*NEJM* 2004) to support using post-op concurrent chemo and RT in patients with SCC of the paranasal sinuses.
- Madani et al. (2009): 73 primary and 11 locally recurrent sinonasal tumors definitively treated by IMRT. No chemo. Sixty-four percent patients had adenocarcinoma histology. Median follow-up 40 m with 5-year LRC, OS, DFS were 71, 58, and 59%, respectively.
- Snyers et al. (2009): 178 patients with sinonasal cancer. Sixty-two percent of long-term survivors had hormonal disturbances and 24% had multiple hormonal deficiencies.

RADIATION TECHNIQUES

SIMULATION AND FIELD DESIGN

- Simulate supine with thermoplastic mask immobilization.
- Eyes open, straight ahead to keep posterior pole away from high dose region.
- Tongue blade/cork to depress tongue out of fields.
- Fill surgical defects with tissue equivalents.
- Recommend 3DCRT or IMRT planning to increase sparing of normal structures.
- GTV = clinical and/or radiographic gross disease. CTV1 = 1 cm margin on primary and/or nodal GTV. CTV2 = high-risk regions (depending on the presence or absence of anatomic boundaries to microscopic spread). CTV3 = elective neck. Individualized planning target volumes are used for the GTV, CTV1, CTV2, and CTV3 tailored to subsite and stage.

DOSE PRESCRIPTIONS

- EBRT 1.8–2 Gy/fx.
- Definitive RT or chemo-RT: CTV1 to 66–70 Gy, CTV2 to 60–63 Gy, CTV3 to 54–57 Gy.
- Post-op RT: CTV1 to 60 Gy with optional boost to 66 Gy to high-risk areas (close/+ margins, ECE, PNI). CTV2 to 50–54 Gy.
- For selected nasal septum tumors, brachytherapy may be appropriate.

DOSE LIMITATIONS

- Lens <10 Gy (cataracts).
- Retina <45 Gy (vision). May go higher if treating bid or partial volume.
- Optic chiasm and nerves <54 Gy at standard fractionation.
- Brain <60 Gy (necrosis).
- Mandible <60 Gy (osteoradionecrosis).
- Parotid mean dose <26 Gy (xerostomia).
- Lacrimal gland <30–40 Gy.
- Pituitary and hypothalamus mean dose <40 Gy.

COMPLICATIONS

- Acute = mucositis, skin erythema, nasal dryness, xerostomia
- Late = xerostomia, chronic keratitis and iritis, optic pathway injury, soft tissue or osteoradionecrosis, cataracts, radiation-induced hypopituitarism

FOLLOW-UP

- H&P, labs, and CXR every 3 months for first year, every 4 months for second year, every 6 months for third year, then annually. Imaging of the H&N at 3 months posttreatment, then as indicated.

Acknowledgment We thank Dr. M. Kara Bucci for her contribution to this chapter in the first edition.

REFERENCES

Allen MW, Schwartz DL, Rana V, et al. Long-term radiotherapy outcomes for nasal cavity and septal cancers. Int J Radiat Oncol Biol Phys 2008;71: 401-406.

Bernier J, Cooper JS, Pajak TF, et al. Defining risk levels in locally advanced head and neck cancers: a comparative analysis of concurrent postoperative radiation plus chemotherapy trials of the EORTC (#22931) and RTOG (# 9501). Head Neck. 2005;27(10):843-850.

Bernier J, Domenge C, Ozsahin M, et al. Postoperative irradiation with or without concomitant chemotheraphy for locally advanced head and neck cancer: N Engl J Med 2004;350: 1945-1952

Bristol IJ, Ahamad, A., Garden AS, et al. Postoperative radiotherapy for maxillary sinus cancer: long-term outcomes and toxicities of treatment. Int J Radiat Oncol Biol Phys 2007;68: 719-730.

Chen AM, Daly ME, Bucci MK, et al. Carcinomas of the paranasal sinuses and nasal cavity treated with radiotherapy at a single institution over five decades: are we making improvement? Int J Radiat Oncol Biol Phys 2007;69:141-147.

Dulguerov P, Jacobsen MS, Allal AS, et al. Nasal and paranasal sinus carcinoma: are we making progress? A series of 220 patients and a systematic review. Cancer 2001;92:3012-3029.

Le QT, Fu KK, Kaplan MJ, et al. Lymph node metastasis in maxillary sinus carcinoma. Int J Radiat Oncol Biol Phys 2000;46:541-549.

Madani I, Bonte K, Vakaet L, et al. Intensity-modulated radiotherapy for sinonasal tumors: Ghent University Hospital update. Int J Radiat Oncol Biol Phys 2009 73:424-432.

Snyers A, Janssens GO, Twickler MB, et al. Malignant tumors of the nasal cavity and paranasal sinuses: long-term outcome and morbidity with emphasis on hypothalamic-pituitary deficiency. Int J Radiat Oncol Biol Phys 2009;73:1343-1351.

FURTHER READING

Ahamad A, Ang KK. Nasal Cavity and Paranasal Sinuses. In: Halperin EC, Perez CA, Brady LW, et al., editors. Principles and Practice of Radiation Oncology. 5th ed. Philadelphia: Lippincott Williams & Wilkins; 2008. pp. 858-873.

National Cancer Institute. Paranasal Sinus and Nasal Cavity Cancer (PDQ): Treatment. Available at: http://cancer.gov/cancertopics/pdq/treatment/paranasalsinus/healthprofessional/. Accessed on May 11, 2009.

National Comprehensive Cancer Network. Clinical Practice Guidelines in Oncology: Head and Neck Cancers. Available at: http://www.nccn.org/professionals/physician_gls/PDF/head-and-neck.pdf. Accessed on May 11, 2009.

Nguyen L, Ang KK. The Nasal Fossa and Paranasal Sinuses. In: Cox JD, Ang KK, editors. Radiation Oncology: Rationale, Technique, Results. 8th ed. St. Louis: Mosby; 2003. pp. 160-177.

Ryu JK. Cancer of the Nasal Cavity and Paranasal Sinuses. In: Leibel SA, Phillips TL, editors. Textbook of Radiation Oncology. 2nd ed. Philadelphia: Saunders; 2004. pp. 731-756.

Chapter 7
Oropharyngeal Cancer

Siavash Jabbari, Kim Huang, and Jeanne Marie Quivey

III

PEARLS

- Approximately 8,500 cases/year in the US with male predominance (3:1).
- Etiologies include consumption of alcohol, tobacco, betal and areca nuts, and HPV infection.
- Recent decrease in the incidence of tobacco-related cancers.
  - Recent increase in HPV-related incidence rates attributed to changing sexual practices.
  - HPV-related cancers appear to occur at a slightly younger age and have better survival rates when treated with radiotherapy and chemotherapy as compared to non-HPV-related cancers.
- Second primary tumors in the upper aerodigestive tract and lung occur in ~25% of patients due to risk factors and lifestyle.
- Risk of second primary cancers is doubled with continued smoking.
- Subsites: soft palate, palatine tonsils, tonsillar pillars, base of tongue (lingual tonsils), pharyngeal wall.
- Anatomic boundaries: superior = plane of superior surface of soft palate; inferior = superior surface of hyoid bone (or floor of vallecula).
- Deep (middle) ear pain may be referred via the tympanic nerve of Jacobson (CN IX) via the petrosal ganglion.
- Histology: 95% SCC, others = adenocarcinoma, mucoepidermoid, adenoid cystic, melanoma, small cell carcinoma of tonsil, non-Hodgkin's lymphoma of tonsil.
- Presentation: sore throat, dysphagia, otalgia, odynophagia, hot potato voice (with base of tongue invasion), hoarseness (with larynx invasion or edema).
- Noninvolved base of tongue may have mild benign enhancement on MRI or FDG uptake on PET.

WORKUP

- H&P. Palpation, indirect mirror exam, fiberoptic endoscopy.
- Panendoscopy with biopsy.
- Labs: CBC, chemistries, BUN, Cr, LFTs including alkaline phosphatase and HPV testing of either the primary or nodal metastases.
- Imaging: MRI with contrast ± CT scan with contrast of head and neck. PET/CT scan. CXR or CT chest. Panorex as indicated.
- Preventive dental care with extractions 10–14 days before RT.
- Speech and swallow evaluation as indicated.

STAGING: OROPHARYNGEAL CANCER

Editors' note: All TNM stage and stage groups referred to elsewhere in this chapter reflect the 2002 AJCC staging nomenclature unless otherwise noted as the new system below was published after this chapter was written.

(AJCC 6TH ED., 2002)

Primary tumor (T)

TX: Primary tumor cannot be assessed
T0: No evidence of primary tumor
Tis: Carcinoma in situ
T1: Tumor 2 cm or less in greatest dimension
T2: Tumor more than 2 cm but not more than 4 cm in greatest dimension
T3: Tumor more than 4 cm in greatest dimension or extension to lingual surface of epiglottis
T4a: Moderately advanced local disease. Tumor invades the larynx, extrinsic muscle of tongue, medial pterygoid, hard palate, or mandible*
T4b: Very advanced local disease. Tumor invades lateral pterygoid muscle, pterygoid plates, lateral nasopharynx, or skull base or encases carotid artery

**Note*: Mucosal extension to lingual surface of epiglottis from primary tumors of the base of the tongue and vallecula does not constitute invasion of larynx.

Regional lymph nodes (N)

NX: Regional lymph nodes cannot be assessed
N0: No regional lymph node metastasis
N1: Metastasis in a single ipsilateral lymph node, 3 cm or less in greatest dimension
N2: Metastasis in a single ipsilateral lymph node, more than 3 cm but not more than 6 cm in greatest dimension, or in multiple ipsilateral lymph nodes, not more than 6 cm in greatest dimension, or in bilateral or contralateral lymph nodes, not more than 6 cm in greatest dimension

(AJCC 7TH ED., 2010)

Primary tumor (T)

TX: Primary tumor cannot be assessed
T0: No evidence of primary tumor
Tis: Carcinoma in situ
T1: Tumor 2 cm or less in greatest dimension
T2: Tumor more than 2 cm but not more than 4 cm in greatest dimension
T3: Tumor more than 4 cm in greatest dimension or extension to lingual surface of epiglottis
T4a: Moderately advanced local disease. Tumor invades the larynx, extrinsic muscle of tongue, medial pterygoid, hard palate, or mandible*
T4b: Very advanced local disease. Tumor invades lateral pterygoid muscle, pterygoid plates, lateral nasopharynx, or skull base or encases carotid artery

**Note*: Mucosal extension to lingual surface of epiglottis from primary tumors of the base of the tongue and vallecula does not constitute invasion of larynx.

Regional lymph nodes (N)

NX: Regional lymph nodes cannot be assessed
N0: No regional lymph node metastasis
N1: Metastasis in a single ipsilateral lymph node, 3 cm or less in greatest dimension
N2: Metastasis in a single ipsilateral lymph node, more than 3 cm, but not more than 6 cm in greatest dimension, or in multiple ipsilateral lymph nodes, not more than 6 cm in greatest dimension, or in bilateral or contralateral lymph nodes, not more than 6 cm in greatest dimension

continued

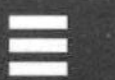

N2a: Metastasis in a single ipsilateral lymph node more than 3 cm but not more than 6 cm in greatest dimension
N2b: Metastasis in multiple ipsilateral lymph nodes, not more than 6 cm in greatest dimension
N2c: Metastasis in bilateral or contralateral lymph nodes, not more than 6 cm in greatest dimension
N3: Metastasis in a lymph node more than 6 cm in greatest dimension

**Note*: Metastases at level VII (upper mediastinum) are considered regional lymph node metastases.

Distant metastases (M)
MX: Distant metastasis cannot be assessed
M0: No distant metastasis

Stage grouping
0: TisN0M0
I: T1N0M0
II: T2N0M0
III: T3N0M0, T1-3N1M0
IVA: T4aN0-1M0, T1-4aN2M0
IVB: T4b, any N, M0; Any T, N3M0
IVC: Any T, any N, M1

Used with the permission from the American Joint Committee on Cancer (AJCC), Chicago, IL. The original source for this material is the AJCC Cancer Staging Manual, Sixth Edition (2002), published by Springer Science+Business Media.

N2a: Metastasis in a single ipsilateral lymph node more than 3 cm but not more than 6 cm in greatest dimension
N2b: Metastasis in multiple ipsilateral lymph nodes, not more than 6 cm in greatest dimension
N2c: Metastasis in bilateral or contralateral lymph nodes, not more than 6 cm in greatest dimension
N3: Metastasis in a lymph node more than 6 cm in greatest dimension

**Note*: Metastases at level VII (upper mediastinum) are considered regional lymph node metastases.

Distant metastases (M)
MX: Distant metastasis cannot be assessed
M0: No distant metastasis

Stage grouping
0: TisN0M0
I: T1N0M0
II: T2N0M0
III: T3N0M0, T1-3N1M0
IVA: T4aN0-1M0, T1-4aN2M0
IVB: T4b, any N, M0; Any T, N3M0
IVC: Any T, any N, M1

Used with the permission from the American Joint Committee on Cancer (AJCC), Chicago, IL. The original source for this material is the AJCC Cancer Staging Manual, Seventh Edition (2010), published by Springer Science+Business Media.

TREATMENT RECOMMENDATIONS

2002 Stage	Recommended treatment
T1-2N0	■ Definitive RT. Alternative, surgery with post-op RT as indicated
III–IV	■ Concurrent chemo-RT (preferred). ■ Alternative, surgery with post-op (chemo-)RT as indicated. For patients not considered candidates for standard chemo-RT (e.g., with cisplatin), consider RT and cetuximab. ■ If unable to tolerate concurrent chemo, altered fractionation RT may be used

III

SURGERY

- For T3-4 primaries, tonsillar lesions require radical tonsillectomy often with partial mandibulectomy; base of tongue lesions require partial or total glossectomy and myocutaneous flap reconstruction. Patients requiring removal of more than 1/2 of tongue or elderly patients with poor pulmonary function often require total laryngectomy to prevent subsequent aspiration. Therefore, for locally advanced oropharyngeal, primary organ preservation approach with radiation or chemo-RT is preferred.
- Types of Neck Dissection
  - Radical neck dissection (RND) removes levels I–V, sternocleidomastoid muscle, omohyoid muscle, internal and external jugular veins, CN XI, and the submandibular gland.
  - Modified RND leaves ≥1 of sternocleidomastoid muscle, internal jugular vein, or CN XI.
  - Selective neck dissection does not remove ≥1 level of levels I–V.
  - Supraomohyoid neck dissection only removes levels I–III.
  - Lateral neck dissection only removes levels II–IV.

POST-OP RT OR CHEMO-RT

- Post-op chemo-RT indications (major risk factors): extracapsular nodal spread, +margin(s)
- Post-op RT indications (minor risk factors): close margin, multiple LN+, PNI, LVSI

STUDIES

PRE-OP VS. POST-OP RT

- *RTOG 73–03* (Kramer et al. 1987; Tupchong et al. 1991): 354 patients with advanced H&N cancer randomized to 2/50 Gy pre-op vs. 2/50/60 Gy post-op. Post-op RT improved LRC (48→65%), and OS for oropharynx lesions (26→38%). Complications not different.

ALTERED FRACTIONATION

- *RTOG 90–03* (Fu et al. 2000): 268 patients with locally advanced H&N cancer randomized to 2/70 Gy vs. 1.2 b.i.d./81.6 Gy vs. split-course 1.6 b.i.d./67.2 Gy (with a 2 weeks break) vs. concomitant boost RT to 72 Gy [with b.i.d. RT for last 12 fractions (1.8 and 1.5 Gy)]. Concomitant boost and hyperfractionated RT improved 2-year LRC (54%), DFS (39%), and OS (53%) compared to standard or split-course accelerated RT. Altered fractionation increased acute side effects.
- *EORTC* (Horiot et al. 1992): 325 patients with T2-3 oropharyngeal cancer randomized to 2/70 Gy vs. 1.15 b.i.d./80.5 Gy. b.i.d. RT increased 5-year LC (40→59%) and OS (31→47%) with benefit primarily for T3 tumors.
- *MARCH metaanalysis* (Bourhis et al. 2006): fifteen phase III trials and 6,515 patients. 3.4% OS benefit at 5 years for altered fractionation vs. conventional fractionation, with most benefit suggested for hyperfractionation. Decreasing benefit with increasing age.

CHEMO-RT ± ALTERED FRACTIONATION

- *GORTEC 94–01* (Denis et al. 2004): 226 patients with stage III/IV oropharyngeal cancer randomized to 2/70 vs. 2/70 Gy + carboplatin/5-FU ×3 cycles. Chemo-RT improved LC (25→48%), DFS (15→27%), and OS (16→23, $p = 0.13$), but increased acute toxicity. Trend for increased late toxicity.
- *Adelstein, Intergroup* (Adelstein et al. 2003): 295 patients with unresectable H&N cancer, randomized to 2/70 Gy vs. 2/70 Gy + cisplatin (100 mg/m^2) ×3 cycles vs. split-course RT (2/30 Gy + 2/30–40 Gy) + cisplatin/5-FU ×3 cycles. Results: chemo-RT improved 3-year OS (23 vs. 37 vs. 27%) and DFS (33 vs. 51 vs. 41%) but did not change DM and it increased toxicity.
- Brizel et al. (2004): 116 patients with advanced H&N cancer randomized to 1.25 b.i.d./75 vs. 1.25 b.i.d./70 Gy (with 1 week break at 40 Gy) + concurrent cisplatin/5-FU ×2 cycles. Both

arms received adjuvant cisplatin/5-FU ×2 cycles. Chemo-RT improved LC (44→70%), DFS (41→61%), and OS (34→55%). No change in DM or toxicity.

- Bonner et al. (2006): 424 patients with locoregionally advanced resectable or unresectable stage III–IV SCC of oropharynx, larynx, or hypopharynx randomized to RT or RT + cetuximab given 1 week before RT and weekly during RT. RT options included 2/70 Gy, 1.2 b.i.d./72–76.8 Gy, or concomitant boost 72 Gy. Cetuximab increased 3-years LRC (34→47%) and OS (45→55%). With the exception of acneiform rash and infusion reactions with cetuximab, toxicity was similar.
- Semrau et al. (2006): 263 patients with stage III–IV oropharynx or hypopharynx cancer randomized to concomitant boost RT (69.9 Gy/38 fxs) alone or concomitant boost chemo-RT. Chemo = concurrent carboplatin/5-FU × 2 cycles. Chemo-RT improved 5-years LRC (12.6→22.7) and OS (15.8→25.6%). Benefit observed in oropharynx patients only, where pretreatment hemoglobin levels (above 12.7 g/dL) predicted for LRC. No difference in late toxicity.
- *GORTEC* (Bourhis, ASTRO 2008): 840 patients with locally advanced head and neck cancer randomized to conventional chemo-RT (70 Gy in 7 weeks + carboplatin/5-FU) vs. accelerated chemo-RT (70 Gy in 6 weeks + carboplatin/5-FU) vs. very-accelerated RT alone (64.8 Gy in 3.5 weeks). Increased mucositis in very-accelerated RT arm, but no difference in overall acute toxicity, LRC, or OS, with a median follow-up of 3.5 years. Improved PFS in conventional chemo-RT arm as compared to very-accelerated RT arm.
- *MACH-NC metaanalysis* (Pignon et al. 2009): 93 phase III trials and 17,346 patients. OS benefit (4.5%) at 5 years when chemotherapy was added to RT, with greater benefit for concurrent chemo-RT vs. induction chemo followed by RT (6.5% OS benefit with concurrent chemo-RT). Similar results in trials with post-op RT, conventional, and altered fractionation. No difference between mono or polychemotherapy regimens, but increased benefit with platinum-based compounds. Decreasing benefit with increasing age, with no benefit observed if ≥71-years old.

POST-OP CHEMO-RT

- *EORTC 22931* (O'Sullivan et al. 2001, Cooper et al., NEJM 2004): 334 patients with operable stage III/IV H&N cancer randomized to post-op 2/66 Gy vs. post-op 2/66 Gy + concurrent cisplatin

(100 mg/m^2) on days 1, 22, and 43. Eligibility: oral cavity, oropharynx, hypopharynx, and larynx with pT3-4N0/+, T1-2N2-3, or T1-2N0-1 with ECE, +margin, or PNI. Chemo-RT improved 3/5-year DFS (41/36→59/47%), OS (49/40→65/53%), and 5-year LRC (69→82%). No difference in DM (21–25%) or second primaries (12%). Chemo-RT increased grade 3/4 toxicities (21→41%).

- *RTOG 95–01* (NEJM 2004): patients (459) with operable H&N cancer who had ≥2 LN, ECE, or + margin randomized to post-op RT (2/60–66 Gy) vs. post-op chemo-RT (2/60–66 + cisplatin ×3 cycles same as EORTC). Chemo-RT improved 2-year DFS (43→54%), LRC (72→82%) and had trend for improved OS (57→63%). No difference in DM (20–23%). Chemo-RT increased grade 3/4 toxicities (34→77%).
- *Combined analysis* (Bernier et al. 2004): chemo-RT improved OS, DFS, and LRC for ECE and/or + margins, but provided only trend for improvements ($p = 0.06$) stage III–IV, PNI, LVI, and/or enlarged LN in levels IV–V for OPX or oral cavity tumors based on EORTC data. Patients with ≥2 LN without ECE as their only factor did not benefit from chemo ($p = 0.73$).

INDUCTION CHEMO

- No published phase III studies have tested induction chemo followed by chemo-RT vs. upfront chemo-RT, and this is the subject of on-going randomized trials.
- *EORTC/TAX 323* (Vermorken et al. 2007): randomized 358 patients with unresectable stage III–IV head and neck cancer to TPF (docetaxol/cisplatin/5-FU) vs. PF (cisplatin/5-FU) induction chemotherapy followed by RT alone, delivered with conventional (66 Gy) or hyperfractionated (74 Gy) RT. Induction TPF increased MS (14.5→18.8 months), but increased hematological toxicity and chemo-related death (2.3 vs. 5.5%). Ten to fifteen percent of patients were unable to receive RT.
- Posner et al. (2007): randomized 501 patients with unresectable stage III–IV head and neck cancer to TPF (docetaxol/cisplatin/5-FU) vs. PF (cisplatin/5-FU) induction chemotherapy followed by carboplatin chemo-RT (70–74 Gy). Induction TPF improved LRC and 3-year OS (48→62%), but not DM. Twenty-one to 25% of patients did not receive concurrent chemo-RT due to progressive disease, adverse events, death, or withdrawal of consent.
- *ECOG 2399* (Fakhry et al. 2009): prospective evaluation of HPV-positive vs. HPV-negative tumors showed 63% HPV-positive rate for oropharynx with higher response to induction chemotherapy

and chemoradiation, as well as overall survival (2-year OS = 95 vs. 62%).

TECHNIQUES

SIMULATION AND FIELD DESIGN

- Simulate patient supine with head hyperextended. Wire neck scars and consider wiring commissure of lips. Shoulders may be pulled down with straps. Immobilize with a thermoplastic head and shoulder mask. Bolus may be needed if skin involved; shield gold crowns with either dental putty or water soaked dental rolls.
- CT planning with fusion to MRI or CT contrast or PET/CT studies.
- 3DCRT or IMRT provides improved normal tissue sparing including parotids, mandible, and larynx.
- Conventional volumes cover the skull base and mastoid to the supraclavicular nodes with a three-field technique (opposed laterals matched to AP lower neck field). Beam-split above larynx at thyroid notch, if possible, to allow laryngeal sparing.
  - Spinal cord is shielded on lateral fields at the matchline if no nodes are present, or on the AP field if larynx is not involved. If cN0, a 1.5–2 cm midline block may spare larynx and cord on AP field. If lateral fields are used, the posterior neck is blocked after 42–45 and boosted with electrons.
  - The anterior border includes a 2 cm margin on the tumor and includes the faucial arch, and a portion of the buccal mucosa and oral tongue. Include level IB if buccal mucosa or N+.
- For BOT, may leave out hard palate.
- Lymph node block coverage: N0 include levels II–IV and retropharyngeal nodes (RPN). N1 include levels IB–IV and RPN; N2-3 include IB–V and lateral RPN. Need for IMRT coverage of medial RPN which has been questioned (Eisbruch et al. 2007) and is controversial.
  - Lateral RPN: medial to internal carotid artery and lateral to prevertebral muscles, at level of C1–C3.
  - Medial RPN: anterior and medial to prevertebral muscles.
- Treat bilateral neck unless T1-2 tonsil or small faucial arch. For T1N0 tonsil, may leave out levels IV–V.
  - O'Sullivan et al. (2001): 228 patients with tonsil carcinoma treated with ipsilateral RT. Most cases T1-2N0. Three-year LRC 77%, CSS 76%. Opposite neck failure occurred in 3.5% overall, all of whom had node + disease (8.5% contralateral failure among LN+ patients). Ten to fifteen percent

contralateral neck failure if palate or BOT involvement, or ~20% if both involved and LN+. No neck failures for N0 patients. Thus, may treat unilaterally for well-lateralized tumors invading ≤1/3 soft palate toward the uvula (≤1 cm).

- Compensating filters may be required.
- Ipsilateral wedged pair may be used for tonsil primaries to reduce dose to contralateral salivary glands.
- Base of tongue implants may be done, but controversial as to whether adds to LRC or decrease in morbidity.

DOSE PRESCRIPTIONS

- Select T1-2N0 patients: definitive conventional fx RT to 70 Gy at 2 Gy/fx.
- Select T1N1 and T2N0-1 patients: definitive altered-fx RT.
  - Six fx/week during weeks 2–6: 70 Gy at 2 Gy/fx to primary and gross adenopathy.
  - Concomitant boost: 72 Gy in 6 weeks (1.8 Gy/fx large field; 1.5 Gy boost as second daily fx during last 12 treatment days).
  - Hyperfractionation: 81.6 Gy in 7 weeks at 1.2 Gy b.i.d.
- Stage III–IV patients: concurrent chemo-RT.
  - Total dose typically 70 Gy in daily fx with cisplatin 100 mg/m^2 q3 weeks × 3c.
  - Altered fractionation and multiagent chemo have been evaluated with no consensus on the optimal approach.
- Elective neck.
  - Uninvolved nodal stations: ≥50–56 Gy at 1.6–2 Gy/fx.
- Post-op RT.
  - 60–66 Gy at 2 Gy/fx to high-risk areas and the postoperative bed.
  - Post-op chemo-RT indicated for nodal ECE and/or +margin(s) and considered for other risk features, including pT3-4, pN2-3, PNI, LVSI. Concurrent single agent cisplatin 100 mg/m^2 q3 weeks recommended.
- IMRT.
  - UCSF volumes.
    - GTV = clinical and/or radiographic gross disease.
    - CTV1 = 0.5–2 cm margin on primary and 3–5mm margin on nodal GTV. (depending on adjacent critical structures).
    - CTV2 = elective neck.
    - Individualized planning target volumes are used for the GTV, CTV1, and CTV2.

- Simultaneous integrated boost ("dose-painting") technique used at UCSF:
  - Thirty-three fx: GTV = 70 Gy at 2.12 Gy/fx, CTV1 = 59.4 Gy at 1.8 Gy/fx, CTV2 = 54 Gy at 1.64 Gy/fx.
- Alternative techniques:
  - Simultaneous integrated boost in 35 fx.
    (a) GTV = 70 Gy at 2 Gy/fx, CTV1 = 63 Gy at 1.8 Gy/fx, CTV2 = 56 Gy at 1.6 Gy/fx.
  - Sequential technique.
    (a) Initial lower-dose phase (weeks 1–5) followed by high-dose boost volume phase (weeks 6 and 7) using 2–3 separate dose plans.
  - Concomitant boost schedule.
    (a) Delivers dose to subclinical targets once daily for 6 weeks, and a separate boost plan as second daily treatment during last 12 treatment days.
- Typically seven nonopposing beam angles are used.
- Extended whole field neck technique is preferred when gross disease extends inferiorly or is close to the glottic larynx. With this technique, lateral fields are typically not used because they would require treating through the shoulder, so these are replaced with anterior oblique fields.
- A split field technique with matched conventional low anterior neck field is sometimes used to reduce the dose to the glottic larynx. In this situation, the matchline is typically just above the arytenoids. A gradient match technique may be used as well.

DOSE LIMITATIONS

- Spinal cord <45 Gy, brainstem <54 Gy, parotid glands mean dose <26 Gy and/or attempt to keep 50% volume of each parotid ≤20 Gy (if possible), mandible <70 Gy, retina <45 Gy, larynx mean dose ≤43.5 Gy, mean (max) cochlea ≤37 (45) Gy, thyroid ≤25–35 Gy depending on adjacent adenopathy.
- When possible, minimizing dose to the larynx and inferior pharyngeal constrictor muscles may reduce the risk of late swallow dysfunction.

COMPLICATIONS

- Acute and chronic mucositis, xerostomia.
- Skin reaction treated with Aquafor, Radiacare, Domeboro's solution for moist desquamation.

- Late toxicity includes skin/soft tissue fibrosis, hyperpigmentation, telangiectasias, swallowing dysfunction, voice alteration, alteration in taste, xerostomia, dental complications, chronic aspiration, acceleration of atherosclerosis, and thromboembolic disease.
- Preventive dental care with extractions before XRT, intensive fluoride treatment, and mouth washing and gargling with antiseptics.
- Severe nutritional problems occur in 10% of patients. Suggest proactive speech and swallowing support. Need minimum 2,000 cal/day diet. Use Ensure or Boost prn. Prophylactic gastrostomy controversial.
- Risk of pharyngocutaneous fistula related to surgery, not RT.
- Flap reconstruction decreases complications.
- Mandibular necrosis uncommon, carotid a rupture <1%.
- Amifostine can be used to decrease acute and late xerostomia.

FOLLOW-UP

- Every 1–2 months for year 1, every 3 months for years 2–3, every 6 months for years 4–5, then annually.
- Surveillance PET/CT and/or MRI optional, routinely performed at UCSF for three years post treatment.
- If recurrence suspected but biopsy is negative, follow up monthly until resolved.
- 85–90% of LRR occur within 3 years.

REFERENCES

Adelstein DJ, Li Y, Adams GL, et al. An intergroup phase III comparison of standard radiation therapy and two schedules of concurrent chemoradiotherapy in patients with unresectable squamous cell head and neck cancer. J Clin Oncol 2003;21:92-98.

Bernier J, Domenge C, Ozsahin M, et al. Postoperative irradiation with or without concomitant chemotherapy for locally advanced head and neck cancer. N Engl J Med 2004;350: 1945-1952.

Bonner JA, Harari PM, Giralt J, et al. Radiotherapy plus cetuximab for squamous-cell carcinoma of the head and neck. N Engl J Med 2006;354:567-578.

Bourhis J, Overgaard J, Audry H, et al. Hyperfractionated or accelerated radiotherapy in head and neck cancer: a meta-analysis. Lancet 2006;368(9538):843-854.

Bourhis J, Sire C, Lapeyre M, et al. Accelerated versus conventional radiotherapy with concomitant chemotherapy in locally advanced head and neck carcinomas: Results of a phase III randomized trial. Int J Radiat Oncol Biol Phys 2008: 72(1 Supplement S): S31-S32.

Brizel DM, Albers ME, Fisher SR, et al. Hyperfractionated irradiation with or without concurrent chemotherapy for locally advanced head and neck cancer. N Engl J Med 1998;338: 1798-1804.

Calais G, Alfonsi M, Bardet E, et al. Randomized trial of radiation therapy versus concomitant chemotherapy and radiation therapy for advanced-stage oropharynx carcinoma. J Natl Cancer Inst 1999;91:2081-2086.

Chaturvedi AK, Engels EA, Anderson WF, Gillison ML. Incidence trends for human papillomavirus-related and -unrelated oral squamous cell carcinomas in the United States. J Clin Oncol 2008;26(4):612-619.

Cooper JS, Pajak TF, Forastiere AA, et al. Postoperative concurrent radiotherapy and chemotherapy for high-risk squamous-cell carcinoma of the head and neck. N Engl J Med 2004;350:1937-1944.

Denis F, Garaud P, Bardet E, et al. Final results of the 94-01 French Head and Neck Oncology and Radiotherapy Group randomized trial comparing radiotherapy alone with concomitant radiochemotherapy in advanced-stage oropharynx carcinoma. J Clin Oncol 2004;22:69-76.

Eisbruch A, Levendag PC, Feng FY, et al. Can IMRT or brachytherapy reduce dysphagia associated with chemoradiotherapy of head and neck cancer? The Michigan and Rotterdam experiences. Int J Radiat Oncol Biol Phys. 2007;69(2 Suppl):S40-S42.

Fu KK, Pajak TF, Trotti A, et al. A Radiation Therapy Oncology Group (RTOG) phase III randomized study to compare hyperfractionation and two variants of accelerated fractionation to standard fractionation radiotherapy for head and neck squamous cell carcinomas: first report of RTOG 9003. Int J Radiat Oncol Biol Phys 2000;48:7-16.

Fakhry C, Westra WH, Sigui L, Cmelak A, Ridge JA, Pinto H, Forastiere A, Gillison ML. Improved survival of patients with human Papillomavirus-positive head and neck squamous cell carcinoma in a prospective clinical trial. J Natl Cancer Inst 2009;100:261-269.

Horiot JC, Le Fur R, N'Guyen T, et al. Hyperfractionation versus conventional fractionation in oropharyngeal carcinoma: final analysis of a randomized trial of the EORTC cooperative group of radiotherapy. Radiother Oncol 1992;25:231-241.

Kramer S, Gelber RD, Snow JB, et al. Combined radiation therapy and surgery in the management of advanced head and neck cancer: final report of study 73-03 of the Radiation Therapy Oncology Group. Head Neck Surg 1987;10:19-30.

Langendijk JA, Bourhis J. Reirradiation in squamous cell head and neck cancer: recent developments and future directions. Curr Opin Oncol 2007;19(3):202-209.

Levendag PC, Teguh DN, Heijmen, BJ. Oropharynx. In: Perez CA, Brady LW, Halperin EC, et al., editors. Principles and practice of radiation oncology. 5th ed. Philadelphia: Lippincott Williams & Wilkins; 2008. pp. 913-957.

O'Sullivan B, Warde P, Grice B, et al. The benefits and pitfalls of ipsilateral radiotherapy in carcinoma of the tonsillar region. Int J Radiat Oncol Biol Phys. Oct 1 2001;51(2):332-343.

Pignon JP, Bourhis J, Domenge C, et al. Chemotherapy added to locoregional treatment for head and neck squamous-cell carcinoma: three meta-analyses of updated individual data. MACH-NC Collaborative Group. Meta-analysis of Chemotherapy on Head and Neck Cancer. Lancet 2000;355:949-955.

Pignon JP, le Maitre A, Bourhis J. Meta-Analyses of chemotherapy in head and neck cancer (MACH-NC): an update. Int J Radiat Oncol Biol Phys 2007;69(2 Suppl):S112-S114.

Pignon JP, le Maitre A, Maillard E, Bourhis J. Meta-analysis of chemotherapy in head and neck cancer (MACH-NC): an update on 93 randomised trials and 17,346 patients. Radiother Oncol. Jul 2009;92(1):4-14.

Posner MR, Hershock DM, Blajman CR, et al. Cisplatin and fluorouracil alone or with docetaxel in head and neck cancer. N Engl J Med 2007;357(17):1705-1715.

Semrau R, Mueller RP, Stuetzer H, et al. Efficacy of intensified hyperfractionated and accelerated radiotherapy and concurrent chemotherapy with carboplatin and 5-fluorouracil: updated results of a randomized multicentric trial in advanced head-and-neck cancer. Int J Radiat Oncol Biol Phys 2006;64(5):1308-1316.

Tupchong L, Scott CB, Blitzer PH, et al. Randomized study of preoperative versus postoperative radiation therapy in advanced head and neck carcinoma: long-term follow-up of RTOG study 73-03. Int J Radiat Oncol Biol Phys 1991;20:21-28.

Vermorken JB, Remenar E, van Herpen C, et al. Cisplatin, fluorouracil, and docetaxel in unresectable head and neck cancer. N Engl J Med 2007;357(17):1695-1704.

III

Chapter 8
Cancer of the Lip and Oral Cavity

Eric K. Hansen, Sue S. Yom, Chien Peter Chen, and Naomi R. Schechter

III

PEARLS

- The oral cavity consists of the upper and lower lips, gingivobuccal sulcus, buccal mucosa, upper and lower gingiva (including alveolar ridge), retromolar trigone, hard palate, floor of mouth, and anterior two-third of the tongue.
- CN XII provides motor innervation of the tongue, and the lingual nerve (CN V) provides sensory innervation. Taste is mediated by the chorda tympani branch of CN VII for the anterior two-third of the tongue and CN IX for the posterior 1/3.
- Risk factors for oral cavity cancer include tobacco, alcohol, poor oral hygiene, and betel and areca nuts. Oral leukoplakia can proceed to cancer (4–18%) as can erythroplakia (30%).
- Neck LN levels: Fig. 8.1. Also see Chap. 13 & Fig. 13.1.
- LN drainage.
  - Upper lip: facial nodes and level IB.
  - Floor of mouth, lower lip, and lower gingiva: levels I, II, and III.
  - Anterior oral tongue: IA, IB, and II, and also directly to levels III–IV.
  - Bilateral node drainage is frequent, especially when the lesion approaches midline.
- Depth of invasion, increasing T size, and grade increase risk of involved LN.
- Approximate risk of LN involvement.
  - Lip: T1/2 5%, T3/4 33%
  - Floor of mouth: T1/2 10–20%, T3/4 33–67%
  - Oral tongue: T1/2 20%, T3/4 33–67%
  - Bucco-gingival mucosa: T1/2 10–20%, T3/4 33–67%
  - Retromolar trigone: 25–40%
- Ninety percent of tumors are SCC. Less common tumors include minor salivary gland cancers (common in the hard palate and include adenoid cystic carcinoma, mucoepidermoid carcinoma, adenocarcinoma). Rarely: lymphoma, melanoma, or sarcoma.

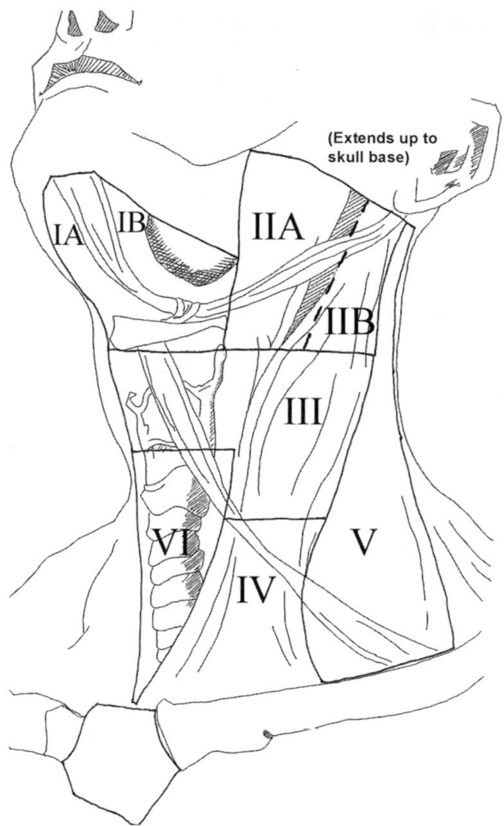

Fig. 8.1 Lymph node levels in the neck

WORKUP

- H&P with palpation. Direct nasopharyngolaryngoscopy. EUA, if indicated.
- Biopsy tumor and/or lymph node(s).
- Labs include CBC, chemistries, BUN/Cr, and LFTs.
- Imaging includes CT and/or MRI of the head and neck. Panorex of mandible for advanced lesions (also helps to rule-out extension through the mental foramen). PET scans may be informative for stage III–IV. CXR or CT chest.
- Preventive dental care and extractions should occur 10–14 days before RT and should include custom fluoride trays.
- Preoperative prosthodontal and psychological evaluation.
- Speech and swallowing and nutrition consultations.

STAGING: CANCER OF THE LIP AND ORAL CAVITY

Editors' note: All TNM stage and stage groups referred to elsewhere in this chapter reflect the 2002 AJCC staging nomenclature unless otherwise noted as the new system below was published after this chapter was written.

(AJCC 6TH ED., 2002)

Primary tumor (T)

TX: Primary tumor cannot be assessed
T0: No evidence of primary tumor
Tis: Carcinoma in situ
T1: Tumor 2 cm or less in greatest dimension
T2: Tumor more than 2 cm, but not more than 4 cm in greatest dimension
T3: Tumor more than 4 cm in greatest dimension
T4a: Moderately advanced local disease.* (lip) Tumor invades through cortical bone, inferior alveolar nerve, floor of mouth, or skin of face, i.e., chin or nose (oral cavity). Tumor invades adjacent structures only (e.g., through cortical bone [mandible or maxilla] into deep [extrinsic] muscle of tongue [genioglossus, hyoglossus, palatoglossus, and styloglossus], maxillary sinus, skin of face)
T4b: Very advanced local disease. Tumor invades masticator space, pterygoid plates, or skull base, and/or encases internal carotid artery

**Note*: Superficial erosion alone of bone/tooth socket by gingival primary is not sufficient to classify a tumor as T4.

Regional lymph nodes (N)

NX: Regional lymph nodes cannot be assessed
N0: No regional lymph node metastasis
N1: Metastasis in a single ipsilateral lymph node, 3 cm or less in greatest dimension
N2a: Metastasis in a single ipsilateral lymph node, more than 3 cm but not more than 6 cm in greatest dimension
N2b: Metastasis in multiple ipsilateral lymph nodes, not more than 6 cm in greatest dimension
N2c: Metastasis in bilateral or contralateral lymph nodes, not more than 6 cm in greatest dimension
N3: Metastasis in a lymph node more than 6 cm in greatest dimension

(AJCC 7TH ED., 2010)

Primary tumor (T)

TX: Primary tumor cannot be assessed
T0: No evidence of primary tumor
Tis: Carcinoma in situ
T1: Tumor 2 cm or less in greatest dimension
T2: Tumor more than 2 cm, but not more than 4 cm in greatest dimension
T3: Tumor more than 4 cm in greatest dimension
T4a: Moderately advanced local disease* (lip) Tumor invades through cortical bone, inferior alveolar nerve, floor of mouth, or skin of face, i.e., chin or nose (oral cavity). Tumor invades adjacent structures only (e.g., through cortical bone [mandible or maxilla] into deep [extrinsic] muscle of tongue [genioglossus, hyoglossus, palatoglossus, and styloglossus], maxillary sinus, skin of face)
T4b: Very advanced local disease. Tumor invades masticator space, pterygoid plates, or skull base, and/or encases internal carotid artery*

**Note*: Superficial erosion alone of bone/tooth socket by gingival primary is not sufficient to classify a tumor as T4.

Regional lymph nodes (N)

NX: Regional lymph nodes cannot be assessed
N0: No regional lymph node metastasis
N1: Metastasis in a single ipsilateral lymph node, 3 cm or less in greatest dimension
N2: Metastasis in a single ipsilateral lymph node, more than 3 cm but not more than 6 cm in greatest dimension; or in multiple ipsilateral lymph nodes, not more than 6 cm in greatest dimension; or in bilateral or contralateral lymph nodes, not more than 6 cm in greatest dimension

continued

Distant metastases (M)

M0: No distant metastasis

M1: Distant metastasis

Stage grouping		~5-Year OS		~LC with EBRT and/or brachy	
0:	TisN0M0	I:	60–90%	T1:	85–100%
I:	T1N0M0	II:	40–70%	T2:	70–95%
II:	T2N0M0	III:	30–40%	T3:	50–90%
III:	T3N0M0, T1-3N1M0	IV:	20–30%	T4:	10–50%
IVA:	T4aN0-1M0, T1-4aN2M0	(Varies by site)		(Varies by site)	
IVB:	Any T, N3M0; T4b, any N, M0				
IVC:	Any T, any N, M1				

Used with permission from the American Joint Committee on Cancer (AJCC), Chicago, IL. The original source for this material is the AJCC Cancer Staging Manual, Sixth Edition (2002), published by Springer Science+Business Media.

N2a: Metastasis in single ipsilateral lymph node more than 3, but not more than 6 cm in greatest dimension

N2b: Metastasis in multiple ipsilateral lymph nodes, not more than 6 cm in greatest dimension

N2c: Metastasis in bilateral or contralateral lymph nodes, not more than 6 cm in greatest dimension

N3: Metastasis in a lymph node more than 6 cm in greatest dimension

Distant metastasis (M)

M0: No distant metastasis

M1: Distant metastasis

Anatomic stage/prognostic groups

0:	Tis N0 M0
I:	T1 N0 M0
II:	T2 N0 M0
III:	T3 N0 M0
	T1-T3 N1 M0
IVA:	T4a N0 M0
	T4a N1 M0
	T1-T3 N2 M0
	T4a N2 M0
IVB:	Any T N3 M0
	T4b Any N M0
IVC:	Any T Any N M1

Used with permission from the American Joint Committee on Cancer (AJCC), Chicago, IL. The original source for this material is the AJCC Cancer Staging Manual, Seventh Edition (2010), published by Springer Science+Business Media.

TREATMENT RECOMMENDATIONS

Stage	Lip
T1-2N0	■ Surgery with reconstruction as necessary (preferred) or RT. ■ Primary RT may consist of EBRT ≥50 Gy and brachytherapy, or EBRT alone ≥60–66 Gy. For +margin only, reexcise if feasible. Post-op RT with treatment of the neck (dissection or RT) indicated for pT3/T4, close margin, multiple nodes, PNI, and/or LVSI, or level IV–V nodes; post-op chemo-RT indicated for +margin, ECE
T3-4N0 or N1-3	■ Preferred: excision of primary and unilateral or bilateral neck dissection (if crosses midline or N2c). Reconstruction as indicated. For +margin only, reexcise if feasible. Post-op RT for pT3/T4, close margin, multiple nodes, PNI, and/or LVSI, or level IV–V nodes; post-op chemo-RT indicated for +margin, ECE ■ Alternatively, concomitant chemo-RT or EBRT/brachytherapy. ■ If primary has < CR, consider salvage surgery and neck dissection. If residual neck mass by CT/MRI or PET at 6–12 weeks, post-RT neck dissection considered

Stage	Oral cavity
T1-2N0	■ Excision of primary (preferred) ± unilateral or bilateral selective neck dissection. Neck treatment (dissection or RT) required for lesions >1.5–3 mm thick. For +margin only, reexcise if feasible. Post-op RT for pT3/T4, close margin, multiple nodes, PNI, and/or LVSI, or level IV–V nodes; post-op chemo-RT indicated for +margin, ECE ■ Alternatively, EBRT ± brachytherapy. Salvage surgery for residual disease
T3N0	■ Excision of primary and unilateral or bilateral selective neck dissection. Reconstruction as indicated. For +margin only, reexcise if feasible. Post-op RT for all; chemo-RT indicated for +margin, ECE
T4a or N1-3	■ Excision of primary and ipsilateral comprehensive neck dissection ± contralateral selective neck dissection, or bilateral neck dissection (for N2c). Reconstruction as indicated. For +margin only, reexcise if feasible. Post-op RT for pT3/T4, close margin, multiple nodes, PNI, and/or LVSI, or level IV–V nodes; may consider post-op RT for N1 as only risk feature; post-op chemo-RT indicated for +margin, ECE
Unresectable	■ Concomitant chemo-RT (preferred). Alternatively, induction chemotherapy followed by chemo-RT, or altered fractionation RT alone if unable to tolerate chemo. If primary has < CR, salvage surgery controversial. If residual neck mass by CT/MRI or PET at 6–12 weeks, post-RT neck dissection considered

STUDIES

POST-OP EBRT AND CHEMO-RT

- *EORTC 22931* (Bernier et al. 2004): 334 patients with operable stage III/IV oral cavity, oropharynx, larynx, and hypopharynx cancer randomized to post-op RT (2/66 Gy) vs. post-op chemo-RT (2/66 Gy and cisplatin 100 mg/m^2 on days 1, 22, 43). All patients received 54 Gy to the low-risk neck. Eligible stages included pT3-4N0/+, T1-2N2-3, and T1-2N0-1 with ECE, +margin, or PNI. Chemo-RT improved 3/5-year DFS (41/36→59/47%), 3/5-year OS (49/40→65/53%), and 5-year LRC (69→82%), but increased grade 3–4 toxicity (21→41%).
- *RTOG 95–01* (Cooper et al. 2004): 459 patients with operable cancer of the oral cavity, oropharynx, larynx, or hypopharynx who had ≥2 involved lymph nodes, nodal extracapsular extension, or a +margin randomized to post-op RT (2/60–66 Gy) vs. post-op chemo-RT (2/60–66 Gy and cisplatin ×3c as in EORTC 22931). Chemo-RT improved 2-year DFS (43→54%), LRC (72→82%), and had a trend for improved OS (57→63%), but increased grade 3–4 toxicity (34→77%).
- *Combined analysis* (Bernier, Head Neck 2005). Chemo-RT improved OS, DFS, and LRC for ECE and/or + margins, but provided only trend for improvements ($p = 0.06$) in stage III–IV, PNI, LVI, and/or enlarged LN in levels IV–V for OPX or oral cavity tumors. Patients with ≥2 LN without ECE as their only factor did not benefit from chemo ($p = 0.73$).
- *Ang et al.* (2001): 213 patients with locally-advanced oral cavity, oropharynx, larynx, and hypopharynx cancers treated with surgery randomized by risk factors to post-op RT. Risk factors included >1 node group, ≥2 nodes, nodes >3 cm, microscopic +margins, PNI, oral cavity site, and nodal extracapsular extension. Low-risk = no risk factors → no RT. Intermediate risk = 1 risk factor (but not ECE) → 1.8/57.6 Gy. High-risk = ECE or ≥2 risk factors → 1.8/63 Gy in 7 weeks or in 5 weeks with a concomitant boost. The 5-year LRC/OS for low-risk was 90/83%, for intermediate risk 94/66%, and for high-risk 68/42%. Overall treatment time <11 weeks increased LRC, and concomitant boost had a trend for improved OS.

ALTERED FRACTIONATION

- *MARCH metaanalysis* (Bourhis et al. 2006). Fifteen phase III trials and 6,515 patients. 3.4% OS benefit at 5 years for altered fractionation vs. conventional fractionation, with most benefit suggested for hyperfractionation (8%). Decreasing benefit with increasing age.

- *RTOG 90–03* (Fu et al. 2000): 268 patients with locally-advanced cancer of the oral cavity, oropharynx, supraglottic larynx, or hypopharynx randomized to 2/70 Gy vs. 1.2 b.i.d./81.6 Gy vs. split-course 1.6 b.i.d./67.2 Gy (with 2-week break) vs. concomitant boost RT to 72 Gy (1.8 Gy/fraction with a 1.5 Gy boost on the last 12 treatment days). Concomitant boost and continuous b.i.d. hyperfractionation improved the 2-year LRC (54%), DFS (38–39%), and OS (51–54%) vs. standard or split-course b.i.d. RT. Altered fractionation increased acute side effects.

III

CHEMORADIATION

- *MACH-NC metaanalysis* (Pignon et al. 2009): 87 phase III trials and 16,485 patients. 4.5% OS benefit at 5 years when chemotherapy was added to RT, with greater benefit for concurrent chemo-RT vs. induction chemo followed by RT (6.5% OS benefit with concurrent chemo-RT). Similar results in trials with post-op RT, conventional, and altered fractionation. No difference between mono or polychemotherapy regimens, but increased benefit with platinum-based compounds. Decreasing benefit with increasing age, with no benefit observed if ≥71 years.
- *Adelstein et al.* (2003): 295 patients with unresectable H&N cancer (13% oral cavity), randomized to 2/70 vs. 2/70 Gy and cisplatin (100 mg/m^2) × 3 cycles vs. split-course RT (2/30 Gy + 2/30–40 Gy) + cisplatin/5-FU × 3 cycles. Results: chemo-RT improved 3-year OS (23 vs. 37 vs. 27%) and DFS (33 vs. 51 vs. 41%), but did not change DM and it increased toxicity.
- *Posner* (NEJM 2007). Randomized 501 patients with unresectable stage II–IV head and neck cancer (14% oral cavity) to TPF (docetaxol/cisplatin/5-FU) vs. PF (cisplatin/5-FU) induction chemotherapy followed by carboplatin chemo-RT (70–74 Gy). Induction TPF improved LRC and 3-year OS (48→62%), but not DM. 21–25% of patients did not receive concurrent chemo-RT due to progressive disease, adverse events, death, or withdrawal of consent.
- No published phase III studies have tested induction chemo followed by chemo-RT vs. upfront chemo-RT, and this is the subject of ongoing randomized trials.

BRACHYTHERAPY

- *Grabenbauer et al.* (2001): 318 patients with primary (74%) and recurrent (26%) oral cavity (63%)/oropharynx (27%) SCC treated with post-op LDR-brachytherapy ± EBRT. Brachytherapy dose was 45–55 Gy when used alone (19% of patients) or 23–25 Gy after 50–60 Gy EBRT (55% of patients). Overall 5-year LC was 74% for primary and 57% for recurrent disease. Among primary patients treated with EBRT and brachytherapy, 5-year LC was 92% for stage I/II and 65% for stage III/IV. A 7.5% of patients developed late soft-tissue necrosis and/or osteoradionecrosis requiring mandibular resection.
- *Melzner et al.* (2007): review of 210 patients with lip/oral cavity (77%) or oropharynx (23%) cancers treated with PDR-brachytherapy either postoperatively or definitively. Median PDR-brachytherapy dose 24 Gy after median 50.4 Gy EBRT (38% of patients), or 56.65 Gy when used alone (62% of patients). With median 2-year follow-up, 7% LF, 11% soft-tissue necrosis, 7.6% osteoradionecrosis, and 83% OS.
- *Martinez-Monge et al.* (2009): phase I–II trial of 40 patients with oral cavity (70%) or oropharynx (30%) cancer treated with perioperative HDR brachytherapy (4 Gy b.i.d. × 4 for R0 resection or × 6 for R1 resection) and 45 Gy EBRT. 7-year LRC was 82%. Seven-year DFS and OS were 50 and 52%, respectively. RTOG grade 3, 4, and 5 perioperative toxicities were 5, 2.5, and 0%, respectively. Late-grade 3, 4, and 5 toxicities were 10, 7.5, and 2.5%, respectively.

RADIATION TECHNIQUES

SIMULATION AND FIELD DESIGN

- In general, simulate the patient supine with the head on a head-rest device. Wire nodes, scars, the oral commissure, and the larynx (thyroid notch). Two to five millimeter bolus may be applied to scars. A cork and tongue blade may be used to depress the tongue away from palate, if appropriate. Shoulders may be pulled down with straps. Immobilize with a thermoplastic head (± shoulder) mask.
- Computed dosimetry should be used to ensure homogeneity and spare normal tissues.

IMRT

- Elective neck
  - Uninvolved nodal stations: ≥50–56 Gy at 1.6–2 Gy/fx.

- Post-op RT
  - 60–66 Gy at 2 Gy/fx to high-risk areas and the postoperative bed.
  - Post-op chemo-RT indicated for nodal ECE and/or + margin(s) and considered for multiple other risk features, including pT3-4, pN2-3, close margins, PNI, LVSI, or level IV–V nodes. Concurrent single agent cisplatin 100 mg/m^2 q3 weeks recommended.
- UCSF IMRT volumes
  - GTV = clinical and/or radiographic gross disease, if present.
  - CTV1 = entire postoperative bed, including at least 0.5–2 cm margin on primary and/or nodal GTV (depending on the presence or absence of anatomic boundaries to microscopic spread).
  - CTV2 = elective neck.
  - Individualized planning target volumes are used for the GTV, CTV1, and CTV2.
- Simultaneous integrated boost ("dose-painting") technique used at UCSF
  - 33 fx: GTV, if present = 70 Gy at 2.12 Gy/fx (definitive), CTV1 = post-op bed/high-risk areas 60–66 Gy at 2 Gy/fx, CTV2 = 54–59.4 Gy at 1.8 Gy/fx.
- Alternative techniques
  - Conedown technique
    - Initial large field phase (weeks 1–5) followed by conedown to boost volume (weeks 6 and 7) using 2–3 separate dose plans.
  - Altered fractionation schedules
    - Either hyperfractionated or concomitant boost schedule can be employed, typically in the absence of chemotherapy.
- Typically 7–9 nonopposing beam angles are used.
- Extended whole field neck technique is preferred when gross disease extends inferiorly or is close to the glottic larynx. With this technique, lateral fields are typically not used because they would require treating through the shoulder, so these are replaced with anterior oblique fields.
- A split field technique with matched conventional low anterior neck field is sometimes used to reduce the dose to the glottic larynx. In this situation, the match line is typically just above the arytenoids. A gradient match technique may be used, as well.
- In combination with chemotherapy and cetuximab, IMRT may be associated with higher toxicity to the oral cavity than 3DCRT.

LIP

- Small lip lesions may be treated with EBRT (100–250 keV orthovoltage or 6–12 MeV electrons), or with brachytherapy, or in combination.
- With EBRT, an appositional field is used and borders are determined clinically with a 1–1.5 cm margin for orthovoltage or a 2–2.5 cm margin for electrons, with bolus for superficial tumors. A lead cut-out is made to outline the treatment volume. Lead shields are placed behind the lip to minimize dose to the mandible and oral cavity.
- The upper neck is treated with opposed lateral fields for T1/2 tumors with commissure involvement, and T3/4, LN+, or poorly differentiated tumors.
- Some institutions use a "moustache field" for elective RT of the perifacial lymphatics (~50 Gy) for advanced upper lip lesions.
- T3/4 tumors are conventionally treated with opposed lateral 4–6 MV fields. The tumor is treated with 1–1.5 cm margin. The inferior border is at the thyroid notch, and the posterior border is at the posterior aspect of the spinous processes.
- When LN+, a low-neck field is matched to the inferior border of the opposed lateral fields. If the posterior chain requires RT, the portals are reduced off-cord at 42–45 Gy and the area is boosted with electrons.
- With conventional 3-field techniques, a small midline block on the AP field is used to shield larynx and spinal cord at the match.
- Complex 3DCRT or IMRT techniques are recommended for more advanced lesions and in order to spare adjacent normal structures.
- Wedges and/or compensating filters may be required.
- Brachytherapy implants typically use Ir-192 seeds or wire in angiocatheters spaced 1 cm apart. A gauze or cotton dental roll is placed between the lip and the gingiva.
- Definitive EBRT dose:
  - T1N0 = 2/50 Gy → boost to 56–60 Gy. T1 lesions may alternatively be treated with 45 Gy at 3 Gy fx.
  - T2N0 = 2/50 Gy → boost to 60–66 Gy.
  - T3N0 = 2/50 Gy → boost to 60–70 Gy and levels I/II are treated.
  - T4 or LN+ = 2/50 Gy → boost to 66–70 Gy and levels I–IV are treated.
- Brachytherapy
  - When used alone for T1-2, LDR-brachytherapy dose is 60–70 Gy at 0.8–1 Gy/h.

- If used 2–4 weeks after EBRT (50–54 Gy), LDR-brachytherapy boost is 15–30 Gy.
- Afterloading HDR brachytherapy may be used instead of LDR.

III

FLOOR OF MOUTH

- The floor of mouth has lower RT tolerance due to increased risk of soft-tissue injury and osteoradionecrosis.
- For early superficial T1-2 lesions, brachytherapy or intraoral cone RT may be used in lieu of surgery.
  - LDR-brachytherapy dose is 60–70 Gy.
  - Intraoral cone dose is 3 Gy/fraction to 45 Gy over 3 weeks.
- For definitive treatment of larger lesions, 3DCRT or IMRT techniques are generally recommended for advanced lesions and in order to spare adjacent normal structures. Brachytherapy or intraoral cone may be used for the boost.
- With opposed laterals, the superior border is 1–1.5 cm above the dorsum of the tongue (2 cm above tumor). A cork should be used between the teeth to exclude palate and if possible, tip of tongue, from field. Level I nodes are always treated, and level II is included for depth of invasion >1.5 mm (with posterior border at the posterior aspect of the spinous processes). The inferior border is at the thyroid notch. The lower lip is excluded when possible. When LN+, a low-neck field is matched to the inferior border of the opposed lateral fields.
- Definitive RT dose for more advanced lesions is 1.8–2 Gy/fx to ≥72 Gy without chemo (altered fractionation recommended).
- With chemo, definitive EBRT dose is 2 Gy/fx to 70 Gy.
- As a boost before or after EBRT (~45 Gy), interstitial brachytherapy (25–30 Gy) or intraoral cone (15–24 Gy) may be used.
- With post-op RT, fields include the primary site and the dissected neck.
- Post-op EBRT dose is 1.8–2 Gy/fx to 50–54 Gy, followed by boost to 60–66 Gy to high-risk areas, including primary surgical bed, and areas of close/+ margins, extranodal extension, nodal involvement, LVSI, or PNI.

ORAL TONGUE

- Brachytherapy or intraoral cone may be used as with floor of mouth lesions.
- A cork and tongue blade is used to keep the tongue down and to exclude the palate.

- Set-up must be very secure due to mobility of the tongue.
- 3DCRT or IMRT techniques are generally recommended for advanced lesions and in order to spare adjacent normal structures. Brachytherapy or intraoral cone may be used for the boost.
- With opposed laterals, the superior border is 1–1.5 cm above the dorsum of the tongue or 2 cm above tumor. The inferior border is at the thyroid notch. The posterior border is placed at the posterior aspect of the spinous processes. The anterior border is 2 cm anterior to the tumor. When N+, a low-neck field is matched to the inferior border of the opposed lateral fields.
- Doses are similar to floor of mouth lesions.

BUCCAL MUCOSA

- Wire ipsilateral commissure. Place intraoral device to displace and shield tongue. May insert metal seeds into the periphery of the tumor for localization.
- Treatment is usually with an ipsilateral mixed photon/electron beam (or wedged photon pair) and a boost is given with brachytherapy or intraoral cone if possible.
- Field borders are: 2-cm anterior and superior to the lesion; the posterior aspect of the spinous processes if nodes are irradiated; inferiorly at the thyroid notch.
- The oral commissures and lips are excluded or shielded if possible.
- Post-op volumes include the tumor bed, scars, and ipsilateral IB and II nodes.
- Patients with + nodes receive bilateral neck RT to the upper and lower neck.
- Doses are similar to other oral cavity lesions.

GINGIVA AND HARD PALATE

- EBRT, rather than brachytherapy, is used due to the risk of osteoradionecrosis.
- For gingival lesions, if PNI is present, the entire hemimandible from mental foramen to the temporomandibular joint is treated; in addition, extension to the buccal mucosa must be carefully evaluated.
- Fields cover the primary with 2 cm margins and the upper neck nodes.
- The low-neck is treated for T3/4 or LN+.
- Definitive RT dose is 60–66 Gy for T1 lesions, 66–70 Gy for T2,

and ≥72 Gy for T3-4 lesions without chemo (concomitant boost used). With chemo, give 2 Gy/fx to 70 Gy.
- Post-op EBRT doses are 1.8–2 Gy/fx to 50–54 Gy followed by boost to 60–66 Gy to high-risk areas.

RETROMOLAR TRIGONE

- An ipsilateral mixed photon/electron beam (or wedged photon pair) is used for lateralized lesions.
- Fields cover the primary with 2 cm margins and the upper neck nodes. The superior border includes the pterygoid plates. The low-neck is treated for T3/4 or LN+.
- Doses are similar to other oral cavity tumors.

DOSE LIMITATIONS

- Spinal cord maximum dose ≤45 Gy. Brainstem maximum dose ≤54 Gy. Keep 50% of the volume of each parotid ≤20 Gy (if possible) and mean dose <26 Gy. Mandible maximum (point) dose ≤70 Gy.

COMPLICATIONS

- Mucositis, dermatitis, xerostomia, dysgeusia, soft-tissue fibrosis, hypothyroidism, and rarely soft tissue or osteoradionecrosis (more common with brachytherapy), pharyngocutaneous fistula, or carotid rupture (more common with reirradiation).
- Perioperative complications of surgery include bleeding, airway obstruction, infection, and wound complications. Post-op complications include webs, stenosis, chondritis, fistulas, aspiration, as well as functional speech and/or swallowing deficits.
- Patients need ≥2,000 calories/day to avoid malnutrition. Supplements (e.g., Boost or Ensure) and/or feeding tubes may be used.
- Amifostine may be considered to possibly reduce xerostomia.

FOLLOW-UP

- H&P every 1–3 months for year 1, every 2–4 months for year 2, every 6 months for years 3–5, then annually. CXR annually. TSH every 6–12 months if neck irradiated.
- If recurrence is suspected but biopsy is negative, follow closely (at least monthly) until resolves.

REFERENCES

Adelstein DJ, Li Y, Adams GL, et al. An intergroup phase III comparison of standard radiation therapy and two schedules of concurrent chemoradiotherapy in patients with unresectable squamous cell head and neck cancer. J Clin Oncol 2003;21:92-98.

Ang KK, Trotti A, Brown BW, et al. Randomized trial addressing risk features and time factors of surgery plus radiotherapy in advanced head-and-neck cancer. Int J Radiat Oncol Biol Phys 2001;51:571-578.

Bernier J, Cooper JS, Pajak TF, et al. Defining risk levels in locally advanced head and neck cancers: a comparative analysis of concurrent postoperative radiation plus chemotherapy trials of the EORTC (#22931) and RTOG (# 9501). Head Neck. 2005;27(10):843-50.

Bernier J, Domenge C, Ozsahin M, et al. Postoperative irradiation with or without concomitant chemotherapy for locally advanced head and neck cancer. N Engl J Med 2004;350:1945-1952.

Bourhis J, Overgaard J, Audry H, et al. Hyperfractionated or accelerated radiotherapy in head and neck cancer: a meta-analysis. Lancet 2006;368:843-854.

Brizel DM, Albers ME, Fisher SR, et al. Hyperfractionated irradiation with or without concurrent chemotherapy for locally advanced head and neck cancer. N Engl J Med 1998;338:1798-1804.

Cooper JS, Pajak TF, Forastiere AA, et al. Postoperative concurrent radiotherapy and chemotherapy for high-risk squamous-cell carcinoma of the head and neck. N Engl J Med 2004;350:1937-1944.

Cooper JS. The Oral Cavity. In: Cox JD, Ang KK, editors. Radiation oncology: rationale, technique, results. 8th ed. St. Louis: Mosby; 2003. pp. 219-255.

de Visscher JG, Grond AJ, Botke G, et al. Results of radiotherapy for squamous cell carcinoma of the vermilion border of the lower lip. A retrospective analysis of 108 patients. Radiother Oncol 1996;39:9-14.

Fu KK, Pajak TF, Trotti A, et al. A Radiation Therapy Oncology Group (RTOG) phase III randomized study to compare hyperfractionation and two variants of accelerated fractionation to standard fractionation radiotherapy for head and neck squamous cell carcinomas: first report of RTOG 9003. Int J Radiat Oncol Biol Phys 2000;48:7-16.

Fujita M, Hirokawa Y, Kashiwado K, et al. Interstitial brachytherapy for stage I and II squamous cell carcinoma of the oral tongue: factors influencing local control and soft tissue complications. Int J Radiat Oncol Biol Phys 1999;44:767-775.

Grabenbauer GG, Rodel C, Brunner T, et al. Interstitial brachytherapy with Ir-192 low-dose-rate in the treatment of primary and recurrent cancer of the oral cavity and oropharynx. Review of 318 patients treated between 1985 and 1997. Strahlenther Onkol 2001;177:338-344.

Greene FL, American Joint Committee on Cancer, American Cancer Society. AJCC cancer staging manual. 6th ed. New York: Springer-Verlag; 2002.

Khuntia D, Harris J, Bentzen S, et al. Increased oral mucositis after IMRT versus non-IMRT when combined with cetuximab and cisplatin or docetaxel for head and neck cancer: preliminary results of RTOG 0234. Int J Radiat Oncol Biol Phys 2008;72:S33-S33.

Lee N, Phillips TL. Cancer of the Oral Cavity. In: Leibel SA, Phillips TL, editors. Textbook of radiation oncology. 2nd ed. Philadelphia: Saunders; 2004. pp. 631-656.

Manon RR, Myers JN, Khuntia D, Harari PM. Oral Cavity Cancer. In: Halperin EC, Perez CA, Brady LW, et al., editors. Principles and practice of radiation oncology. 5th ed. Philadelphia: Lippincott Williams & Wilkins; 2008. pp. 913-957.

Martinez-Monge R, Gomez-Iturriaga A, Cambeiro M, et al. Phase I-II trial of perioperative high-dose-rate brachytherapy in oral cavity and oropharyngeal cancer. Brachytherapy 2009;8:26-33.

Mazeron JJ, Ardiet JM, Haie-Meder C, et al. GEC-ESTRO recommendations for brachytherapy for head and neck squamous cell carcinomas. Radiother Oncol 2009;91:150-156.

Melzner WJ, Lotter M, Sauer R, et al. Quality of interstitial PDRbrachytherapy-implants of head-and-neck-cancers: predictive factors for local control and late toxicity? Radiother Oncol 2007;82:167-173.

National Comprehensive Cancer Network. Clinical Practice Guidelines in Oncology: Head and Neck Cancers. Available at: http://www.nccn.org/professionals/physician_gls/PDF/head-and-neck.pdf. Accessed on June 1, 2009.

Pignon JP, le Maitre A, Maillard E, et al. Meta-analysis of chemotherapy in head and neck cancer (MACH-NC): an update on 93 randomized trials and 17,346 patients. Radiother Oncol 2009;92:4-14.

Posner MR, Hershock DM, Blajman CR, et al. Cisplatin and fluorouracil alone or with docetaxel in head and neck cancer. N Engl J Med. 2007;357(17):1705-15.

Chapter 9

Larynx and Hypopharynx Cancer

Sunanda Pejavar, Eric K. Hansen, Sue S. Yom, and Naomi R. Schechter

III

PEARLS

LARYNX

- Larynx cancer is the most common cancer of the head and neck.
- Risk factors include tobacco, alcohol, betel and areca nuts, and deficiencies of iron, vitamin B12, and vitamin C.
- Larynx subsites:
  - Supraglottis: suprahyoid and infrahyoid epiglottis, aryepiglottic folds, arytenoids, and false cords.
  - Glottis: true vocal cords (TVCs) including the anterior and posterior commissures.
  - Subglottis: extends from the lower boundary of the glottis to the inferior aspect of the cricoid cartilage.
- TVCs attach to the thyroid cartilage at the center of the "figure of 8" on a lateral X-ray.
- LN drainage is common from the supraglottis (to levels II–V) and subglottis [to pretracheal (Delphian), paratracheal, and inferior jugular nodes]. Glottic tumors rarely spread to LN when ≤T1–2 (<3%), but more commonly spread to LN when T3–4 (~20–30%).
- Superior laryngeal nerve innervates the cricothyroid muscles that produce tension and elongation of the vocal cords. All other laryngeal muscles are innervated by the recurrent laryngeal nerve.

HYPOPHARYNX

- Portion of the pharynx extending from the plane of the superior border of the hyoid bone to the inferior border of the cricoid cartilage.
- Hypopharynx subsites:
  - Pyriform sinuses.

    - Posterior and lateral hypopharyngeal walls.
    - Postcricoid area.
- LN drainage from the hypopharynx is to levels II–V, the retropharyngeal LN, and to paratracheal and paraesophageal LN (when tumor involves the lowest portion of the hypopharynx and the postcricoid area).
- Ninety five percent of tumors of the larynx and hypopharynx are SCC.
- External auditory canal pain may be referred via the superior laryngeal nerve through the auricular nerve of Arnold (branch of CN X).
- A "hot potato" voice may be due to the involvement of the base of tongue.

WORKUP

- H&P, including hoarseness, pain, dysphagia, odynophagia, otalgia, trismus.
- All patients should have nasopharyngolaryngoscopy. Fixation of the true cord may be caused by invasion of the cricoarytenoid muscle or joint, or from recurrent laryngeal nerve injury.
- Esophagoscopy for hypopharnx tumors or if clinically indicated for laryngeal tumors.
- Bronchoscopy if clinically indicated.
- Biopsy tumor and/or lymph node(s).
- Labs include CBC, chemistries, BUN/Cr, LFTs, baseline TSH.
- Imaging includes thin-cut CT and/or MRI of the head and neck and a CXR. PET scans may be informative for stage III–IV.
- Preventive dental care and extractions should occur 10–14 days before RT.
- Baseline speech, swallowing, and nutrition evaluations. If locally-advanced, consider baseline audiometry too.

STAGING: LARYNX AND HYPOPHARYNX CANCER

Editors' note: All TNM stage and stage groups referred to elsewhere in this chapter reflect the 2002 AJCC staging nomenclature unless otherwise noted as the new system below was published after this chapter was written.

(AJCC 6TH ED., 2002)

Primary tumor (T)

Larynx and hypopharynx

TX: Primary tumor cannot be assessed
T0: No evidence of primary tumor
Tis: Carcinoma in situ

Supraglottis

T1: Tumor limited to one subsite of supraglottis with normal vocal cord mobility
T2: Tumor invades mucosa of more than one adjacent subsite of supraglottis or glottis or region outside the supraglottis (e.g., mucosa of the base of tongue, vallecula, medial wall of pyriform sinus), without fixation of the larynx
T3: Tumor limited to larynx with vocal cord fixation and/or invades any of the following: postcricoid area, preepiglottic tissues, paraglottic space, and/or minor thyroid cartilage erosion (e.g., inner cortex)
T4a: Moderately advanced local disease. Tumor invades through the thyroid cartilage and/ or invades tissues beyond the larynx (e.g., trachea, soft tissues of neck including deep extrinsic muscle of the tongue, strap muscles, thyroid, or esophagus)
T4b: Very advanced local disease. Tumor invades prevertebral space, encases carotid artery, or invades mediastinal structures

Glottis

T1: Tumor limited to the vocal cord(s) (may involve anterior or posterior commissure) with normal mobility
  T1a: Tumor limited to one vocal cord
  T1b: Tumor involves both vocal cords
T2: Tumor extends to supraglottis and/or subglottis, and/or with impaired vocal cord mobility
T3: Tumor limited to the larynx with vocal cord fixation and/or invasion of paraglottic space, and/or inner cortex of the thyroid cartilage

(AJCC 7TH ED., 2010)

Primary tumor (T)

Larynx

TX: Primary tumor cannot be assessed
T0: No evidence of primary tumor
Tis: Carcinoma in situ

Supraglottis

T1: Tumor limited to one subsite of supraglottis with normal vocal cord mobility
T2: Tumor invades mucosa of more than one adjacent subsite of supraglottis or glottis or region outside the supraglottis (e.g., mucosa of the base of tongue, vallecula, medial wall of pyriform sinus) without fixation of the larynx
T3: Tumor limited to larynx with vocal cord fixation and/or invades any of the following: postcricoid area, preepiglottic space, paraglottic space, and/or inner cortex of thyroid cartilage
T4a: Moderately advanced local disease. Tumor invades through the thyroid cartilage and/ or invades tissues beyond the larynx (e.g., trachea, soft tissues of neck including deep extrinsic muscle of the tongue, strap muscles, thyroid, or esophagus)
T4b: Very advanced local disease. Tumor invades prevertebral space, encases carotid artery, or invades mediastinal structures

Glottis

T1: Tumor limited to the vocal cord(s) (may involve anterior or posterior commissure) with normal mobility
  T1a: Tumor limited to one vocal cord
  T1b: Tumor involves both vocal cords
T2: Tumor extends to supraglottis and/or subglottis, and/or with impaired vocal cord mobility
T3: Tumor limited to the larynx with vocal cord fixation and/or invasion of paraglottic space, and/or inner cortex of the thyroid cartilage

continued

T4a: Moderately advanced local disease. Tumor invades through the outer cortex of the thyroid cartilage and/or invades tissues beyond the larynx (e.g., trachea, soft tissues of neck including deep extrinsic muscle of the tongue, strap muscles, thyroid, or esophagus)
T4b: Very advanced local disease. Tumor invades prevertebral space, encases carotid artery, or invades mediastinal structures

Subglottis
T1: Tumor limited to subglottis
T2: Tumor extends to vocal cord(s) with normal or impaired mobility
T3: Tumor limited to larynx with vocal cord fixation
T4a: Moderately advanced local disease. Tumor invades cricoid or thyroid cartilage and/or invades tissues beyond the larynx (e.g., trachea, soft tissues of neck including deep extrinsic muscles of the tongue, strap muscles, thyroid, or esophagus)
T4b: Very advanced local disease. Tumor invades prevertebral space, encases carotid artery, or invades mediastinal structures

Hypopharynx
T1: Tumor limited to one subsite of hypopharynx and/or 2 cm cr less in greatest dimension
T2: Tumor invades more than one subsite of hypopharynx or an adjacent site, or measures more than 2 cm, but not more than 4 cm in greatest dimension, without fixation of hemilarynx
T3: Tumor more than 4 cm in greatest dimension or with fixation of hemilarynx or extension to esophagus
T4a: Moderately advanced local disease. Tumor invades thyroid/cricoid cartilage, hyoid bone, thyroid gland, or central compartment soft tissue*
T4b: Very advanced local disease. Tumor invades prevertebral fascia, encases carotid artery, or involves mediastinal structures.

**Note*: Central compartment soft tissue includes prelaryngeal strap muscles and subcutaneous fat.

Regional lymph nodes (N)
Larynx and hypopharynx
NX: Regional lymph nodes cannot be assessed
N0: No regional lymph node metastasis

T4a: Moderately advanced local disease. Tumor invades through the outer cortex of the thyroid cartilage and/or invades tissues beyond the larynx (e.g., trachea, soft tissues of neck including deep extrinsic muscle of the tongue, strap muscles, thyroid, or esophagus)
T4b: Very advanced local disease. Tumor invades prevertebral space, encases carotid artery, or invades mediastinal structures

Subglottis
T1: Tumor limited to the subglottis
T2: Tumor extends to vocal cord(s) with normal or impaired mobility
T3: Tumor limited to larynx with vocal cord fixation
T4a: Moderately advanced local disease. Tumor invades cricoid or thyroid cartilage and/ or invades tissues beyond the larynx (e.g., trachea, soft tissues of neck including deep extrinsic muscles of the tongue, strap muscles, thyroid, or esophagus)
T4b: Very advanced local disease. Tumor invades prevertebral space, encases carotid artery, or invades mediastinal structures

Hypopharynx
T1: Tumor limited to one subsite of hypopharynx and/or 2 cm or less in greatest dimension
T2: Tumor invades more than one subsite of hypopharynx or an adjacent site, or measures more than 2 cm, but not more than 4 cm in greatest dimension without fixation of hemilarynx
T3: Tumor more than 4 cm in greatest dimension or with fixation of hemilarynx or extension to esophagus
T4a: Moderately advanced local disease. Tumor invades thyroid/cricoid cartilage, hyoid bone, thyroid gland, or central compartment soft tissue*
T4b: Very advanced local disease. Tumor invades prevertebral fascia, encases carotid artery, or involves mediastinal structures

**Note*: Central compartment soft tissue includes prelaryngeal strap muscles and subcutaneous fat.

Regional lymph nodes (N)*
Larynx and hypopharynx
NX: Regional lymph nodes cannot be assessed N0; no regional lymph node metastasis
N1: Metastasis in a single ipsilateral lymph node, 3 cm or less in greatest dimension

continued

N1: Metastasis in a single ipsilateral lymph node, 3 cm or less in greatest dimension
N2a: Metastasis in a single ipsilateral lymph node, more than 3 cm but not more than 6 cm in greatest dimension
N2b: Metastasis in multiple ipsilateral lymph nodes, not more than 6 cm in greatest dimension
N2c: Metastasis in bilateral or contralateral lymph nodes, not more than 6 cm in greatest dimension
N3: Metastasis in a lymph node more than 6 cm in greatest dimension

**Note*: Metastases at level VII are considered regional lymph node metastases.

Distant metastases (M)
Larynx and hypopharynx
M0: No distant metastasis
M1: Distant metastasis

Stage Grouping		**~2/5-Year OS**	*Larynx*	*Hypopharynx*
0:	TisN0M0			
I:	T1N0M0	I:	65/35%	65/35%
II:	T2N0M0	II:	80/60%	60/30%
III:	T3N0M0, T1-3N1M0	III:	70/50%	50/30%
IVA:	T4aN0-1M0, T1-4aN2M0	IV:	60/35%	35/15%
IVB:	T4b any N M0, any T N3 M0			
IVC:	Any T, any N, M1			

Used with permission from the American Joint Committee on Cancer (AJCC), Chicago, IL. The original source for this material is the AJCC Cancer Staging Manual, Sixth Edition (2002), published by Springer Science+Business Media.

N2: Metastasis in a single ipsilateral lymph node, more than 3 cm but not more than 6 cm in greatest dimension, or in multiple ipsilateral lymph nodes, not more than 6 cm in greatest dimension, or in bilateral or contralateral lymph nodes, not more than 6 cm in greatest dimension
N2a: Metastasis in a single ipsilateral lymph node, more than 3 cm but not more than 6 cm in greatest dimension
N2b: Metastasis in multiple ipsilateral lymph nodes, not more than 6 cm in greatest dimension
N2c: Metastasis in bilateral or contralateral lymph nodes, not more than 6 cm in greatest dimension
N3: Metastasis in a lymph node, more than 6 cm in greatest dimension

**Note*: Metastases at level VII are considered regional lymph node metastases.

Distant metastasis (M)
Larynx and hypopharynx
M0: No distant metastasis
M1: Distant metastasis

Anatomic stage/prognostic groups
Larynx and hypopharynx
0: Tis N0 M0
I: T1 N0 M0
II: T2 N0 M0
III: T3 N0 M0
T1-T3 N1 M0
IVA: T4a N0 M0
T4a N1 M0
T1-T3 N2 M0
T4a N2 M0
IVB: T4b Any N M0
Any T N3 M0
IVC: Any T Any N M1

Used with permission from the American Joint Committee on Cancer (AJCC), Chicago, IL. The original source for this material is the AJCC Cancer Staging Manual, Seventh Edition (2010), published by Springer Science+Business Media.

continued

SURGICAL OPTIONS

Operation	Indications	Removes	Contraindications/notes
Limited surgery (stripping or CO_2 laser)	Carcinoma in situ	Mucosa of cord	Can lead to thickened or harsh voice. Difficult to determine if invasive CA present
Cordectomy	Early T1a lesions of middle 1/3 of one TVC	Transoral laser excision of part of one cord. Afterwards, pseudocord forms and patient has useful (but harsh) voice	
Vertical partial (hemi) laryngectomy	Voice preservation for TVC lesions involving one and <1/3 (<5 mm) of other TVC	Bisects larynx and removes 1/2 of thyroid cartilage, a portion or all of one TVC and up to 1/3 (5 mm) of other TVC	Contraindicated if TVC fixation, >5 mm posterior or >10 mm anterior subglottic extension (because must preserve cricoid), or supraglottic extension to false cord or interarytenoid area
Supraglottic (horizontal partial) laryngectomy (SGL)	Early supraglottic lesions for voice preservation	Removes epiglottis, aryepiglottic folds, false cords, upper 1/3–1/2 of thyroid cartilage, ± hyoid bone (if epiglottic space involvement). Preserves one or both arytenoids and both TVCs	Contraindicated if exolaryngeal spread, vocal cord fixation, involvement of arytenoids, <3 mm between tumor and anterior commissure, thyroid/cricoid cartilage invasion, and/or inadequate pulmonary function (due to high aspiration risk)

continued

Extended SGL	Supraglottic lesion with <1 cm base of tongue invasion	Same as SGL with removal of ipsilateral BOT up to circumvalate papillae	
Total laryngectomy	Indicated for advanced lesions with transglottic or extensive subglottic extension, most pyriform sinus lesions, and/or cartilage invasion	Removes hyoid, thyroid, and cricoid cartilages, epiglottis, strap muscles. Patient left with a permanent tracheostoma and pharynx reconstruction (by suturing to the base of tongue)	Most frequent sites of failure include tracheal stoma, base of tongue, and neck nodes. Rehabilitation options include tracheoesophageal speech, artificial electronic larynx, esophageal speech
Partial laryngopharyngectomy	Used for small medial and anterior pyriform sinus lesions	Removes false cords, epiglottis, aryepiglottic fold, and pyriform sinus, but TVCs are preserved	Contraindicated if transglottic extension, cartilage invasion, vocal fold paralysis, pyriform apex invasion (b/c below level of TVCs), postcricoid invasion, exolaryngeal spread, or poor pulmonary reserve
Total laryngopharyngectomy	For more advanced hypopharyngeal lesions	TL plus removal of varying amount of pharyngeal wall	Requires flap or gut graft if total pharyngectomy

III

TREATMENT RECOMMENDATIONS

2002 Stage	Larynx
Tis	■ Endoscopic removal (stripping/laser) or definitive RT
T1-2N0 glottic	■ Definitive RT. Advantage of RT is that failures can be salvaged with partial laryngectomy and still have third chance with salvage total laryngectomy. Alternative, cordectomy or partial laryngectomy ± selective neck dissection. Post-op RT for close/+ margin, PNI, LVSI
T1-2N0 supraglottic	■ Definitive RT. Or, partial supraglottic laryngectomy ± selective neck dissection. Post-op chemo-RT for + margin; post-op RT for close margin, PNI, LVSI
Resectable T1-2N+, T3N0/+ requiring total laryngectomy	■ Concurrent chemo-RT as in RTOG 91–11 (preferred). ■ If < complete response, salvage surgery and neck dissection may be performed. If residual neck mass or initial N2-3, post-RT neck dissection considered ■ Alternative is total laryngectomy, and ipsilateral or bilateral neck dissection (N0-1) or bilateral comprehensive neck dissection (N2-3). Post-op chemo-RT for + margin or nodal ECE. Post-op RT (or chemo-RT with multiple factors) for pT3-4, pN2-3, close margin, PNI, LVSI, ≥1 cm subglottic extension, and/or cartilage invasion ■ Induction chemo × 3c may be considered. If CR or PR, proceed with concurrent chemo-RT as above. If < PR or progression, proceed to surgery and neck dissection as indicated
Resectable T4N0/+	■ Total laryngectomy and ipsilateral or bilateral neck dissection followed by post-op chemo-RT ■ Alternative for selected patients is definitive concurrent chemo-RT as in RTOG 91–11. Induction chemotherapy may be considered
Unresectable T3-4 or N+	■ Concurrent chemo-RT. If unable to tolerate chemo, definitive RT with concomitant boost (CB) and consider concurrent cetuximab

2002 Stage	Hypopharynx
Early T1-2 not requiring total laryngectomy (T1N0-1, small T2N0, T1N2)	■ Definitive RT. If < complete response, salvage surgery and neck dissection as indicated. If complete response, neck dissection considered for N2-3

continued

	■ Alternatively, partial laryngopharyngectomy and ipsilateral or bilateral selective neck dissection (N0) or comprehensive neck dissection (N+). Post-op chemo-RT for + margin or nodal ECE. Post-op RT (or chemo-RT if multiple factors) for pN2-3, close margin, PNI, LVSI, cartilage invasion
T2-4N0/+ requiring total laryngectomy	■ Concurrent chemo-RT as extrapolated from RTOG 91–11. Or, induction chemo ×2c (with a third cycle if PR). If CR at primary site, proceed with definitive RT (≥70 Gy). If primary site has only PR, proceed with concurrent chemo-RT. Nonresponders to induction chemo should undergo surgery → post-op RT or chemo-RT as indicated. If residual neck mass after definitive RT or initial N2-3, post-RT neck dissection considered ■ Or, laryngopharyngectomy and selective (N0) or comprehensive neck dissection (N+ or T4). Post-op chemo-RT for + margin or nodal ECE. Post-op RT (or chemo-RT if multiple factors) for pT3-4, pN2-3, close margin, PNI, LVSI, cartilage invasion
Unresectable T3-4 or N+	■ Concurrent chemo-RT. If unable to tolerate chemo, definitive RT with CB

STUDIES

RT DOSE FRACTIONATION

- Yamazaki et al. (2006): 180 patients with T1N0 glottic carcinoma randomized to 2 Gy/fx to 60 Gy (if ≤2/3 TVC involved) or 66 Gy (if >2/3 TVC involved) vs. 2.25 Gy/fx to 56.25–63 Gy. The 2.25 Gy/fx arm improved 5-year LC (77→92%), but not CSS (97 vs. 100%) or toxicity.
- *RTOG 95–12* (Trotti et al. 2006, abstract): Randomized 250 patients with T2 glottic cancer to 70 Gy in 35 fx vs. 79.2 Gy at 1.2-Gy b.i.d. b.i.d. arm had nonsignificant trend for improved 5-year LC (70→79%, $p>0.11$), DFS (37→51%, $p>0.07$), and OS (62→73%, $p>0.19$), but trial was underpowered.
- Le et al. (1997) reviewed 398 patients with T1–2 glottic cancer treated with RT alone. On multivariate analysis, overall treatment time ≤43 days, fraction size ≥2.25 Gy, and total dose ≥65 Gy improved LC for T2 lesions. Anterior commissure involvement decreased T1 LC, and impaired cord mobility and subglottic extension decreased T2 LC.

- Garden et al. (2003) reviewed 230 patients treated with RT alone for T2 glottic cancer. Treatment with ≤2 Gy/fraction had decreased 5-year LC (68%) compared to >2 Gy/fraction (82%) or b.i.d. RT (79%).
- *RTOG 90–03* (Fu et al. 2000; update ASTRO 2005): 268 patients with locally-advanced cancer of the oral cavity, oropharynx, supraglottic larynx, or hypopharynx randomized to 2/70 Gy (standard) vs. 1.2 b.i.d./81.6 Gy (HFX) vs. split-course 1.6 b.i.d./67.2 Gy (with 2 week break) vs. CB-RT to 72 Gy (1.8 Gy/fraction with a 1.5-Gy boost on the last 12 treatment days). On update, 5-year LRF and DFS improved w/ HFX and CB vs. standard fx and split-course. LRF: 60% standard, 58% split-course, 52% CB, 51% HFX. DFS: 21% standard, 27% split-course, 29% CB, 31% HFX. No difference in DM (27–29%), CSS (40–46%). Trend for improved OS with HFX (37 vs. 29–34%).

CHEMO-RT FOR LARYNX PRESERVATION

- Larynx preservation rates:
  - RT alone: ~60–70%.
  - Induction chemo → RT: ~65–75%.
  - Concurrent chemo-RT: ~80–85%.
- *VA Larynx Trial* (Department of Veterans Affairs Laryngeal Cancer Study Group 1991): 332 patients with III/IV larynx (T1N1 excluded), randomized to surgery and post-op RT (50–74 Gy) vs. induction cisplatin/5-FU × 2c (with a third cycle if PR/CR) → RT (66–76 Gy). No routine neck dissection for N+ patients. Chemo allowed 64% larynx preservation at 2 years. There was no difference in 2-year OS (68%). Chemo-RT decreased distant recurrences, but had higher LF (12 vs. 2%). Organ preservation improved quality of life. Salvage laryngectomy was required for 56% of T4 patients.
- *EORTC 24891* (Lefebvre et al. 1996; update ASCO 2004): 202 patients with operable pyriform sinus tumors randomized to surgery → post-op RT (50–70 Gy) vs. induction cisplatin/5-FU × 2c (with a third cycle if PR/CR) → RT (70 Gy). Nonresponders to chemo underwent surgery → RT. Fifty-one to fifty-four percent of patients had a CR after chemo. There was no difference in LRF, and chemo decreased DM (36→25%). The 3/5-year functional intact larynx rates were 42/35% with chemo. On update, no difference in 5- or 10-year OS and PFS.

- *RTOG 91–11* (Forastiere et al. 2003; update ASCO 2006): 547 patients with stage III/IV larynx (T2–3 or low-volume T4 without gross cartilage destruction or >1 cm base of tongue invasion, or LN+) randomized to one of three arms: RT alone, chemo → RT, or concurrent chemo-RT. RT was 2/70 Gy in all arms. Induction chemo was cisplatin/5-FU × 2c → reassessment. If progression or <PR, treated with laryngectomy and post-op RT. If PR/CR → third cycle chemo → RT. Concurrent chemo was cisplatin × 3c. All patients with cN2 had neck dissection within 8 weeks after RT. On update, concurrent chemo-RT improved 5-year larynx preservation (84%) vs. induction chemo (71%) and RT alone (66%), and LRC (69%) vs. induction chemo (55%) and RT alone (51%). Chemo reduced the rate of DM (13% concurrent, 14% induction vs. 22% RT alone) and improved DFS (39% with chemo vs. 27% with RT alone). No difference in OS (55% concurrent, 59% induction, 54% RT alone).
- *GORTEC 2000–01* (Pointreau et al. 2009): 220 patients with locally-advanced larynx or hypopharynx cancer that required total laryngectomy randomized to 3c of TPF (docetaxel, cisplatin, 5-FU) vs. PF (cisplatin, 5-FU) chemo. If CR, PR, and larynx mobility, patients received RT with or without additional chemo; if no response, patients had surgery and post-op RT with or without additional chemo. TPF improved overall response (80 vs. 59%) and 3-year larynx preservation rate (70 vs. 58%), but had more neutropenia.
- *TAX 324* (Posner et al. 2007): Randomized 501 patients with unresectable stage III/IV head and neck SCC (33% were larynx or hypopharynx) to induction TPF chemo (docetaxel, cisplatin, 5-FU) vs. PF (cisplatin, 5-FU) every 3 weeks for 3 cycles. Patients then had concurrent weekly carboplatin and RT to 70 Gy. TPF improved 3-year OS (48→62%) and LRC (62→70%), but not DM. TPF increased neutropenia (54→84%). Twenty-one percent of patients who got TPF induction were not able to receive subsequent concurrent chemo-RT.
- *EORTC 24954* (Lefebvre et al. 2009): 450 patients with resectable T3–T4 larynx or T2–T4 hypopharynx, N0–N2 randomized to sequential arm (2c cisplatin/5-FU → if >50% tumor reduction, 2 more cycles cisplatin/5-FU → 70 Gy) vs. alternating arm (4 c cisplatin/5-FU in weeks 1, 4, 7, and 10 alternating with 20 Gy RT during 2-week interval to 60 Gy total). No difference in larynx preservation, PFS, OS, or acute and late toxicity.

- *Cetuximab* (Bonner et al. 2006): 424 patients with locoregionally advanced resectable or unresectable stage III–IV SCC of oropharynx, larynx, or hypopharynx randomized to RT or RT + cetuximab given 1 week before RT and weekly during RT. RT options included 2/70 Gy, 1.2 b.i.d./72–76.8 Gy, or CB 72 Gy. Cetuximab increased 3-year LRC (34→47%) and OS (45→55%). With the exception of acneiform rash and infusion reactions with cetuximab, toxicity was similar.
- See Oropharynx chapter 7 for list of other key trials of chemo-RT, most of which included patients with larynx or hypopharynx cancer.

POST-OP RT AND POST-OP CHEMO-RT

- *RTOG 95–01* (Cooper et al. 2004): 459 patients with operable cancer of the oral cavity, oropharynx, larynx, or hypopharynx who had ≥2 involved lymph nodes, nodal extracapsular extension, or a + margin randomized to post-op RT (2/60–66 Gy) vs. post-op chemo-RT (2/60–66 Gy and cisplatin ×3 c as in EORTC 22931). Chemo-RT improved 2-year DFS (43→54%), LRC (72→82%), and had a trend for improved OS (57→63%), but increased grade 3–4 toxicity (34→77%).
- *EORTC 22931* (Bernier et al. 2004): 334 patients with operable stage III/IV oral cavity, oropharynx, larynx, and hypopharnx cancer randomized to post-op RT (2/66 Gy) vs. post-op chemo-RT (2/66 Gy and cisplatin 100 mg/m^2 on days 1, 22, 43). All patients received 54 Gy to the low-risk neck. Eligible stages included pT3–4N0/+, T1–2N2–3, and T1–2N0–1with ECE, +margin, or PNI. Chemo-RT improved 3/5-year DFS (41/36→59/47%), 3/5-year OS (49/40→65/53%), and 5-year LRC (69→82%), but increased grade 3–4 toxicity (21→41%).
- *Combined RTOG/EORTC analysis* (Bernier 2005): Chemo-RT improved OS, DFS, and LRC for ECE and/or + margins, but provided only trend for improvements ($p > 0.06$) for stage III–IV, PNI, LVSI, and/or enlarged LN in levels IV–V for OPX or oral cavity tumors based on EORTC data. Patients with ≥2 LN without ECE as their only factor did not benefit from chemo ($p > 0.73$).
- Ang et al. (2001): 213 patients with locally-advanced oral cavity, oropharynx, larynx, and hypopharynx cancers treated with surgery randomized by risk factors to post-op RT. Risk factors included >1 node group, ≥2 nodes, nodes >3 cm, microscopic +margins, PNI, oral cavity site, and nodal extracapsular extension.

Low-risk: no risk factors → no RT. Intermediate risk: 1 risk factor (but not ECE) → 1.8/57.6 Gy. High-risk: ECE or ≥2 risk factors → 1.8/63 Gy in 7 weeks or in 5 weeks with a CB. The 5-year LRC/OS for low-risk was 90/83%, for intermediate risk 94/66%, and for high-risk 68/42%. Overall treatment time <11 weeks increased LRC, and CB had a trend for improved OS.

META-ANALYSES

- *Altered fractionation* (Bourhis 2006): Meta-analysis of 15 trials with 6,515 patients, 74% with stage III–IV disease, mostly of oropharynx and larynx, treated with conventional RT (1.8–2/65–70 Gy), hyperfractionated RT (higher dose, same time), accelerated RT (same dose, shorter time), or accelerated RT with reduced total dose. Altered fractionation improved 5-year OS by 3.4%, with greatest benefit for hyperfractionated RT (8% benefit) vs. accelerated RT (1.7–2% benefit). Five-year LRC benefit 6.4% overall, mainly for local as opposed to regional failure. Benefit highest for youngest patients (<50–60 years). No effect of altered fractionation on DM.
- *MACH-NC meta-analysis* (Pignon et al. 2009): 93 phase III trials and 17,346 patients. OS benefit (4.5%) at 5 years when chemotherapy was added to RT, with greater benefit for concurrent chemo-RT vs. induction chemo followed by RT (6.5% OS benefit with concurrent chemo-RT). Similar results in trials with post-op RT, conventional, and altered fractionation. No difference between mono or polychemotherapy regimens, but increased benefit with platinum-based compounds. Decreasing benefit with increasing age, with no benefit observed if ≥71 years.

RADIATION TECHNIQUES

SIMULATION AND FIELD DESIGN

- Simulate the patient supine with the head hyperextended. Wire neck scars and the tracheostoma (if present). Shoulders may be pulled down with straps. Immobilize with a thermoplastic head and shoulder mask. Bolus may be needed for anterior commissure tumors and over the tracheostoma (if present).
- A 3D conformal or IMRT plan should be used for any but simple opposed-lateral fields in order to spare normal tissues.
- Computed dosimetry should be used in all cases. Wedges and/or compensating filters may be required.

- Use fluoroscopy if available to evaluate superior motion of larynx with swallowing to ensure appropriate location of superior border.
- Glottic larynx traditional field design.
  - For T1N0, use a 5×5-cm field with the superior border at the top of the thyroid cartilage, the inferior border at the bottom of the cricoid, a 1-cm skin flash anteriorly, and a 2-cm margin posteriorly (or the anterior edge of the vertebral body) (Fig. 9.1).
  - For glottic T2N0, the field size is increased to 6×6 cm with the inferior border one tracheal ring below the cricoid.
  - For T3–4N0, extend the superior border to 2 cm above the angle of the mandible, the posterior border behind the spinous processes, and the inferior border to include 1.5–2 cm margin on the subglottic extent of the tumor. Match the lateral fields to the low-neck AP field. Treat the lateral fields to 42–45 Gy with a small cord block, then move the posterior border off-cord and use an electron boost to treat the elective posterior neck to 50 Gy. Boost the primary with a 1.5-cm margin to 70 Gy with chemo or to 72 Gy with a CB if chemo not used.

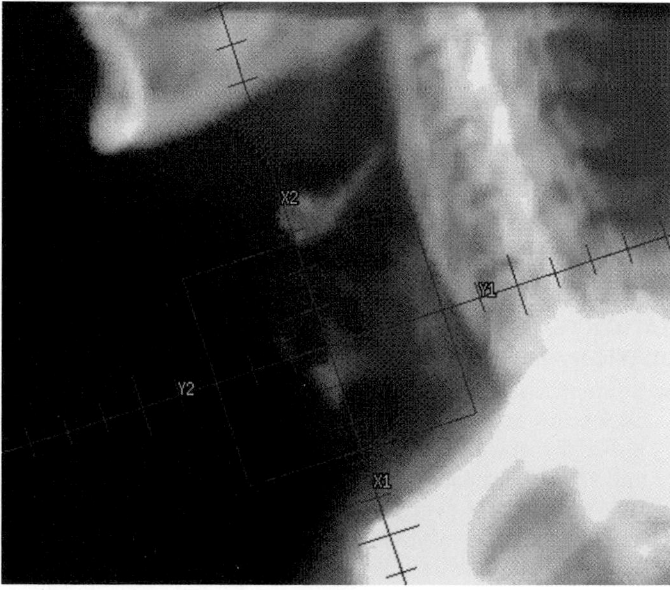

Fig. 9.1 Lateral DRR of a field used to treat a T1 glottic carcinoma

- Supraglottic larynx
  - For T1N0 treat the primary and levels II–III.
  - For T2–3, also treat low-neck because of increased risk of microscopic nodal disease.
  - For advanced cases, treat as described above for glottic.
- Hypopharynx
  - Treat primary and levels II–V and retropharyngeal nodes in all cases.
  - With traditional field design, the superior border is the skull base and mastoid. The inferior border is 1 cm below the inferior extent of disease (or 1 cm below cricoid) on the laterals and matched to the AP low-neck field. With posterior pharyngeal wall tumors, the anterior border does not need to flash the skin. A clothespin may be used to spare the skin anteriorly.
- Post-op
  - With traditional fields, use 3-field technique with stoma in low-neck AP field. Lateral fields cover neopharynx, adenopathy, and 1.5–2 cm margin on preoperative extent of disease.
  - With conventional three-field techniques, the spinal cord is shielded on the lateral fields at the matchline if no gross disease is present. If gross disease is present at the matchline, angling the lateral fields to match the divergence of the AP field may help. A small midline block on the AP field may be necessary.
  - Indications to boost tracheal stoma to 60–66 Gy: emergent tracheostomy, subglottic extension, tumor invasion to soft tissues of neck, extranodal extension in level VI, close/+ margin, scar crosses stoma.
- For low-lying high-risk areas in which matchline would go through the area, extended-field IMRT may be used.
  - Alternatively, may consider caudal tilt technique in which the lateral field gantry is moved 10° anterior and the couch is kicked 10° away from the beam and the SCV field is included in these lateral fields. At 42-Gy, posterior border is brought off-cord and this long strip is supplemented with electrons.
- IMRT
  - IMRT is not recommended for T1–2N0 glottic cancers, but may be considered for more advanced lesions.
  - GTV: clinical and/or radiographic gross disease.
  - CTV1: 0.5–2 cm margin on primary and/or nodal GTV (depending on the presence or absence of anatomic boundaries to microscopic spread).

- CTV2: elective neck.
- Individualized planning target volumes are used for the GTV, CTV1, and CTV2.

DOSE PRESCRIPTIONS

- T1–2N0 glottic larynx
  - >2 Gy/fx preferred. If 2 Gy/fx is used, total dose >66 Gy.
  - UCSF uses 2.25 Gy/fx.
    - Tis: 56.25–58.5 Gy.
    - T1N0: 63 Gy.
    - T2N0: 65.25 Gy.
- T3–4 and LN+ patients
  - Concurrent chemo-RT.
    - Total dose typically 70 Gy in daily fx with cisplatin 100 mg/m^2 q3 weeks ×3c.
    - Altered fractionation and multiagent chemo have been evaluated with no consensus on the optimal approach.
  - With definitive RT, use altered fractionation. Options:
    - Six fx/week during weeks 2–6: 70 Gy at 2 Gy/fx to primary and gross adenopathy.
    - CB: 72 Gy in 6 weeks (1.8 Gy/fx large field; 1.5 Gy boost as second daily fx during last 12 treatment days).
    - Hyperfractionation: 81.6 Gy in 7 weeks at 1.2 Gy b.i.d.
- Post op RT
  - 60–66 Gy at 2 Gy/fx to high-risk areas and the postoperative bed.
  - Post-op chemo-RT indicated for nodal ECE and/or +margin(s) and considered for other risk features, including pT3–4, pN2–3, PNI, LVSI. Concurrent single agent cisplatin 100 mg/m^2 q3 weeks recommended.
- Elective neck
  - Uninvolved nodal stations: ≥50–56 Gy at 1.6–2 Gy/fx.
- IMRT
  - IMRT has been shown to reduce long-term toxicity in oropharyngeal, paranasal sinus, and nasopharyngeal cancers by reducing dose to salivary glands, temporal lobes, auditory structures, and the optic apparatus. The use of IMRT for laryngeal and hypopharyngeal cancers is evolving and may be used at the discretion of the treating physician.
  - Simultaneous integrated boost ("dose-painting") technique used at UCSF.

  - 33 fx: GTV = 70 Gy at 2.12-Gy/fx, CTV1 = 59.4 Gy at 1.8-Gy/fx, CTV2 = 54 Gy at 1.64-Gy/fx.
- Alternative techniques.
  - Simultaneous integrated boost in 35 fx.
    (a) GTV = 70 Gy at 2-Gy/fx, CTV1 = 63 Gy at 1.8-Gy/fx, CTV2 = 56 Gy at 1.6-Gy/fx.
  - Sequential technique.
    (a) Initial lower-dose phase (weeks 1–5) followed by high-dose boost volume phase (weeks 6 and 7) using two to three separate dose plans.
  - CB schedule.
    (a) Delivers dose to subclinical targets once daily for 6 weeks, and a separate boost plan as second daily treatment during last 12 treatment days.
- Typically, seven nonopposing beam angles are used.
- Extended whole field neck technique is typically preferred for larynx and hypopharynx as the glottic larynx is considered a target or when gross disease extends inferiorly and close to the glottic larynx. With this technique, lateral fields are typically not used because they would require treating through the shoulder, so these are replaced with anterior oblique fields.
- A split field technique with matched conventional low anterior neck field is sometimes used for nasopharynx and oropharynx lesions to reduce the dose to the glottic larynx. In this situation, the matchline is typically just above the arytenoids. A gradient match technique may be used as well.

DOSE LIMITATIONS

- Spinal cord maximum dose ≤45–50 Gy. Brainstem maximum dose ≤54 Gy. Keep 50% of the volume of each parotid ≤20 Gy (if possible) and mean dose <26 Gy. Mandible maximum dose ≤70 Gy. Brachial plexus dose <60 Gy.
- Tracheostomas are limited to ≤50 Gy unless (1) significant subglottic extension, (2) emergent tracheostomy, (3) extranodal extension in neck level VI, or (4) close/+ margin, in which case it is boosted to 60–66 Gy.
- For other head and neck primary sites, the goal mean dose to the larynx is <35–45 Gy and 2/3 should be kept below 50 Gy.
- 70 Gy carries 5% risk of laryngeal cartilage necrosis.

COMPLICATIONS

- Complications of RT include mucositis, dermatitis, xerostomia, dysgeusia, soft-tissue fibrosis, hypothyroidism, and rarely radionecrosis, pharyngocutaneous fistula, or carotid rupture.
- Perioperative complications of surgery include bleeding, airway obstruction, infection, and wound complications. Post-op complications include webs, stenosis, chondritis, fistulas, and aspiration.
- Patients need ≥2,000 calories/day to avoid malnutrition. Supplements (e.g., Boost or Ensure) and/or feeding tubes may be used.
- Amifostine may decrease xerostomia and mucositis, but it may be associated with significant side effects (e.g., hypotension, N/V).

FOLLOW-UP

- H&P every 1–3 month for year 1, every 2–4 month for year 2, every 4–6 month for years 3–5, and every 6–12 months thereafter. Posttreatment baseline imaging recommended, and thereafter, as clinically indicated. CXR annually. TSH every 6–12 month if neck irradiated. Speech, swallow, dental, and hearing evaluations and rehabilitation as indicated. Smoking cessation counseling.
- If recurrence is suspected but biopsy is negative, follow closely (at least monthly) until it resolves.

REFERENCES

Ang KK, Trotti A, Brown BW, et al. Randomized trial addressing risk features and time factors of surgery plus radiotherapy in advanced head-and-neck cancer. Int J Radiat Oncol Biol Phys 2001;51:571-578.

Bernier J, Cooper JS, Pajak TF, et al. Defining risk levels in locally advanced head and neck cancers: a comparative analysis of concurrent postoperative radiation plus chemotherapy trials of the EORTC (#22931) and RTOG (# 9501). Head Neck. 2005;27(10):843-50.

Bernier J, Domenge C, Ozsahin M, et al. Postoperative irradiation with or without concomitant chemotherapy for locally advanced head and neck cancer. N Engl J Med 2004;350:1945-1952.

Bonner JA, Harari PM, Giralt J, et al. Radiotherapy plus cetuximab for squamous-cell carcinoma of the head and neck. N Engl J Med 2006; 354: 567-578.

Bourhis J, Overgaard J, Audry H, et al. Hyperfractionated or accelerated radiotherapy in head and neck cancer: a meta-analysis. Lancet. Sep 2 2006;368(9538):843-854.

Cooper JS, Pajak TF, Forastiere AA, et al. Postoperative concurrent radiotherapy and chemotherapy for high-risk squamous-cell carcinoma of the head and neck. N Engl J Med 2004;350:1937-1944.

Forastiere AA, Goepfert H, Maor M, et al. Concurrent chemotherapy and radiotherapy for organ preservation in advanced laryngeal cancer. N Engl J Med 2003;349:2091-2098.

Fu KK, Pajak TF, Trotti A, et al. A Radiation Therapy Oncology Group (RTOG) phase III randomized study to compare hyperfractionation and two variants of accelerated fractionation to standard fractionation radiotherapy for head and neck squamous cell carcinomas: first report of RTOG 9003. Int J Radiat Oncol Biol Phys 2000;48:7-16.

Garden AS. The Larynx and Hypopharynx. In: Cox JD, Ang KK, editors. Radiation oncology: rationale, technique, results. 8th ed. St. Louis: Mosby; 2003. pp. 255-281.

Induction chemotherapy plus radiation compared with surgery plus radiation in patients with advanced laryngeal cancer. The Department of Veterans Affairs Laryngeal Cancer Study Group. N Engl J Med 1991;324:1685-1690.

Le QT, Fu KK, Kroll S, et al. Influence of fraction size, total dose, and overall time on local control of T1-T2 glottic carcinoma. Int J Radiat Oncol Biol Phys 1997;39:115-126.

Lefebvre JL, Rolland F, Tesselaar M et al. Phase 3 randomized trial on larynx preservation comparing sequential vs alternating chemotherapy and radiotherapy. J Natl Cancer Inst. 2009;101(3):142-52.

Lefebvre JL, Chevalier D, Luboinski B, et al. Larynx preservation in pyriform sinus cancer: preliminary results of a European Organization for Research and Treatment of Cancer phase III trial. EORTC Head and Neck Cancer Cooperative Group. J Natl Cancer Inst 1996;88:890-899.

Pignon JP, Maître AL, Maillard E, et al. Meta-analysis of chemotherapy in head and neck cancer (MACH-NC): An update on 93 randomised trials and 17,346 patients. Radiother Oncol. 2009 May 14. [Epub ahead of print].

Pointreau Y, Garaud P, Chapet S, et al. Randomized trial of induction chemotherapy with cisplatin and 5-fluorouracil with or without docetaxel for larynx preservation. J Natl Cancer Inst 2009;101(7):498-506.

Posner MR, Hershock DM, Blajman CR, et al. Cisplatin and fluorouracil alone or with docetaxel in head and neck cancer. N Engl J Med 2007;357:1705-1715.

Trotti A, Pajak T, Emami B, et al. A randomized trial of hyperfractionation versus standard fractionation in T2 squamous cell carcinoma of the vocal cord. Int J Radiat Oncol Biol Phys 2006;66(3):S15.

Yamazaki H, Nishiyama K, Tanaka E, et al. Radiotherapy for early glottic carcinoma (T1N0M0): results of prospective randomized study of radiation fraction size and overall treatment time. Int J Radiat Oncol Biol Phys 2006;64(1):77-82

FURTHER READING

Adelstein DJ, Li Y, Adams GL, et al. An intergroup phase III comparison of standard radiation therapy and two schedules of concurrent chemoradiotherapy in patients with unresectable squamous cell head and neck cancer. J Clin Oncol 2003;21:92-98.

Brizel DM, Albers ME, Fisher SR, et al. Hyperfractionated irradiation with or without concurrent chemotherapy for locally advanced head and neck cancer. N Engl J Med 1998;338: 1798-1804.

Forastiere A, Maor M, Weber R, et al. Long-term Results of Intergroup RTOG 91-11: A Phase III Trial to Preserve the Larynx -Induction Cisplatin/5-FU and Radiation Therapy versus Concurrent Cisplatin and Radiation Therapy versus Radiation Therapy, ASCO National Proceedings, 2006.

Garden AS, Forster K, Wong PF, et al. Results of radiotherapy for T2N0 glottic carcinoma: does the "2" stand for twice-daily treatment? Int J Radiat Oncol Biol Phys 2003;55:322-328.

Greene FL, American Joint Committee on Cancer., American Cancer Society. AJCC cancer staging manual. 6th ed. New York: Springer; 2002.

Lee N, Phillips TL. Cancer of the Larynx. In: Leibel SA, Phillips TL, editors. Textbook of radiation oncology. 2nd ed. Philadelphia: Saunders; 2004. pp. 679-698.

Lefebvre JL, Ang KK. Larynx preservation consensus panel. Larynx preservation clinical trial design: key issues and recommendations-a consensus panel summary. Int J Radiat Oncol Biol Phys. 2009;73(5):1293-1303.

Lefebvre JL, Chevalier D, Luboinski B et al. Is laryngeal preservation (LP) with induction chemotherapy (ICT) safe in the treatment of hypopharyngeal SCC? Final results of the phase III EORTC 24891 trial. Journal of Clinical Oncology, 2004 ASCO Annual Meeting Proceedings (Post-Meeting Edition). Vol 22, No 14S (July 15 Supplement), 2004: 5531

Mendenhall WM, Hinerman RW, Amdur RJ, et al. Larynx. In: Perez CA, Brady LW, Halperin EC, et al., editors. Principles and practice of radiation oncology. 4th ed. Philadelphia: Lippincott Williams & Wilkins; 2004. pp. 1094-1116.

National Comprehensive Cancer Network. Clinical Practice Guidelines in Oncology: Head and Neck Cancers. Available at: http://www.nccn.org/professionals/physician_gls/PDF/head-and-neck.pdf. Accessed on May 19, 2009.

Shah HK, Khuntia D, Hoffman HT, Harari PM. Hypopharynx. In: Halperin EC, Perez CA, Brady LW, et al., editors. Principles and practice of radiation oncology. 5th ed. Philadelphia: Lippincott Williams & Wilkins; 2008. pp. 958-974.

Zelefsky MJ. Cancer of the Hypopharynx. In: Leibel SA, Phillips TL, editors. Textbook of radiation oncology. 2nd ed. Philadelphia: Saunders; 2004. pp. 657-678.

III

Chapter 10

Salivary Gland Tumors

Chien Peter Chen and Naomi R. Schechter

III

PEARLS

- Salivary gland neoplasms account for ~3–5% of H&N cancers.

ANATOMY

- Major salivary glands consist of the paired parotid, submandibular, and sublingual glands.
- Minor salivary glands located throughout oral cavity, pharynx, and paranasal sinuses.
- Parotid glands located lateral to the mandibular ramus and masseter muscle.
  - Facial nerve divides parotid gland into superficial and deep lobes.
  - Parotid gland drains into oral cavity through Stensen's duct adjacent to upper second molar.
  - Lymphatic drainage from parotid gland is to intraparotid and periparotid nodes, followed by ipsilateral level I, II, and III nodes.
- Submandibular gland is located under the horizontal mandibular ramus.
  - Submandibular gland is lateral to and abuts lingual (V3) and hypoglossal nerves and is medial to mandibular and cervical branches of CN VII.
  - Submandibular glands drain into oral cavity through Wharton's duct.
  - Submandibular lymphatic drainage is to levels I, II, III.
  - Drainage from parotid and submandibular glands to contralateral nodes is rare.
- Sublingual gland located superior to mylohyoid muscle and deep to mucous membrane.
  - Sublingual glands drain into oral cavity through Rivinus ducts or Bartholin's duct.

- Incidence of LN involvement varies according to histology and site.
- Overall risk of lymph node involvement is less common than for SCC.
- Adenoid cystic carcinoma has the lowest frequency of cervical node metastasis (5–8%), but the highest propensity for perineural spread.
- LN metastases are most common with minor salivary gland tumors followed by submandibular gland tumors followed by parotid tumors.

HISTOLOGY

- Majority of salivary gland neoplasms are benign.
- Inverse relationship exists between size of parotid gland and ratio of malignant to benign cancer.
- For tumors of the parotid gland, 80% are benign and 20% malignant.
- Most parotid tumors present as painless swelling.
- Pleomorphic adenoma is most common benign salivary gland neoplasm.
- Salivary gland cancer is notable for its remarkable histologic diversity.
- Most common malignant histology of parotid gland is mucoepidermoid carcinoma.
- Most common malignant histology of submandibular and minor salivary glands is adenoid cystic carcinoma.
- Acinic cell carcinoma usually occurs only in the parotid gland.

OTHER

- Prognostic variables include grade, postsurgical residual disease, and LN status.
- Larger tumor size and cranial nerve involvement associated with poor prognosis.
- Patterns of failure generally dominated by high rates of distant metastases.
- Most likely sites for DM is lung, followed by bone and liver.
- Adenoid cystic, ductal, and undifferentiated carcinoma have highest rates of DM.
- Loss of salivary function is permanent and complete after 35 Gy with standard fx.

- Despite high DM rate, there is generally no role for chemotherapy.

WORKUP

- H&P with bimanual palpation. Carefully examine cranial nerves and for trismus.
- CT and/or MRI of head and neck. PET scan is still investigational for salivary gland cancers.
- Fine-needle aspiration biopsy.
- Chest X-ray.
- Dental evaluation prior to the start of RT.
- Note that minor salivary gland cancer is staged according to systems for the anatomic site of origin (e.g., oral cavity, sinuses, etc.)

STAGING: MAJOR SALIVARY GLAND

Editors' note: All TNM stage and stage groups referred to elsewhere in this chapter reflect the 2002 AJCC staging nomenclature unless otherwise noted as the new system below was published after this chapter was written.

(AJCC 6TH ED., 2002)

Primary tumor (T)

- TX: Primary tumor cannot be assessed
- T0: No evidence of primary tumor
- T1: Tumor 2 cm or less in greatest dimension without extraparenchymal extension*
- T2: Tumor more than 2 cm but not more than 4 cm in greatest dimension without extraparenchymal extension*
- T3: Tumor more than 4 cm and/or having extraparenchymal extension
- T4a: Moderately advanced disease. Tumor invades skin, mandible, ear canal, and/or facial nerve
- T4b: Very advanced disease. Tumor invades skull base and/or pterygoid plates and/or encases carotid artery

**Note*: Extraparenchymal extension is clinical or macroscopic evidence of invasion of soft tissues. Microscopic evidence alone does not constitute extraparenchymal extension for classification purposes.

Regional lymph nodes (N)

- NX: Regional lymph nodes cannot be assessed
- N0: No regional lymph nodes metastasis
- N1: Metastasis in a single ipsilateral lymph node, 3 cm or less in greatest dimension
- N2: Metastasis in a single ipsilateral lymph node, more than 3 cm but not more than 6 cm in greatest dimension, or in multiple ipsilateral lymph nodes, not more than 6 cm in greatest dimension, or in bilateral or contralateral lymph nodes, not more than 6 cm in greatest dimension
- N2a: Metastasis in single ipsilateral lymph node, more than 3 cm but not more than 6 cm in greatest dimension

(AJCC 7TH ED., 2010)

Primary tumor (T)

- TX: Primary tumor cannot be assessed
- T0: No evidence of primary tumor
- T1: Tumor 2 cm or less in greatest dimension without extraparenchymal extension*
- T2: Tumor more than 2 cm but not more than 4 cm in greatest dimension without extraparenchymal extension*
- T3: Tumor more than 4 cm and/or tumor having extraparenchymal extension*
- T4a: Moderately advanced disease. Tumor invades skin, mandible, ear canal, and/or facial nerve
- T4b: Very advanced disease. Tumor invades skull base and/or pterygoid plates and/or encases carotid artery

**Note*: Extraparenchymal extension is clinical or macroscopic evidence of invasion of soft tissues. Microscopic evidence alone does not constitute extraparenchymal extension for classification purposes

Regional lymph nodes (N)

- NX: Regional lymph nodes cannot be assessed
- N0: No regional lymph node metastasis
- N1: Metastasis in a single ipsilateral lymph node, 3 cm or less in greatest dimension
- N2: Metastasis in a single ipsilateral lymph node, more than 3 cm but not more than 6 cm in greatest dimension, or in multiple ipsilateral lymph nodes, not more than 6 cm in greatest dimension, or in bilateral or contralateral lymph nodes, not more than 6 cm in greatest dimension

continued

N2b: Metastasis in multiple ipsilateral lymph nodes, not more than 6 cm in greatest dimension
N2c: Metastasis in bilateral or contralateral lymph nodes, not more than 6 cm in greatest dimension
N3: Metastasis in a lymph node, more than 6 cm in greatest dimension

Distant metastasis (M)
M0: No distant metastasis
M1: Distant metastasis present

Stage grouping		~2/5-Year OS	
I:	T1N0M0	I:	88/75%
II:	T2N0M0	II:	77/59%
III:	T3N0M0, T1-3N1M0	III:	68/47%
IVA:	T4aN0-2M0, T1-3N2M0	IV:	47/28%
IVB:	T4b any N M0, any T N3 M0		
IVC:	Any T, any N, M1		

Used with the permission from the American Joint Committee on Cancer (AJCC), Chicago, IL. The original source for this material is the AJCC Cancer Staging Manual, Sixth Edition (2002), published by Springer Science+Business Media.

N2a: Metastasis in a single ipsilateral lymph node, more than 3 cm but not more than 6 cm in greatest dimension
N2b: Metastasis in multiple ipsilateral lymph nodes, not more than 6 cm in greatest dimension
N2c: Metastasis in bilateral or contralateral lymph nodes, not more than 6 cm in greatest dimension
N3: Metastasis in a lymph node, more than 6 cm in greatest dimension

Distant metastasis (M)
M0: No distant metastasis
M1: Distant metastasis

Anatomic stage/prognostic groups
I: T1 N0 M0
II: T2 N0 M0
III: T3 N0 M0
T1-T3 N1 M0
IVA: T4a N0 M0
T4a N1 M0
T1-T3 N2 M0
T4a N2 M0
IVB: T4b Any N M0
Any T N3 M0
IVC: Any T Any N M1

Used with the permission from the American Joint Committee on Cancer (AJCC), Chicago, IL. The original source for this material is the AJCC Cancer Staging Manual, Seventh Edition (2010), published by Springer Science+Business Media.

III

TREATMENT RECOMMENDATIONS

GENERAL POINTS

- Surgery forms the mainstay of definitive treatment for salivary gland malignancies.
- Complications of surgery include facial nerve dysfunction and Frey's syndrome.
- Frey's syndrome consists of gustatory flushing, sweating, auriculotemporal syndrome.
- Superficial parotidectomy can generally be performed for low-grade parotid tumors.
- Facial nerve-sparing approaches can often be performed to preserve function, cosmesis.
- Neck dissection recommended for clinically + LN or high-grade histology.
- Indications for post-op RT are currently controversial as there is no randomized data analyzing the role of post-op RT.
- Consider post-op RT for PNI, close/+ margins, high-grade tumors, and T3-4 tumors.
- Patients with pathological LN involvement should receive post-op RT.
- RT alone is indicated for medically inoperable and unresectable tumors. LC rates with RT alone range from 20 to 80%.
- Neutron therapy may achieve better LC for unresectable or inoperable tumors.
- Brachytherapy or intraoperative RT can be considered for recurrent tumors.
- IMRT reduces mean doses to normal structures and allows dose-escalation to tumor.
- Chemotherapy is considered investigational.

2002 Stage	Recommended treatment
Resectable T1-2N0, superficial	■ Surgery followed by observation if low-grade. ■ Consider post-op RT if adenoid cystic or intermediate to high grade
Resectable, T3-4 or N+	■ Surgery with neck dissection for LN+ or high grade followed by post-op RT for close/+ margins, intermediate–high grade, adenoid cystic, PNI, LVSI. RT to neck for pN+, T3-4, and/or high grade to reduce local/regional failure (>20–50% down to 5–10%)

continued

Unresectable

- Definitive RT. LRC may be higher with neutrons than photons

Pleomorphic adenoma

- If total parotidectomy, LR <1 vs. ~20% after simple enucleation. Post-op RT controversial and sometimes indicated if multifocal, PNI, or residual disease. Post-op RT LRC is 90–95%

STUDIES

- Fu et al. (1977): retrospective analysis of 100 cases of major and minor salivary gland cancer treated with surgery or surgery + RT. The addition of post-op RT significantly improved LC for patients with adenoid cystic carcinoma, locally advanced (stage III/IV) disease, and + margins.
- Garden et al. (1997): retrospective analysis of 166 patients with parotid gland malignancies treated with surgery + RT. On multivariate analysis, facial nerve sacrifice and pathologic cervical nodal disease were associated with LF. The actuarial 5-, 10-, and 15-year LC rates were 92, 90, and 90%, respectively.
- Garden et al. (1995): retrospective analysis of 198 patients with adenoid cystic carcinoma of the H&N treated with surgery + RT. Five- and 10-year LC was 95 and 86%, respectively. Patients with positive margins and major (named) nerve involvement were at significantly increased risk of LR.
- Armstrong et al. (1990): matched-pair analysis of 92 patients treated with surgery vs. surgery and post-op RT. The addition of post-op RT improved outcome for patients with stage III/IV disease and for patients with pathological + LN.
- Armstrong et al. (1992): retrospective review of 474 previously untreated patients with major salivary gland cancers in an attempt to define indications for elective treatment of the neck. Overall, clinically occult, pathologically + LN occurred in only 12% of patients. On multivariate analysis, only primary tumor size and grade were significant risk factors.
- Chen et al. (2007a, b): retrospective analysis of 251 patients with clinically N0 salivary gland carcinomas treated with surgery and postoperative radiation therapy. Ten-year regional (neck) failure was 13%. Median time to neck relapse was 1.4 year. Ten-year actuarial rates of nodal failure for T1, T2, T3, and T4 disease were 7, 5, 12, and 16%, respectively. ENI reduced 10-year estimated nodal failure from 26 to 0%.
- North et al. (1990): retrospective analysis of 87 patients with major salivary gland cancer treated with surgery or surgery +

post-op RT. The addition of post-op RT significantly improved 5-year OS (59→75%) LF (26→4%).

- Storey et al. (2001): retrospective analysis of 83 patients treated with surgery and postoperative RT for submandibular gland malignancies. Actuarial 10-year LRC was 88%, 10-year DFS was 53%, and OS was 55%.
- Terhaard et al. (2005): retrospective analysis of 538 patients treated for major salivary gland tumors. Post-op RT improved 10-year LC compared with surgery alone for patients with T3-4 tumors (18→84%), close (55→95%) and incomplete resection (44→82%), bone invasion (54→86%), and PNI (60→88%).
- Chen et al. (2007a, b): retrospective analysis of 207 patients with major salivary gland carcinomas treated with definitive surgery without postoperative radiation therapy. Five and 10-year LRC were 86 and 74%, respectively. Pathologic lymph node metastasis, high histologic grade, positive margins, and T3-4 disease were independent predictors of LRR. Presence of any one of these factors had associated 10-year LRC of 37–63%.
- Spiro et al. (1993): retrospective analysis of 62 patients with parotid gland malignancies treated with surgery and post-op RT. Actuarial 5/10-year LC was 95/84%. Patients with larger tumors, recurrent disease, or facial nerve involvement had lower DFS.
- Boahene et al. (2004): retrospective analysis of 89 patients with mucoepidermoid carcinoma of parotid gland treated predominantly with surgery alone. DFS at 5, 15, and 25 years were 99, 97, and 97%, respectively.
- Garden et al. (1994): retrospective analysis of 160 patients treated with surgery and post-op RT for minor salivary gland cancer. Fifteen-year LC, DFS, and OS were 78, 54, and 43%, respectively. On multivariate analysis, paranasal primary site associated with increased risk of LF.
- Loh et al. (2009): retrospective analysis of 171 patients treated by surgery alone (30.7%), surgery and post-op RT (30.7%), or RT alone (38.6%) for minor salivary gland cancer. Ten-year DFS, DSS, and OS were 48, 67, and 58%, respectively. LR and DM were 27 and 19%, respectively. On multivariate analysis, grade of tumor associated with DSS.
- RTOG/MRC (Laramore et al. 1993): randomized trial of 32 patients with inoperable primary or recurrent salivary gland cancer compared fast neutron RT vs. conventional RT with photons and/or electrons. Trial was stopped early due to advantage

with neutrons [improved 10-year LRC, but not OS (15–25%)]. Distant metastases accounted for most failures.

- Wang and Goodman (1991): retrospective analysis of 24 patients treated with RT alone for salivary gland malignancies. All lesions were irradiated by accelerated hyperfractionated photons (bid) with 1.6 Gy per fraction, intermixed with various boost techniques including electron beam, intraoral cone, interstitial implant, and/or submental photons for a total of 65–70 Gy. Five-year LC for parotid gland lesions was 100% with 65% OS. For minor salivary gland tumors, the 5-year LC was 78% and OS was 93%.
- Mendenhall et al. (2004): retrospective analysis of 101 patients treated with RT for adenoid cystic carcinoma of the H&N. Ten-year LC was 43% for patients treated with RT alone compared to 91% for patients treated with surgery and post-op RT. On multivariate analysis, T stage and clinical nerve invasion influenced CSS.

RADIATION TECHNIQUES

SIMULATION AND FIELD DESIGN

- Simulate supine with customized immobilization devices.
- Head secured in holder with face mask and neck hyperextended.
- All incisional scars and masses are wired for visualization.
- Bite block used to facilitate immobilization and reduce amount of normal tissue in field.
- Shoulder pull board can be employed to maximally depress shoulders.
- CT-planning allows for more accurate dose distribution.
- Various techniques have been described for salivary gland radiation.
- Post-op tumor volume includes operative bed with at least 2 cm margin.
- Mixed photon/electron beam can be used en face to cover target volume with margin. Weighting is generally 50–80% weighting toward electrons. Electron energy depends on distance from skin of ipsilateral cheek to oral mucosa. Typically, 12–16 MeV electrons are used in combination with 4–6-MV photons.
- Wedge pair technique with photons can also be used with anterior/posterior obliques. To avoid exit dose through contralateral eye, slightly angle beams inferiorly. Include entire surgical bed in irradiated tumor volume with bolus over the scar.

- Consider neutron therapy for unresectable or medically inoperable tumors.
- IMRT may be used to spare normal tissues and dose-escalate.
- Elective RT to the neck depends on histology, primary site, and presentation.
- Treatment of contralateral lymph nodes is unnecessary since failure there is rare.
- Using photons, AP/PA, or direct AP fields can be used.
- Neck field is angled obliquely to keep off spinal cord.
- With neck RT, attention to geometric match with primary field is essential.
- Half-beam block is used for the cranial edge of the neck field to eliminate divergence.
- For adenoid cystic carcinoma, irradiate pathways of cranial nerves to base of skull.

DOSE PRESCRIPTIONS

- Post-op RT, negative margins: 60–63 Gy at 1.8–2 Gy/fx
- Post-op RT, +margins 66 Gy at 1.8–2 Gy/fx
- RT alone or post-op RT for gross residual disease: 70 at 1.8–2 Gy/fx
- Elective neck RT: 50–54 Gy at 1.8–2 Gy/fx

DOSE LIMITATIONS

- Spinal cord ≤45 Gy, brainstem ≤54 Gy, optic chiasm and nerves ≤54 Gy, cochlea ≤50 Gy, mandible ≤60–70 Gy, temporal brain ≤60 Gy, uninvolved salivary glands ≤24 Gy.

COMPLICATIONS

- Xerostomia, trismus, otitis media, hair loss, skin erythema and desquamation, dental problems, taste loss, hypothyroidism, mucositis, oral candidiasis, esophagitis, CN palsy, second malignancy.

FOLLOW-UP

- H&P every 1–3 months for 1 year, every 2–4 months for second year, every 4–6 months for years 3–5, and annually thereafter. Regular head imaging with MRI and CXR as indicated. TSH every 6–12 months if neck irradiated.

Acknowledgement We thank Allen Chen for his contribution to this chapter in the first edition.

REFERENCES

Armstrong JG, Harrison LB, Thaler HT, et al. The indications for elective treatment of the neck in cancer of the major salivary glands. Cancer 1992; 69: 615-619.

Armstrong JG, Harrison LB, Spiro RH, et al. Malignant tumors of major salivary gland origin. A matched-pair analysis of the role of combined surgery and postoperative radiotherapy. Arch Otolaryngol Head Neck Surg 1990; 116:290-293.

Boahene DK, Olsen KD, Lewis, JE, et al. Mucoepidermoid carcinoma of the parotid gland. Arch Otolaryngol Head Neck Surg 2004; 130: 849-856.

Chen AM, Granchi PJ, Garcia J, et al. Local-regional recurrence after surgery without postoperative irradiation for carcinomas of the major salivary glands: implications for adjuvant therapy. Int J Radiat Oncol Biol Phys 2007;67:982-987.

Chen AM, Garcia J, Lee NY, Bucci MK, Eisele DW. Patters of nodal relapse after surgery and postoperative radiation therapy for carcinomas of the major and minor salivary glands: what is the role of elective neck irradiation? Int J Radiat Oncol Biol Phys 2007; 67: 988-994.

Fu KK, Leibel SA, Levine ML, et al. Carcinoma of the major and minor salivary glands. Cancer 1977; 40: 2882-2890.

Garden AS, El-Naggar AK, Morrison WH, et al. Postoperative radiotherapy for malignant tumors of the parotid gland. Int J Radiat Oncol Biol Phys 1997; 37:79-85.

Garden AS, Weber RS, Ang KK, et al. Postoperative radiation therapy for malignant tumors of minor salivary glands. Cancer 1994;73:2563-2569.

Garden AS, Weber RS, Morrison WH, et al. The influence of positive margins and nerve invasion in adenoid cystic carcinoma of the head and neck treated with surgery and radiation. Int J Radiat Oncol Biol Phys 1995;32:619-626.

Laramore GE, Krall JM, Griffin TW, et al. Neutron versus photon irradiation for unresectable salivary gland tumors: final report of an RTOG-MRC randomized clinical trial. Radiation Therapy Oncology Group. Medical Research Council. Int J Radiat Oncol Biol Phys 1993;27:235-240.

Loh KS, Barker E, Bruch G, et al. Prognostic factors in malignancy of the minor salivary glands. Head Neck 2009;31:58-63.

Mendenhall WM, Morris CG, Amdur RJ, et al. Radiotherapy alone or combined with surgery for adenoid cystic carcinoma of the head and neck. Head Neck 2004;26:154-162.

North CA, Lee DJ, Piantadosi S, et al. Carcinoma of the major salivary glands treated by surgery or surgery plus postoperative radiotherapy. Int J Radiat Oncol Biol Phys 1990;18:1319-1326.

Spiro IJ, Wang CC, Montgomery WW. Carcinoma of the parotid gland. Analysis of treatment results and patterns of failure after combined surgery and radiation therapy. Cancer 1993;71:2699-2705.

Storey MR, Garden AS, Morrison WH, et al. Postoperative radiotherapy for malignant tumors of the submandibular gland. Int J Radiat Oncol Biol Phys 2001;51:952-958.

Terhaard CH, Lubsen H, Rasch CR, et al. The role of radiotherapy in the treatment of malignant salivary gland tumors. Int J Radiat Oncol Biol Phys 2005;61:103-111.

Wang CC, Goodman M. Photon irradiation of unresectable carcinomas of salivary glands. Int J Radiat Oncol Biol Phys 1991;21:569-576.

FURTHER READING

Bragg CM, Conway J, Robinson MH. The role of intensity-modulated radiotherapy in the treatment of parotid tumors. Int J Radiat Oncol Biol Phys 2002;52:729-738.

Douglas JG, Koh WJ, Austin-Seymour M, et al. Treatment of salivary gland neoplasms with fast neutron radiotherapy. Arch Otolaryngol Head Neck Surg 2003;129:944-948.

Chapter 11
Thyroid Cancer

Jennifer S. Yu, Joy Coleman, and Jeanne Marie Quivey

III

PEARLS

- Thyroid cancer is rare – 1% of malignancies and 0.2% of cancer deaths in the US. Incidence is increasing, which may, in part, be related to increased detection of subclinical disease by extensive use of ultrasound and FNA. Female:male ratio of 3:1. Incidence begins increasing in teenage years, peaking in the fifth decade.
- Prior radiation exposure is the main environmental factor linked to development. It can result in benign (goiter, nodular disease) and malignant thyroid disease. Radiation induced tumors are usually well-differentiated and behave similar to spontaneous thyroid cancer. Periodic clinical and biochemical testing (serum thyroglobulin) is prudent for those who have undergone prior thyroid irradiation (including incidental irradiation during mantle or head and neck radiation). No evidence to support increased incidence of medullary or anaplastic thyroid cancer in patients previously exposed to radiation.
- Pathology – listed in order of declining prognosis:
  - Papillary thyroid carcinoma (several variants; all arise from follicular cells).
    - Solid papillary thyroid carcinoma – good prognosis.
    - Follicular variant, formerly called mixed papillary-follicular, but not to be confused with follicular carcinoma (demonstrates biologic and prognostic characteristics of papillary carcinoma). Good prognosis.
    - Diffuse sclerosing, tall cell, columnar cell – all have poor prognosis.
    - Takes up RAI.
  - Follicular thyroid carcinoma (arises from follicular cells).
    - No cytologic features distinguish minimally invasive carcinomas from benign follicular adenomas. Therefore, cannot diagnose on FNA.
    - Takes up RAI.

- Hürthle Cell (oncocytic carcinoma).
  - Cell of origin unclear: historically thought to be follicular variant, but molecular studies suggest it may be more similar to papillary.
  - Can be benign or malignant – if they do not demonstrate evidence of microscopic invasion, they behave like adenomas. If they have histologic evidence of malignancy, they are usually more aggressive than ordinary follicular/papillary carcinomas (10-year survival 76 vs. 85%).
  - Takes up RAI.
- Medullary thyroid cancer.
  - Arises from the parafollicular/C cells that produce calcitonin.
  - Often multifocal or bilateral, lymph nodes commonly involved.
  - Monitor disease by calcitonin levels.
  - Twenty to thirty percent familial so work up for MEN.
  - MEN 2 is autosomal dominant; it involves the RET proto-oncogene on chromosome 10. MEN 2A – pheochromocytoma, parathyroid tumors, medullary thyroid cancer. MEN 2B – Marfanoid habitus, ganglioneuromas of the mucosa and GI tract, pheochromocytomas, mucosal neuromas of tongue and lips, medullary thyroid cancer. Lifetime risk for carriers ~90%. It is codon dependent and age dependent. Prophylactic total thyroidectomy produces cure rate >90%.
  - C cells do not take up RAI, but may consider treating with RAI in inoperable cases as nearby follicular cells will take up RAI and may kill adjacent medullary thyroid cancer cells in thyroid bed. Note: RAI would not treat involved LN or distant sites of disease.
- Anaplastic thyroid carcinoma.
  - Rare; aggressive.
  - Must be distinguished from poorly differentiated medullary carcinoma, lymphoma, and poorly differentiated follicular carcinoma (all have different treatment and better prognosis).
  - Poor prognostic markers: older age, male gender, tumor >7 cm, extent of disease, LN involvement, metastasis, leukocytosis, poor performance status, presence of acute symptoms.
  - Does not take up RAI.

- Lymphatic drainage initially to the central compartment, nodes in the tracheo-esophageal groove, and the nodes anterior to the larynx just above the isthmus (Delphian nodes). Cervical nodes also frequently involved; less commonly the anterior mediastinum, and occasionally, the supraclavicular and retropharyngeal nodes. All of these sites must be considered in treatment planning.

- Sites of DM: lung > bone > liver.
- Prognostic factors: age is the most important prognostic factor determining survival in well-differentiated thyroid cancers and is reflected in staging criteria. Poor prognostic factors: old age, large tumor size, extrathyroidal extension (ETE), higher histologic grade, postoperative macroscopic residual disease, male sex, and distant metastases.
- Treatment modalities: surgery (total thyroidectomy or near-total thyroidectomy preferred, prophylactic central neck and lateral neck dissection controversial), thyroid hormone suppression, RAI. Consider EBRT ± chemotherapy if high risk (multiple recurrences, positive margins, no RAI uptake, or anaplastic cell type).

III

WORKUP

- Many present with asymptomatic palpable thyroid nodule. Advanced cases can present with larger masses, hoarseness caused by recurrent laryngeal nerve paralysis, or invasion into the larynx, pharynx, or esophagus. Can also present in a thyroglossal duct cyst (rare) or with cervical nodal mets. Occasionally, can present with DM in lung or skeleton.
- FNA is the most important diagnostic tool. Sensitivity 98%, specificity 99%, accuracy 98%. Results can be benign, suspicious, malignant, or unsatisfactory/indeterminant. A negative FNA still requires careful consideration of all clinical factors before a decision to perform repeat FNA or advance to an excisional bx/lobectomy can be made. A suspicious or indeterminate finding on FNA does not exclude follicular carcinoma.
- Radionuclide scintigraphy and thyroid ultrasound are complementary tests that can help provide additional information. Should be performed after FNA (if FNA is positive, they are superfluous and not cost effective for evaluating the thyroid gland).
- US of the neck or MRI are useful to detect adenopathy. Do not use iodinated contrast with CT scan as this will block treatment with I-131 for up to 6 months (24 h urinary iodine measurement will indicate when RAI treatment possible).
- Blood tests: T3, T4, TSH, thyroglobulin.

- If FNA indicates medullary carcinoma, check serum calcitonin, CEA, and calcium as well as urine and serum catecholamines (to screen for pheochromocytoma). If positive for pheochromocytoma, this should be treated first. With more advanced disease, medullary carcinoma can present with diarrhea from calcitonin production. This carries a poor prognosis. Medullary carcinoma can be a finding in MEN 2 patients, and families must be screened for the RET proto-oncogene. If a RET proto-oncogene germline mutation is detected, other family members should undergo codon oriented prophylactic surgery (COPS). The specific codon involved will dictate the appropriate timing of surgery for other family members.
- Check TSH levels prior to initiating RAI therapy. It should be high for maximal efficacy.

STAGING: THYROID CANCER

Editors' note: All TNM stage and stage groups referred to elsewhere in this chapter reflect the 2002 AJCC staging nomenclature unless otherwise noted as the new system below was published after this chapter was written.

(AJCC 6TH ED., 2002)

Primary tumor (T)

Note: All categories may be subdivided: (a) solitary tumor and (b) multifocal tumor (the largest determines the classification)

TX: Primary tumor cannot be assessed
T0: No evidence of primary tumor
T1: Tumor 2 cm or less in greatest dimension limited to the thyroid
T2: Tumor more than 2 cm but not more than 4 cm in greatest dimension limited to thyroid
T3: Tumor more than 4 cm in greatest dimension limited to thyroid or any tumor with minimal extrathyroid extension (e.g., extension to sternothyroid muscle or perithyroid soft tissues)
T4a: Tumor of any size extending beyond the thyroid capsule to invade subcutaneous soft tissues, larynx, trachea, esophagus, or recurrent laryngeal nerve
T4b: Tumor invades prevertebral fascia or encases carotid artery or mediastinal vessels

All anaplastic carcinomas are considered T4 with T4a being surgically resectable and T4b being surgically unresectable

T4a: Intrathyroidal anaplastic carcinoma – surgically resectable
T4b: Extrathyroidal anaplastic carcinoma – surgically unresectable

Regional lymph nodes (N)

Regional lymph nodes are the central compartment, lateral cervical, and upper mediastinal lymph nodes

NX: Regional lymph nodes cannot be assessed.
N0: No regional lymph node metastasis
N1: Regional lymph node metastasis
- N1a: Metastasis to Level VI LN (pretracheal, paratracheal, and prelaryngeal/Delphian lymph nodes)

(AJCC 7TH ED., 2010)

Primary tumor (T)

Note: All categories may be subdivided: (s) solitary tumor and (m) multifocal tumor (the largest determines the classification)

TX: Primary tumor cannot be assessed
T0: No evidence of primary tumor
T1: Tumor 2 cm or less in greatest dimension limited to the thyroid
- T1a: Tumor 1 cm or less, limited to the thyroid
- T1b: Tumor more than 1 cm but not more than 2 cm in greatest dimension, limited to the thyroid

T2: Tumor more than 2 cm but not more than 4 cm in greatest dimension limited to the thyroid
T3: Tumor more than 4 cm in greatest dimension limited to the thyroid or any tumor with minimal extrathyroid extension (e.g., extension to sternothyroid muscle or perithyroid soft tissues)
T4a: Moderately advanced disease. Tumor of any size extending beyond the thyroid capsule to invade subcutaneous soft tissues, larynx, trachea, esophagus, or recurrent laryngeal nerve
T4b: Very advanced disease. Tumor invades prevertebral fascia or encases carotid artery or mediastinal vessels

All anaplastic carcinomas are considered T4 tumors

T4a: Intrathyroidal anaplastic carcinoma
T4b: Anaplastic carcinoma with gross extrathyroid extension

Regional lymph nodes (N)

Regional lymph nodes are the central compartment, lateral cervical, and upper mediastinal lymph nodes

NX: Regional lymph nodes cannot be assessed
N0: No regional lymph node metastasis
N1: Regional lymph node metastasis

continued

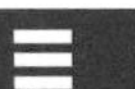

N1b: Metastasis to unilateral, bilateral, or contralateral cervical or superior mediastinal lymph nodes

Distant metastases (M)
MX: Distant metastasis cannot be assessed
M0: No distant metastasis
M1: Distant metastases

Stage grouping
Separate stage grouping is recommended for papillary or follicular, medullary, and anaplastic (undifferentiated) carcinoma
Papillary or follicular: under age 45
I: Any T any N M0
II: Any T any N M1
Papillary or follicular: age 45 years and older or Medullary carcinoma
I: T1 N0 M0
II: T2 N0 M0
III: T3 N0 M0
T1-3 N1a M0
IVA: T4a N0-1b M0
T1-3 N1b M0
IVB: T4b any N M0
IVC: Any T any N M1
Anaplastic carcinomas
IVA: T4a any N M0
IVB: T4b any N M0
IVC: Any T any N M1

Survival
Follicular and papillary: 95–97% DSS at 20 years (follicular and papillary, respectively)
Tumor size >1.5 cm, male, and age >45 have increased mortality
Medullary: 60–80% DSS at 10 years
Anaplastic: 25% 1-year DSS

N1a: Metastasis to Level VI (pretracheal, paratracheal, and prelaryngeal/Delphian lymph nodes)
N1b: Metastasis to unilateral, bilateral, or contralateral cervical (Levels I, II, III, IV, or V) or retropharyngeal or superior mediastinal lymph nodes (Level VII)

Distant metastasis (M)
M0: No distant metastasis
M1: Distant metastasis

Anatomic stage/prognostic groups
Separate stage groupings are recommended for papillary or follicular (differentiated), medullary, and anaplastic (undifferentiated) carcinoma
Papillary or follicular (differentiated)
Under 45 years
I: Any T Any N M0
II: Any T Any N M1
45 Years and older
I: T1 N0 M0
II: T2 N0 M0
III: T3 N0 M0
T1-T3 N1a M0
IVA: T4a N0 M0
T4a N1a M0
T1-T3 N1b M0
T4a N1b M0
IVB: T4b Any N M0
IVC: Any T Any N M1
Medullary carcinoma (all age groups)
I: T1 N0 M0
II: T2-T3 N0 M0
III: T1-T3 N1a M0
IVA: T4a N0 M0
T4a N1a M0
T1-T3 N1b M0
T4a N1b M0

continued

IVB: T4b Any N M0
IVC: Any T Any N M1
Anaplastic carcinoma
All anaplastic carcinomas are considered Stage IV
IVA: T4a Any N M0
IVB: T4b Any N M0
IVC: Any T Any N M1

Used with the permission from the American Joint Committee on Cancer (AJCC), Chicago, IL. The original source for this material is the AJCC Cancer Staging Manual, Seventh Edition (2010), published by Springer Science+Business Media.

III

TREATMENT RECOMMENDATIONS

Papillary/follicular/Hürthle cell	Recommended treatment
Low-risk disease Well differentiated, age 15–45 years, no prior RT, no LN or DM, no extrathyroidal extension, no FH of thyroid cancer, and tumor <4 cm in diameter	■ Total thyroidectomy. At 4–6 weeks post-op, TSH, thyroglobulin, and anti-thyroglobulin antibodies measured along with total body RAI scan →RAI treatment if indicated. Common indications include elevated thyroglobulin >1 ng/mL or a positive RAI scan ■ Lobectomy + isthmusectomy with no RAI is an option for low-risk patients, but not considered standard because it makes follow-up with TSH, thyroglobulin, and RAI difficult/impossible ■ Incidental micropapillary carcinoma (≤1 cm). Slow-growing. Treatment is controversial-observation vs. unilateral lobectomy ± levothyroxine therapy. Consider more aggressive treatment (total thyroidectomy ± neck dissection, RAI) if multifocal, N+ or M+
High-risk disease Age <15 year or >45 years, RT history, known regional or DM, multifocal tumor, ECE, tumor >4 cm, or +FH	■ Thyroidectomy with LN dissection followed by RAI scan and tx. If LN+, then post-op RAI ± EBRT
Local/regional recurrence	■ LN recurrence: neck dissection followed by RAI. Small volume disease in the superior mediastinum: RAI alone. Large volume mediastinal disease: superior mediastinal dissection followed by RAI. EBRT used for persistent/recurrent disease after surgery and RAI. Other indications include patients with unresectable disease or patients with no uptake on RAI
Metastatic disease	■ Can have long survival so treat aggressively with RAI and EBRT, depending on site of metastasis. Survival times longest for patients with diffuse, small-lung metastases that concentrate RAI. Chemo not very effective. Most effective is single agent doxorubicin. Total thyroidectomy important even in the face of DM to allow for treatment with RAI

Medullary carcinoma	Recommended treatment
Local/regional disease	■ Total thyroidectomy with central Level VI LN dissection. Consider ipsilateral cervical Level II–V. Contralateral cervical LN dissection only if ipsilateral nodes are positive. EBRT for patients with gross/microscopic residual disease after surgery, extensive regional LN involvement, T4a disease, or unresectable disease. Check serum calcitonin and CEA post-op to help determine if residual/metastatic disease is present. No role for chemo
Metastatic disease	■ Palliative chemo (doxorubicin ± cisplatin), hormonal therapy (octreotide), and/or local RT. Consider a clinical trial: EGFR receptors being tested in phase II clinical trials
Anaplastic	■ Complete surgical resection gives only chance of cure. If GTR not possible, then radical surgery is not indicated but airway management is needed. EBRT used for LC and to palliate symptoms. Altered fractionation and concurrent chemo-RT is under investigation due to poor LC with EBRT alone. Clinical trials preferred. No role for RAI

EBRT TRIALS

- No major prospective, randomized trials have been successful in enrolling adequate patient numbers. However, large international groups are studying the incidence, biology, and treatment of thyroid cancers, such as EUROMEN and the International RET Mutation Consortium for MTC.

DIFFERENTIATED THYROID CANCER

- *PMH experience* (Brierley et al. 2005): retrospective review of 729 patients with papillary or follicular thyroid cancer treated with surgery and/or RAI and/or EBRT. Median follow-up 11 years. Overall 10-year CSS 87.3%, 10-year local-regional relapse-free rate (LRFR) 84.9%. RAI improved overall LRFR (HR 0.5, $p = 0.007$). No benefit of RAI in low-risk, Stage I patients ≤45 years. EBRT improved 10-year LRFR (85.4 vs. 95.9%, $p = 0.03$), but not CSS (98.2 vs. 100%, $p = 0.09$) among patients <60 years. EBRT improved both 10-year CSS (81 vs. 64.4%, $p = 0.04$) and LRFR (86.4 vs. 65.7%, $p = 0.01$) in high risk, elderly patients (age >60 years, ETE but no gross residual disease).

- *Hong Kong experience* (Chow et al. 2002): retrospective review of 842 patients with papillary thyroid cancer treated with surgery and/or RAI, and/or RT. Mean follow-up 9.2 years. Distribution of patients by stage (1/2/3/4/unknown) 59%/9.6%/26%/2.3%/3.4%. Ten-year CSS by stage: 99.8%/91.8%/77.4%/37.1%. If M0 and no post-op LR disease, RAI improved LRC (RR = 0.29) and DM (RR = 0.2), but not CSS. EBRT improved LRC, particularly in patients with gross residual disease [10-year LRC 56% (+RT) vs. 24% (no RT)].
- *Hurthle cell carcinoma* (Foote et al. 2003): retrospective review of 18 patients receiving RT for Hurthle cell carcinoma of the thyroid gland between 1943 and 1995. Five patients received adjuvant RT, seven received salvage RT for unresectable recurrent disease, and 6 received palliative RT for DM. Five-year OS and CSS rates were 66.7 and 71.8%, respectively. Adjuvant and salvage RT prevented recurrence in 4/5 and 3/5 patients, respectively. Salvage RT was successful in 3 of 5 patients treated with EBRT.
- *Incidental papillary microcarcinoma*, Mayo Clinic experience (Hay et al. 2008): review of 900 patients status postsurgery (85% with bilateral lobar resection, 50% nodal resection – 27% with "node picking," 23% compartment dissection). Mean follow-up 17.2 years. Ninety-eight percent intrathyroidal, 30% with neck nodal involvement, 0.3% with DM at diagnosis. Seventeen percent received RAI. OS similar to age-matched controls. Only 0.3% died of disease. Multifocal disease and LN+ at higher risk of recurrence, but overall risk of recurrence was low, 6%/8% at 20/40 years. No difference in recurrence rate if total thyroidectomy or RAI vs. unilateral lobectomy alone.

MEDULLARY THYROID CANCER

- *MDACC experience* (Schwartz et al. 2008): retrospective review of 34 patients with advanced medullary cancer (Stage IVa–c) treated with surgery and post-op RT. Median RT dose for all patients 60 Gy/30 fx (66 Gy if gross disease, 50.5 Gy if metastatic at time of presentation). Five-year locoregional relapse-free survival 87%, DSS 62%, OS 56%.

ANAPLASTIC THYROID CARCINOMA

- *SEER analysis* (Kebebew et al. 2005): 516 patients diagnosed between 1973 and 2000 drawn from the SEER database. Sixty-four percent of patients underwent resection of their tumor, and 63% received EBRT. The overall CSS was 68.4% at 6 months and 80.7% at 12 months. On multivariate analysis, only age <60 years, an intrathyroidal tumor, and the combined use of surgery and EBRT were independent predictors of lower cause-specific mortality.
- *SEER reanalysis* (Chen, Am J Clin Oncol 2008): 261 patients with anaplastic thyroid cancer treated with surgery with or without adjuvant RT. In contrast to Kebebew analysis, excluded patients with <1 month survival after diagnosis and all patients were operable candidates. Thirty-eight percent patients presented with DM. MS 4 months. RT improved survival for patients with ETE involving adjacent tissues, but not patients with disease confined to capsule, further extension, or DM. Poor prognostic factors on multivariate analysis: disease extension beyond thyroid, DM, older age, tumor size >7 cm, no treatment.

RADIATION TECHNIQUES

SIMULATION AND FIELD DESIGN

- Simulate patient supine with neck extended using an aquaplast mask to immobilize head and shoulders.
- Must decide when to treat thyroid bed alone (for differentiated thyroid carcinoma without extensive extrathyroidal disease) vs. thyroid, neck, and superior mediastinum (essentially all other definitive treatment).
- When treating the thyroid alone, treat from the hyoid superiorly to just below the suprasternal notch. CT treatment planning is encouraged to ensure adequate coverage of substernal thyroid. Can use an anterior electron beam vs. anterolateral wedged pair.
- For large volume treatment, there are many different treatment possibilities, but 3DCRT or IMRT is essential due to the target volume's size, shape, and proximity to other critical structures (including the spinal cord, larynx, and lungs). In general, low-risk CTV includes uninvolved bilateral cervical nodes (Levels II–IV, VI, ± retropharyngeal nodes) and superior mediastinal nodes. Volume typically extends from mastoid tip to aortic arch. High-risk CTV includes primary tumor bed and central nodal compartment, areas with involved nodes.

- Boost gross residual disease or any areas of ETE to doses listed below.

DOSE PRESCRIPTIONS

- Papillary/follicular/medullary: treat low-risk CTV to 54 Gy, higher-risk areas for microscopic disease to 59.4–63 Gy, positive margins to 63–66 Gy, and macroscopic disease to 66–70 Gy.
- Anaplastic: conventional fractionation to ≥65 Gy. Due to poor response with standard fractionation, some use 1.5 Gy b.i.d. to 60 Gy ± chemo. For patients with poor KPS or known metastasis, a palliative approach can be used.

DOSE LIMITATIONS

- From EBRT: esophagus <50–60 Gy. Salivary gland <24 Gy mean dose (consider RAI also affects salivary function). Spinal cord ≤45–50 Gy. Brachial plexus <60 Gy. Lung 2/3 <20 Gy.
- From RAI: total dose to bone marrow is 2 Gy.

NUCLEAR MEDICINE

- The details of treatment with RAI are beyond the scope of this book. Readers are referred to nuclear medicine literature for details about the procedure.
- RAI indicated for papillary, follicular, and some medullary thyroid cancers.
- Treatment with ^{131}I requires preparation with thyroxine withdrawal and a low iodine diet in order to maximize uptake of RAI. Synthyroid (T4) is stopped for 6 weeks and cytomel (T3) given for the first 3 weeks prior to scanning and treatment. For the last 2–3 weeks, patients are given no replacement at all and started on a low iodine diet.
- Recombinant TSH (rhTSH, thyrogen) – alternative to thyroid hormone withdrawal. Allows scanning without thyroxine withdrawal, which does not require induced hypothyroidism, and thus is better tolerated by patients, but its use is relatively new and it is still gaining acceptance. The patient still needs to be on the low iodine diet.
- RAI scan is performed first to determine if treatment is appropriate and to determine the appropriate therapeutic dose. Treat with 100–200 mCi within 5 days of the diagnostic scan. Some physicians skip the diagnostic scan for fears of blunting uptake

at the time of treatment and prescribe a fixed dose of 100 mCi. Others standardly prescribe 30 mCi as this is easier to deal with from a nuclear regulatory commission perspective, but this lower dose is much less effective. Rescan 7–10 days after treatment to identify additional foci of uptake undetected on the diagnostic scan and to document sites of disease treated.

- Repeat diagnostic RAI scan ~4–6 months later if the first scan is positive. If repeat scan is positive, can retreat or rescan in 6 months. Continue rescanning and retreating until all detectable tumor cells has disappeared by I-131 scan. Once scan is negative, repeat in 1–2 years. If this is negative, then follow clinically.
- Never use iodinated contrast in a patient who will need RAI within 3–6 months.

COMPLICATIONS

- From EBRT: acute – skin breakdown, esophagitis, mucositis, changes in taste, xerostomia, laryngitis. Late – skin changes, fibrosis, lymphedema under chin, xerostomia, dental carries, esophageal stenosis.
- From RAI: acute – sialadenitis, xerostomia, cystitis (encourage good hydration), radiation gastritis (nausea, vomiting), diarrhea, pain (from localized tumor picking-up RAI very well), transient leucopenia/thrombocytopenia. Transient oligospermia in males. Rarely, thyrotoxicosis during the first 1–2 weeks due to tumor lysis and release or thyroid hormone. Manage with propranolol. Acute radiation pneumonitis if extensive pulmonary metastases are present.
- Chronic side effects – increased risk of leukemia with cumulative doses >800 mCi, increased risk of breast and bladder cancer with doses >1,000 mCi; late pulmonary fibrosis in patients with diffuse pulmonary metastases. No increased incidence of infertility, miscarriages, stillbirth, prematurity, and congenital anomalies, although most advise that patients wait 6 months before attempting pregnancy.

FOLLOW-UP

- H&P, labs (thyrotropin, free T3, thyroglobulin, TSH), US of the neck every 6 months. MRI neck increasing in use. Frequency of RAI scans controversial. Disadvantage is the requirement for thyroxine withdrawal and resultant hypothyroidism, but use of recombinant TSH (thyrogen) may allow scanning without thyroxine withdrawal. PET/CT scans are sometimes useful in patients with elevation of thyroglobulin, but no uptake with RAI. Serum calcitonin useful for following medullary thyroid carcinoma.

REFERENCES

Brierley J, Tsang R, Panzarella T, et al. Prognostic factors and the effect of treatment with radioactive iodine and external beam radiation on patients with differentiated thyroid cancer seen at a single institution over 40 years. Clin Endocrinol (Oxf) 2005;63(4):418-427.

Chen J, Tward J, Shrieve DC, et al. Surgery and radiotherapy improves survival in patients with anaplastic thyroid carcinoma: analysis of the surveillance, epidemiology, and end results 1983-2002. Am J Clin Oncol 2008: 460-464.

Chow SM, Law SCK, Mendenhall WM, et al. Papillary thyroid carcinoma: prognostic factors and the role of radioiodine and external radiotherapy. IJROBP 2002;52(3):784-795.

Foote RL, Brown PD, Garces YI, et al. Is there a role for radiation therapy in the management of Hurthle cell carcinoma? Int J Radiat Oncol Biol Phys 2003;56(4):1067-1072.

Hay ID, Hutchinson ME, Gonzalez-Losada T, et al. Papillary thyroid microcarcinoma: a study of 900 cases observed in a 60-year period. Surgery 2008;144(6):980-987.

Kebebew E, Greenspan FS, Clark OH, et al. Anaplastic thyroid carcinoma. Treatment outcome and prognostic factors. Cancer 2005;103(7):1330-1335.

Schwartz DL, Rana V, Shaw S, et al. Postoperative radiotherapy for advanced medullary thyroid cancer- local disease control in the modern era. Head Neck 2008;30:883-888.

FURTHER READING

Biermann M, Pixberg MK, Schuck A, Heinecke A, Kopcke W, Schmid KW, Dralle H, Willich N, Schober O. Multicenter study differentiated thyroid carcinoma (MSDS). Diminished acceptance of adjuvant external beam radiotherapy. Nuklearmedizin. 2003;42(6):244-250.

Fraker DL, Skarulis M, Livolsi V. Thyroid Tumors. In: Davita VT, Hellman S, and Rosenberg SA, editors. Cancer: Principles and practice of oncology. 6th ed. Philadelphia: Lippincott Williams & Wilkins. pp. 1740-1763.

Leenhardt L, Grosclaude P, Cherie-Challine L; Thyroid Cancer Committee. Increased incidence of thyroid carcinoma in France: a true epidemic or thyroid nodule management effects? Report from the French Thyroid Cancer Committee. Thyroid 2004;14(12):1056-1060.

Machens A, Ukkat J, Brauckhoff M, et al. Advances in the management of hereditary medullary thyroid cancer. J Intern Med 2005;257(1):50-59.

Nahas Z, Goldenberg D, Fakhry C, et al. The role of positron emission tomography/computed tomography in the management of recurrent papillary thyroid carcinoma. Laryngoscope 2005;115(2):237-243.

NCCN Physician Guidelines. http://www.nccn.org/professionals/physician_gls/PDF/thyroid.pdf. Accessed May 8, 2009.

Posner MD, Quivey JM, Akazawa PF, et al. Dose optimization for the treatment of anaplastic thyroid carcinoma: a comparison of treatment planning techniques. Int J Radiat Oncol Biol Phys 2000;48:475-483.

Reynolds RM, Weir J, Stockton DL, Brewster DH, et al. Changing trends in incidence and mortality of thyroid cancer in Scotland. Clin Endocrinol (Oxf) 2005;62(2):156-162.

Rosenbluth BD, Serrano V, Happersett L, et al. Intensity-modulated radiation therapy for the treatment of nonanaplastic thyroid cancer. Int J Radiat Oncol Biol Phys 2005;63(5):1419-1426.

Swift PS, Larson S, Price DC. Cancer of the Thyroid. In: Leibel SA, Phillips TL, editors. Textbook of radiation oncology. 2nd ed. Philadelphia: Saunders; 2004. pp. 757-778.

Tsang RW, Brierly JD. The Thyroid. In: Cox JD, Ang KK, editors. Radiation oncology: Rationale, techniques, results. 8th ed. St. Louis: Mosby; 2003. pp. 310-330.

Tubiana M. Role of radioiodine in the treatment of local thyroid cancer. Int J Radiat Oncol Biol Phys 1996;36(1):263-265.

Wilson PC, Millar BM, Brierley JD. The management of advanced thyroid cancer. Clin Oncol (R Coll Radiol) 2004;16(8):561-568.

Yutan E, Clark OH. Hurthle cell carcinoma. Curr Treat Options Oncol 2001;2(4):331-335.

Chapter 12

Unusual Neoplasms of the Head and Neck

Sunanda Pejavar, Eric K. Hansen, and Sue Yom

III

PEARLS

- *Chloromas* (also called *granulocytic sarcomas* or *myeloid sarcomas*) are solid extramedullary tumors consisting of early myeloid precursors associated with AML. The name derives from the green color of affected tissues. They are more frequent with AML M4 and M5 subtypes, and are associated with t(8;21). They may herald AML relapse after remission. They present in the CNS with increased intracerebral pressure, or in the orbit with exophthalmos.
- *Chordomas* originate from the primitive notochord. Fifty percent occur in the sacrococcygeal area, 35% in the base of skull, and 15% in cervical vertebrae. The most common age is in the range of 50–60. They are more common in men (2–3:1). They are locally invasive with slow growth. Metastases occur in up to 25% of patients, but lymph node spread is uncommon. Gross total resection is accomplished in only 10–20% of patients. Protons offer improved local control.
- *Chondrosarcomas* are malignant primary bone tumors that arise in cartilaginous elements. They frequently arise in the base of skull, commonly in the sphenoid bone. They can be either high or low grade, with the majority being low grade.
- *Esthesioneuroblastomas* arise in the olfactory receptors of the nasal mucosa or cribiform plate. They present most commonly at ages 11–20 or 40–60 years, and the most common symptoms are epistaxis and nasal blockage. LN spread is ≤10% for early-stage disease, but is as high as 50% for Kadish stage C disease.
- *Glomus tumors* are also called *paragangliomas*, *chemodectomas* (when nonchromaffin producing), or *carotid body tumors* (when chromaffin producing). They arise from the carotid body, jugular bulb, or middle ear from the tympanic nerve (of Jacobson) or auricular nerve (of Arnold). They rarely spread to

nodes or metastasize (<5%). The mean age is in the 40s. They are more common in women (3:1). They present with ear pain, pulsations, tinnitus, cranial nerve palsies, or a painless mass. Biopsies may cause severe bleeding. They are associated with neurofibromatosis, MEN syndromes, and thyroid CA.

- *Hemangioblastomas* are benign vascular tumors. The most common age is in the 20–30s. Most are found in the cerebellum. It is the most common cerebellar tumor in adults. It is associated with von-Hippel Lindau disease (cerebellar and retinal hemangioblastomas, pancreatic and renal cysts, renal cell carcinoma).
- *Hemangiopericytomas* are sarcomatous lesions arising from the smooth muscle around vessels. They most commonly present in the base of the skull. They grow slowly and are locally invasive and hypervascular. They may be confused for meningioma. In the nose, they present with epistaxis. In the orbit, they present as painless proptosis. Meningeal hemangiopericytomas have >80% LR. Late metastases occur in 50–80% of patients.
- *Juvenile nasopharyngeal angiofibromas* arise most frequently in pubertal boys, but age ranges from 9 to 30 years. They present with nasal obstruction or epistaxis. They have a pronounced tendency for hemorrhage, so biopsy is contraindicated. They often contain androgen receptors and may regress with estrogen therapy. Less than 4% of patients are female.
- *Nasal NK/T cell lymphoma* (called also *lethal midline granuloma* or midline polymorphic reticulosis) presents with progressive ulceration and necrosis of midline facial tissues, and is associated with EBV. The differential diagnosis includes Wegener's granulomatosis, polymorphic reticulosis, cocaine abuse, sarcoidosis, and infection. Pathology reveals nonspecific acute and chronic inflammation with necrosis. The cause is idiopathic. It is more common in men, and presents most commonly in the nasal cavity and paranasal sinuses. The most common age is in the 50s. Must rule out Wegener's because it responds to steroids.

WORKUP

- H&P, CT, MRI, angiogram (optional), CBC, chemistries, audiogram (to establish baseline hearing), visual testing (optional), neurosurgical consultation with biopsy only as indicated (radiographic appearance may be pathognomonic).
- For hemangioblastoma, MRI brain ± CT angiography ± MRI spine (if VHL+).

- For hemangiopericytoma, consider CT chest abdomen pelvis to rule out metastases.
- For NK/T cell lymphoma, CT of abdomen and pelvis and/or whole body PET/CT, and bone marrow biopsy.

STAGING

- AML has three stages: untreated, in remission, or recurrent.
- Chordomas and chondrosarcomas are staged like sarcomas.
- *Esthesioneuroblastoma* is staged according to the *Kadish System* (A = confined to nasal cavity; B = extends to ≥1 of the paranasal sinuses; C = extends beyond nasal cavity or paranasal sinuses; D = distant metastasis).
- *Glomus tumors* are staged according to the Glassock-Jackson classification or the McCabe-Fletcher classification based on anatomic location, extension, and tumor volume.
- *Hemangiopericytomas* are staged as localized or metastatic.
- *Nasopharyngeal angiofibromas* are staged according to one of two systems: *Chandler* (I = confined to nasopharynx; II = extends to nasal cavity or sphenoid sinus; III = extends to antrum, ethmoid, pterygomaxillary and infratemporal fossa, orbit, and/or cheek; IV = intracranial extension) or *Sessions* (Ia = limited to nasopharynx and posterior nares; Ib = extends to paranasal sinuses; IIa/b/c = extends to other extracranial locations; III = intracranial extension).
- *NK/T cell lymphomas* are currently staged in the Ann Arbor lymphoma staging system.

TREATMENT RECOMMENDATIONS

Stage	Recommended treatment	Results
Chloroma	■ Often respond to systemic therapy for AML ■ Definitive RT (1.5/30 Gy) with 2–3 cm margin	>80–90% LC
Chordoma and chondrosarcoma	■ Maximal safe resection. If gross total resection, post-op RT (50–54 Gy). If subtotal resection, post-op RT (60 Gy). ■ For small tumors, may use SRS. ■ Protons beneficial, if available due to sharp dose gradient and ability to dose escalate	Chordoma: LC ~ 40%. DFS 10–20% (some long-term survivors) Chondrosarcoma: LC 50–100% (depends on extent resection and dose)

continued

Esthesioneuroblastoma	■ Surgery or RT alone (65–70 Gy) for small, low-grade tumors confined to ethmoids. Usually, combine surgery, with pre-op RT (50 Gy) or post-op RT (60 Gy), and chemo	LC: Stage A 70%, Stage B 50–65%, Stage C 30–50%
Glomus tumor	■ Pre-op embolization → maximal safe resection → post-op RT (50 Gy). Alternative SRS 12–14 Gy or EBRT (IMRT) 45–54 Gy	LC > 90%
Hemangioblastoma	■ Maximal safe resection. If GTR, observe. If STR/unresectable, SRS or EBRT (50–60 Gy) with 1–2 cm margin	LC 60–90%
Hemangiopericytoma	■ Pre-op embolization → maximal safe resection + post-op RT (60–65 Gy) with wide margins up to 5 cm. SRS may be used (12–20 Gy). Need long-term follow-up due to DM	LC ~70–90%
Nasopharyngeal angiofibroma	■ If extracranial and resectable, surgery ± embolization. Residual disease may be observed, or treated with RT if symptoms develop. If intracranial, orbital, or pterygopalatine extension, treat with RT (30–50 Gy in 2–3 Gy fractions)	RT LC ~80% but tumors regress slowly (up to 2 years)
NK/T cell lymphoma	■ Definitive RT (54 Gy) with 2–3 cm margin and treat adjacent structures (e.g., paranasal sinuses for nasal) ± doxorubicin-based chemotherapy	OS 50–60%

RADIATION TECHNIQUES

- Depend on histology and location. Refer to primary literature for details.

COMPLICATIONS

- Depend on the location, and they are in common with other head and neck sites described in this Handbook.

FOLLOW-UP

- Regular H&P, and follow-up imaging. Long-term follow-up may be needed due to late recurrences.

Acknowledgment We thank Dr. M. Kara Bucci for her contribution to this chapter in the first edition.

FURTHER READING

Carew JF, Singh B, Kraus DH. Hemangiopericytoma of the head and neck. Laryngoscope 1999;109:1409-1411.

Chao KS, Kaplan C, Simpson JR, et al. Esthesioneuroblastoma: the impact of treatment modality. Head Neck 2001;23:749-757.

Chen HH, Fong L, Su IJ, et al. Experience of radiotherapy in lethal midline granuloma with special emphasis on centrofacial T-cell lymphoma: a retrospective analysis covering a 34-year period. Radiother Oncol 1996;38:1-6.

Hinerman RW, Mendenhall WM, Amdur RJ. Definitive radiotherapy in the management of chemodectomas arising in the temporal bone, carotid body, and glomus vagale. Head Neck 2001;23:363-371.

Khairi S, Ewend MG. Chordoma. Curr Treat Options Neurol 2002;4:167-173.

Lee JT, Chen P, Safa A, et al. The role of radiation in the treatment of advanced juvenile angiofibroma. Laryngoscope 2002;112:1213-1220.

Pellitteri PK, Rinaldo A, Myssiorek D, et al. Paragangliomas of the head and neck. Oral Oncol 2004;40:563-575.

Perez CA, Thorstad WL. Unusual Neonepithelial Tumors of the Head and Neck. In: Halperin EC, Perez CA, Brady LW, editors. Principles and practice of radiation oncology. 5th ed. Philadelphia: Lippincott Williams & Wilkins; 2008. pp. 996-1034.

Tsao MN, Wara WM, Larson DA. Radiation therapy for benign central nervous system disease. Semin Radiat Oncol 1999;9:120-133.

Chapter 13

Management of the Neck and Unknown Primary of the Head and Neck

Tania Kaprealian and Sue S. Yom

III

LEVELS OF THE NECK (Fig. 13.1)

- IA: submental
  - Bounded anteriorly by mandible, posteriorly by body of hyoid bone, superiorly by inferior edge of mandible, inferiorly by midhyoid bone, laterally by medial edge of anterior belly of digastric
- IB: submandibular
  - Bounded anteriorly by mandible, posteriorly by posterior edge of the submandibular gland, superiorly by superior edge of submandibular gland, inferiorly by midhyoid bone, laterally by inner side of mandible, and medially by lateral edge of anterior belly of digastric muscle
- II: upper jugular
  - Bounded superiorly by the inferior edge of lateral process of C1, inferiorly by inferior edge of hyoid, laterally by medial edge of sternocleidomastoid muscle (SCM), and medially by medial edge of carotid and paraspinal muscles
  - IIA: bounded anteriorly by posterior edge of submandibular gland and anterior carotid; posteriorly by posterior border of internal jugular v
  - IIB: bounded anteriorly by posterior border of internal jugular v and posteriorly by posterior border of SCM
- III: midjugular
  - Bounded superiorly by inferior edge of hyoid, inferiorly by inferior edge of cricoid, anteriorly by anterior edge of SCM, posteriorly by posterior edge of SCM, laterally by medial edge of SCM, and medially by medial edge of carotid and paraspinal muscles
- IV: inferior jugular
  - Bounded superiorly by inferior edge of cricoid, inferiorly at a plane 2 cm above the sternoclavicular joint, anteriorly by anteromedial edge of SCM, posteriorly by posterior edge of SCM, laterally by medial edge of SCM, and medially by medial edge of carotid and paraspinal muscles

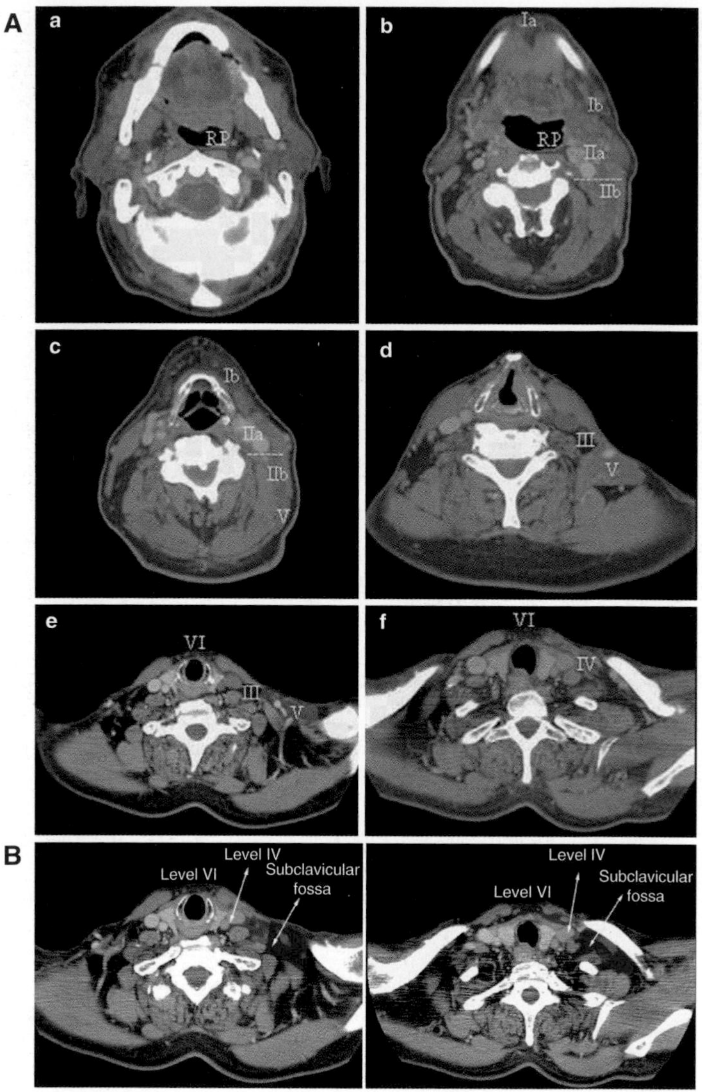

Fig. 13.1 (**A**) Neck nodal CTVs. Consensus guidelines for the N0 neck. (Reprinted by permission of Elsevier from Gregoire et al., 2003). (**B**) Neck nodal CTVs. Consensus guidelines for the supraclavicular fossa. (Reprinted by permission of Elsevier from Gregoire et al. 2006). (**C**) Neck nodal CTVs. Consensus guidelines for the retropharyngeal nodes and retrosyloid space. (Reprinted by permission of Elsevier from Gregoire et al. 2006)

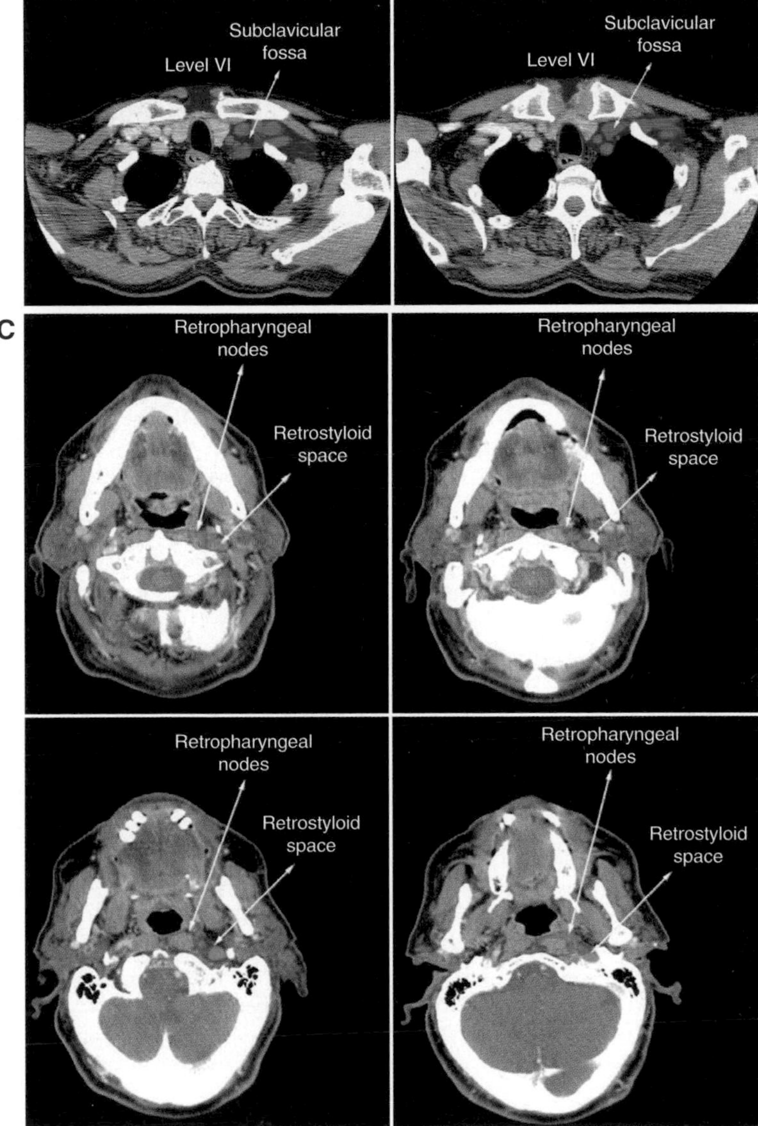

Fig. 13.1 (continued)

- V: posterior triangle spinal accessory nodes
  - Bounded superiorly by superior edge of hyoid, inferiorly by CT slice with transverse cervical vessels, anteriorly by posterior edge of SCM, posteriorly by anterior border of trapezius, laterally by platysma muscle and skin, and medially by paraspinal muscles
- VI: anterior neck nodes, including paratracheal, pretracheal, prelaryngeal (Delphian), and tracheoesophageal nodes
  - Bounded superiorly by inferior edge of thyroid cartilage, inferiorly by manubrium, anteriorly by skin and platysma muscle, posteriorly between the trachea and esophagus, and laterally by the medial edge of the thyroid gland and anteromedial SCM
- Retropharyngeal
  - Bounded superiorly by the base of skull, inferiorly by superior edge of hyoid bone, posteriorly by the prevertebral muscles, medially by midline, and laterally by the medial edge of the internal carotid
- Retrostyloid space
  - Bounded superiorly by base of skull (jugular foramen), inferiorly by inferior edge of lateral process of C1, anteriorly by parapharyngeal space, posteriorly by the vertebral body and base of skull, laterally by the parotid space, and medially by the medial edge of the internal carotid
- Supraclavicular fossa
  - Bounded superiorly by the plane 2 cm above the sternoclavicular joint (inferior level IV) and the CT slice with the transverse cervical vessels (inferior level V), inferiorly by the sternoclavicular joint, anteriorly by the SCM and clavicle, posteriorly by the anterior edge of the posterior scalene muscle, medially by the thyroid gland and trachea, and laterally by the lateral edge of the posterior scalene muscle
- VII: upper mediastinal
- Other groups = suboccipital, peri- and intraparotid, facial, buccinator, and preauricular nodes

APPROXIMATE RISK OF LYMPH NODE INVOLVEMENT BY SITE

Subsite	cN+ (%)	Bilateral (%)	cN0, occult LN+ (%)	Retropharyngeal LN+ (%)
Nasopharynx	80–90	50	90	75 N0: 40 N+: 85
Nasal cavity/ethmoid	10–15			
Esthesioneuroblastoma	20		A–B: <10–15 C: up to 44	
Nasal vestibule	5–10		10–15	
Maxillary sinus	SCC, poorly diff: 15–20 Nonsquamous: <5		SCC, poorly diff: 40 nonsquamous: <10	
Oropharynx	65			
Soft palate	55	15	20	10–15 N0: 5 N+: 20
Tonsillar pillar	45	5	10–15	
Tonsillar fossa	76	10	50–60	10 N0: 4 N+: 12
Base of tongue	75	30	40–50	4 N0: 0 N+: 6

continued

III

Oral tongue	35 T1/2: 20–30 T3/4: >30 (70–80%) Skip mets: 15% III/IV	5	30	
Retromolar trigone	30		15–25	
Floor of mouth	30	4	10–35	
Lip	5			
Buccal mucosa	10–30		15	
Lower gingiva	18–52		15–20	
Upper gingiva/hard palate	10–25		20–25	
Supraglottic larynx	55	15	15–25	2 N0: 0 N+: 4
Glottic larynx	T1: 2 T2: 5 T3/4: 20–30			
Subglottic larynx	10			
Hypopharynx	70			
Hypoharyngeal wall	60	15–20		20 N0: 15 N+: 20
Pyriform sinus	75	10	60–65	5N0: 0 N+: 10
Carotid body	5			

continued

Salivary gland	High-grade: 30 SCC: 50–60 High-grade mucoep: 45 Anapl: 40–80 CA ex pleo: 25–40 Adeno: 20–55 Adenoid cystic: <10% at dx (<20% overall) Acinic: <5–15 Low-grade mucoep: few	
Thyroid	Papillary: 30 Follicular: 5–10	35–50

NECK STAGING

- Most subsites of the head and neck use the same AJCC neck staging system, including the lip, oral cavity, oropharynx, hypopharynx, larynx, and major salivary glands.
- Nasopharyngeal cancer has a different neck staging system.
- Please refer to these other chapters for details of neck staging.

TREATMENT RECOMMENDATIONS FOR MANAGEMENT OF THE NECK

- These are general; specific guidelines for primary site, histology, and stage should be followed
- Clinically negative neck:
  - If risk of occult metastasis exists
    - Surgery for primary with elective neck dissection
      - (a) If N0, follow
      - (b) If N1 with no extracapsular extension (ECE), follow
      - (c) If >pN1 and/or ECE, postoperative RT or chemo-RT
    - Alternatively, RT or chemo-RT for primary with elective neck RT; surgery for persistent disease
- Clinically positive neck:
  - N1
    - Surgery for primary with selective or modified radical neck dissection
      - (a) If pN0, follow
      - (b) If pN1 with no ECE, follow
      - (c) If >pN1 and/or ECE, postoperative RT or chemo-RT
    - Alternatively, RT or chemo-RT for primary and involved neck with elective neck RT; surgery and/or neck dissection for persistent disease
  - >N1
    - Surgery for primary with modified radical, radical, or extended radical neck dissection
      - (a) If pN1 with no ECE, follow
      - (b) If >pN1 and/or ECE, postoperative RT or chemo-RT
    - Alternatively, RT or chemo-RT for primary with comprehensive RT for neck; surgery and/or neck dissection for persistent disease and/or node >3 cm

- Neck control with RT:
  - cN0: >90–95%
  - N1: 85%
  - N2A: 80%
  - N2B: 70%
  - N3: 35%

III

STUDIES OF POSTRADIOTHERAPY NECK DISSECTION

- Clayman et al. (2001): nonrandomized controlled trial. Sixty-six patients with stage ≥N2a SCC of oropharynx treated with sequential platinum-based induction chemotherapy, radiation therapy followed by selective neck dissections 6–10 weeks post-RT in patients with radiographic evidence of residual neck disease. Twenty-four of sixty-six (36%) patients had complete response in primary oropharyngeal tumor and regional neck lymphadenopathy, both clinically and radiographically. Significantly improved DSS and OS and nonsignificant lower rates of LRR in patients with CR vs. patients with PR or no response. Ten of eighteen (56%) patients who underwent neck dissection had pathological evidence of residual tumor. Significantly improved OS in patients with no response or PR who underwent neck dissection vs. patients with no response or PR who did not undergo neck dissection.
- Narayan et al. (1999): 52 patients with ≥1 node, ≥3 cm (94% stage N2–3). Most common primary tumor was oropharyngeal carcinoma (56%). Sixty percent had T2 or T3 primaries and all patients were AJCC stage IV. Patients were treated with high-dose RT (various fractionation schemes) followed by radical or modified radical neck dissection after confirmation of CR at primary site. Five-year actuarial overall neck control rate was 83% and in-field control rate was 88%. Only 1/28 with pathologically negative neck specimens had an in-field failure vs. 5/24 patients with pathologic evidence of residual disease. Five-year actuarial DFS was 57% and OS was 38%. Seventeen percent had significant postoperative complications. Conclusion: due to significant morbidity of routine neck dissection, recommend observation in patients with CR to high-dose RT ± chemotherapy.
- Brizel (IJROBP 2004): 154 patients with LN+ head and neck cancer treated with concurrent chemotherapy/hyperfractionated

RT. Modified neck dissection performed within 8 weeks for 43% of N1 and 66% of N2-3. For N1, NPV of a clinical CR after RT was 92%, PPV of less than clinical CR was 100%. For N2-3, NPV was 74%, PPV was 44%. Four-year OS/DFS for N2-3 patients with clinical CR was 77/75%, with neck dissection vs. 50/53% without neck dissection.

- Liauw et al. (2006): 550 patients with LN+ head and neck cancer treated with RT ± chemotherapy (24%). Three hundred and forty-one of these patients underwent planned post-RT neck dissection. Thirty day post-RT CT in 211 was correlated with neck dissection pathology to determine criteria associated with a low likelihood of having residual disease. Radiographic CR (rCR) defined as absence of large (>1.5 cm) or focally abnormal lymph node. NPV of 77% for clinical exam CR and 94% for rCR. There was no significant difference in the 5-year neck control rate (100%) and CSS (72%) in 32 rCR patients who did not undergo neck dissection vs. patients with negative post-RT neck dissection.
- Yao et al. (2007): 90 patients with ≥ stage N2a head and neck SCC were treated with definitive IMRT (three clinical target volumes: 70–74, 60, 54 Gy). Thirteen patients with residual lymphadenopathy underwent post-RT neck dissection. Six of thirteen had residual tumor. Seventy-four of ninety patients were observed and only 1 had regional failure. Among all patients, 3-year LC was 96.3% and LRC was 95.4%. PET was useful in selecting patients for neck dissection. Five of eighty with + PET scans had residual viable tumor. Four patients with negative PET had negative pathological results. Sixty-four of seventy-three observed patients had PET scan and only 1 had + uptake and FNA revealed reactive changes. Post-IMRT PET prediction of pathologic status has sensitivity of 88.9%, specificity of 94.3%, PPV of 66.7%, and NPV of 98.5%.
- Van der Putten et al. (2009): 61/540 patients with advanced head and neck cancer treated with concomitant chemoradiation had suspicion of regional residual or recurrent disease and underwent 68 salvage neck dissections. Note: 68 patients also had suspicion, but were deemed unresectable. Forty-three percent (26/61) had specimens with viable tumor. US guided FNA of suspicious lymph nodes had sensitivity of 80% and specificity of 42%. Five-year regional control 79% and 5-year OS 36%. Significant prognostic factors for OS were surgical margins and "residual vs. recurrent disease."

UNKNOWN PRIMARY OF THE HEAD AND NECK

III

PEARLS

- Definition = metastatic carcinoma with no primary site evident after history, physical exam, and initial imaging.
- Most unknown primary = adenocarcinoma originating below the clavicles; SCC of cervical nodes <10% of all unknown primary.
- Most likely head and neck primary site: tonsil 45% > base of tongue 40% > pyriform sinus 10%.
- Patients with upper neck lymphadenopathy have much better prognosis than those with low cervical or supraclavicular lymphadenopathy.
- Lymphadenopathy in low internal jugular chain or supraclavicular fossa may be associated with primary lesions below the clavicles, with much worse prognosis, so workup should proceed accordingly.
- Pathology
  - Most are squamous cell carcinoma or poorly differentiated (undifferentiated) carcinoma.
  - Adenocarcinoma in the neck is almost always associated with a primary lesion below the clavicles but must rule out salivary gland, thyroid, or parathyroid primary tumors.
  - Other = lymphoma, sarcoma.

WORKUP

- Specialist examination, CT and/or MRI, and panendoscopy identify primary site >50% of the time.
- H&P including nasopharyngolaryngoscopy with examination of oral cavity, pharynx, and larynx.
- Imaging:
  - Chest roentgenogram
  - CT and/or MRI of head and neck
  - PET/CT useful in prebiopsy setting
  - Chest CT for N stage ≥N2b, or low neck or bulky lymphadenopathy to evaluate for pulmonary metastases
- Labs:
  - CBC
  - Chemistries including electrolytes, BUN/Cr, LFTs

- EUA with panendoscopy and biopsies of nasopharynx, both tonsils, base of tongue, both pyriform sinuses, and any other suspicious areas seen during examination.
  - Identifies 40% of primaries (but only 25% if no CT or MRI)
- Ipsilateral or bilateral tonsillectomy may also be performed in those with adequate lymphoid tissue in tonsillar fossae.
  - Evaluate for EBV DNA via PCR in geographic regions where nasopharyngeal primary tumors are common
  - Detects 30% of primaries
  - Bilateral tonsillectomy identifies contralateral tonsillar primary in 10%; may make surveillance exam easier
- If lymphoma is suspected: core needle or excisional biopsy of node preferred; staging per lymphoma guidelines.
- Dental examination and cleaning; extractions done before any RT.

TREATMENT RECOMMENDATIONS

- Typically irradiate nasopharynx, oropharynx, and both sides of neck
  - Hypopharynx and larynx were irradiated historically; eliminated more recently because they are rarely the primary site and including these sites greatly increases morbidity of treatment
  - Consider hypopharyngeal and laryngeal irradiation for adenopathy centered in level III/IV
  - Oral cavity is not irradiated unless submandibular lymphadenopathy is present
    - If submandibular lymphadenopathy: perform neck dissection and observe, or irradiate oral cavity and oropharynx but not nasopharynx
- If only 1 cN+
  - Selective or modified radical neck dissection first (benefit = directs pathology and post-op RT dose is lower, but disadvantage is more surgical morbidity)
  - If no additional lymphadenopathy or extracapsular extension (ECE), may observe
  - If ≥2 LN or ECE: post-op RT or chemo-RT
- If ≥2 cN+
  - Early N2 disease (N2A, early N2B): RT
  - Advanced N2-N3: chemo-RT
  - PET/CT 8 weeks after RT or chemo-RT
    - Risk of residual disease ≤5%: observe

    - Risk of residual disease >5% (nodes >15 mm, focal lucency, or enhancement or calcification in lymph node, ECE or nodal rupture): neck dissection

- Alternative: Definitive RT or chemo-RT with follow-up PET/CT in 8–12 weeks with salvage surgery
- Neck control rates
  - N1-N2a: 90–100%
  - N2b-N2c: 80%
  - N3: 50–60%
- Rate of DM
  - N1-N2a: <10%
  - N2b-N2c: 15%
  - N3: 25%
- Five-year OS: 40–60% depending on the extent of disease
- Ten percent have emergence of a head and neck SCC primary after treatment

Most common location for mucosal site failure is oropharynx, particularly the base of the tongue

RADIATION TECHNIQUES

SIMULATION AND FIELD DESIGN

- Patient set-up: supine, hyperextend head, wire neck scars, may need bolus, consider wiring oral commissures, shoulders pulled down with straps, immobilization with thermoplastic mask or bite block
- Volumes
  - Nasopharynx, oropharynx, bilateral retropharyngeal nodes and levels IB-IV, ipsilateral $\pm$ contralateral supraclavicular nodes
  - Include oral cavity only if submandibular adenopathy present, and may eliminate nasopharynx in that case
- Conventional borders
  - Parallel-opposed lateral fields at 1.8–2 Gy/fraction
    - Superior = covers nasopharynx and level Ib and V to base of tongue
    - Posterior = behind spinous processes to C2
    - Anterior = 2 cm margin on nasopharynx and the base of tongue; shield skin and subcutaneous tissue of submentum as much as possible
    - Inferior = thyroid notch

    - Reduction of spinal cord at 42–45 Gy; supplement posterior neck with 9–12 MeV electron fields
    - Advanced lymphadenopathy receives additional boost with anteroposterior or oblique beams to 66–70 Gy
    - Anterior supraclavicular field
        - Five to ten millimeter wide larynx block splits thyroid cartilage and is tapered inferiorly to stop at cricoid
        - Cover ipsilateral ± contralateral supraclavicular fossa (very low risk of recurrence)
- IMRT: spare contralateral parotid gland in patients with ipsilateral neck lymphadenopathy; low neck may be treated with a separate anterior field using isocentric match to upper IMRT fields

DOSE PRESCRIPTIONS

- Definitive = 42–45 Gy followed by off-cord boost to 70 Gy, or if using concomitant boost, 72 Gy
- UCSF IMRT doses
    - GTV 2.12/69.96 Gy, high-risk CTV 2/66 Gy, intermediate-risk CTV 1.8/59.4 Gy, low-risk CTV 1.64/54 Gy
- Postoperative
    - With no adverse features = 50–54 Gy to primary and bilateral necks
    - Otherwise 60–66 Gy (e.g., for perineural invasion, ECE, close/+ margin)

DOSE LIMITATIONS

- IMRT limits
    - Mandible <70 Gy, spinal cord <45 Gy, brainstem <54 Gy, mean parotid dose <26 Gy, optic nerves and chiasm 54 Gy, retina 45 Gy

COMPLICATIONS

- Surgical
    - Operative mortality 2–3%
    - Morbidity = infection, hematoma/seroma, lymphedema, wound dehiscence, chyle fistula, pharyngocutaneous fistula, cranial nerve VII, X, XI, XII injury, carotid exposure, or rupture
    - Incidence of complications is greater with RT doses >60 Gy
- Radiation therapy
    - Acute and chronic mucositis, xerostomia
    - Skin reaction
    - Subcutaneous fibrosis

    - Lymphedema of larynx and submentum
    - Mandibular necrosis uncommon, carotid artery rupture <1%
- Amifostine may reduce acute ± late xerostomia, but associated with nausea, vomiting and hypotension (Peters IJROBP 1992 and Brizel et al., 2000)

III

FOLLOW-UP

- Every 1–2 months first year, every 3 month for years 2–3, every 6 months for years 4–5, then every year.
- If recurrence suspected but biopsy negative, follow-up every 1 month until resolved.
- Eighty-five to ninety percent of LRR occur within 3 years.

REFERENCES

Brizel DM, Wasserman TH, Henke M, et al. Phase III randomized trial of amifostine as a radioprotector in head and neck cancer. J Clin Oncol. 2000;18(19):3339-3345.

Brizel DM, Prosnitz RG, Hunter S, et al. Necessity for adjuvant neck dissection in setting of concurrent chemoradiation for advanced head-and-neck cancer: IHYPERLINK "javascript:AL_get(this,%20'jour',%20'Int%20J%20Radiat%20Oncol%20Biol%20Phys.');" \o "International journal of radiation oncology, biology, physics." Int J Radiat Oncol Biol Phys. 2004;58(5). 1418-1423.

Brizel DM, Prosnitz RG, Hunter S, et al. Necessity for adjuvant neck dissection in setting of concurrent chemoradiation for advanced head-and-neck cancer. Int J Radiat Oncol Biol Phys 2004; 58(5): 1418-23.

Clayman GL, Johnson CJ II, Morrison W, Ginsberg L, Lippman SM. The role of neck dissection after chemoradiotherapy for oropharyngeal cancer with advanced nodal disease. Arch Otolaryngol Head Neck Surg. 2001;127(2): 135-139.

Gregoire V, et al. CT-based delineation of lymph node levels and related CTVs in the node-negative neck: DAHANCA, EORTC, GORTEC, NCIC, RTOG consensus guidelines. Radiother Oncol. 2003;69(3):227-236

Gregoire V, et al. Proposal for the delineation of the nodal CTV in the node-positive and the postoperative neck. Radiother Oncol. 2006;79(1):15-20

Liauw SL, Mancuso AA, Amdur RJ, et al. Postradiotherapy neck dissection for lymph node-positive head and neck cancer: the use of computed tomography to manage the neck. J Clin Oncol. 2006;24(9):1421-1427.

Narayan K, Crane CH, Kleid S, Hughes PG, Peters LJ. Planned neck dissection as an adjunct to the management of patients with advanced neck disease treated with definitive radiotherapy: for some or for all? Head Neck. 1999; 21(7):606-613.

Peters GJ, van der Wilt CL, Gyergyay F, et al. Protection by WR-2721 of the toxicity induced by the combination of cisplatin and 5-fluorouracil: Int J Radiat Oncol Biol Phys. 1992;22(4):785-789.

van der Putten L, van den Broek GB, de Bree R, et al. Effectiveness of salvage selective and modified radical neck dissection for regional pathologic lymphadenopathy after chemoradiation. Head Neck. 2009;31(5):593-603.

Yao M, Hoffman HT, Chang K, et al. Is planned neck dissection necessary for head and neck cancer after intensity-modulated radiotherapy? Int J Radiat Oncol Biol Phys. 2007;68(3):707-713.

FURTHER READING

Gregoire V, Duprez T, Lengele B, Hamoir M. Management of the neck. In: Gunderson L, Tepper J, editors. Clinical Radiation Oncology, 2nd ed. Philadelphia: Churchill Livingstone; 2007. pp. 827-852.

Mendenhall WM, Mancuso AA, Parsons JT, Stringer SP, Cassisi NJ. Diagnostic evaluation of squamous cell carcinoma metastatic to cervical lymph nodes from an unknown head and neck primary site. Head Neck. 1998;20(8): 739-744.

Mendenhall WM, Mancuso AA, Villaret DB. Unknown head and neck primary site. In: Gunderson L, Tepper J, editors. Clinical Radiation Oncology, 2nd ed. Philadelphia: Churchill Livingstone; 2007. pp. 819-826.

IV

PART IV
Thorax

Chapter 14
Small Cell Lung Cancer

R. Scott Bermudez, Brian Missett, and Daphne A. Haas-Kogan

IV

PEARLS

- SCLC accounts for 15–20% of lung cancer cases with decreasing incidence.
- Approximately 1/3 of patients present with limited stage disease and the remainder present with extensive stage disease.
- More than 95% of cases are associated with a history of tobacco exposure.
- Ten to 15% of patients present with brain metastases and 2 year incidence after chemo-RT is 50–80%.
- SCLC is the most common solid tumor associated with paraneoplastic syndromes: SIADH, ACTH production syndrome, and Eaton–Lambert syndrome.
- Histopathologic hallmarks include dense sheets of small, round to fusiform cells with scant cytoplasm, extensive necrosis, and a high mitotic rate.
- Pathologic subtypes (pure or classic, variant, and mixed) carry the same prognosis.
- Most important prognostic factors are stage and performance status.

WORKUP

- H&P.
- Labs: CBC, chemistries, BUN/Cr, LFTs, LDH. Consider bone marrow aspirate/biopsy if LDH elevated.
- Diagnosis: sputum, FNA, bronchoscopic biopsy, or CT-guided biopsy. No need for invasive mediastinal staging after SCLC diagnosis made due to limited role of surgical resection.
- Imaging: CT chest and abdomen, bone scan, and MRI brain (preferred over CT brain). PET optional.
- Additional: PFTs, pathology review, smoking cessation intervention.

STAGING

- See Chap. 15 for details of the AJCC 7th Ed Staging for Lung Cancer.
- In practice, SCLC has been divided into limited stage and extensive stage disease.

Limited stage (LS): disease confined to one hemithorax and regional nodes (historically defined as fitting into a single radiation port)
Extensive stage (ES): any disease not meeting limited stage criteria

TREATMENT RECOMMENDATIONS

Stage	Recommended treatment	Outcome
Limited	Concurrent cisplatin and etoposide (4c every 3 weeks) with early RT during cycle 1 or 2 (45 Gy/1.5 Gy b.i.d. preferred). If CR or near-CR, prophylactic cranial RT (25 Gy in 10 fx) For <5% of patients with cT1-2N0 disease with negative mediastinoscopy (or endoscopic biopsy), lobectomy and mediastinal node dissection/sampling may be performed initially. If pN0, chemotherapy along. If pN+, concurrent chemoradiation as above	MS 20 months, 5-year OS 20–26%
Extensive	Combination platinum-based chemotherapy ± palliative RT to symptomatic sites. For patients with PR or CR to chemotherapy, consider prophylactic cranial RT (25 Gy in 10 fx). If brain metastases present, WBRT (30–37.5 Gy in 10–15 fx)	MS 12 months, 5-year OS <5–10%

STUDIES

LIMITED STAGE (LS-SCLC)

- Pignon et al. (1992): metaanalysis of 13 trials and 2,140 patients with LS-SCLC treated with chemo ± thoracic RT. Thoracic RT improved 3-year OS by 5.4% vs. chemo alone (14.3 vs. 8.9%).
- Metaanalyses of randomized controlled trials performed on LS-SCLC patients receiving chemo and early vs. late timing of thoracic RT demonstrate improved survival for early concurrent integration of RT with platinum-based chemo (Fried et al. 2004; De Ruysscher et al. 2006).
- *INT 0096* (Turrisi et al. 1999): 417 patients with LS-SCLC randomized to concurrent cisplatin/etoposide with either 45 Gy/1.8 Gy QD or 45 Gy/1.5 Gy b.i.d. Twice daily arm decreased local failure

(36 vs. 52%) and increased 5-year OS (26 vs. 16%) compared to QD arm. Grade 3 esophagitis more frequent with b.i.d. regimen (27 vs. 11%).

- *RTOG 0239* (Komaki et al. 2009): phase II trial using accelerated high-dose thoracic RT (AHTRT) with concurrent etoposide/cisplatin. RT was given to large field to 28.8 Gy /1.8 Gy QD, then 14.4 Gy/1.8 Gy b.i.d. (1.8 Gy AP/PA in am; 1.8 Gy boost in pm). Total RT dose 61.2 Gy in 5 weeks. Two-year OS 37%, 2-year LC 80%, and 18% acute severe esophagitis, improved compared to INT 0096. One of three arms in ongoing randomized trial of LS-SCLC RTOG0538/CALGB30610.
- Auperin et al. (1999): metaanalysis of seven trials of SCLC patients in CR comparing prophylactic cranial irradiation (PCI) vs. no PCI. PCI reduced the 3-year incidence of brain metastases (59 vs.33%) and increased 3-year OS (15.3 vs. 20.7). Neurocognitive function not assessed.
- Le Pechoux et al. (2003): 720 LS-SCLC patients in CR to chemo-RT randomized to standard dose (25 Gy/2.5 Gy QD) vs. higher dose (36 Gy/2 Gy QD or 36 Gy/1.5 Gy b.i.d.) PCI. No significant difference in 2-year incidence of brains metastases. Reduced 2-year OS in higher dose group (37 vs. 42%) probably due to increased cancer-related mortality.

IV

EXTENSIVE STAGE (ES-SCLC)

- Jeremic et al. (1999): 210 ES-SCLC patients treated with three cycles cisplatin/etoposide with local PR or CR and distant CR randomized to accelerated hyperfractionated RT (54 Gy/1.5 Gy b.i.d.) and chemo vs. four cycles chemo alone. Patients receiving chemo-RT had improved 5-year OS (9.1 vs. 3.7%) and MS (17 vs. 11 months) vs. those treated with chemo alone.
- *EORTC* (Slotman et al. 2007): 286 patients with ES-SCLC with response to chemotherapy randomized to PCI vs. no further treatment. PCI reduced 1-year incidence of symptomatic brain mets (14.6 vs. 40.4%) and improved OS (27.1 vs. 13.3%) compared to the control group.

RADIATION TECHNIQUES

SIMULATION AND FIELD DESIGN

- High-dose volume to GTV + 1.5 cm margin. Include ipsilateral hilum, and bilateral mediastinum from thoracic inlet to subcarinal region (5 cm below carina or adequate margin on subcarinal disease). Exclude contralateral hilum or SCV unless involved.

- If RT is preceded by chemotherapy, target volumes should be defined on the RT planning CT scan. However, the prechemotherapy originally involved lymph node regions should be included.

DOSE PRESCRIPTIONS

- 45 Gy in 1.5 b.i.d. fx (preferred) or 50–70 Gy at 1.8–2.0 Gy QD (Miller et al. 2003; Roof et al. 2003; Schild et al. 2004)
- PCI: 25 Gy in 10 fx
- Brain metastases: 30–37.5 Gy in 10–15 fx

DOSE LIMITATIONS

- Spinal cord: limit maximum dose to ≤36 Gy with 1.5 Gy b.i.d. RT or ≤46 Gy at 1.8–2 Gy/fx QD.
- Lung: limit volume receiving ≥20 Gy (V20) to <20–30%. Pneumonitis rates increase rapidly with V20 >25–30%.
- Esophagus: limit 1/3 to 60 Gy, entire esophagus to 55 Gy.
- Heart: limit 50% of volume of heart to <25–40 Gy.
- Brachial plexus: limit maximum dose to <60 Gy.

COMPLICATIONS

- Acute: esophagitis, dermatitis, cough, fatigue.
- Subacute/late: radiation pneumonitis, pulmonary fibrosis, esophageal stricture or perforation, pericarditis, coronary artery disease, Lhermitte's syndrome, brachial plexopathy, rib fracture.

FOLLOW-UP

- Clinic visits every 2–3 months initially (H&P, chest imaging, and blood work at each visit), then decrease frequency to every 3–6 months, then annually.

REFERENCES

Auperin A, Arriagada R, Pignon JP, et al. Prophylactic cranial irradiation for patients with small-cell lung cancer in complete remission. Prophylactic Cranial Irradiation Overview Collaborative Group. N Engl J Med 1999; 341:476-484.

Chang JY, Bradley JD, Govindan R, Komaki R. Lung. In: Halperin EC, Perez CA, Brady LW, et al., editors. Principles and practice of radiation oncology. 5th ed. Philadelphia: Lippincott Williams & Wilkins; 2008. pp. 1076-1108.

De Ruysscher D, Pijls-Johannesma M, Vansteenkiste J, et al. Systematic Review and meta-analysis of randomised, controlled trials of the timing of chest radiotherapy in patients with limited-stage, small-cell lung cancer. Ann Oncol 2006;17:543-552.

De Ruysscher D, Pijls-Johannesma M, Bentzen S, et al. Time between the first day of chemotherapy and the last day of chest radiation is the most important predictor of survival in limited-disease small cell lung cancer. J Clin Oncol 2006;24:1057-1063.

Fried DB, Morris DE, Poole C, et al. Systematic review evaluating the timing of thoracic radiation therapy in combined modality therapy for limited-stage small-cell lung cancer. J Clin Oncol 2004;22:4837-4845.

Huncharek M, McGarry R. A meta-analysis of the timing of chest irradiation in the combined modality treatment of limited-stage small cell lung cancer. Oncologist 2004;9:665-672.

Jeremic B, Shibamoto Y, Nikolic N. Role of radiation therapy in the combined-modality treatment of patients with extensive disease small-cell lung cancer: a randomized study. J Clin Oncol 1999;17:2092-2099.

Komaki R, Travis EL, Cox JD. The Lung and Thymus. In: Cox JD, Ang KK, editors. Radiation oncology: rationale, technique, results. 8th ed. St. Louis: Mosby; 2003. pp. 399-427.

Komaki R, Paulus R, Ettinger DS, Videtic GM, Bradley JD, Glisson BS, Choy H. A phase II study of accelerated high-dose thoracic radiation therapy (AHTRT) with concurrent chemotherapy for limited small cell lung cancer: RTOG 0239. J Clin Oncol 2009;27:7s (suppl; abstr 7527).

Le Pechoux C, Dunant A, Senan S, et al. Standard-dose versus higher-dose prophylactic cranial irradiation (PCI) in patients with limited-stage small-cell lung cancer in complete remission after chemotherapy and thoracic radiotherapy (PCI 99-01, EORTC 2203-08004, RTOG 0212, and IFCT 99-01): a randomised clinical trial. Lancet Oncol 2009;10:467-474.

Miller KL, Marks LB, Sibley GS, et al. Routine use of approximately 60 Gy once daily thoracic irradiation for patients with limited-stage small-cell lung cancer. Int J Radiat Oncol Biol Phys 2003;56:355-359.

National Comprehensive Cancer Network Clinical Practice Guidelines in Oncology: Small Cell Lung Cancer. Available at: http://www.nccn.org/professionals/physician_gls/PDF/sclc.pdf. Accessed on May 19, 2009.

Pignon JP, Arriagada A, Ihde DC, et al. A meta-analysis of thoracic radiotherapy for small-cell lung cancer. N Engl J Med 1992;3:1618-1624.

Roof KS, Fidias P, Lynch TJ, et al. Radiation dose escalation in limited-stage small cell lung cancer. Int J Radiat Oncol Biol Phys 2003;57:701-708.

Rosenzweig KE, Krug LM. Tumors of the Lung, Pleura, and Mediastinum. In: Leibel SA, Phillips TL, editors. Textbook of radiation oncology. 2nd ed. Philadelphia: Saunders; 2004. pp. 779-810.

Schild SE, Bonner JA, Shanahan TG, et al. Long-term results of a phase III trial comparing once-daily radiotherapy with twice-daily radiotherapy in limited-stage small-cell lung cancer. Int J Radiat Oncol Biol Phys 2004;59:943-951.

Schild SE, Curran WJ. Small Cell Lung Cancer. In: Gunderson LL, Tepper JE, et al., editors. Clinical radiation oncology, 2nd ed. Philadelphia: Churcill Linigstone; 2007. pp. 897-909.

Slotman B, Faivre-Finn C, Kramer G, et al. Prophylactic cranial irradiation in extensive small-cell lung cancer. N Engl J Med 2007;357:664-672.

Turrisi AT III, Kim K, Blum R, et al. Twice-daily compared with once-daily thoracic radiotherapy in limited small-cell lung cancer treated concurrently with cisplatin and etoposide. N Engl J Med 1999;340:265-271.

IV

Chapter 15
Non-small Cell Lung Cancer

Siavash Jabbari, Eric K. Hansen, and Daphne A. Haas-Kogan

IV

PEARLS

- Most common noncutaneous cancer in the world.
- Second most common cancer in the US, behind prostate in men and breast in women.
- No. 1 cause of cancer death in the US and worldwide.
- >90% of cases are associated with smoking or involuntary smoking.
- Second most common cause in the US is radon.
- Asbestos exposure is associated with 3–4% of cases.
- Risk of tobacco-induced second primary is ~2–3% per year.
- The surgical lymph node levels 1–9 correspond to N2 nodes, and levels 10–14 correspond to N1 nodes.
  - 1 = high mediastinal, 2 = upper paratracheal, 3 = pre and retrotracheal, 4 = lower paratracheal, 5 = AP window, 6 = paraaortic, 7 = subcarinal, 8 = paraesophageal below carina, 9 = pulmonary ligament, 10 = hilar, 11 = interlobar, 12 = lobar, 13 = segmental, and 14 = subsegmental.
- Adenocarcinoma comprises 40–50% of cases. It tends to be peripherally located; it has a high propensity to metastasize (frequently to the brain).
- TTF-1 helps to distinguish primary lung (and thyroid) adenocarcinoma from metastatic adenocarcinoma.
- Bronchioalveolar carcinoma is a subtype of adenocarcinoma that is not associated with smoking, but is associated with prior lung disease. Can present as solitary nodule, multifocal disease, or pneumonitic form. Spreads along alveoli without invasion of basement membrane. May be sensitive to EGFR tyrosine kinase inhibitors (gefitinib, erlotinib).
- Squamous cell carcinoma tends to be centrally located with lower propensity for brain metastasis.
- Large cell carcinoma tends to be peripherally located. It has a high propensity to metastasize, especially to brain.

- EGFR is overexpressed in 60–70% of NSCLC, mainly SqCC (80–90%) vs. adenocarcinoma (30–35%).
- Pancoast tumor = apical tumor + either chest wall (rib) invasion or Pancoast syndrome (shoulder pain or brachial plexus palsy, ±Horner's syndrome (ptosis, meiosis, and ipsilateral anhidrosis))
- Carcinoid tumors are rare, and they tend to be endobronchial. Most common site is in the GI tract, but 25% occur in the lung. Seventy to ninety percent are typical carcinoids, which rarely metastasize and are not associated with smoking. Ten to thirty percent are atypical carcinoids, which more frequently metastasize and are associated with smoking, and have poorer prognosis. Only 10–15% of patients with carcinoid tumors present with carcinoid syndrome (flushing, diarrhea, and wheezing), but up to two-third may eventually develop these symptoms.
- Presentation: stage I 10%, II 20%, III 30%, IV 40%.
- Prognostic factors: stage, weight loss (>10% body weight over 6 months), KPS, pleural effusion, Kras ongogene activation.
  - RTOG RPA analysis (Werner-Wasik et al. 2000): Prognostic factors include KPS <90, use of chemo, age >70 years, pleural effusion, and N stage. Worst survival in patients with malignant pleural effusion (5 months).

WORKUP

- H&P, including performance status, weight loss, and smoking status.
  - Cough, dyspnea, hemoptysis, postobstructive pnuemonia, pleural effusion, pain, hoarseness (left recurrent laryngeal nerve), SVC syndrome, clubbing, superior sulcus (Pancoast) tumor triad = shoulder pain, brachial plexus palsy, and Horner's syndrome.
- Laboratories: CBC, BUN, Cr, LFTs, alkaline phosphatase, and LDH.
- Imaging.
  - CT chest and abdomen (to rule out adrenal or liver metastasis).
    - Mediastinal LN sensitivity ~60%, specificity ~80% (Gould et al. 2003).
    - Approximately 10–20% false negative rate for CT depending on T stage and size.
  - PET scan.
    - +PET scan should have pathologic confirmation because up to 20% false + rate due to inflammation.

    - Mediastinal LN sensitivity 85%, specificity 90%.
    - Addition of PET-CT decreased the total number of thoracotomies and futile thoracotomies in a randomized controlled trial of conventional staging (including CT and mediastinoscopy) ± whole-body PET–CT (Fischer et al. 2009).
  - MRI of brain for LN + nonsquamous and all stage III–IV, or for neurologic symptoms.
  - MRI of the thoracic inlet for superior sulcus tumors to assess vertebral body and/or brachial plexus invasion.
  - Octreotide scan for carcinoid tumor.
- Pathology: thoracentesis for pleural effusions. For central lesions, perform bronchoscopy because sputum cytology has only ~65–80% sensitivity. For peripheral lesions, perform CT-guided biopsy.
- Mediastinoscopy or bronchoscopic biopsy should be performed to confirm any CT + or PET + nodes, and for all superior sulcus tumors. If T3 or central T1–2, perform mediastinoscopy to evaluate superior mediastinal nodes (95% accurate).
  - Cervical mediastinoscopy assesses nodal levels 1–4R.
  - Anterior (Chamberlain) mediastinoscopy assesses levels 4 L (left lower paratracheal), 5, 6, and 7.
- Pulmonary function testing for presurgical and/or preradiotherapy evaluation.
  - Desire FEV1 ≥1.2–2 L (if pneumonectomy >2.5 L, if lobectomy >1.2 L) or >75% predicted or predicted post-op FEV1 >0.8 L; also DLCO >60%.
  - Medically inoperable is generally FEV1 <40% or <1.2 L, DLCO <60%, FVC <70%.
- Paraneoplastic syndromes.
  - Hypercalcemia (SqCC).
  - Hypertrophic pulmonary osteoarthropathy (adenocarcinoma).
  - Hypercoagulable (adenocarcinoma).
  - Gynecomastia (large cell).
  - Carcinoid = VIP diarrhea.

IV

STAGING: NON-SMALL CELL LUNG CANCER

Editors' note: All TNM stage and stage groups referred to elsewhere in this chapter reflect the 2002 AJCC staging nomenclature unless otherwise noted as the new system below was published after this chapter was written.

(AJCC 6TH ED., 2002)

Primary tumor (T)

TX: Primary tumor cannot be assessed, or tumor proven by the presence of malignant cells in sputum or bronchial washings but not visualized by imaging or bronchoscopy

T0: No evidence of primary tumor

Tis: Carcinoma in situ

T1: Tumor 3 cm or less in greatest dimension, surrounded by lung or visceral pleura, without bronchoscopic evidence of invasion more proximal than the lobar bronchus (i.e., not in the main bronchus)

T2: Tumor with any of the following features of size or extent: more than 3 cm in greatest dimension; involves main bronchus, 2 cm or more distal to the carina; invades visceral pleura; associated with atelectasis or obstructive pneumonitis that extends to the hilar region but does not involve the entire lung

T3: Tumor of any size that directly invades any of the following: chest wall (including superior sulcus tumors), diaphragm, mediastinal pleura, and parietal pericardium; or tumor in the main bronchus less than 2 cm distal to the carina, but without involvement of the carina; or associated atelectasis or obstructive pneumonitis of the entire lung

T4: Tumor of any size that invades any of the following: mediastinum, heart, great vessels, trachea, esophagus, vertebral body, and carina; or separate tumor nodules in the same lobe; or tumor with malignant pleural effusion

**Note*: The uncommon superficial tumor of any size with its invasive component limited to the bronchial wall, which may extend proximal to the main bronchus, is classified T1.

(AJCC 7TH ED., 2010)

Primary tumor (T)

TX: Primary tumor cannot be assessed, or tumor proven by the presence of malignant cells in sputum or bronchial washings, but not visualized by imaging or bronchoscopy

T0: No evidence of primary tumor

Tis: Carcinoma in situ

T1: Tumor 3 cm or less in greatest dimension, surrounded by lung or visceral pleura, without bronchoscopic evidence of invasion, more proximal than the lobar bronchus (i.e., not in the main bronchus)*

- T1a: Tumor 2 cm or less in greatest dimension
- T1b: Tumor more than 2 cm but 3 cm or less in greatest dimension

T2: Tumor more than 3 cm but 7 cm or less or tumor with any of the following features (T2 tumors with these features are classified T2a if 5 cm or less); involves main bronchus, 2 cm or more distal to the carina; invades visceral pleura (pl1 or pl2); associated with atelectasis or obstructive pneumonitis that extends to the hilar region but does not involve the entire lung

- T2a: Tumor more than 3 cm but 5 cm or less in greatest dimension
- T2b: Tumor more than 5 cm but 7 cm or less in greatest dimension

T3: Tumor more than 7 cm or one that directly invades any of the following: parietal pleural (PL3) chest wall (including superior sulcus tumors), diaphragm, phrenic nerve, mediastinal pleura, and parietal pericardium; or tumor in the main bronchus (less than 2 cm distal to the carina*) but without involvement of the carina; or associated atelectasis or obstructive pneumonitis of the entire lung or separate tumor nodule(s) in the same lobe

T4: tumor of any size that invades any of the following: mediastinum, heart, great vessels, trachea, recurrent laryngeal nerve, esophagus, vertebral body, carina, separate tumor nodule(s) in a different ipsilateral lobe

continued

Regional lymph nodes (N)
NX: Regional lymph nodes cannot be assessed
N0: No regional lymph node metastasis
N1: Metastasis to ipsilateral peribronchial and/or ipsilateral hilar nodes, and intrapulmonary nodes including involvement by direct extension of the primary tumor
N2: Metastasis to ipsilateral mediastinal and/or subcarinal lymph node(s)
N3: Metastasis to ontralateral mediastinal, contralateral hilar, ipsilateral or contralateral scale or supraclavicular or lymph node(s)

Distant metastases (M)
MX: Distant metastasis cannot be assessed
M0: No distant metastasis
M1: Distant metastasis present

Note: M1 includes separate tumor nodule(s) in a different lobe (ipsilateral or contralateral).

Used with the permission from the American Joint Committee on Cancer (AJCC), Chicago, IL. The original source for this material is the AJCC Cancer Staging Manual, Sixth Edition (2002), published by Springer Science+Business Media.

*The uncommon superficial spreading tumor of any size with its invasive component limited to the bronchial wall, which may extend proximally to the main bronchus, is also classified as T1a.

Regional lymph nodes (N)
NX: Regional lymph nodes cannot be assessed
N0: No regional lymph node metastases
N1: Metastasis in ipsilateral peribronchial and/or ipsilateral hilar lymph nodes and intrapulmonary nodes, including involvement by direct extension
N2: Metastasis in ipsilateral mediastinal and/or subcarinal lymph node(s)
N3: Metastasis in contralateral mediastinal, contralateral hilar, ipsilateral or contralateral scalene, or supraclavicular lymph node(s)

Distant metastasis (M)
M0: No distant metastasis
M1: Distant metastasis
M1a: Separate tumor nodule(s) in a contralateral lobe tumor with pleural nodules or malignant pleural (or pericardial) effusion*
M1b: Distant metastasis

Anatomic stage/prognostic groups
Occult carcinoma: TX N0 M0
0: Tis N0 M0
IA: T1a N0 M0
T1b N0 M0
IB: T2a N0 M0
IIA: T2b N0 M0
T1a N1 M0
T1b N1 M0
T2a N1 M0
IIB: T2b N1 M0
T3 N0 M0

continued

IV

IIIA: T1a N2 M0
T1b N2 M0
T2a N2 M0
T2b N2 M0
T3 N1 M0
T3 N2 M0
T4 N0 M0
T4 N1 M0
IIIB: T1a N3 M0
T1b N3 M0
T2a N3 M0
T2b N3 M0
T3 N3 M0
T4 N2 M0
T4 N3 M0
IV: Any T Any N M1a
Any T Any N M1b

SURVIVAL ESTIMATES WITH NEW STAGING SYSTEM*

~5-Year survival	~Median survival
IA: 50–70%	IA: 5–10 years
IB: 40–60%	IB: 3–7 years
IIA: 55%	IIA: 3–4 years
IIB: 40%	IIB: 1.5–3 years
IIIA: 20–25%	IIIA: 14–23 months
IIIB: 7–9%	IIIB: 10–16 months
IV: 2–13%	IV: 6–18 months (best supportive care 3–6 months; 8–10 months with chemo)
Superior sulcus: 3 year 50%	

*Range represents clinical vs. pathologic staging

IV

TREATMENT RECOMMENDATIONS

2002 Stage	Recommended treatment	Outcome
Operable I–II	■ Lobectomy (~2–3% mortality) preferred over pneumonectomy (~5–7% mortality) if anatomically feasible. ■ Wedge resection only if physiologically compromised. LN sampling or resection generally indicated b/c ~15% of cT1–2N0 found to have +LN ■ For completely resected T1–2N1, give adjuvant chemo (NCIC BR.10). ■ Consider adjuvant chemo for T2N0, especially if >4 cm (CALGB) ■ For completely resected T3N0, give adjuvant chemo (IALT) ■ For close/+margin, re-resect or consider post-op RT	LRF: lobectomy 6%, wedge 18% 5-years OS and CSS stage I: 50–70%
I–II marginally operable	■ Pre-op chemo → surgery → chemo (van Meerbeeck et al. 2005 (EORTC metaanalysis)). Chemo = cisplatin combination or carboplatin-paclitaxel ■ For close/+margin, re-resect or consider post-op RT	5-year OS N1: ~50%
I–II inoperable	■ Definitive RT to primary and involved nodes ■ Conventional fractionation is 2 Gy/fraction to ~66 Gy (Dosoretz et al. 1996; Sibley, 1998) ■ If peripheral tumor or poor PS, may hypofractionate with 4 Gy/fraction to 48 Gy to primary tumor only (Slotman et al. 1996, Cheung et al. 2002)	Std RT 5-year OS T1N0: 30–50% T2N0: 15–20% Hypofx: 2–3-year OS 40–50% SBRT: 2–3-year LC 85–95%, OS 55%

continued

	■ However, dose escalation >70 Gy and SBRT techniques (~60 Gy/3 fx) appear in phase I/II trials to provide improved LC compared to conventional techniques and doses ■ If patient can tolerate it, give chemo (induction, concurrent, and/or consolidation) if T3N0 or N1. Off trial, chemotherapy should be avoided concurrently with dose-escalated RT or SBRT until further data are available	
IIIA operable or marginally operable	■ Concurrent chemo-RT (45 Gy) → restage* → if no progression → surgery → chemo (Int 0139) (especially if initially bulky or multiple N2 nodes) ■ Alternatively, chemo alone → restage* → if no progression → surgery → chemo and post-op RT for close (<5 mm) or + margin, nodal ECE, or N2 disease (Depierre et al. 2002; Roth et al. 1994; Rosell et al. 1994; Crowley et al. 2005; (van Meerbeeck et al. 2005 (EORTC metaanalysis)) ■ *If unresectable after restaging → complete definitive concurrent chemo-RT (63 Gy)	5-year OS 20–25%, MS 16–17 months Induction chemo-RT pCR rate 15–20% Post-op RT possible 5–10% OS benefit for N2 (LCSG, MRC, SEER, and ANITA)
IIIA inoperable	■ Concurrent chemo-RT (63 Gy) → adjuvant chemo (LAMP, RTOG 9410; French and Japanese) (preferred) ■ If unacceptable risk of pneumonitis with upfront RT, consider induction chemo for down-staging → concurrent chemo-RT (to postchemo volume) if no progression (CALGB 39801)	~5-year OS and MSConcurrent chemo-RT: 20–25%, 16–17 months Sequential chemo-RT: 20%, 13–15 months RT alone: <10%, 10–12 months
IIIB (no pleural effusion)	■ Concurrent chemo-RT (61–63 Gy) (LAMP, RTOG 9410) (preferred) ■ If unacceptable risk of pneumonitis with upfront RT, consider induction chemo for down-staging → concurrent chemo-RT (to postchemo volume) if no progression (CALGB 39801)	

continued

	■ If T4N0-1, may treat with surgery → chemo ± RT (if residual or + margins), or chemo ± RT → surgery → chemo	
Typical chemo	<u>Postsurgery</u> ■ Cisplatin 100 mg/m² d1 and etoposide 100 mg/m² d1–3 every 4 weeks × 4 cycles ■ Other cisplatin combinations with vinorelbine, vinblastine, gemcitabine, and docetaxel may be considered ■ Alternative if not able to tolerate cisplatin: carboplatin, Paclitaxel every 3 weeks for 4 cycles <u>Concurrent with RT</u> ■ Cisplatin 50 mg/m² d1, 8, 29, and 36 and etoposide 50 mg/m² d1–5 and 29–33 ■ Alternatives: cisplatin week 1 and 4, vinblastine weekly; or, carboplatin and paclitaxel weekly <u>Sequential chemo → RT</u> ■ Cisplatin 100 mg/m² d1, 29 and vinblastine 5 mg/m² weekly × 5 weeks ■ Alternative: carboplatin and paclitaxel every 3 weeks × 2 cycles <u>Consolidation chemo after chemo-RT</u> ■ Carboplatin and paclitaxel every 3 weeks × 2 cycles	
IIIB (pleural effusion)	■ Local treatment as necessary (e.g., pleurodesis) and treat as stage IV	
IV	■ ECOG PS 0–2: platinum-based chemo ± bevacizumab ± palliative RT. First-line chemo uses 2 agents with response assessment after each cycle, for up to 4–6 cycles or until progression. ■ ECOG PS 3–4: best supportive care	
Superior sulcus	■ If operable, concurrent chemo-RT (45 Gy) → surgery → chemo (preferred). Or, surgery → post-op chemo + RT (60–66 Gy) for close or + margins, nodal ECE ■ If marginally resectable, concurrent chemo-RT (45 Gy) → restage → if no	50% pCR or minimal microscopic residual disease after initial chemo-RT

continued

	progression → surgery → chemo (INT 0160) ■ If unresectable (initially or after restaging), complete definitive concurrent chemo-RT (63–66 Gy)	5-year OS 45%. Most common site failure in brain (40%)
Pulmonary carcinoid	■ For stage I–III, surgery preferred (lobectomy or other anatomic re-section with mediastinal LN dis-section or sampling). Adjuvant RT considered for atypical histology, involved LN, +margin, subtotal re-section. No definite role for chemo since response rate is only 20–30% (mainly with doxorubicin), but many institutions consider cisplatin/etoposide with RT. ■ For stage III, if surgery is not feasible, definitive RT (typical) or chemo-RT (atypical) is used ■ For stage IV, systemic therapy is used. Octreotide considered if octreotide scan positive or symptoms of carcinoid syndrome. Palliative RT may be used as well	5-year OS: Resected typical carcinoid >70–90% Resected atypical carcinoid: 25–70% Metastatic carcinoid: 20–40%

STUDIES

SCREENING

- IELCAP (NEJM 2006): 31,567 asymptomatic persons at risk for lung CA screened with low-dose CT. Screening diagnosed 484 patients, 85% of which had stage I disease with 88–92% survival rate.
- Bach et al. (2007): 3,246 current or former smokers screened in one of three single-arm annual CT scan screening programs. CT screening increased the rate of lung CA diagnosis by 3× and surgery by 10×, but there was no decline in the number of advanced cases diagnosed nor in deaths from lung CA (observed vs. predicted). Criticized because of short (3 years) follow-up which may lead to bias because more years may be needed to confirm that death is prevented.
- National Lung Screening Trial (closed): 50,000 current or former smokers randomized to annual CXR vs. CT × 3 years to determine reduction in lung cancer mortality.

SURGERY

- For T1–2N0, surgery has ≥80% LC and 50–70% CSS. Twenty-five to thirty-five percent pathologic upstaging from clinical stage.
- Video-assisted thoracoscopic surgery (VATS) + lymphadenectomy may have equivalent oncologic results as open thoracotomy in properly selected cases.
- LCSG 821 (Ginsberg and Rubinstein 1995): 247 patients with peripheral T1N0 randomized to lobectomy vs. wedge resection with a 2 cm margin of normal lung. Wedge resection tripled LRF (6 → 18%).

IV

RT ALONE

Standard fractionation

- SEER (Chest 2005): 4,300 patients with unresected stage I–II NSCLC. RT improved MS vs. no RT (stage I 14 → 21 months, stage II 9 → 14 months), but not 5-year lung CA specific survival (stage I 15%, stage II 10%).
- Dosoretz et al. (1996): review of T1–3N0 medically inoperable patients treated with RT alone. RT >64 Gy improved PFS and increasing field size did not improve outcomes.
- Sibley (1998): review of ten studies of medically inoperable T1–2N0 patients treated with RT alone 60–66 Gy. Five-year OS was ~15%. Approximately 50% of failures were local only vs. ~5% regional-only failure. Approximately 30% of patients died of DM, ~30% of patients died after LF, and ~25% died of intercurrent disease.
- RTOG 73–01 (Perez et al. 1980): 375 patients with IIIA/IIIB treated with RT alone randomized to 2/40 Gy vs. 2/50 Gy vs. 2/60 Gy vs. 4/40 Gy (split-course). Clinical LC was improved with dose escalation. However, 75–80% of patients developed DM in all arms and 2-year OS was only 14–18% in continuous RT arms.

Dose escalation

- RTOG 93-11 (Bradley et al. 2005): 179 patients with medically inoperable or unresectable I–III disease stratified into RT dose escalation levels of 70.9, 77.4, 83.8, or 90.3 Gy at 2.15 Gy/fx depending on V20. Concurrent chemo not allowed. Twenty-five patients received neoadjuvant chemo. The PTV included the GTV (primary and involved LN) +1 cm margin. RT was generally well tolerated except in 90.3 Gy group (with two dose-related deaths). LRC ranged from 50 to 78%.

SBRT and hypofractionation

- Indiana (Fakiris et al. 2009; Timmerman et al. 2006): 70 patients with T1–3N0 (≤7 cm) treated with 60–66 Gy in 3 fx over 1–2 weeks. Three-year LC 88%, CSS 82%, OS 43%, regional failure 9%, and distant failure 13%. Patients with central tumors had increased risk of grade 3–5 toxicity (27 vs. 10%).
- Onishi et al. (2004): 245 patients with T1–2N0 treated with 18–75 Gy in 1–22 fx. LF was 8% for BED ≥100 Gy vs. 26% for BED <100 Gy. Three-year OS was 88% for BED ≥100 Gy vs. 69% for BED <100 Gy.
- Slotman et al. (1996): review of 31 patients with T1–2N0 treated with 4 Gy/fraction to the tumor +1.5 cm margin to 40 Gy → conedown to tumor +0.5 cm margin to 48 Gy. Three-year OS 40%, DFS 76%. Only 6% regional failure.
- Cheung et al. (2002): 33 patients with T1–2N0 treated with 4 Gy × 12. Two-year OS 46%, CSS 54%, RFS 40%.
- RTOG 0236 (ASTRO 2009 abstract): patients with T1–3N0 (≤5 cm) medically inoperable tumors >2 cm from proximal bronchial tree treated with SBRT 20 Gy × 3 over 1.5–2 weeks, (54 Gy with proper heterogeneity correction). GTV = CTV. PTV = 0.5 cm axial margin and 1 cm superior/inferior margin, Two yr LC 94%, 15% DM, DFS 67%, OS 72%.

INDUCTION CHEMO VS. SURGERY ALONE

Study	Patients	Randomization	Outcome	Comment
(van Meerbeeck et al. 2005 (EORTC metaanalysis))/MRC LU22 (Gilligan et al. 2007)	519 patients Stage cI (61%), cII (31%), and cIII (7%)	3c platinum-based chemo over ~9 weeks → surgery vs. surgery alone Most common chemo regimen was cisplatin vinorelbine	No benefit for 2-year PFS (52–53%) or 5-year OS (44–45%) Updating of metaanalysis: chemo improved 5year OS by 5%	Underpowered study given large number of cT1 patients (few events). Combined data for metaanalysis
S9900 (Pisters et al. ASCO 2005 and 2007)	335 patients Stage cT2N0, T1–2N1, and T3N0–1	Carboplatin–paclitaxel × 3c → surgery vs. surgery alone	Trend in favor of induction chemo: 5-year PFS (32 vs. 41%, $p = 0.10$) and OS (42 vs. 48%, $p = 0.24$)	pCR to chemo was 10%

continued

Depierre et al. (2002)	355 patients Resectable stage cIB–IIIA	Pre-op chemo × 3c → surgery → chemo × 2c vs. no pre-op chemo Chemo was mitomycin C, ifosfamide, cisplatin Patients with pT3 or pN2 received 60 Gy RT	Pre-op chemo increased DFS (13 → 27 months, $p = 0.03$)	On subset analysis, benefit only for N0–1 patients and not for N2 patients
Rosell et al. (1994)	60 patients Stage cIIIA	Pre-op chemo × 3c → surgery → 50 Gy to mediastinum vs. no pre-op chemo Pre-op chemo was MMC, ifosfamide, cisplatin	Induction chemo improved MS (8 months → 26 months) and 2-year OS (0 → 30%)	
Roth et al. (1994)	60 patients Stage cIIIA	Pre-op chemo × 3c → surgery → chemo × 3c vs. surgery alone Chemo was cytoxan, etoposide, cisplatin RT given for unresectable or residual disease	Chemo improved MS (11 → 64 months) and 3-year OS (15 → 56%)	
NATCH (Felip et al. 2009)	618 patients Stage cI (>2 cm), II, and T3N1	Surgery alone; induction carboplatin/ paclitaxel × 3c → surgery;	No difference in 5-year DFS (39–40.5%) in preliminary analysis with median	

continued

	or surgery → adjuvant carboplatin/ paclitaxel × 3c	follow-up of 43 months, but more patients in induction arm received planned chemotherapy

INDUCTION CHEMO FOLLOWED BY SURGERY VS. DEFINITIVE RT

- EORTC 08941 (JNCI 2007): 579 patients with initially unresectable pIIIA(N2) disease treated with induction cisplatin-based chemo. Three hundred and thirty-two patients (61%) with a response randomized to surgery or definitive RT. Post-op RT (2/56 Gy) given to 40% of patients with an incomplete resection. pCR was 5%, and 47% had pneumonectomy. Four percent surgical mortality. Definitive RT was to tumor and involved mediastinum to 60–62 Gy with 46 Gy to uninvolved mediastinum. One RT patient died of RT pneumonitis. No difference in MS (16–18 months) or PFS (9–11 months). Fewer local/regional failures (32 vs. 55%), but more distant metastases (61 vs. 39%) with surgery. patients with pneumonectomy, incomplete resection or persistent pN2 disease did worse.

INDUCTION CHEMO FOLLOWED BY CHEMO-RT AND SURGERY VS. SURGERY AND POST-OP RT

- German trial (Thomas et al. 2008): 524 patients with IIIA/IIIB treated with neoadjuvant cisplatin/etoposide × 3c, then randomized to pre-op hyperfractionated chemo-RT vs. immediate surgery → post-op RT. Pre-op chemo-RT was 1.5 b.i.d./45 Gy with carboplatin/vindesin × 3c → surgery if possible → RT boost (1.5 b.i.d./24 Gy) if inoperable or R1/R2 resection. Post-op RT was 1.8/54 Gy or 1.8/68.4 Gy if inoperable or R1/R2 resection. There was no difference in 5-year OS or PFS (16 vs. 14%). Pre-op hyperfractionated RT increased complete resection rates (37 vs. 32%), and in those with complete resection, increased mediastinal down-staging (46 vs. 29%).

INDUCTION CHEMO-RT VS. DEFINITIVE CHEMO-RT

- Intergroup/RTOG 0139 (Lancet 2009; ASCO 2005 abstr.): 396 patients with T1–3pN2M0 treated with concurrent chemo × 2c + 45 Gy → restaging → randomized to (surgery (if no progression) → chemo × 2c] vs. [concurrent chemo-RT to 61 Gy (no surgery)) → chemo × 2c. Chemo was cisplatinum and etoposide. Eighteen percent of patients in surgery arm had pCR to induction chemo. Surgery improved 5-year PFS (11 → 22%) and median PFS (10.5 → 12.8 months) with fewer local-only relapses (10 vs. 22%). There was no significant difference in MS (23.6 vs. 22.2 months, $p = 0.24$), although there was a 5-year OS trend in favor of surgery (20 vs. 27%, $p = 0.1$). Increased treatment-related deaths with surgery (8 vs. 2%), particularly when pneumonectomy required.

IV

PRE-OP RT

- There is no improvement in survival with pre-op RT alone (without chemo) as noted in two collaborative studies from 1970s (VA and NCI).

POST-OP CHEMO

Study	Patients	Randomization	Primary outcome	Comment
ANITA (Lancet Oncol 2006)	840 patients with resected IB–IIIA	Cisplatinum vinorelbine × 4c vs. observation	Chemo increased 5-year OS by 8.6%	On subset analysis, benefit limited to *N* + patients (II–IIIA)
ALPI (JNCI 2003)	1,209 patients with resected I–IIIA	MMC/cisplatin/vindesine × 3c vs. observation	No difference in OS or PFS	Poor compliance with MVP chemo
NCIC JBR.10 (Winton et al. 2005, Vincent 2009)	482 patients with completely resected pIB–II	Cisplatin/vinorelibine × 4c vs. observation. No RT	Chemo improved 5-year OS (54 → 69%) and RFS (49 → 61%). Long-term survival benefit limited to N1 patients after a median follow-up of 9.3 years	0.8% of patients died due to chemo toxicity
CALGB 9633 (Strauss et al. 2004	344 patients with completely	Carbo/taxol × 4c vs. observation	No significant difference in OS and DFS with chemo	On subset analysis, OS and DFS benefit for

continued

	resected T2N0		with a median follow-up of 74 months	tumors ≥4 cm. No treatment-related deaths
Kato et al. (2004)	980 patients with pT1–2N0 (adenocarcinoma only)	Daily uracil-tegafur (UFT) for 2 years vs. observation	UFT improved 5-year OS (85 → 88%)	Most benefit for T2 (74 → 85%) but not T1 (89 → 90%)
IALT (Arriagada et al. 2004; Le Chevalier, 2008 abstract 7507)	1,867 patients with pI (36%), pII (25%), and pIII (39%)	3–4c adjuvant cisplatinum-based chemo (most platinum/ etoposide) vs. obs. Post-op RT (60 Gy) to the mediastinum was given to ~1/3 of N1 patients and ~2/3 of N2 patients	Chemo improved 5-year OS (40 → 45%) and DFS (34 → 39%)	0.8% of patients died due to chemo toxicity. With 7.5-year follow-up, there were more deaths in chemo group
LACE (Pignon et al. 2008)	Metaanalysis of five largest trials of 4,584 patients	Cisplatin-based chemo after complete resection vs. observation	5-year OS benefit 5.4% with chemo, greatest for stage II and III	No difference among chemo regimens

POST-OP RT

- *SEER* (JCO 2006): >7,400 patients with stage II–III resected NSCLC. PORT used most often for patients <50 years, T3–4, larger T size, increased N stage, more than number and percent involved LN. PORT improved 5-year OS for N2 patients (20→27%, HR 0.85), but reduced OS for N0 (41 → 31%, HR 1.2), and N1 (34 → 30%, HR 1.1) patients.
- *LCSG 773* (NEJM 1986): 210 patients with pII–IIIA (squamous cell carcinoma only) randomized to observation vs. post-op RT to the mediastinum (50 Gy). RT decreased LR overall (41 → 3%) and for N2 patients, but there were no differences in OS.

- MRC (Stephens et al. 1996): 308 patients with pII–IIIA randomized to observation vs. post-op RT (2.67/40 Gy). Subgroup analysis demonstrated a 1 month survival advantage and improved LRC for N2 (but not N1) patients.
- Sawyer et al. (1997): regression tree analysis of pN2 patients treated with and without post-op RT. RT improved LRC and OS for patients with more than or equal to two N2 nodes or T3–4 tumors with one N2 node.
- PORT Metaanalysis Trialists Group (1998): 9 trials of surgery ± post-op RT. For N0–1 patients, RT produced a 7% absolute OS decrement, but there was no OS difference for N2 patients. Analysis criticized because 25% of patients were N0, many patients were treated with Co-60, older studies used inadequate staging, and unpublished data were included.
- Van Houtte et al. (1980): pI–II randomized to observation vs. post-op 60 Gy to mediastinum. RT improved local-regional control, but 5-year OS was worse (24% RT vs. 43% with observation) due to increased pneumonitis. Study criticized because used Co-60 machines, large field size, and no CT planning.

IV

POST-OP RT ± CHEMO

- INT 0115/ECOG 3590 (Keller et al. 2000): 488 patients with completely resected pII–IIIA randomized to RT (1.8/50.4 Gy) ± concurrent cisplatin/etoposide chemo × 4c. RT boost given for ECE (10.8 Gy). Addition of chemo did not change MS (38–39 months) or LF (12–13%).

POST-OP CHEMO ± RT

- ANITA (Douillard et al. 2008): see details above under post-op chemo trials. Post-op RT (45–60 Gy) was given to 28% of patients (8% of N0, 35% of N1, and 52% of N2). RT increased 5-year OS by 5–13% for all N2 patients and by 12% for N1 patients not given chemo. RT reduced OS for N1 patients given chemo. PORT reduced local/regional failure (first site) for both N1 and N2 patients.
- *CALGB 9734* (Strauss et al. 2004): randomized patients with resected N2 disease treated with 4c adjuvant carbo-taxol to observation vs. post-op mediastinal RT. Closed early after only 40 patients enrolled. Median FFS increased with RT (16→26 months), but no difference in OS.
- French IFCT 0503 (ongoing): randomizes patients with resected N2 disease to post-op -conformal RT 54 Gy. Pre-op or post-op chemo allowed before RT, but not concurrent with RT.

SEQUENCING AND TIMING OF DEFINITIVE CHEMO AND RT

- RT alone: MS 10–12 months, 5-year OS 7%
- Sequential chemo → RT: MS 13–15 months, 5-year OS 20%
- Concurrent chemo-RT: MS 16–17 months, 5-year OS 20–30

RT ± INDUCTION CHEMO

- CALGB 8433 (Dillman et al. 1990): 155 patients with T3 or N2 randomized to RT alone (2/60 Gy) vs. sequential cisplatin/vinblastine → RT (60 Gy). Induction chemo improved MS (10 → 14 months) and 2/5-year OS (13/7 → 26/19%).
- *RTOG 8808* (Sause et al. 2000): 458 patients with cII, IIIA, IIIB randomized to RT alone (2/60 Gy) vs. sequential cisplatin/vinblastine → 2/60 Gy vs. b.i.d. RT alone (1.2/69.6 Gy). Induction chemo improved MS (13.2 months) vs. RT alone, and there was no difference for qd RT (11.4 months) vs. b.i.d. RT (12 months).

SEQUENTIAL VS. CONCURRENT CHEMO-RT

- *RTOG 9410* (Curran et al. 2003 abstr.): 610 patients with unresectable or medically inoperable II–III randomized to chemo → 1.8/63 Gy (seq) vs. concurrent 1.8/63 Gy + chemo (con-qd) vs. concurrent 1.2 b.i.d./69.6 Gy + chemo (con-b.i.d.). Chemo was cisplatin/vinblastine, but cisplatin/etoposide for b.i.d. arm. Concurrent chemo improved MS (seq = 14.6 months, con-qd = 17 months, con-b.i.d. = 15.2 months) and 4y OS, but increased toxicity, especially with b.i.d. RT.
- *French NPC 95-01* (Fournel et al. 2005): randomized 205 patients with unresectable stage III to sequential cisplatin/vinorelbine → RT (2/66 Gy) vs. concurrent cisplatin/etoposide ×2c + RT (2/66 Gy) → consolidation cisplatin/vinorelbine. Although not statistically significant, concurrent chemo-RT had improved MS (14.5 → 16.3 months) and 2–4-year OS (by 7–13%). Esophageal toxicity was more frequent with concurrent.
- Huber et al. (2006): 214 patients with IIIA/B received induction carbo/paclitaxel × 2 cycles and if no progression randomized to 60 Gy with or without weekly paclitaxel. Trend for improved MS with chemo-RT (14→19 months) and significantly improved MPFS (6→12 months). No difference in toxicity.
- LAMP (Belani et al. 2005): randomized phase II study of 276 patients with unresectable IIIA/IIIB randomized to sequential chemo ×2c → 63 Gy (arm 1) vs. induction chemo ×2c → concurrent 63 Gy + chemo × 7c (arm 2) vs. concurrent 63 Gy + chemo × 7c → adjuvant chemo ×2c (arm 3). Chemo was carboplatin and

paclitaxel. Med follow-up 40 months. Upfront concurrent chemo-RT improved MS (arm 1 = 13 months, arm 2 = 12.7 months, arm 3 = 16.3 months). Arm 2 was stopped early because 20% of patients did not get chemo with RT. G3–4 esophagitis 19–28% arm 2–3.

- Furuse et al. (1999): 320 patients treated with 56 Gy (split-course) and concurrent vs. sequential cisplatin, vindesine, and mitomycin. Concurrent chemo improved MS 13→17 months and 5-year OS 9→16% vs. sequential.

CONCURRENT CHEMO-RT ± INDUCTION CHEMO

- CALGB 39801 (Vokes et al. 2007): 366 patients with unresectable IIIA/IIIB randomized to concurrent weekly carbo-taxol chemo + RT (66 Gy) vs. induction carbo-taxol q3 weeks ×2c → same concurrent chemo-RT. No difference in MS (12–14 months) or OS. Induction chemo increased toxicity (20% grade 3–4 neutropenia).
- Also see arm two of LAMP (above).

CONCURRENT CHEMO REGIMENS

- CALGB 9431 (Vokes 2002): phase II trial of 175 patients with unresectable stage III disease treated with chemo ×2c → concurrent chemo-RT to 66 Gy randomized to three different cisplatin-based chemo regimens (with gemcitabine, paclitaxel, or vinorelbine). Median OS was 18 months for gemcitabine and vinorelbine and 15 months for paclitaxel, but no difference in 3-year OS.
- CALGB 30105 (Blackstock 2006): 69 patients randomized to induction carbo/paclitaxel → concurrent carbo-paclitaxel and RT vs. induction carbo-gemcitabine → concurrent gemcitabine 2×/week during RT. RT 2/74 Gy. MS 24 months for carbo-paclitaxel vs. 17 months for carbo-gemcitabine.

CONSOLIDATION THERAPIES

- HOG (Hanna et al. 2008): randomized 203 unresectable IIIA/B patients without progression after concurrent cisplatin/etoposide × 2c and RT to 59.4 Gy to docetaxel 75 mg/m^2 q3 weeks × 3 vs. no additional treatment. Interim analysis demonstrated no differences in OS (MS 21–23 months) or PFS and more toxicity with docetaxel.
- SWOG 0023 (Kelly et al. 2008): 243 IIIA/B patients treated with cisplatin-etoposide × 2c and concurrent 61 Gy → docetaxel × 3c randomized to observation vs. maintenance gefitinib (Iressa). Worse MS (23 vs. 35 months) and trend for worse PFS with gefitinib.

SUPERIOR SULCUS

- Int 0160 (Rusch et al. 2007): phase II trial of 111 patients with T3–4N0–1 superior sulcus tumors treated with concurrent chemo-RT (45 Gy) → restaging → surgery (if no progression) → chemo ×2c. Chemo was platinum/etoposide. If progression on restaging, complete definitive chemoRT to 63Gy without surgery. Eighty-six percent of patients had surgery. Fifty-six percent had pCR or minimal microscopic residual disease. The most common site of relapse was in the brain.

PROPHYLACTIC CRANIAL RT (PCI)

- Brain is the site of failure for ~15% of early-stage patients and >15% for advanced stage patients. Three older randomized trials have investigated PCI in advanced NSCLC. PCI delayed and reduced the incidence of brain failure, but had no impact on OS. Extracranial disease was the cause of death for most patients, and may be a source of CNS re-seeding after PCI.
- RTOG 0214 (Gore 2009): randomized patients with definitively treated stage IIIA/B disease to prophylactic cranial RT (30 Gy/15 fractions) or observation. No difference in 1-year OS or DFS, but PCI improved rates of brain metastasis at 1 year (7.7 vs. 18%).

RADIATION TECHNIQUES

SIMULATION AND FIELD DESIGN

- Simulate patient supine with arms up so that arms do not block the tattoos on the sides of the patient.
- Immobilize with a wingboard or with an alpha cradle (with arms up).
- Use a 3D conformal or IMRT plan throughout treatment so that beams passing through normal tissues have lower doses per fraction throughout treatment.
- Wedges and/or compensating filters may be needed.
- Favor 6–10 MV photons with 3D planning over higher energies because underdosing of tumor can occur in regions of electronic disequilibrium such as the tumor/lung interface with higher energies.
- GTV: gross primary and nodal disease including LN(s) ≥1 cm or hypermetabolic on PET scan or harboring tumor cells per mediastinoscopy.
- CTV: typically includes the GTV plus 1–1.5 cm margin.
- PTV: add 0.5–1.5 cm margin on CTV to account for set-up uncertainties and respiratory motion.

- Respiratory tracking or gating systems or 4D planning may allow for decreased PTV margins.
- Elective nodal RT.
  - The rationale against elective nodal RT for early-stage disease is that there are high rates of local recurrence with current doses and techniques. If gross disease cannot be controlled, then why enlarge the volume and increase complications by including areas that might harbor microscopic disease that will frequently be addressed by chemo.
  - Rosenzweig et al. (2007): 524 patients with NSCLC treated with 3DCRT to only tumor and histologically or radiographically involved LN regions. No elective nodal RT. Only 6% of patients developed failure in an initially uninvolved LN region in the absence of local failure. Many patients experienced treatment failure in multiple LN regions simultaneously.
  - Only consider treating the supraclavicular fossa if an upper lobe primary or gross upper mediastinal disease because it is the first site of failure in only ~3% of patients.
  - Contralateral hilar or supraclavicular treatment is discouraged unless involved.
- Post-op RT.
  - If N2 and margins are negative, adjuvant chemo for 2–4c → mediastinal RT.
    - Involved LN region ± ipsilateral hilum ± subcarinal LN region to 50.4 Gy depending on the extent of node dissection, number, bulk, and location of mediastinal disease and primary tumor.
    - 10–16 Gy boost if extranodal extension.
  - If + margin: favor initial post-op RT → adjuvant chemo or post-op concurrent chemo-RT (e.g., carbo/taxol with RT). Limit field to area of + margin if N0–1 disease (i.e., no elective mediastinal nodal coverage).
  - If gross residual disease → favor concurrent chemo-RT.
- "Classic" post-op mediastinal field borders.
  - Superior border = Apex of lung. SCV fossa included for bulky N2 disease and T3 upper lobe lesions.
  - Inferior = 5 cm below carina (more if subcarinal originally involved).
  - Lateral = 2 cm on trachea and ipsilateral hilum.

DEFINITIVE RT DOSE PRESCRIPTIONS

- Primary and involved LN: generally, 63–66 Gy at 1.8–2 Gy per fraction with or without chemo. May consider treating up to 77.4 Gy without concurrent chemo (keep V20≤35%) or up to 74 Gy with concurrent chemo (mainly carboplatin and paclitaxel).

- For peripheral lesions, may hypofractionate at 4 Gy/fraction to tumor +1.5 cm margin to 40 Gy followed by conedown to tumor +0.5 cm to 48 Gy.
- Various radiosurgical techniques have been reported.
- Commonly used radiosurgical technique for peripheral tumors <5 cm.
  - 20 Gy per fraction for three fractions to the 60–90% isodose line covering the PTV (54 Gy with proper heterogeneity correction).
  - Delivered over 1.5–2 weeks with 2–8 days between fractions.
  - Uses 7–10 nonopposing, noncoplanar beams.
  - To reduce internal motion, abdominal compression, respiratory gating, or active breath holding techniques may be used.
  - For planning, the GTV = CTV. PTV = 0.5 cm axial and 1 cm superior/inferior margin.

POST-OP RT DOSE PRESCRIPTIONS

- If N2: 50.4 Gy with consideration of 10–16 Gy boost for extranodal extension.
- If + margin, 60–66 Gy to area of + margin.

DOSE LIMITATIONS

- Spinal cord:
  - RT alone: maximum dose <50 Gy.
  - Chemo-RT: maximum dose <46 Gy at 1.8–2 Gy/fx QD or <36 Gy with b.i.d. RT.
- Lung:
  - Combined volume of both normal lungs receiving ≥20 Gy (V20): RT alone <40%, chemo-RT <35%.
  - Mean lung dose: RT alone <20 Gy, chemo-RT <16.5–20 Gy.
  - V5: chemo-RT <42%.
  - Pneumonitis grading.
    - Grade 1: asymptomatic radiographic changes.
    - Grade 2: changes requiring steroids or diuretics; dyspnea on exertion
    - Grade 3: requires oxygen; shortness of breath at rest
    - Grade 4: requires assisted ventilation
    - Grade 5: death
- Esophagus:
  - Maximum dose <75 Gy.
  - Without chemo: V60 Gy <50%, V55 Gy <65%.
  - With chemo: V55 Gy <50%.

- Heart: V40 Gy <50%.
- Pacemakers/internal cardiac defibrilators (ICD).
  - Can malfunction at ≤2.5 Gy, depending on manufacturer and model. Attempt to get RT tolerance specifications from manufacturer. Always keep out of field. Estimate dose. If >2 Gy, move out of field.
  - ICDs can be more sensitive and critical than pacemakers. Consider deactivating ICD during RT and replace with ECD (external cardiac defibrillator, temporary).
  - Cardiologist should evaluate and interrogate pacemaker/ICD before, weekly during RT, and monthly after RT.
  - Have CPR equipment available.
  - Observe patient after initial ports and each treatment.
- Brachial plexus: maximum dose <60 Gy.
  - If superior sulcus, inform of increased risk with concurrent chemo if 60–63 Gy.
- Liver: V30 Gy <40%.
- Kidney: V20 Gy <50% of combined volume or <25% of one side if one kidney is not functional.
- Chemo agents that may increase lung toxicity = busulfan, cyclophosphamide, IFN, bleomycin, MMC, MTX, nitrosureas.

IV

COMPLICATIONS

- Acute RT complications include esophagitis, dermatitis, and/or cough.
- Subacute and late complications include pneumonitis, pulmonary fibrosis, pericarditis, brachial plexopathy, and Lhermitte's syndrome.
- Radiation pneumonitis occurs ~6 weeks after RT. It presents with cough, dyspnea, hypoxia, and fever. Treat symptomatic radiation pneumonitis with prednisone (1 mg/kg/d) or 60 mg/day and trimethoprim/sulfamethaxazole for PCP prophylaxis. Often produces dramatic and quick response in symptoms, but very gradual and prolonged taper is critical for durable symptom resolution.
- Lhermitte's syndrome (sudden electric-like shocks extending down the spine with head flexion) usually resolves spontaneously. Not predictive for late myelopathy.

FOLLOW-UP

- H&P and CXR every 3–4 months for 2 years, then every 6 months for 3 years, then annually. CT chest annually. PET scans optional.

REFERENCES

Arriagada R, Bergman B, Dunant A, et al. Cisplatin-based adjuvant chemotherapy in patients with completely resected non-small-cell lung cancer. N Engl J Med 2004;350:351-360

Bach PB, Jett JR, Pastorino U, Tockman MS, Swensen SJ, Begg CB. Computed tomography screening and lung cancer outcomes. Jama. Mar 7 2007;297(9):953-961.

Belani C, Choy H, Bonomi P, et al. Combined chemoradiotherapy regimens of paclitaxel and carboplatin for locally advanced non-small-cell lung cancer: a randomized phase II locally advanced multi-modality protocol. J Clin Oncol 2005;23:5883-5891.

Bradley J, Graham MV, Winter K. Toxicity and outcome results of RTOG 9311: A phase I-II dose escalation study using three-dimensional conformal radiation therapy in patients with inoperable non-small cell lung carcinoma. Int J Radiat Oncol Biol Phys 2005;61:318-328.

Cheung PC, Yeung LT, Basrur V, Ung YC, Balogh J, Danjoux CE. Accelerated hypofractionation for early-stage non-small-cell lung cancer. Int J Radiat Oncol Biol Phys. Nov 15 2002;54(4): 1014-1023.

Crowley R, Ginsberg P, Ellis B, et al. S9900: A phase III trial of surgery alone or surgery plus preoperative (preop) paclitaxel/carboplatin (PC) chemotherapy in early stage non-small cell lung cancer (NSCLC): Preliminary results. J Clin Oncol, 2005; ASCO Annual Meeting Proceedings, 2005;23;16S (1 Supplement):624S.

Curran WJ, Scott CB, Langer CJ, et al. Long-term benefit is observed in a phase III comparison of sequential vs concurrent chemo-radiation for patients with unresected stage III nsclc: RTOG 9410. Proc Am Soc Clin Oncol 2003 (abstr 2499);22:621.

Depierre A, Milleron B, Moro-Sibilot D, et al. Preoperative chemotherapy followed by surgery compared with primary surgery in resectable stage I (except T1N0), II, and IIIa non-small-cell lung cancer. J Clin Oncol 2002;20:247-253.

Dillman RO, Seagren SL, Propert KJ, et al. A randomized trial of induction chemotherapy plus high-dose radiation versus radiation alone in stage III non-small-cell lung cancer. N Engl J Med 1990;323:940-945.

Douillard JY, Rosell R, De Lena M, Riggi M, Hurteloup P, Mahe MA. Impact of postoperative radiation therapy on survival in patients with complete resection and stage I, II, or IIIA non-small-cell lung cancer treated with adjuvant chemotherapy: the adjuvant Navelbine International Trialist Association (ANITA) Randomized Trial. Int J Radiat Oncol Biol Phys. Nov 1 2008;72(3):695-701.

Dosoretz DE, Katin MJ, Blitzer PH, et al. Medically Inoperable Lung Carcinoma: The Role of Radiation Therapy. Semin Radiat Oncol 1996;6:98-104.

Felip E, Garrido P, Trigo JM, et al. SEOM guidelines for the management of non-small-cell lung cancer (NSCLC). Clin Transl Oncol. May 2009;11(5):284-289.

Fournel P, Robinet G, Thomas P, et al. Randomized phase III trial of sequential chemoradiotherapy compared with concurrent chemoradiotherapy in locally advanced non-small-cell lung cancer: Groupe Lyon-Saint-Etienne d'Oncologie Thoracique- Groupe Français de Pneumo-Cancérologie NPC 95-01 Study. J Clin Oncol 2005;23: 5910-5917.

Fakiris AJ, McGarry RC, Yiannoutsos CT, et al. Stereotactic Body Radiation Therapy for Early-Stage Non-Small-Cell Lung Carcinoma: Four-Year Results of a Prospective Phase II Study. Int J Radiat Oncol Biol Phys. Feb 27 2009.

Fischer B, Lassen U, Mortensen J, et al. Preoperative staging of lung cancer with combined PET-CT. N Engl J Med. 2009;361(1):32-39.

Gilligan D, Nicolson M, Smith I, et al. Preoperative chemotherapy in patients with resectable non-small cell lung cancer: results of the MRC LU22/NVALT 2/EORTC 08012 multicentre randomised trial and update of systematic review. Lancet. Jun 9 2007;369(9577):1929-1937.

Ginsberg RJ, Rubinstein LV. Randomized trial of lobectomy versus limited resection for T1 N0 non-small cell lung cancer. Lung Cancer Study Group. Ann Thorac Surg 1995;60:615-622; discussion 622-613.

Gould MK, Kuschner WG, Rydzak CE, et al. Test performance of positron emission tomography and computed tomography for mediastinal staging in patients with non-small-cell lung cancer: a meta-analysis. Ann Intern Med. Dec 2 2003;139(11):879-892.

Gore E. Prophylactic cranial irradiation versus observation in stage III non-small-cell lung cancer. Clin Lung Cancer. Jan 2006;7(4):276-278.

Huber RM, Flentje M, Schmidt M, et al. Simultaneous chemoradiotherapy compared with radiotherapy alone after induction chemotherapy in inoperable stage IIIA or IIIB non-small-cell lung cancer: study CTRT99/97 by the Bronchial Carcinoma Therapy Group. J Clin Oncol. Sep 20 2006;24(27):4397-4404.

Kato H, Ichinose Y, Ohta M, et al. A randomized trial of adjuvant chemotherapy with uracil-tegafur for adenocarcinoma of the lung. N Engl J Med 2004;350:1713-1721.

Keller SM, Adak S, Wagner H, et al. A randomized trial of postoperative adjuvant therapy in patients with completely resected stage II or IIIA non-small-cell lung cancer. Eastern Cooperative Oncology Group. N Engl J Med 2000;343:1217-1222.

Kelly K, Chansky K, Gaspar LE, et al. Phase III trial of maintenance gefitinib or placebo after concurrent chemoradiotherapy and docetaxel consolidation in inoperable stage III non-small-cell lung cancer: SWOG S0023. J Clin Oncol. May 20 2008;26(15):2450-2456.

Onishi H, Araki T, Shirato H, et al. Stereotactic hypofractionated high-dose irradiation for stage I nonsmall cell lung carcinoma: clinical outcomes in 245 subjects in a Japanese multiinstitutional study. Cancer. Oct 1 2004;101(7):1623-1631.

Perez CA, Stanley K, Rubin P, et al. A prospective randomized study of various irradiation doses and fractionation schedules in the treatment of inoperable non-oat-cell carcinoma of the lung. Preliminary report by the Radiation Therapy Oncology Group. Cancer 1980;45: 2744-2753.

Pisters KM, Evans WK, Azzoli CG, et al. Cancer Care Ontario and American Society of Clinical Oncology adjuvant chemotherapy and adjuvant radiation therapy for stages I-IIIA resectable non small-cell lung cancer guideline. J Clin Oncol. Dec 1 2007;25(34):5506-5518.

PORT Meta-analysis Trialists Group. Postoperative radiotherapy in non-small-cell lung cancer: systematic review and meta-analysis of individual patient data from nine randomised controlled trials. Lancet 1998;352:257-263.

Rosell R, Gomez-Codina J, Camps C, et al. A randomized trial comparing preoperative chemotherapy plus surgery with surgery alone in patients with non-small-cell lung cancer. N Engl J Med 1994;330:153-158.

Rosenzweig KE, Sura S, Jackson A, Yorke E. Involved-field radiation therapy for inoperable non small-cell lung cancer. J Clin Oncol. Dec 10 2007;25(35):5557-5561.

Roth JA, Fossella F, Komaki R, et al. A randomized trial comparing perioperative chemotherapy and surgery with surgery alone in resectable stage IIIA non-small-cell lung cancer. J Natl Cancer Inst 1994;86:673-680.

Rusch VW, Giroux DJ, Kraut MJ, et al. Induction chemoradiation and surgical resection for non-small cell lung carcinomas of the superior sulcus: Initial results of Southwest Oncology Group Trial 9416 (Intergroup Trial 0160). J Thorac Cardiovasc Surg 2001;121:472-483.

Rusch VW, Giroux DJ, Kraut MJ, et al. Induction chemoradiation and surgical resection for superior sulcus non-small-cell lung carcinomas: long-term results of Southwest Oncology Group Trial 9416 (Intergroup Trial 0160). J Clin Oncol. 2007;25(3):313-318

Sandler AB, Gray R, Brahmer J, et al. Randomized phase II/III trial of paclitaxel (P) plus carboplatin (C) with or without bevacizumab (NSC#704865) in patients with advanced non-squamous non-small cell lung cancer (NSCLC): An Eastern Cooperative Oncology Group (ECOG) Trial – E4599. J Clin Oncol, 2005 ASCO Annual Meeting Proceedings, 2005; 23; 16S (June 1 Supplement):2S.

Sause W, Kolesar P, Taylor SI, et al. Final results of phase III trial in regionally advanced unresectable non-small cell lung cancer: Radiation Therapy Oncology Group, Eastern Cooperative Oncology Group, and Southwest Oncology Group. Chest 2000;117:358-364.

Sawyer TE, Bonner JA, Gould PM, et al. Effectiveness of postoperative irradiation in stage IIIA non-small cell lung cancer according to regression tree analyses of recurrence risks. Ann Thorac Surg 1997;64:1402-1407; discussion 1407-1408.

Sibley GS. Radiotherapy for patients with medically inoperable Stage I nonsmall cell lung carcinoma: smaller volumes and higher doses--a review. Cancer 1998;82:433-438.

Slotman BJ, Antonisse IE, Njo KH. Limited field irradiation in early stage (T1-2N0) non-small cell lung cancer. Radiother Oncol 1996;41:41-44.

Stephens RJ, Girling DJ, Bleehen NM, et al. The role of post-operative radiotherapy in non-small-cell lung cancer: a multicentre randomised trial in patients with pathologically staged T1-2, N1-2, M0 disease. Medical Research Council Lung Cancer Working Party. Br J Cancer 1996;74:632-639.

Strauss GM, Herndon J, Maddaus MA, et al. Randomized clinical trial of adjuvant chemotherapy with paclitaxel and carboplatin following resection in Stage IB non-small cell lung cancer (NSCLC): Report of Cancer and Leukemia Group B (CALGB) Protocol 9633. Journal of Clinical Oncology, 2004 ASCO Annual Meeting Proceedings (Post-Meeting Edition) 2004; 22;14S (July 15 Supplement):7019.

Thomas M, Rube C, Hoffknecht P, et al. Effect of preoperative chemoradiation in addition to preoperative chemotherapy: a randomised trial in stage III non-small-cell lung cancer. Lancet Oncol. 2008;9(7):636-648.

Timmerman R, McGarry R, Yiannoutsos C, et al. Excessive toxicity when treating central tumors in a phase II study of stereotactic body radiation therapy for medically inoperable early-stage lung cancer. J Clin Oncol. Oct 20 2006;24(30):4833-4839.

Timmerman RD, Paulus R, Galvin J, et al. Stereotactic Body Radiation Therapy for Medically Inoperable Early-stage Lung Cancer Patients: Analysis of RTOG 0236. Int J Radiat Oncol Biol Phys 2009; 75(3S): S3.

Turrisi III AT (2004). Updates and Issues in Lung Cancer. Presented at American Society of Therapeutic Radiology and Oncology Spring Refresher Course, Chicago, IL.

Van Houtte P, Rocmans P, Smets P, et al. Postoperative radiation therapy in lung cancer: a controlled trial after resection of curative design. Int J Radiat Oncol Biol Phys 1980;6:983-986.

van Meerbeeck JP, Kramer G, van Schil PE, et al. A randomized trial of radical surgery (S) versus thoracic radiotherapy (TRT) in patients (pts) with stage IIIA-N2 non-small cell lung cancer (NSCLC) after response to induction chemotherapy (ICT) (EORTC 08941). J Clin Oncol, 2005 ASCO Annual Meeting Proceedings, 2005;23;16S (June 1 Supplement): 624S.

Vokes EE, Herndon JE, Kelley MJ, et al. Induction chemotherapy followed by concomitant chemoradiotherapy (CT/XRT) versus CT/XRT alone for regionally advanced unresectable non-small cell lung cancer (NSCLC): Initial analysis of a randomized phase III trial. Journal of Clinical Oncology, 2004 ASCO Annual Meeting Proceedings (Post-Meeting Edition) 2004; 22;14S (July 15 Supplement):7005.

Wagner H. Non-Small Cell Lung Cancer. In: Gunderson LL, Tepper JE, editors. Clinical radiation oncology. 2nd ed. Philadelphia: Churchill Livingstone; 2007. pp. 911-950.

Winton TL, Livingston R, Johnson D, et al. Vinorelbine plus cisplatin vs. observation in resected non-small-cell lung cancer. N Engl J Med 2005; 352:2589-2597.

FURTHER READING

Albain KS, Swann RS, Rusch VR, et al. Phase III study of concurrent chemotherapy and radiotherapy (CT/RT) vs CT/RT followed by surgical resection for stage IIIA(pN2) non-small cell lung cancer (NSCLC): Outcomes update of North American Intergroupl 0139 (RTOG 9309). J Clin Oncol, 2005 ASCO Annual Meeting Proceedings, 2005;23;16S(1 Supplement):624S.

Albain KS, Swann RS, Rusch, VW, et al. Radiotherapy plus chemotherapy with or without surgical resection for stage III non-small-cell lung cancer: a phase III randomised controlled trial. Lancet 2009;374:379-386.

Albain KS, Swann RS, Rusch VW, et al. Radiotherapy plus chemotherapy with or without surgical resection for stage III non-small-cell lung cancer: a phase III randomised controlled trial. Lancet. Aug 1 2009;374(9687):379-386.

Blackstock AW, Bogart JA, Matthews C, et al. Split-course versus continuous thoracic radiation therapy for limited-stage small-cell lung cancer: final report of a randomized phase III trial. Clin Lung Cancer. Mar 2005;6(5):287-292.

Chang J, Bradley J, Govindan R, et al. Lung. In: Perez CA, Brady LW, Halperin EC, et al., editors. Principles and practice of radiation oncology. 5th ed. Philadelphia: Lippincott Williams & Wilkins; 2008. pp. 1076-1108.

Choy H, Jr. WJC, Scott CB, et al. Preliminary report of locally advanced multimodality protocol (LAMP): ACR 427: a randomized phase II study of three chemo-radiation regimens with paclitaxel, carboplatin, and thoracic radiation (TRT) for patients with locally advanced non small cell lung cancer (LA-NSCLC). Presented at American Society of Clinical Oncology, 2002.

Field JK, Smith RA, Duffy SW, et al. The Liverpool Statement 2005: priorities for the European Union/United States spiral computed tomography collaborative group. J Thorac Oncol. Jun 2006;1(5):497-498.

Furuse K, Fukuoka M, Kawahara M, et al. Phase III study of concurrent versus sequential thoracic radiotherapy in combination with mitomycin, vindesine, and cisplatin in unresectable stage III non-small-cell lung cancer. J Clin Oncol. Sep 1999;17(9):2692-2699.

Gandara DR, Chansky K, Albain KS, et al. Consolidation docetaxel after concurrent chemoradiotherapy in stage IIIB non-small-cell lung cancer: phase II Southwest Oncology Group Study S9504. J Clin Oncol 2003;21:2004-2010.

Greene FL, American Joint Committee on Cancer. American Cancer Society. AJCC cancer staging manual. 6th ed. New York: Springer; 2002.

Gore E. RTOG 0214: a phase III comparison of prophylactic cranial irradiation versus observation in patients with locally advanced non-small cell lung cancer. Clin Adv Hematol Oncol. Aug 2005;3(8):625-626.

Hanna N, Neubauer M, Yiannoutsos C, et al. Phase III study of cisplatin, etoposide, and concurrent chest radiation with or without consolidation docetaxel in patients with inoperable stage III non-small-cell lung cancer: the Hoosier Oncology Group and U.S. Oncology. J Clin Oncol. Dec 10 2008;26(35):5755-5760.

Henschke CI, Yankelevitz DF, Libby DM, Pasmantier MW, Smith JP, Miettinen OS. Survival of patients with stage I lung cancer detected on CT screening. N Engl J Med. Oct 26 2006;355(17):1763-1771.

Komaki R, Lee JS, Milas L, et al. Effects of amifostine on acute toxicity from concurrent chemotherapy and radiotherapy for inoperable non-small cell lung cancer: report of a randomized comparative trial. Int J Radiat Oncol Biol Phys 2004;58:1369-1377.

Komaki R, Travis EL, Cox JD. The Lung and Thymus. In: Cox JD, Ang KK, editors. Radiation oncology: rationale, technique, results. 8th ed. St. Louis: Mosby; 2003. pp. 399-427.

Lally BE, Zelterman D, Colasanto JM, Haffty BG, Detterbeck FC, Wilson LD. Postoperative radiotherapy for stage II or III non-small-cell lung cancer using the surveillance, epidemiology, and end results database. J Clin Oncol. Jul 1 2006;24(19):2998-3006.

Langer C, Rosenzweig KE (2004). Lung Cancer Part I: Non-Small Cell (#204). Presented at American Society of Therapeutic Radiology and Oncology Annual Meeting, Atlanta, GA

Movsas B, Scott C, Langer C, et al. Randomized trial of amifostine in locally advanced non-small-cell lung cancer patients receiving chemotherapy and hyperfractionated radiation: radiation therapy oncology group trial 98-01. J Clin Oncol. Apr 1 2005;23(10):2145-2154.

National Comprehensive Cancer Network. Clinical practice guidelines in oncology: non-small cell lung cancer. Available at: http://www.nccn.org/professionals/physician_gls/f_guidelines.asp. Accessed on May 14, 2009.

Pignon JP, Tribodet H, Scagliotti GV, et al. Lung adjuvant cisplatin evaluation: a pooled analysis by the LACE Collaborative Group. J Clin Oncol. Jul 20 2008;26(21):3552-3559.

Rosenzweig KE, Krug LM. Tumors of the Lung, Pleura, and Mediastinum. In: Leibel SA, Phillips TL, editors. Textbook of radiation oncology. 2nd ed. Philadelphia: Saunders; 2004. pp. 779-810.

Ruebe C, Riesenbeck D, Semik M, et al. (2004). Neoadjuvant chemotherapy followed by preoperative radiochemotherapy (hfRTCT) plus surgery or surgery plus postoperative radiotherapy in stage III non-small cell lung cancer: Results of a randomized phase III trial of the German Lung Cancer Cooperative Group. Presented at American Society of Therapeutic Radiology and Oncology 46th Annual Meeting, Atlanta, GA.

Sarna L, Swann S, Langer C, et al. Clinically meaningful differences in patient-reported outcomes with amifostine in combination with chemoradiation for locally advanced non-small-cell lung cancer: an analysis of RTOG 9801. Int J Radiat Oncol Biol Phys. Dec 1 2008;72(5):1378-1384.

Sandler HM, Curran WJ, Jr., Turrisi AT, 3rd. The influence of tumor size and pre-treatment staging on outcome following radiation therapy alone for stage I non-small cell lung cancer. Int J Radiat Oncol Biol Phys. Jul 1990;19(1):9-13.

Socinski MA, Blackstock AW, Bogart JA, et al. Randomized phase II trial of induction chemotherapy followed by concurrent chemotherapy and dose-escalated thoracic conformal radiotherapy (74 Gy) in stage III non-small-cell lung cancer: CALGB 30105. J Clin Oncol. May 20 2008;26(15):2457-2463.

Strauss GM, Herndon JE, 2nd, Maddaus MA, et al. Adjuvant paclitaxel plus carboplatin compared with observation in stage IB non-small-cell lung cancer: CALGB 9633 with the Cancer and Leukemia Group B, Radiation Therapy Oncology Group, and North Central Cancer Treatment Group Study Groups. J Clin Oncol. Nov 1 2008;26(31):5043-5051.

The Lung Cancer Study Group. Effects of postoperative mediastinal radiation on completely resected stage II and stage III epidermoid cancer of the lung. N Engl J Med 1986;315: 1377-1381.

Timmerman R, Paulus R, Galvin J, et al. Stereotactic body radiation therapy for inoperable early stage lung cancer. Jama. Mar 17;303(11):1070-1076.

Vokes EE, Herndon JE, 2nd, Kelley MJ, et al. Induction chemotherapy followed by chemoradiotherapy compared with chemoradiotherapy alone for regionally advanced unresectable stage III Non-small-cell lung cancer: Cancer and Leukemia Group B. J Clin Oncol. May 1 2007;25(13):1698-1704.

Wisnivesky JP, Bonomi M, Henschke C, Iannuzzi M, McGinn T. Radiation therapy for the treatment of unresected stage I-II non-small cell lung cancer. Chest. Sep 2005;128(3): 1461-1467.

Werner-Wasik M, Scott C, Cox JD, et al. Recursive partitioning analysis of 1999 Radiation Therapy Oncology Group (RTOG) patients with locally-advanced non-small-cell lung cancer (LA-NSCLC): identification of five groups with different survival. Int J Radiat Oncol Biol Phys. Dec 1 2000;48(5):1475-1482.

Zinner RG, Fossella FV, Gladish GW, et al. Phase II study of pemetrexed in combination with carboplatin in the first-line treatment of advanced nonsmall cell lung cancer. Cancer. Dec 1 2005;104(11):2449-2456.

Chapter 16

Mesothelioma and Thymic Tumors

Fred Y. Wu, Brian Lee, and Joycelyn L. Speight

IV

MESOTHELIOMA

PEARLS

- Rare: only 2,000–3,000 cases per year in the US.
- Eighty percent cases involve asbestos exposure.
- Strong causal rclationship exists with cigarette smoking.
- Can affect visceral pleura, parietal pleura, and peritoneum.
- May mimic adenocarcinoma on pathologic examination; immunohistochemical staining required for definitive diagnosis.

WORKUP

- H&P, CXR, CT/MRI chest, PET/CT, pulmonary function tests.
- On CT, look for pleural thickening, effusions, contraction of ipsilateral hemithorax.
- Functional imaging important because prior talc pleurodesis results in pleural thickening, which may be indistinguishable from disease-related plaques.
- Circumferential pleural thickening, mediastinal/chest wall/diaphragm involvement, and/or irregular pleural contour are most likely malignant.

STAGING (AJCC 7TH ED., 2010): MESOTHELIOMA

Editors' note: All TNM stage and stage groups referred to elsewhere in this chapter reflect the 2002 AJCC staging nomenclature unless otherwise noted as the new system below was published after this chapter was written.

Primary tumor (T)

TX: Primary tumor cannot be assessed
T0: No evidence of primary tumor
T1: Tumor limited to the ipsilateral parietal pleura with or without mediastinal pleura and with or without diaphragmatic pleural involvement
  T1a: No involvement of the visceral pleura
  T1b: Tumor also involving the visceral pleura
T2: Tumor involving each of the ipsilateral pleural surfaces (parietal, mediastinal, diaphragmatic, and visceral pleura) with at least one of the following:
  Involvement of diaphragmatic muscle
  Extension of tumor from visceral pleura into the underlying pulmonary parenchyma
T3: Locally advanced but potentially resectable tumor. Tumor involving all of the ipsilateral pleural surfaces (parietal, mediastinal, diaphragmatic, and visceral pleura) with at least one of the following:
  Involvement of the endothoracic fascia
  Extension into the mediastinal fat
  Solitary, completely resectable focus of tumor
  Extending into the soft tissues of the chest wall
  Nontransmural involvement of the pericardium
T4: Locally advanced technically unresectable tumor. Tumor involving all of the ipsilateral pleural surfaces (parietal, mediastinal, diaphragmatic, and visceral pleura) with at least one of the following:
  Diffuse extension or multifocal masses of tumor in the chest wall, with or without associated rib destruction
  Direct transdiaphragmatic extension of tumor to the peritoneum
  Direct extension of tumor to the contralateral pleura
  Direct extension of tumor to mediastinal organs
  Direct extension of tumor into the spine
  Tumor extending through to the internal surface of the pericardium with or without a pericardial effusion or tumor involving the myocardium

Regional lymph nodes (N)

NX: Regional lymph nodes cannot be assessed
N0: No regional lymph node metastases
N1: Metastases in the ipsilateral bronchopulmonary or hilar lymph nodes
N2: Metastases in the subcarinal or the ipsilateral mediastinal lymph nodes including the ipsilateral internal mammary and peridiaphragmatic nodes
N3: Metastases in the contralateral mediastinal, contralateral internal mammary, ipsilateral or contralateral supraclavicular lymph nodes

Distant metastasis (M)

M0: No distant metastasis
M1: Distant metastasis present

Anatomic stage/prognostic groups

I: T1 N0 M0
IA: T1a N0 M0
IB: T1b N0 M0
II: T2 N0 M0
III: T1, T2 N1 M0
  T1, T2 N2 M0
  T3 N0, N1, N2 M0
IV: T4 Any N M0
  Any T N3 M0
  Any T Any N M1

continued

TREATMENT RECOMMENDATIONS

2002 Stage	Recommended treatment	~MS
I–II	■ If resectable/N0: extrapleural pneumonectomy (EPP) → 4–6 week break → RT 1.8/54 Gy ■ If resectable/N + or medically unsuitable for EPP consider pleurectomy/decortication → 4–6 week break → RT 1.8/54 Gy ■ If surgically inoperable → neoadjuvant chemo and reevaluate for resection; if remains unresectable, continue chemo	Stage I: 35 months Stage II: 16 months
III–IV	■ Primary EPP followed by adjuvant RT ± chemo vs. Neoadjuvant chemo → resection → RT 1.8/54 Gy ± adjuvant CT	Stage III: 12 months Stage IV: 6 months

STUDIES

- Rusch (2001): phase II trial of 88 patients treated with EPP and adjuvant hemithoracic RT (54 Gy). MS 34 months for Stage I–II and 10 months for late stage. Toxicity included fatigue and esophagitis.
- Vogelzang et al. (2003): phase III single-blinded study of pemetrexed and cisplatin vs. cisplatin alone in chemo naïve patients with malignant pleural mesothelioma. Addition of pemetrexed improved response rate (17→41%) and MS (9→12 months).
- Flores et al. (2006): phase II trial of stage III or IV patients treated with induction chemo (gemcitabine/cisplatin), EPP, and adjuvant radiotherapy (54 Gy). MS: resectable patients 33.5 months, unresectable patients 9 months, all patients 19 months.
- Lucchi et al. (2008): phase II study of stage II–III patients treated with intrapleural pre-op IL-2, pleurectomy/decortication, adjuvant intrapleural epidoxorubicin/IL-2, adjuvant radiotherapy (30 Gy), systemic chemotherapy (cisplatin/gemcitabine), and long-term IL-2. MS is 26 months, 2- and 5-year OS 60.2 and 23.3%, respectively.
- Allen et al. (2007a): retrospective review of outcomes associated with moderate dose hemithoracic RT (MDRT) vs. high dose

hemithoracic RT (HDRT) in 39 patients after EPP. (MDRT = 30 Gy to hemithorax, 40 Gy to mediastinum, and boost to positive margins or nodes to 54 Gy with concurrent CT; HDRT = 54 Gy with sequential CT). Median OS 19 months. HDRT yield lower LF rate (27%) vs. MDRT (50%; p = ns). RT technique was not predictive of local failure, distant failure, or OS.

- Perrot et al. (2009): retrospective review of 60 patients treated with trimodality therapy with induction chemo followed by EPP and adjuvant hemithoracic RT (≥50 Gy). Type of induction chemo did not impact survival. For N0 patients, MS 59 months, 5-year DFS 53%. Pathologic nodal status is a good predictor of survival.
- Rice et al. (2007): review of 100 consecutive patients treated with EPP. Sixty-three patients received IMRT (median dose 45 Gy). Chemo not routinely administered. Overall MS 10 months. For IMRT patients, MS 14 months (28 months if pN0), 3-year OS 20% (41% if pN0). Only 5% recurrence within irradiated field. Fifty-four percent developed distant recurrences.
- Krayenbuehl (2007): retrospective planning comparison of 17 patients treated with adjuvant 3D-CRT (n = 8) or IMRT (n = 9) following EPP. IMRT improved coverage and homogeneity vs. 3D-CRT (p < 0.01) through an increase in mean lung dose to ipsilateral and contralateral lung.
- Miles et al. (2008): retrospective review of 13 patients treated with IMRT to entire ipsilateral hemithorax and nodes (median dose 45 Gy) after EPP. With 9.5 months median follow-up, 23% had grade 2 or greater pulmonary toxicity; 46% developed LR and/or DM, and 46% were alive and NED. Authors describe dosimetric parameters for pulmonary toxicity.
- Sterzing et al. (2008): retrospective planning comparison of step and shoot IMRT and helical tomotherapy for 10 patients treated with adjuvant RT (54 Gy) following neoadjuvant chemo and EPP. Tomotherapy had improved coverage and homogeneity and decreased mean lung dose.
- Boutin (Chest 1995): randomized study of 40 patients treated with 7 Gy × 3 fx with electrons to drain sites vs. observation. RT to drain sites decreased LF 40–0%.
- O'Rourke (Radiother Oncol 2007). Randomized study of 61 patients after chest drain or pleural biopsy treated with 21 Gy in 3 fx to drain site vs. best supportive care. No difference in the risk of tract metastases between arms (<10%).
- Plathow et al. (2008): computed tomography, positron emission tomography, positron emission tomography/computed tomography, and magnetic resonance imaging for staging of limited pleural mesothelioma: initial results. Accuracy for detecting

stage II: CT 77%, PET 86%, MRI 80%, PET/CT 100%. Stage III: CT 75%, PET 83%, MRI 90%, and PET/CT 100%.

RADIATION TECHNIQUES

SIMULATION AND FIELD DESIGN

- Hemithoracic RT 4–8 weeks post resection.
- Simulate and CT pt supine, arms overhead, immobilization.
- Favor image-based (e.g., CT) planning.
- Earlier study by Allen et al. suggested IMRT may be associated with increased complications and/or deaths (Allen et al. 2006). However, later studies by the same group (Allen et al., 2007a, b) and others (Krayenbuhl, 2007) have shown decreased toxicity with careful planning.
- Conventional AP/PA borders: superior = top of T1; inferior = bottom L2; medial = contralateral edge of vertebral body (if mediastinum negative) or 1.5 cm beyond contralateral edge of vertebral body (if mediastinum involved), lateral = flash.
- Blocks: liver and stomach (covers diaphragm/abdomen interface), humerus, heart (after 20 Gy), spinal cord (after 41.4 Gy, shift medial border to ipsilateral edge of vertebral body).
- Scar: include in field, bolus, or boost to scar may be needed.
- Electron boost to areas of chest wall blocked for abdominal or cardiac protection.

DOSE PRESCRIPTIONS

- 1.8 Gy/fx to 54 Gy (off-cord after 41.4 Gy)
- Electrons: give concurrent with photon treatment, 1.53 Gy/fx (15% scatter under blocks from photon fields). Choose energy so that chest wall is covered by 90% IDL

DOSE LIMITATIONS

- Spinal cord: ≤45 Gy
- Lung: mean lung dose ≤8–10 Gy; V20 ≤4–10 Gy; V5 ≤75%
- Heart: limit 50% <25–40 Gy
- Esophagus: limit 1/3 to <60 Gy; 2/3 to <55 Gy; 3/3 to <45 Gy

COMPLICATIONS

- Acute: may include skin reactions, fatigue, nausea, vomiting, dysphagia, odynophagia, cough, dyspnea, L'hermitte's syndrome (radiationmyelitis), acute pneumonitis, pneumonia.

- Late: may include pericarditis, restrictive cardimyopathy, myocardial infarction, CHF, radiation myelopathy, radiation pneumonitis, pulmonary fibrosis.

THYMIC TUMORS

PEARLS

- Thymoma has an indolent, predominantly locally invasive growth pattern, but can metastasize.
- Thymoma accounts for 20% of mediastinal tumors and 50% of anterior mediastinal masses in adults; most common age at diagnosis = 40–60 years.
- Most common presentation is as an anterior mediastinal mass on CXR performed for other reasons; 40–50% are asymptomatic.
- Thymomas are often associated with immune and nonimmune mediated paraneoplastic syndromes: myasthenia gravis (MG; ~30%), pure red cell aplasia (PRCA; 5–10%), and hypogammaglobulinemia (Good's syndrome, 3–6%).
- Only 10–15% of patients with MG have a thymoma; 50% of patients with PRCA have a thymoma.
- Common presenting symptoms include fatigue, chest pain, cough, dyspnea, hoarseness, symptoms of superior vena cava syndrome, and/or paraneoplastic symptoms (i.e., MG: muscle weakness, dysphagia, blurred vision).
- Prognosis is related to stage and completeness of resection; on multivariate analysis, treatment dose ≥50 Gy is a prognostic factor (Zhu et al. 2004).
- Thymomas are chemosensitive tumors; complete and partial response rates = 1/3 and 2/3, respectively.
- Other histologies.
  - Thymic carcinoma: more locally-aggressive with ~30% LN and DM.
  - Thymic carcinoid: more locally-aggressive with 30% LN and 30–40% DM, associated with MEN, Cushing's, Eaton–Lambert, SIADH, and hypercalcemia paraneoplastic syndromes.

WORKUP

- H&P, CXR, and preoperative chest imaging, mainly CT chest with contrast; MRI and PET–CT have been used.

- Monden et al. (1985): 127 patients treated with surgery ± RT. RT reduced recurrence from 30 to 15%.

COMBINED MODALITY

- Mornex (1995): retrospective review of 90 patients treated with surgery and RT (30–70 Gy) ± chemo (cisplatin based). Five out of ten-year OS was 51/39%. Extent of surgery impacted 10-year OS (43% for partial resection vs. 31% for biopsy only). Stage, histology, and chemo were not prognostic.
- Kim et al. (2004): phase II study of a multidisciplinary approach with induction chemotherapy, followed by surgical resection, radiation therapy, and consolidation chemotherapy for unresectable malignant thymomas. Induction chemo 77% response rate. OS rates 95% (5-year) and 79% (7-year). PFS rates 77% (5-year) and 77% (7-year).
- Wright et al. (2008): 10 patients with stage III–IVA thymoma tread with 2 cycles of cisplatin and etoposide with concurrent RT followed by surgery. Four patients had >90% necrosis in resected specimen. Eight patients had R0 resection. Seven patients received 2 more cycles of chemo. Five-year OS 69%.

IV

RADIATION TECHNIQUES

SIMULATION AND FIELD DESIGN

- Simulate patient supine with arms overhead and adequate immobilization.
- Conformal, image-based planning techniques are preferred (IMRT, 3D-CRT, tomotherapy) to minimize dose to surrounding normal structures.
- Surgical clips denoting the extent of surgical resection and/or regions of residual disease are important for design of post-op fields.
- Volumes.
  - PTV = GTV/tumor bed and clips +1.5–2.0 cm margin.
- No need for SCV field(s) unless involved.
- Heterogeneity corrections are likely necessary.

DOSE PRESCRIPTIONS

- Pre-op RT: 1.8 Gy/fx to 45 Gy
- Stage II post-op: 1.8 Gy/fx to 45–50 Gy
- Stage III post-op: 1.8 Gy/fx to 50–54 Gy
- Gross residual disease: 1.8 Gy/fx to 54–60 Gy

DOSE LIMITATIONS

- Spinal cord: ≤45 Gy
- Lung: limit the volume receiving >20 Gy (V20) to <20–30%
- Heart: limit 50% <25–40 Gy
- Esophagus: limit 1/3 to <60 Gy; 2/3 to <55 Gy; 3/3 to <45 Gy

COMPLICATIONS

- Acute: may include skin reactions,fatigue, dysphagia, odynophagia, cough, dyspnea, L'hermitte's syndrome (radiationmyelitis), acute pneumonitis, pneumonia.
- Late: may include pericarditis, restrictive cardimyopathy, myocardial infarction, CHF, radiation myelopathy, radiation pneumonitis, pulmonary fibrosis.

FOLLOW-UP

- Late recurrences are not uncommon; long-term follow-up is indicated.
- Post-op RT has no impact on the incidence of subsequent pleural spread (outside of one RT field).

REFERENCES

Allen AM, Czerminska M, Janne PA, et al. Fatal pneumonitis associated with intensity-modulated radiation therapy for mesothelioma. Int J Radiat Oncol Biol Phys. 2006;65(3):640-645.

Allen AM, Den R, Wong JS, et al. Influence of radiotherapy technique and dose on patterns of failure for mesothelioma patients after extrapleural pneumonectomy. Int J Radiat Oncol Biol Phys. 2007;68(5):1366-1374.

Allen AM, Schoenfield MS, Hacker F et al. Restricted field IMRT dramatically enhances IMRT planning for mesothelioma. Int J Radiat Oncol Biol Phys. 2007;69(5):1587-1592.

Batata M. Thymomas: Clinicopathologic features, therapy, and prognosis. Cancer 1974;34:389-396.

Berghmans T, Lafitte J, Paesmans M et al. A phase II study evaluating the cisplatin and epirubicin combination in patients with unresectable malignant pleural mesothelioma. Lung Cancer 2005;50:75-82.

Boutin C, Rey F, Viallat R et al. Prevention of malignant seeding after invasive diagnostic procedures in patients with pleural mesothelioma. A randomized trial of local radiotherapy. Chest 1995;108(3):754-758.

Bruin M, Burgers J, Baas P, et al. Malignant mesothelioma following radiation treatment for Hodgin's lymphoma. Blood 2009;113(16):3679-3681.

Ceresoli G, Zucali P, Favaretto A, et al. Phase II study of pemetrexed plus carboplatin in malignant pleural mesothelioma. J Clin Oncol. 2006;24:1443-1448.

Ciernik IF, Meier U, Lutolf UM. Prognostic factors and outcome of incompletely resected invasive thymoma following radiation therapy. J Clin Oncol. 1994;12:1484-1490.

Curran WJ Jr., Kornstein MJ, Brooks JJ, et al. Invasive thymoma: the role of mediastinal irradiation following complete or incomplete surgical resection. J Clin Oncol. 1988;6:1722-1727.

Eng TY, et al. Mediastinum and Trachea. In: Perez CA, Brady LW, Halperin ED, Schmidt-Ullrich RK, editors. Principles and practice of radiation oncology. 4th ed. Philadelphia: Lippincott Williams & Wilkins; 2004. pp 1244-1281.

Flores R, Krug L, Rosenzweig K, et al. Induction chemotherapy, extrapleural pneumonectomy, and postoperative high-dose radiotherapy for locally advanced malignant pleural mesothelioma: a Phase II trial. J Thorac Oncol. 2006;1:289-295.

Forquer JA, Rong N, Fakiris AJ, et al. Postoperative radiotherapy after surgical resection of thymoma: differing roles in localized and regional disease. Int J Radiat Oncol Biol Phys. 2010;76(2):440-445.

Hillerdal G, Sorensen J, Sundstrom S, et al. Treatment of malignant pleural mesothelioma with carboplatin, liposomized doxorubicin, and gemcitabine: a phase II study. J Thorac Oncol. 2008;3:1325-1331.

Janne P, Simon G, Langer C, et al. Phase II trial of pemetrexed and gemcitabine in chemotherapy-naïve malignant pleural mesothelioma. J Clin Oncol. 2008;26:1465-1471.

Kalmadi S, Rankin C, Kraut M, et al. Gemcitabine and cisplatin in unresectable malignant mesothelioma of the pleura: a phase II study of the Southwest Oncology Group (SWOG 9810). Lung Cancer 2008;60:259-263.

Kim E, Putnam J, Komaki R, et al. Phase II study of a multidisciplinary approach with induction chemotherapy, followed by surgical resection, radiation therapy, and consolidation chemotherapy for unresectable malignant thymomas: final report. Lung Cancer 2004;44:369-379.

Kondo K, Monden Y. Therapy for thymic epithelial tumors: a clinical study of 1,320 patients from Japan. Ann Thorac Surg. 2003;76(3):878-884.

Krayenbuhl J, OErtel S, Davis JB, et al. Combined photon and electron three-dimensional conformal versus intensity-modulated radiotherapy with integrated boost for adjuvant treatment of malignant pleural mesothelioma after pleuropneumectomy. Int J Radiat Oncol Biol Phys. 2007;69(5):1593-1599.

Komaki R, Travis EL, Cox JD. The Lung and Thymus. In: Cox JD, Ang KK, editors. Radiation oncology: rationale, technique, results. 8th ed. St. Louis: Mosby; 2003. pp. 399-427.

Loehrer Sr P, Wang W, Johnson D, et al. Octreotide alone or with prednisone in patient with advanced thymoma and thymic carcinoma: an Eastern Cooperative Oncology Group Phase II trail. J Clin Oncol. 2004;22:293-299.

Lu C, Perez-Soler R, Piperdi B, et al. Phase II study of a liposome-entrapped cisplatin analog (L-NDDP) administered intrapleurally and pathologic response rates in patients with malignant pleural mesothelioma. J Clin Oncol. 2005;23:3495-3501.

Lucchi M, Chella A, Dini P, et al. Four-modality therapy in malignant pleural mesothelioma: a phase II study. J Thorac Oncol. 2008;2:237-242.

Masaoka A, Monden Y, Nakahara K, et al. Follow-up study of thymomas with special reference to their clinical stages. Cancer 1981;48:2485.

Miles EF, Larrier NA, Kelsey CR, et al. Intensity modulated radiotherapy for restricted mesothelioma: the Duke Experience. Int J Radiat Oncol Biol Phys. 2008;71(4):1143-1150.

Monden Y, Nakahara K, Iioka S, et al. Recurrence of thymoma: clinicopathological features, therapy, and prognosis. Ann Thorac Surg. 1985;39:165-169.

Mornex F. Radiotherapy and chemotherapy for invasive thymomas: a multicentric retrospective review of 90 cases. Int J Radiation Oncology Biol Phys. 1995;2:651-659.

Ohara K, Okumura T, Sugahara S, et al. The role of preoperative radiotherapy for invasive thymoma. Acta Oncol. 1990;29:425-429.

Okuno S, Delaune, Sloan J, et al. A phase 2 study of gemcitabine and epirubicin for the treatment of pleural mesothelioma. Cancer 2008;112:1772-1779.

O'Rourke N, Garcia JC, Paul J et al. A randomized controlled trial of intervention site radiotherapy in malignant pleural mesothelioma. Radiother Oncol 2007;84(1):18-22.

Palmieri G, Montella L, Martignetti A, et al. Somatostatin analogs and prednisone in advanced refractory thymic tumors. Cancer 2002;94:1414-1420.

Perrot M, Feld R, Cho B, et al. Trimodality therapy with induction chemotherapy followed by extrapleural pneumonectomy and adjuvant high-dose hemithoracic radiation for malignant pleural mesothelioma. J Clin Oncol. 2009;27(9):1413-1418.

Plathow C, Staab A, Schmaehl A, et al. Computed tomography, positron emission tomography, positron emission tomography/computed tomography, and magnetic resonance imaging for staging of limited pleural mesothelioma: initial results. Invest Radiol. 2008;43:737-744.

Rice DC, Stevens CW, Correa AM, et al. Outcomes after extrapleural pneumonectomy and intensity-modulated radiation therapy for malignant pleural mesothelioma. Ann Thorac Surg. 2007;84(5):1685-1692.

Rosenzweig KE KL. Tumors of the Lung, Pleura, and Mediastinum. In Leibel SA, Phillips TL, editors. Textbook of radiation oncology. 2nd ed. Philadelphia: Saunders; 2004. pp. 779-810.

Rosenzweig K, Fox J, Zelefsky M, et al. A pilot trial of high-dose-rate intraoperative radiation therapy for malignant pleural mesothelioma. Brachytherapy 2005;4:30-33.

Rusch VW, Rosenzweig K, Venkatraman E, et al. A phase II trial of surgical resection and adjuvant high-dose hemithoracic radiation for malignant pleural mesothelioma. J Thorac Cardiovasc Surg. 2001;122:788-795.

IV

Scagliotti G, Shin D, Kindler H, et al. Phase II study of pemetrexed with and without folic acid and vitamin B12 as front-line therapy in malignant pleural mesothelioma. J Clin Oncol. 2003;21:1556-1561.

Sterzing F, Sroka-Perez G, Schubert K, et al. Evaluating taget coverage and normal tissue sparing in the adjuvant radiotherapy of malignant pleural mesothelioma: helical tomotherapy compared with step and shoot IMRT. Radiother Oncol. 2008;86(2):251-257.

Urgesi A, Monetti U, Rossi G, et al. Role of radiation therapy in locally advanced thymoma. Radiother Oncol. 1990;19:273-280.

van Meerbeeck JP, Baas P, Debruyne C, et al. A Phase II study of gemcitabine in patients with malignant pleural mesothelioma. European Organization for Research and Treatment of Cancer Lung Cancer Cooperative Group. Cancer 1999;85:2577-2582.

Vogelzang NJ, Rusthoven JJ, Symanowski J, et al. Phase III study of pemetrexed in combination with cisplatin versus cisplatin alone in patients with malignant pleural mesothelioma. J Clin Oncol. 2003;21:2636-2644.

Wright CD, Choi NC, Wain JC, et al Induction chemoradiotherapy followed by resection for locally advanced Masaoka stage III and IVA thymic tumors. Ann Thoracic Surg. 2008;85(2):385-389.

Zhu G, He S, Fu X, et al. Radiotherapy and prognostic factors for thymoma: a retrospective study of 175 patients. Int J Radiat Oncol Biol Phys. 2004;60(4):1113-1119.

Zucali P, Ceresoli G, Garassino I, et al. Gemcitabine and vinorelbine in pemetrexed-pretreated patients with malignant pleural mesothelioma. Cancer 2008;112:1555-1561.

PART V
Breast

V

Chapter 17
Breast Cancer

Siavash Jabbari, Catherine Park, and Barbara Fowble

V

PEARLS
EPIDEMIOLOGY

- Most common cancer (excluding skin) among women in the United States, with a lifetime risk of ~13.4%.
- Approximately 184,450 invasive and 67,770 in situ cases/year in the United States.
- Recent decline in incidence attributed in part to decreased use of postmenopausal hormone replacement therapy.
- Second leading cause of cancer deaths in women (40,500 deaths/year in the United States).
  - Decreased incidence and increased mortality rates in African-Americans as compared to whites.
- Most important risk factor for breast cancer development is age.
- Risk also affected by age at menarche, first pregnancy, menopause, family history, and mammographic breast density.
- Use of exogenous estrogen increases risk for breast cancer.

GENETICS

- Approximately 10% of breast cancer cases are associated with germline mutation, including p53 (Li Fraumeni), BRCA1, and BRCA2.
- BRCA mutation carriers have 40–85% lifetime risk of breast and 25–65% life-time risk of ovarian cancer.
  - BRCA2 mutation carriers have a similar risk of breast cancer as BRCA1, and 10–15% lifetime risk of ovarian cancer.
  - Prophylactic bilateral salpingo-oophorectomy decreases ovarian/fallopian tube cancers by 80%, and breast cancers by 50% (Rebbeck et al. 2009).
  - Prophylactic mastectomy nearly eliminates the risk of breast cancers, but does not alter the risk of ovarian/fallopian tube cancer.

- Chemoprevention with tamoxifen is an alternative strategy.
- MRI may have an increasing role in the screening and diagnosis of breast cancer in BRCA mutation carriers.

CHEMOPREVENTION

- Selective estrogen receptor modulators (SERMS), e.g., tamoxifen, can be considered in high risk cohorts, including strong immediate family history, history of LCIS, confirmed adverse gene carrier, or deemed high risk by various risk assessment tools (Gail model).

- *NSABP P-1* (Fisher et al. 1998c): 13,388 patients at elevated risk for breast cancer (>60 years old, 35–59 years old with 5-year predicted risk of at least 1.66% based on Gail model, history of LCIS) randomized to placebo vs. tamoxifen × 5 years. At 69 months follow-up, tamoxifen reduced relative risk of invasive breast cancer by 49% and noninvasive breast cancer by 50%. However, reductions in absolute risk were only 2 and 0.9%, respectively. Increased risk of Stage I uterine cancer (HR = 2.53). Individuals with ADH had the greatest benefit, 4–5X.
- *NSABP-P2 STAR* (vogel et al 2006). Randomized 19,747 postmenopausal women at increased risk of breast CA to Tamoxifen 20 mg qd vs. Raloxifene 60 mg qd × 5 years. Incidence of invasive breast CA 0.4% both arms, but fewer noninvasive cases (DCIS/LCIS) with Tamoxifen (0.15 vs. 0.21%). Raloxifene reduced risk of uterine cancer (absolute 0.7→0.5%), cataracts, and thromboembolic events. Similar number of osteoporotic fractures, other cancers, stroke, and heart disease.

ANATOMY

- Medial and lateral borders of breast tissue: typically the sternum and midaxillary line.
- Cranial and caudal borders: typically the second anterior rib and sixth anterior rib.
- Primary lymphatic drainage is to axillary, internal mammary, and SCV nodes.
- Axillary lymph nodes divided into three levels by relation to pectoralis minor muscle.
- Level I (low axillary) = nodes inferior/lateral to pectoralis minor muscle.

- Level II (midaxillary) = nodes directly beneath the pectoralis minor muscle.
  - Rotter's (interpectoral) nodes considered level II and are located between pectoralis major and minor muscles.
- Level III (apical or infraclavicular) = nodes superior/medial to pectoralis minor muscle.
- Internal mammary LN (IMLN) located in first to fifth intercostal spaces (first to third most commonly involved), 3–3.5 cm from midline.

IMAGING

Screening

- Screening yields 20–35% decrease in breast cancer mortality between the ages of 50–69, with slightly less impact for ages 40–49.
- Approximately 10% of all breast cancers are mammographically occult.
- Clinical breast exam every 1–3 years and periodic self-exam is generally recommended beginning in young adulthood.
- Annual clinical breast exam and screening mammography are generally recommended to begin at age 40–50 in the United States.
- Screening mammography (± adjunct MRI) should begin earlier in high-risk populations, such as prior thoracic RT (e.g., mantle-field RT), genetic predisposition or strong family history, or prior history of LCIS/atypical hyperplasia.
- For specific guidelines, please see National Comprehensive Cancer Network (www.nccn.org) and/or American College of Radiology (www.acr.org).
- Breast Imaging Reporting and Data System (BI-RADS) provides a standardized classification for mammographic studies, and demonstrates good correlation with the likelihood of malignancy.

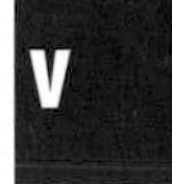

BREAST IMAGING REPORTING AND DATA SYSTEM (BI-RADS)

BI-RADS category	Assessment	Clinical management recommendation(s)
0	Assessment incomplete	Need to review prior studies and/ or complete additional imaging
1	Negative	Continue routine screening
2	Benign finding	Continue routine screening
3	Probably benign finding	Short-term follow-up mammogram at 6 months, then every 6–12 months for 1–2 years

continued

4	Suspicious abnormality	Perform biopsy, preferably needle biopsy
5	Highly suspicious of malignancy; appropriate action should be taken	Biopsy and treatment, as necessary
6	Known biopsy-proven malignancy, treatment pending	Assure that treatment is completed

Adapted from: American College of Radiology (ACR). ACR BI-RADS®–4th Edition. ACR Breast Imaging Reporting and Data System, Breast Imaging Atlas; BI-RADS. Reston. American College of Radiology; 2003. *Reprinted with permission from the American College of Radiology. No other representation of this material is authorized without expressed, written permission from the American College of Radiology.*

- Annual screening using MRI (in addition to mammography) is recommended by the American Cancer Society for women who:
  - Have a BRCA 1 or 2 mutation
  - Have a first-degree relative with a BRCA 1 or 2 mutation and are untested
  - Have a lifetime risk of breast cancer of 20–25% or more using standard risk assessment models (BRCAPRO, Claus, Tyrer-Cuzick)
  - Received radiation treatment to the chest between ages 10 and 30, such as for Hodgkin's Disease
  - Carry or have a first-degree relative who carries a genetic mutation in the TP53 or PTEN genes (Li-Fraumeni syndrome and Cowden and Bannayan-Riley-Ruvalcaba syndromes)

Saslow et al. 2007. Copyright 2007 American Cancer Society. This material is reproduced with the permission from Wiley-Liss, Inc., a subsidiary of John Wiley & Sons, Inc.

Diagnostic studies

- Bilateral diagnostic mammography (including magnification and compression views as indicated).
  - Sensitivity and specificity ≥90%
  - Note masses, areas of architectural distortion, suspicious calcifications (calcs present in 85–90% of DCIS)
  - Postlumpectomy mammogram should be routinely obtained to rule out residual microcalcifications if mammographic presentation associated with malignant appearing calcifications (for both invasive and in situ disease)

- Ultrasound of breast (especially in young and/or dense breasts) and axilla.
- Breast MRI is under investigation. Associated with high false-positive rates, but may have utility in select patients (i.e., invasive lobular cancers, axillary adenopathy with occult breast primary, Paget's disease without evidence of underlying tumor, assessing response to neoadjuvant chemotherapy, young women with dense breasts, and BRCA 1/2 mutation careers).

PATHOLOGY

- Ductal carcinoma in situ (DCIS) comprises 15–20% of all breast cancer
  - DCIS represents confinement of malignant cells within basement membrane
  - One-third of patients with DCIS develop invasive disease within 10 years
  - Mortality risk from DCIS ≈ 10% of recurrence risk after breast conserving surgery
  - Prognostic variables for DCIS include tumor size, margins, nuclear grade, necrosis, multifocality, and age
  - High-grade DCIS: tend to be continuous, 25% ER+
  - Low-grade DCIS: increased multifocality and multicentricity, 90% ER +
- Lobular carcinoma in situ (LCIS) is marker for bilateral breast cancer
  - Approximately 15% of in situ disease
  - Approximately 20–25% lifetime risk for developing ipsilateral or contralateral cancer; risk dependent on age of diagnosis of LCIS
  - Often mammographically silent
  - Usually ER/PR+ Her2neu–
  - Twenty-two to twenty-six percent associated with DCIS or invasive disease, treat according to DCIS or invasive disease indications
- Invasive (infiltrating) ductal carcinoma (IDCA) is the most common type of breast cancer (85% of invasive cases)
- Invasive lobular carcinoma (ILCA) has prognosis similar to that of ductal carcinoma
  - Associated with increased risk of bilateral, multifocal breast cancer
- E-cadherin distinguishes DCIS/IDCA (E-cadherin +) from LCIS/ILCA (E-cadherin–)
- Tubular, medullary, and mucinous carcinomas generally have better prognosis

V

- Medullary carcinoma is typically high grade, and associated with BRCA1/2
- Paget's disease is nipple involvement associated with an underlying cancer
  - Pathologically, tumor cells can be seen involving the epidermis
  - Treat per underlying tumor characteristics; not a contraindication to breast conserving therapy (BCT), but the nipple-areolar complex must be excised
- Multicentricity is disease in multiple quadrants and is a contraindication to BCT
- Multifocality is multiple foci within same quadrant and is not a contraindication to BCT
- Pathological status of axillary lymph nodes is the most important prognostic variable
  - T1–2: 10–40% pLN+
  - Predictors for pLN+ status: size >1 cm, G2–3, high S-phase ratio, +LVSI
- Risk of IMLN+ ranges from 1 to 10% if axilla pLN0 vs. 20–50% if axilla pLN+ based on older radical mastectomy series of locoregionally advanced disease
  - Risk of clinical IMLN failure in modern series is ≤1%
  - Approximately 5% of sentinel lymph node biopsy (SLNB) procedures localize to IMLN as first echelon drainage
- Extensive intraductal component (EIC) is defined as 25% or more of primary invasive tumor is DCIS, and DCIS is present in surrounding normal breast tissue

GENE EXPRESSION PROFILING AND MOLECULAR SUBTYPES

- Molecular subtypes approximated by receptor status include:
  - *Luminal A:* ER/PR+ Her2neu–
  - *Luminal B:* ER/PR+ Her2neu +
  - *Basal like:* ER/PR – Her2neu – (triple negative)
  - *Her2neu+:* ER/PR – Her2neu +
    - Her2neu + amplification is a negative prognosticator in both mastectomy and BCT cohorts
- Commercially available gene expression profiling assays include Oncotype Dx® and MammaPrint®
  - MammaPrint® predicts prognostic category (low vs. high risk) in terms of DMFS and OS in treated and untreated, ER positive and negative, and LN positive and negative patients.

Requires fresh-frozen tissue (and on-site) processing (van der Vijver and He 2002).

- Oncotype Dx® predicts prognostic category (low vs. intermediate vs. high risk) in terms of DMFS and OS and magnitude of chemotherapy benefit in tamoxifen treated, ER+, LN negative patients, and can assay a fixed specimen (obviating need for on-site testing).

- Paik et al. 2004. Twenty-one gene assay (Oncotype Dx®) of Tamoxifen alone arm of NASBP B-14 (below) was highly predictive for OS and DM, independent of tumor size or age. Ten-year risk of recurrence for Tamoxifen-treated, ER+, pLN– tumors according to gene assay recurrence score (RS): <18 (low risk), 6.8%; 18–30 (intermediate risk), 14.3%; ≥31 (high risk), 30.5%.
- Paik et al. 2006. Analysis of 21-gene assay (Oncotype Dx®) RS for 651 ER+, pLN– patients treated with tamoxifen ± chemotherapy on NASBP B-20 (below). RS predicts magnitude of chemotherapy benefit in terms of 10-year distant recurrence rates, with largest benefit seen in high-RS patients, uncertain benefit in intermediate-risk patients, and small to no benefit in low-RS patient.

V

WORKUP

- Breast cancer specific history including risk factors, gynecologic history, menopausal status, and general physical exam.
- Breast exam (tumor size, satellites, skin/chest wall, nipple changes, symmetry).
- Lymph node exam (axillary, supraclavicular/infraclavicular).
- Biopsy with estrogen and progesterone receptor studies; Her-2-neu status, ki-67.
- CBC, blood chemistries, liver function labs.
- CXR.
- Breast imaging as above.
- Bone scan, head imaging (MRI preferred to CT), PET–CT when clinically indicated.
- Careful histologic assessment of breast specimens.
- Consider ultrasound-guided FNA of suspicious nodes (especially if neoadjuvant chemo considered).
  - cN0 axilla: 30% pN+
  - cN+ axilla: 20–40% pN0

STAGING : BREAST CANCER

Editors' note: All TNM stage and stage groups referred to elsewhere in this chapter reflect the 2002 AJCC staging nomenclature unless otherwise noted as the new system below was published after this chapter was written.

(AJCC 6TH ED., 2002)

Primary tumor (T)

TX: Primary tumor cannot be assessed
T0: No evidence of primary tumor
Tis: Carcinoma in situ
Tis (DCIS): Ductal carcinoma in situ
Tis (LCIS): Lobular carcinoma in situ
Tis (Paget's): Paget's disease of the nipple with no tumor
T1: Tumor 2 cm or less in greatest dimension
- T1mic: Microinvasion 0.1 cm or less in greatest dimension
- T1a: Tumor more than 0.1 cm, but not more than 0.5 cm in greatest dimension
- T1b: Tumor more than 0.5 cm, but not more than 1 cm in greatest dimension
- T1c: Tumor more than 1 cm, but not more than 2 cm in greatest dimension

T2: Tumor more than 2 cm, but not more than 5 cm in greatest dimension
T3: Tumor more than 5 cm in greatest dimension
T4: Tumor of any size with direct extension to (a) chest wall or (b) skin
- T4a: Extension to chest wall, not including pectoralis muscle
- T4b: Edema (including peau d'orange) or ulceration of the skin of the breast, or satellite skin nodules confined to the same breast
- T4c: Both T4a and T4b
- T4d: Inflammatory carcinoma

Regional lymph nodes (N)

Clinical

NX: Regional lymph nodes cannot be assessed (e.g., previously removed)
N0: No regional lymph node metastasis

(AJCC 7TH ED., 2010)

Primary tumor (T)

The T classification of the primary tumor is the same regardless of whether it is based on clinical or pathologic criteria, or both. Size should be measured to the nearest millimeter. If the tumor size is slightly less than or greater than a cut-off for a given T classification, it is recommended that the size be rounded to the millimeter reading that is closest to the cut-off. For example, a reported size of 1.1 mm is reported as 1 mm, or a size of 2.01 cm is reported as 2.0 cm. Designation should be made with the subscript "c" or "p" modifier to indicate whether the T classification was determined by clinical (physical examination or radiologic) or pathologic measurements, respectively. In general, pathologic determination should take precedence over clinical determination of T size.

TX: Primary tumor cannot be assessed
T0: No evidence of primary tumor
Tis: Carcinoma in situ
Tis (DCIS): Ductal carcinoma in situ
Tis (LCIS): Lobular carcinoma in situ
Tis (Paget's): Paget's disease of the nipple not associated with invasive carcinoma and/or carcinoma in situ (DCIS and/or LCIS) in the underlying breast parenchyma. Carcinomas in the breast parenchyma associated with Paget's disease are categorized based on the size and characteristics of the parenchymal disease, although the presence of Paget's disease should still be noted
T1: Tumor ≤20 mm in greatest dimension
T1mi: Tumor ≤1 mm in greatest dimension
T1a: Tumor >1 mm, but ≤5 mm in greatest dimension
T1b: Tumor >5 mm, but ≤10 mm in greatest dimension
T1c: Tumor >10 mm, but ≤20 mm in greatest dimension
T2: Tumor >20 mm, but ≤50 mm in greatest dimension

continued

T3: Tumor >50 mm in greatest dimension
T4: Tumor of any size with direct extension to the chest wall and/or to the skin (ulceration or skin nodules). Note: Invasion of the dermis alone does not qualify as T4
- T4a: Extension to the chest wall, not including only pectoralis muscle adherence/invasion
- T4b: Ulceration and/or ipsilateral satellite nodules and/or edema (including peau d'orange) of the skin, which do not meet the criteria for inflammatory carcinoma
- T4c: Both T4a and T4b
- T4d: Inflammatory carcinoma (see "Rules for Classification")

Posttreatment ypT. Clinical (pretreatment) T will be defined by clinical and radiographic findings, while y pathologic (posttreatment) T will be determined by pathologic size and extension.

The ypT will be measured as the largest single focus of invasive tumor, with the modifier "m" indicating multiple foci. The measurement of the largest tumor focus should not include areas of fibrosis within the tumor bed. The inclusion of additional information in the pathology report, such as the distance over which tumor foci extend, the number of tumor foci present, or the number of slides/blocks in which tumor appears, may assist the clinician in estimating the extent of disease. A comparison of the cellularity in the initial biopsy to that in the posttreatment specimen may also aid in the assessment of response.

Note : If a cancer was designated as inflammatory before neoadjuvant chemotherapy, the patient will be designated to have inflammatory breast cancer throughout, even if the patient has complete resolution of inflammatory findings.

Regional lymph nodes (N)

Clinical

NX: Regional lymph nodes cannot be assessed (e.g., previously removed)
N0: No regional lymph node metastases
N1: Metastases to movable ipsilateral level I, II axillary lymph node(s)

continued

V

N1: Metastasis to moveable ipsilateral axillary lymph node(s)
N2: Metastases in ipsilateral axillary lymph nodes fixed or matted, or in clinically apparent ipsilateral internal mammary nodes in the absence of clinically evident axillary lymph node metastasis
- N2a: Metastasis in ipsilateral axillary lymph nodes fixed to one another (matted) or to other structures
- N2b: Metastasis in clinically apparent ipsilateral internal mammary nodes and in the absence of clinically evident axillary lymph node metastasis

N3: Metastasis in ipsilateral infraclavicular lymph node(s) with or without axillary lymph node involvement, or in clinically apparent ipsilateral internal mammary lymphnode(s) and in the presence of clinically evident axillary lymph node metastasis; or metastasis in ipsilateral supraclavicular lymph node(s) with or without axillary or internal mammary lymph node involvement
- N3a: Metastasis in ipsilateral infraclavicular lymph node(s)
- N3b: Metastasis in ipsilateral internal mammary lymph node(s) and axillary lymph node(s)
- N3c: Metastasis in ipsilateral supraclavicular lymph node(s)

*Clinically apparent is defined as detected by imaging studies (excluding lymphoscintigraphy) or by clinical examination or grossly visible pathologically.

Pathologic (pN)

pNX: Regional lymph nodes cannot be assessed (e.g., previously removed, or not removed for pathologic study)
pN0: No regional lymph node metastasis histologically, no additional examination for isolated tumor cells (ITC)
- pN0(i–): No regional lymph node metastasis histologically, negative IHC
- pN0(i+): No regional lymph node metastasis histologically, positive IHC, no IHC cluster greater than 0.2 mm
- pN0(mol–): No regional lymph node metastasis histologically, negative molecular findings (RT-PCR)
- pN0(mol+): No regional lymph node metastasis histologically, positive molecular findings (RT-PCR)

pN1: Metastasis in 1–3 axillary lymph nodes, and/or in internal mammary nodes with microscopic disease detected by sentinel lymph node dissection, but not clinically apparent

- pN1mi: Micrometastasis (greater than 0.2 mm, not greater than 2.0 mm)
- pN1a: Metastasis in 1–3 axillary lymph nodes
- pN1b: Metastasis in internal mammary nodes with microscopic disease detected by sentinel lymph node dissection, but not clinically apparent
- pN1c: Metastasis in 1–3 axillary lymph nodes and in internal mammary nodes with microscopic disease detected by sentinel lymph node dissection, but not clinically apparent. (If associated with greater than three positive axillary lymph nodes, the internal mammary nodes are classified as pN3b to reflect increased tumor burden)

pN2: Metastasis in 4–9 axillary lymph nodes, or in clinically apparent internal mammary lymph nodes in the absence of axillary lymph node metastasis

- pN2a: Metastasis in 4–9 axillary lymph nodes (at least one tumor deposit greater than 2.0 mm)
- pN2b: Metastasis in clinically apparent internal mammary lymph nodes in the absence of axillary lymph node metastasis

pN3: Metastasis in ten or more axillary lymph nodes, or in infraclavicular lymph nodes, or in clinically apparent ipsilateral internal mammary lymph nodes in the presence of one or more positive axillary lymph nodes; or in more than three axillary lymph nodes with clinically negative microscopic metastasis in internal mammary lymph nodes; or in ipsilateral supraclavicular lymph nodes

- pN3a: Metastasis in ten or more axillary lymph nodes (at least one tumor deposit greater than 2.0 mm), or metastasis to the infraclavicular lymph nodes
- pN3b: Metastasis in clinically apparent ipsilateral internal mammary lymph nodes in the presence of one or more positive axillary lymph nodes; or in more than three axillary lymph nodes and in internal mammary lymph nodes with microscopic disease detected by sentinel lymph node dissection, but not clinically apparent
- pN3c: Metastasis in ipsilateral supraclavicular lymph nodes

N2: Metastases in ipsilateral level I, II axillary lymph nodes that are clinically fixed or matted; or in clinically detected* ipsilateral internal mammary nodes in the *absence* of clinically evident axillary lymph node metastases

- N2a: Metastases in ipsilateral level I, II axillary lymph nodes fixed to one another (matted) or to other structures
- N2b: Metastases only in clinically detected* ipsilateral internal mammary nodes and in the *absence* of clinically evident level I, II axillary lymph node metastases

N3: Metastases in ipsilateral infraclavicular (level III axillary) lymph node(s) with or without level I, II axillary lymph node involvement; or in clinically detected* ipsilateral internal mammary lymph node(s) with clinically evident level I, II axillary lymph node metastases; or metastases in ipsilateral supraclavicular lymph node(s) with or without axillary or internal mammary lymph node involvement

- N3a: Metastases in ipsilateral infraclavicular lymph node(s)
- N3b: Metastases in ipsilateral internal mammary lymph node(s) and axillary lymph node(s)
- N3c: Metastases in ipsilateral supraclavicular lymph node(s)

**Note* : *Clinically detected* is defined as detected by imaging studies (excluding lymphoscintigraphy) or by clinical examination and having characteristics highly suspicious for malignancy or a presumed pathologic macrometastasis based on fine needle aspiration biopsy with cytologic examination. Confirmation of clinically detected metastatic disease by fine needle aspiration without excision biopsy is designated with an (f) suffix, for example, cN3a(f). Excisional biopsy of a lymph node or biopsy of a sentinel node, in the absence of assignment of a pT, is classified as a clinical N, for example, cN1. Information regarding the confirmation of the nodal status will be designated in site-specific factors as clinical, fine needle aspiration, core biopsy, or sentinel lymph node biopsy. Pathologic classification (pN) is used for excision or sentinel lymph node biopsy only in conjunction with a pathologic T assignment.

continued

Note: Isolated tumor cells (ITC) are defined as single tumor cells or small cell clusters not greater than 0.2 mm, usually detected only by immunohistochemical (IHC) or molecular methods, but which may be verified on H&E stains. ITCs do not usually show evidence of malignant activity, e.g., proliferation or stromal reaction.

Classification is based on axillary lymph node dissection with or without sentinel lymph node dissection. Classification solely based on sentinel lymph node dissection without subsequent axillary lymph node dissection is designated (sn) for "sentinel node," e.g., pN0(i+) (sn).

Distant metastasis (M)

MX: Distant metastasis cannot be assessed
M0: No distant metastasis
M1: Distant metastasis

*Rules: The pathologic tumor size is a measure of only the invasive component. For multiple ipsilateral primaries, use largest primary to designate T stage. Do not assign separate T stage for smaller tumor. Enter into the record that it is a case of multiple ipsilateral primaries. For bilateral disease, each primary is staged separately. If surgery occurs after neoadjuvant chemotherapy, hormonal therapy, immunotherapy, or radiation therapy, the prefix "y" should be used with the TNM classification, e.g., ypTNM

Stage grouping		~5-Year survival
0:	TisN0M0	100%
I:	T1N0M0	98%
IIA:	T2N0M0, T0-1N1M0	88%
IIB:	T3N0M0, T2N1M0	76%
IIIA:	T3N1M0, T0-3N2M0	56%
IIIB:	T4N0-2M0	49%
IIIC:	Any T, N3 M0	16%
IV:	Any T, any N, M1	

Used with the permission from the American Joint Committee on Cancer (AJCC), Chicago, IL. The original source for this material is the AJCC Cancer Staging Manual, Sixth Edition (2002), published by Springer Science+Business Media.

Pathologic (pN)*

pNX: Regional lymph nodes cannot be assessed (e.g., previously removed, or not removed for pathologic study)
pN0: No regional lymph node metastasis identified histologically

Note : Isolated tumor cell clusters (ITC) are defined as small clusters of cells not greater than 0.2 mm, or single tumor cells, or a cluster of fewer than 200 cells in a single histologic cross-section. ITCs may be detected by routine histology or by immunohistochemical (IHC) methods. Nodes containing only ITCs are excluded from the total positive node count for purposes of N classification, but should be included in the total number of nodes evaluated.

pN0(i–): No regional lymph node metastases histologically, negative IHC
pN0(i+): Malignant cells in regional lymph node(s) no greater than 0.2 mm (detected by H&E or IHC including ITC)
pN0(mol–): No regional lymph node metastases histologically, negative molecular findings (RT-PCR)
pN0(mol+): Positive molecular findings (RT-PCR), **but no regional lymph node metastases detected by histology or IHC
pN1: Micrometastases; or metastases in 1–3 axillary lymph nodes; and/or in internal mammary nodes with metastases detected by sentinel lymph node biopsy, but not clinically detected***
pN1mi: Micrometastases (greater than 0.2 mm and/or more than 200 cells, but none greater than 2.0 mm)
pN1a: Metastases in 1–3 axillary lymph nodes, at least one metastasis greater than 2.0 mm
pN1b: Metastases in internal mammary nodes with micrometastases or macrometastases detected by sentinel lymph node biopsy, but not clinically detected***
pN1c: Metastases in 1–3 axillary lymph nodes and in internal mammary lymph nodes with micrometastases or macrometastases detected by sentinel lymph node biopsy, but not clinically detected
pN2: Metastases in 4–9 axillary lymph nodes; or in clinically detected**** internal mammary lymph nodes in the *absence* of axillary lymph node metastases

continued

- pN2a: Metastases in 4–9 axillary lymph nodes (at least one tumor deposit greater than 2.0 mm)
- pN2b: Metastases in clinically detected**** internal mammary lymph nodes in the *absence* of axillary lymph node metastases

pN3: Metastases in ten or more axillary lymph nodes; or in infraclavicular (level III axillary) lymph nodes; or in clinically detected**** ipsilateral internal mammary lymph nodes in the *presence* of one or more positive level I, II axillary lymph nodes; or in more than three axillary lymph nodes and in internal mammary lymph nodes with micrometastases or macrometastases detected by sentinel lymph node biopsy, but not clinically detected***; or in ipsilateral supraclavicular lymph nodes

- pN3a: Metastases in ten or more axillary lymph nodes (at least one tumor deposit greater than 2.0 mm); or metastases to the infraclavicular (level III axillary lymph) nodes
- pN3b: Metastases in clinically detected**** ipsilateral internal mammary lymph nodes in the *presence* of one or more positive axillary lymph nodes; or in more than three axillary lymph nodes and in internal mammary lymph nodes with micrometastases or macrometastases detected by sentinel lymph node biopsy, but not clinically detected***
- pN3c: Metastases in ipsilateral supraclavicular lymph nodes

Notes: *Classification is based on axillary lymph node dissection with or without sentinel lymph node biopsy. Classification based solely on sentinel lymph node biopsy without subsequent axillary lymph node dissection is designated (sn) for "sentinel node," for example, pN0(sn).
**RT-PCR: reverse transcriptase/polymerase chain reaction.
***"Not clinically detected" is defined as not detected by imaging studies (excluding lymphoscintigraphy) or not detected by clinical examination.
****"Clinically detected" is defined as detected by imaging studies (excluding lymphoscintigraphy) or by clinical examination and having characteristics highly suspicious for malignancy or a presumed pathologic macrometastasis based on fine needle aspiration biopsy with cytologic examination.

continued

Posttreatment ypN

Posttreatment yp "N" should be evaluated as for clinical (pretreatment) "N" methods above. The modifier "sn" is used only if a sentinel node evaluation was performed after treatment. If no subscript is attached, it is assumed that the axillary nodal evaluation was by axillary node dissection (AND).

The X classification will be used (ypNX) if no yp posttreatment SN or AND was performed

N categories are the same as those used for pN.

Distant metastases (M)

M0: No clinical or radiographic evidence of distant metastases

cM0(i+): No clinical or radiographic evidence of distant metastases, but deposits of molecularly or microscopically detected tumor cells in circulating blood, bone marrow, or other nonregional nodal tissue that are no larger than 0.2 mm in a patient without symptoms or signs of metastases

M1: Distant detectable metastases as determined by classic clinical and radiographic means and/or histologically proven larger than 0.2 mm

Posttreatment yp M classification. The M category for patients treated with neoadjuvant therapy is the category assigned in the clinical stage, prior to the initiation of neoadjuvant therapy.

Identification of distant metastases after the start of therapy in cases where pretherapy evaluation showed no metastases is considered progression of disease. If a patient was designated to have detectable distant metastases (M1) before chemotherapy, the patient will be designated as M1 throughout.

Anatomic stage/prognostic groups

0: Tis N0 M0
IA: T1* N0 M0
IB: T0 N1mi M0
T1 * N1mi M0
IIA: T0 N1** M0
T1 * N1 ** M0
T2 N0 M0

V

continued

IIB:	T2 N1 M0
	T3 N0 M0
IIIA:	T0 N2 M0
	T1 * N2 M0
	T2 N2 M0
	T3 N1 M0
	T3 N2 M0
IIIB:	T4 N0 M0
	T4 N1 M0
	T4 N2 M0
IIIC:	Any T N3 M0
IV:	Any T Any N M1

Notes: * T1 includes T1mi
** T0 and T1 tumors with nodal micrometastases only are excluded from Stage IIA and are classified Stage IB

- M0 includes M0(i+)
- The designation pM0 is not valid; any M0 should be clinical
- If a patient presents with M1 prior to neoadjuvant systemic therapy, the stage is considered Stage IV and remains Stage IV regardless of response to neoadjuvant therapy
- Stage designation may be changed if postsurgical imaging studies reveal the presence of distant metastases, provided that the studies are carried out within 4 months of diagnosis in the absence of disease progression and provided that the patient has not received neoadjuvant therapy
- Postneoadjuvant therapy is designated with "yc" or "yp" prefix. Of note, no stage group is assigned if there is a complete pathologic response (CR) to neoadjuvant therapy, for example, ypT0ypN0cM0

continued

TREATMENT RECOMMENDATIONS

SURGICAL CONSIDERATIONS

- Breast conservation surgery (BCS) may consist of (in order of decreasing tissue removed): quadrantectomy, wide excision, lumpectomy (local excision).
- Variations of mastectomy.
  - Radical mastectomy: removal of breast, pectoralis minor and major muscles, axillary LN dissection (ALND) (levels I–III)
  - Modified radical mastectomy: removal of breast to the level of pectoralis minor muscle, ALND (levels I–II), pectoralis major is spared
  - Total (simple) mastectomy: removal of breast to the level of pectoralis minor muscle with no lymph node dissection
  - Skin sparing mastectomy preserves skin of breast for enhanced reconstructive cosmetic outcomes
  - Total skin sparing mastectomy preserves skin and nipple/areolar complex for enhanced reconstructive outcome
- Reconstructive options postmastectomy include delayed vs. immediate, and autologous tissue vs. expander/implant.
- Surgical evaluation/treatment of axilla:
  - Axillary LN dissection (ALND)
  - Level I/II axillary node dissection performed with modified radical mastectomy

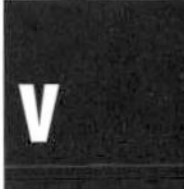

- *NSABP B-04* (NEJM 2002): 1,079 patients with clinically negative axillary LN randomized to 1 of 3 arms: radical mastectomy vs. total mastectomy (TM) without axillary dissection but with post-op RT vs. total mastectomy plus axillary dissection if LN pathologically positive. Also 586 patients with clinically + axillary LN randomized to 1 of 2 arms (radical mastectomy vs. total mastectomy without axillary dissection but with post-op RT). No systemic therapy. At 25-year follow-up, no significant differences in DFS, or OS among the three groups of patients with clinically negative LN or the two groups of patients with clinically + LN. The use of systemic therapy in modern cohorts likely alters patterns of distant vs. LR recurrence, increasing the need for LR control. Approximately 40% of cN0 patients were found to be pLN+ after ALND. Among cN0 patients, axillary failure was <4% if addressed surgically or with RT vs. 19% in TM alone arm.
- Louis-Sylvestre, C (Louis-Sylvestre et al. 2004): 658 cN0 patients with <3 cm primary randomized to ALND or axillary

continued

RT. All had wide excision of primary and breast RT, and <10% had systemic therapy. Twenty-one percent of the patients in the axillary dissection group were pN+. Five-year survival benefit in ALND group, but identical OS at 15 years (73.8 vs. 75.5%). Decreased isolated axillary recurrences in ALND group at 15 years (1 vs. 3%; $p = 0.04$). No difference in breast, supraclavicular, and distant recurrence.

- Sentinel lymph node biopsy (SLNbx) has replaced ALND for the clinically negative axilla
  - Performed with injection of radiotracer and/or methylene blue dye into breast skin and/or tumor
  - False negative rate is similar to ALND (~2–12%) and likely not increased with neoadjuvant chemotherapy (Buchholz et al. 2008)
  - Completion of ALND indicated in the case of involved SLNB (controversial in case of pN1mi+ or low risk disease, nomograms can be used to assess risk for nonsentinel node positivity and ALND may be omitted if <10% risk: http://www.mskcc.org/mskcc/html/15938.cfm)

- *NSABP B-32* (Cancer Oncology 2007): Randomized trial of SLNbx (with ALND if +) vs. upfront ALND. SLNbx had an overall accuracy of 97.1%, false negative rate of 9.8%, and negative predictive value of 96.1%. Only 1.4% of SLN specimens were outside of axillary levels I and II. Survival and recurrence outcomes pending.
- Kim (Kim et al. 2006). Metaanalysis of 69 trials of SLNbx. Average false negative rate of 7.3%. Forty-eight percent nonsentinel node positivity in setting of positive sentinel lymph nodes.

SYSTEMIC THERAPY

- *Chemotherapy* has traditionally been delivered in the adjuvant setting.
  - Generally recommended for >1 cm tumors or node positive disease.
  - Consider for all triple negative tumors, given high rates of recurrence and lack of options for targeted or endocrine therapies.
  - The omission of chemotherapy in LN− ER+ tumors treated with hormonal therapy, and an intermediate Oncotype Dx® RS (11–25) is investigational and is the subject of an ongoing phase III (Tailor Rx) trial.

- Adjuvant chemotherapy reduces LR after lumpectomy + RT.
- Anthracycline (doxorubicin)-based regiments (± taxanes for high-risk disease) have been associated with superior outcomes as compared to nonanthracyclin containing regimens.
- Recent evidence suggests increased DFS and OS with taxane-based therapy as compared to anthracyclin-based therapy (USOT 9735, Jones et al. 2009).
- Agents: CMF (lowest incidence of alopecia)= cyclophosphamide, methotrexate, and 5-fluorouracil; FAC = 5-fluorouracil, adriamycin, cyclophosphamide; AC= adriamycin and cyclophosphamide; AC-Taxol= AC followed by paclitaxel; TAC= taxotere (docetaxel), adriamycin, and cyclophosphamide; FEC = 5-fluorouracil, epirubicin, and cyclophosphamide; TC= taxotere and cyclophosphamide.
- Dose-dense regimens may have increased efficacy in high-risk patients.

V

- *EBCTCG chemo/HT* (2005a). Metaanalysis of 194 randomized trials with ~150,000 women. Approximately 6 months of anthracycline-based polychemotherapy reduced annual breast cancer death rate by 38% for women <50 years (15-year absolute gain: 10/15% for LN–/LN+) and by 20% for women 50–69 years (15-year absolute gain: 5/6% for LN–/LN+). Anthracycline regimens were significantly more effective than CMF chemo. Tamoxifen × 5 years for ER+ (any age) reduced annual breast cancer death rate by 31% (5-year absolute gains: without chemo 12%, in addition to chemo 11%, <50 years 10%, ≥50 years 12%, LN– 9%, LN+ 16%). Five-year tamoxifen significantly better than 1–2 years of tamoxifen.
- *NSABP B-20* (Fisher et al. 2004): 2,306 patients status post surgery with pathologically LN–, ER+ breast ca randomized to tamoxifen alone vs. tamoxifen + MF chemotherapy vs. tamoxifen + CMF chemotherapy. The addition of chemotherapy to tamoxifen improved 12-year DFS (HR = 0.52) and OS (HR = 0.78, $p = 0.068$).
- *NSABP-B28* (Mamounas et al. 2005): 3,060 LN+ patients randomized to AC × 4 ± Paclitaxel. Addition of taxane improved 5-year DFS (72→76%) and LRR, despite delay of RT (9.7 vs. 3.7%).
- *CALGB 9344* (Sartor et al. 2005; Henderson et al. 2003) 3 × 2 randomization: Standard dose AC vs. dose escalation of doxorubicin ± sequential addition of paclitaxel. The sequential

continued

addition of adjuvant paclitaxel to AC for LN+ patients improves DFS and OS vs. adjuvant AC alone, and further improves 5-year LRC in patients treated with BCS+RT despite delaying RT delivery. No DFS or OS improvement with dose escalation of doxorubicin.

- *CALGB 9741* (Citron et al. 2003). Four arm randomized trial: sequential vs. concurrent addition of paclitaxel (T) to AC chemotherapy, every 3 weeks vs. every 2 week (dose dense) dosing. Increased 4-year DFS with dose-dense chemo (82 vs. 75%), no difference between sequential or concurrent delivery.
- *USOT* (Jones et al. 2009): 1,016 Stage I–III patients randomized to AC × 4 vs. TCx4. With a median of 7-year follow-up, TC improved DFS (81 vs. 75%) and OS (87% TC v 82). TC improved outcomes regardless of age, hormone receptor, or HER2 expression status.

- *Neoadjuvant chemotherapy* is considered standard of care in high-risk populations such as young patients and/or advanced-stage disease, and has been evaluated in Stage II–IIIa breast cancer in randomized trials.
  - Typically, similar indications as adjuvant chemotherapy
  - Advantages of neoadjuvant chemotherapy: assessment of disease response, increased rate of BCT
  - Neoadjuvant chemotherapy converts 20–30% of patients initially ineligible for BCT to eligible
  - Complete clinical (cCR) and pathological response rates (pCR) depend on initial extent of disease
  - For advanced-stage disease, 20–40% achieve cCR after neoadjuvant chemotherapy and 10–20% achieve pCR
  - Clinical response frequently does not correlate with pathological response
    - Approximately 1/3 with a cCR found to have pathological residual disease.
    - If Initially cLN+, full ALND should be considered regardless of response to neoadjuvant chemo
    - Diminished response noted in ER+, low grade, or invasive lobular cancers

- *NSABP B-18* (J Natl Cancer Inst Monogr 2001; Rastogi et al. 2008): 1,523 patients with breast ca randomized to AC chemo × 4 pre-op vs. AC chemo × 4 post-op. At 9-year follow-up, no significant difference in DFS, DM-free survival, or OS. Patients

continued

assigned to pre-op group underwent more BCT than post-op patients (60–80%), especially among patients with tumors >5 cm at study entry. Neoadjuvant chemo associated with increased LR post-BCS vs. mastectomy (10.7 vs. 7.6%). LR increased twofold if planned mastectomy was changed to BCS postneoadjuvant chemo as compared to preplanned BCS (15.7 vs. 9.6%).

- Kuerer (Kuerer et al. 1999). Retrospective review of 372 patients with locally advanced breast cancer treated with neoadjuvant AC × 4. With median follow-up 58 months, 12% of patients had a pCR in both primary tumor and axillary nodes. Five-year OS was significantly higher in patients with a pCR vs. those with less than pCR (89 vs. 64%).
- *Metaanalysis of neoadjuvant chemotherapy* (Mieog et al. 2007): Fourteen studies randomizing 5,500 patients. Equivalent OS and LRC when excluding neoadjuvant trials that omitted surgery. Lower mastectomy rates (relative risk 0.71) and chemotherapy-induced infectious and cardiac toxicity with neoadjuvant chemotherapy.

V

- *Trastuzumab (Herceptin),* a humanized monoclonal antibody for HER2/neu, indicated for patients with HER2 overexpression
  - IV administration concurrent with nonanthracycline chemo and for 1-year postchemo
  - Concurrent administration with anthracyclines contraindicated given synergistic cardiac toxicity
  - Concurrent administration with left-sided RT does not appear to increase cardiac risk

- *NSABP B-31 & NCCTG N9831* (Romond et al. 2005): 3,351 patients with resected LN+ or high-risk LN−, HER2+ breast cancer randomized to ACT chemo (doxorubicin, cyclophosphamide, and paclitaxel) vs. chemo + trastuzumab (ACT-H). Trastuzumab increased 3-year DFS (75→87%) and OS (92→94%), but was associated with increased risk of heart failure or cardiac death (3–4%).
- *HERA BIG 01-01* (Piccart-Gebhart et al. 2005): 5,090 patients status postsurgery ± RT and neoadjuvant or adjuvant chemo ± HT (if ER/PR+) with HER2 overexpression randomized to observation, 1-year trastuzumab (q3 week), or 2-year trastuzumab. On interim analysis, trastuzumab × 1 year improved 2-year DFS (77→86%), but no difference in OS (95–96%).

- *Adjuvant hormonal therapy* generally recommended for all ER-positive tumors.
- The need for complete ovarian suppression/ablation in premenopausal women is currently under investigation.
- SERMS (e.g., tamoxifen) indicated for both pre and postmenopausal women.
  - Associated with increased bone mineral density, hot flashes, increased risk of thromboembolic disease, and endometrial proliferation/uterine cancer
- Aromatase inhibitors (AI) indicated for postmenopausal patients, preceding or in place of SERMS, and have shown increased efficacy as compared to tamoxifen alone.
  - Commonly associated with arthralgia

- *NSABP B-14* (Fisher et al. 2004): 2,644 patients status-post surgery for breast ca (pathologically LN−, ER+) randomized to tamoxifen × 5 years vs. placebo. Adjuvant tamoxifen improved 15-year DFS (HR = 0.58) and OS (HR = 0.80).
- *ATAC Trial* (2002; Lancet 2005): 9,366 postmenopausal patients (both ER +/-) status-post definitive therapy for early-stage breast ca randomized to anastrozole, tamoxifen, or both given concurrently. Anastrozole alone improved 3-year DFS compared with tamoxifen (89 vs. 87%) or both (87%). Benefit observed only in ER+ patients. Anastrozole better tolerated with respect to side-effects.
- *Goss* (Goss et al. 2003): 5,187 postmenopausal patients (98% ER+) status-post definitive therapy and adjuvant tamoxifen × 5 years for early-stage breast ca randomized to letrozole (2.5 mg) or placebo daily × 5 years. Addition of letrozole improved 4-year DFS (87→93%).

- Bisphosphonates may play a role in preventing skeletal events and improving DFS.

- *Gnant* (Gnant et al. 2009): 1,803 premenopausual ER/PR+ patients randomized to endocrine therapy ± zoledronic acid. With a median follow-up of 47.8 months, Zoledronic acid improved DFS 90.8→94%.

- Various targeted therapies, such as antiangiogenic agents (bevacizumab), appear promising and are currently under investigation.

IN-SITU DISEASE

Stage	Recommended treatment
DCIS	■ BCT with lumpectomy ± RT. RT generally indicated for all patients to reduce LR, but some patients may have small absolute benefit and may choose to omit RT [e.g., older women, with small (<0.5 cm), unicentric, low-grade tumors excised with wide (≥1 cm) negative margins]. Alternative is total mastectomy (TM) with or without SLN bx. TM indicated for diffuse malignant microcalcifications, multicentric disease, persistently +margins, or patient desire. Consider adjuvant tamoxifen for ER+ tumors
LCIS	■ Lifelong close observation ± tamoxifen for risk reduction (decrease invasive cancer rate by 56%). If young and strong FH, diffuse disease, or genetic predisposition, consider prophylactic bilateral mastectomy

- DCIS treatment is individualized based on clinical and pathological features, and patient preference.
- Margins ≤1–2 mm post-BCS require reexcision as up to 1/2 will have residual DCIS.
- Tamoxifen for ER/PR+ DCIS reduces local recurrence after lumpectomy and RT, although absolute benefit may be small and diminishes with increased follow-up.

SELECT COOPERATIVE GROUP DCIS TRIAL OF BCS ± RT ± TAMOXIFEN

Study	Patients	Randomization	Outcome	Comments
NSABP B-17 (Fisher et al. 1998c, 2001b)	818 patients with DCIS (negative margins)	Lumpectomy ±50 Gy RT	12-year follow-up: RT reduced noninvasive LF 15→8% and invasive LF 17→8% (total LF: 32→16%). No difference on DM or OS	Increased LR with: + margins (borderline significance), moderate-marked comedonecrosis, and microcalcs ≥1 cm
EORTC 10853 (Julien et al. 2000; Bijker et al. 2006)	1,010 patients with DCIS (negative margins)	Lumpectomy ±50 Gy RT	10-year follow-up: RT improved noninvasive local recurrence-free rate 86→93% and invasive LR-free rate 87→92% (total LR-free rate: 74→85%). No difference on DM or OS	Increased LR with: age ≤40 years old, sxtic presentation, G2–3, cribriform or solid growth pattern, positive margins (with or without RT), omission of RT
South Sweden (Holmberg et al. 2008)	1,046 patients with DCIS	Lumpectomy ±50 Gy RT	5-year follow-up: RT reduced noninvasive LF 13→4% and invasive LF 9→3% (total LF: 22→7%). No difference on DM or OS	

NSABP B-24 (Fisher et al. 1999, 2001b, 2002b, 2007; Allred, Breast Cancer Res 2003)	1,804 patients with DCIS (16% + margins; all unknown ER status)	Lumpectomy and 50 Gy ±tamoxifen (20 mg daily × 5 years)	10.5-year follow-up: addition of tamoxifen reduced incidence of IBTR from 14.9% (49.5% invasive) to 11% (43.8% invasive) and contralateral events from 5.4 to 4.5% (64–68% invasive). No difference on DM or OS	On secondary analysis, benefit only seen for ER+ patients (50% risk reduction)
UKCCR (2003)	1,701 patients with DCIS status postlumpectomy (negative margins)	randomized to: 50 Gy RT, tamoxifen × 5 years, neither; or both	median follow-up 53 months: rates of all breast events were 8, 18, 22, and 6%, respectively. When analyzing those randomized to RT vs. no RT, RT reduced LF (invasive or noninvasive) in ipsilateral breast from 14 to 6%	Tamoxifen had no apparent benefit in IBTR if given with RT, but did decrease contralateral breast tumor recurrence
ECOG 5194, NCCTG (Hughes et al. 2009)	711 patients with DCIS (median age 60) post local excision	Two cohorts: G1–2, <2.5 cm G3, <1 cm ER/PR status unknown	Group 1: 5 year IBTR 6.1% (53% invasive) Group 2: 5 year IBTR 15.3% (35% invasive)	Margins ≥ 3 mm. No RT

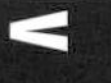

SELECT NONRANDOMIZED DCIS STUDIES OF BCS ± RT

- VNPI (Silverstein 2003). Retrospective review of 706 patients status post-BCT with or without RT scored based on four parameters: tumor size (≤1.5, 1.6–4.0, ≥4.1 cm); pathology (nonhigh-grade without necrosis, nonhigh-grade with necrosis, high grade); margins (≥1, 0.1–0.9, <0.1 cm); and age (>60, 40–60, <40 years). For low-risk (score 4, 5, 6), no significant difference in 12-year local RFS (>90–95%) with or without RT. For intermediate-risk (score 7, 8, 9), addition of RT provided 12–15% 12-year local RFS benefit. For high-risk (score 10, 11, 12), mastectomy recommended due to high 5-year LR (~50%) with or without RT. Generalizability of study questioned given unique and intensive surgical/pathological specimen preparation techniques.
- Wong et al. (2006). Phase II trial of 158 women with predominantly grade 1–2 DCIS measuring ≤2.5 cm on mammography with final margins ≥1 cm observed after lumpectomy (no RT or Tamoxifen). Twelve percent LF at 5 years.

Meta-analysis

- Cochrane Meta-analysis (Goodwin et al. 2009). Four randomized trials of BCS ±RT, and 3,925 patients. Confirmed benefit of RT on all ipsilateral breast events (HR 0.49) and ipsilateral DCIS recurrence (HR 0.64). All subgroups benefited from RT, with no significant long-term toxicity with RT.

INVASIVE DISEASE ELIGIBLE FOR UPFRONT BREAST CONSERVING THERAPY

Stage	Recommended treatment
I–IIB(± T3N0)	BCT with lumpectomy and surgical axillary staging + RT. Some consider RT optional for patients ≥70 years of age with T1N0, ER+, low grade, no LVI tumors who receive adjuvant hormone therapy (HT). Alternative: TM with surgical axillary staging ± RT as indicated. Adjuvant chemo, HT, and/or trastuzumab as indicated

- BCT is equivalent to mastectomy for early-stage disease in appropriately selected patients.
- BCT with lumpectomy + whole breast RT is considered standard of care.
- Repeat excision generally indicated for close/positive margins, especially in young, EIC+, ILC, multiple or diffusely positive margins.
- Mastectomy reserved for patients ineligible for BCT due to medical or surgical contraindications, or patient preference.
  - See below for postmastectomy RT indications
- Contraindications to BCT include multicentricity, ratio of tumor size to breast, diffuse microcalcifications, persistently close/positive margins despite reasonable number of repeat excisions (especially in the setting of EIC, ILCA, <35–40 years old, diffuse or multiple close/+ margins), previous breast RT, pregnancy, and scleroderma (lupus is a relative contraindication).
- Lymph node involvement not a contraindication to BCT.
- EIC is not an independent risk factor for recurrence post-BCT when margins are considered, but true negative margins may be more difficult to be achieved in the presence of EIC.
- Younger patients are generally at higher risk for LR.
- Positive margins, close margins (≤1–2 mm), and lymphatic invasion are associated with increased LR post-BCT.
- High grade associated with increased LR in some, but not all series.

SEVEN PHASE III TRIALS HAVE DEMONSTRATED EQUIVALENT OS AND DFS WITH BCS + RT VS. MASTECTOMY FOR INVASIVE DISEASE. SELECT TRIALS:

Study	Patients	Randomization	Outcome	Comments
NSABP B-06 (NEJM 2002)	1,851 patients with Stage I/II breast ca (<4 cm, negative margins)	Total mastectomy vs. lumpectomy alone vs. lumpectomy + 50 Gy RT	20-year follow-up: no significant differences observed among three groups with respect to DFS, OS, or DM-free survival. Addition of RT to lumpectomy reduced LF 39→14%	N+ patients had 5-FU based chemo
EORTC 10801 (Van Dongen et al. 2000)	902 patients with Stage I/II breast ca	Modified radical mastectomy vs. lumpectomy + 50 Gy RT + boost	10-year follow-up: Decreased LF with MRM (12 vs. 20%, $p = 0.01$). No difference in OS (66 vs. 65%)	48% in lumpectomy group had + margins
Milan I (NEJM 2002)	701 patients with T1N0 breast ca	Radical mastectomy vs. quadrantectomy + 60 Gy RT	Median follow-up 20 years: LF 2.3 vs. 8.8% in favor of RM ($p < 0.001$). No difference in OS (59 vs. 58%) or breast ca-specific survival (76 vs. 74%)	N+ patients had CMF chemo

SELECT PHASE III TRIALS OF BCS ± RT FOR INVASIVE DISEASE

Study	Patients	Randomization	Outcome	Comments
NSABP B-06 (NEJM 2002)	1,851 Patients with Stage I/II <4 cm negative margins	Total mastectomy vs. lumpectomy alone vs. lumpectomy + 50 Gy RT	20-year follow-up: no significant differences observed among three groups with respect to DFS, OS, or DM-free survival. Addition of RT to lumpectomy reduced LF 39→14%	N+ patients had 5-FU based chemo
Milan III (Ann Oncol 2001)	570 Patients <70 years old with ≤2.5 cm	Surgery alone (quadrantectomy + axillary dissection) vs. surgery + 60 Gy RT	10-year follow-up: addition of RT reduced LF (23.5→5.8%), but no difference in OS. patients <45 years had highest LF, but also derived most benefit from RT. Subset: N0-1, ≥66 year old, and margin negative: 4% LF with no RT	All patients received systemic therapy (tamoxifen if ER+ and postmenopausal; CMF if ER– and/or premenopausal)
Swedish Trial (Liljegren et al. 1999)	1,187 patients ≤3 cm Negative margins	Lumpectomy vs. lumpectomy – 50 Gy RT	5-year follow-up: LR 14→4%No OS difference	No systemic therapy

continued

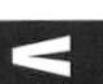

Study	Patients	Randomization	Outcome	Comments
Scottish Trial (Lancet 1996)	585 patients with Stage I/II tumors <4 cmgross margins >1 cm	Lumpectomy vs. lumpectomy + 50 Gy RT	LF was 24.5% with adjuvant systemic therapy alone vs. 5.8% with addition of RT ($p<0.01$)	All patients received systemic therapy (tamoxifen if ER+ or CMF if ER–) Microscopic Margins not specified
Finnish Trial (Holli et al. 2009)	264 T1N0 patients > 40 year old, ≥ 1 cm tumor-free margin, PR+, G1-2, unifocal, no EIC, low cell proliferation rate (S-phase fraction ≤7% or nuclear Ki-67 expression <10%)	Lumpectomy vs. lumpectomy + 50 Gy RT	Median follow-up 12.1 years: 11.6 vs. 27.2% LR in favor of RT. No difference in OS, DFS, or CSS	No systemic therapy

PHASE III TRIALS OF BCS AND TAMOXIFEN ±RT FOR INVASIVE DISEASE

Study	Patients	Randomization	Outcome	Comments
PMH/Canada (Fyles et al. 2004)	769 patients (median age 68 years), Stage I/II (pN0) ER/PR±	Tamoxifen + RT vs. tamoxifen alone	RT reduced 8-year LR (12.2 vs. 4.1%, $p < 0.05$) and improved DFS (82 vs. 76%, $p < 0.05$)	No difference in breast ca-specific survival or OS
CALGB C9343/ INT Trial (NEJM 2004, SABCS 2006).	636 patients (>70 years) pT1N0, ER+	Tamoxifen + RT vs. tamoxifen alone	Addition of RT to tamoxifen improved 7.9-year LF (1 vs. 7%, $p < 0.05$)	No difference in breast ca-specific survival or OS
NSABP B-21 (JCO 2002, Cancer 2007)	1,009 pN0 patients with tumors ≤1 cm (both ER/PR ±)	Three arm trial: Tamoxifen vs. RT + placebo vs. RT + tamoxifen	At 8-year follow-up, both tamoxifen and RT independently reduced LF (16.5, 9.3, and 2.8%), but effect of tamoxifen on IBTR had disappeared at 14-year follow-up (Tam still decreased contralateral breast primaries) 14-Year follow-up / LR-free survival (%) / DFS% / OS % Tam / 80.5 / 61.5 / 82.2 RT / 89.2 / 60.6 / 82.1 Tam +RT / 89.9 / 56 / 77.8	No difference in OS and DM-free survival

V

ADVANCED INVASIVE DISEASE NOT ELIGIBLE FOR UPFRONT BCT

- Incidence is decreasing with mammography
- Multimodality approach for all patients
- With standard therapy, OS is 40–60% at 5 years and 20–40% at 10 years
- Current standard is to treat with upfront chemotherapy
- Can be divided into operable and inoperable disease
  - Signs of inoperability: arm edema, satellite skin nodules, inflammatory, and SCV disease
- Haagensen's Grave Signs: skin edema, ulceration, chest fixation, fixed/matted nodes
- Metastatic workup is important because high percentage develop distant disease
- Most common site of LRF is the chest wall
- IMLN involvement more likely with medial tumors, axillary nodes +
- Prognostic variables include tumor size and extent of lymph node involvement
- Inflammatory carcinoma is a clinical diagnosis
  - Confirmed by pathological findings of cancer cells in dermal lymphatics
  - Pathologic findings in the absence of clinical signs/symptoms are not diagnostic of inflammatory carcinoma
  - Presents with rapid onset of erythema, warmth, and edema of breast
  - Underlying mass often cannot be appreciated for inflammatory carcinoma
  - Localized inflammatory changes do not qualify for inflammatory carcinoma

RECOMMENDED TREATMENT

Stage	Recommended Treatment
IIB (T3N0) and IIIA	■ Neoadjuvant chemo → surgery (mastectomy or BCT) with surgical axillary staging + RT as indicated. Alternative: TM with surgical axillary staging + RT as indicated. Adjuvant chemo, HT, and/or trastuzumab as indicated

IIIB–IIIC	■ Neoadjuvant chemo → surgery (mastectomy or BCT [except T4d: BCT contraindicated]) with surgical axillary staging + RT. Adjuvant chemo, HT, and/or trastuzumab as indicated
IV	■ HT, chemo, and/or trastuzumab as indicated. Consider bisphosphonates for bone metastases. Palliative RT may be needed. Role of surgical resection of primary disease in selected Stage IV patients is under investigation

POSTMASTECTOMY RT (PMRT)

- Early PMRT trials limited by selection, technique, and no systemic therapy. Survival detriment attributed to RT in early trials due to cardiac/pulmonary toxicity.
- Contemporary randomized trials have shown OS benefit for PMRT in patients receiving systemic therapy.
- *PMRT indications:* T3/4 (T3N0 controversial), + margins, gross ECE, and ≥4+ nodes.
- For T1–2 and 1–3 axillary lymph nodes involved, indications for PMRT unclear.
- Consider percent positive nodes (>20%, not applicable if SLNB only), tumor size, margins, LVSI, petient age, histological grade
- Percent nodes positive ≥20% may be better predictor of LRR and OS than absolute number of positive nodes (Vinh-Hung et al. 2009; Truong et al. 2007).
- PMRT generally not indicated for T1–2N0 if adequate surgical axillary staging performed. Consider PMRT for close/positive margins, age ≤ 35 years, LVI + and/or grade 3.

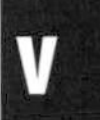

- *ASTRO postmastectomy consensus* (IJROBP 1999). Practice guidelines issued by multidisciplinary expert panel recommend PMRT for patients with ≥4 LN+. Patients with 1–3 LN+ should be enrolled on protocol. Controversy regarding sites requiring RT.
- *ASCO postmastectomy consensus* (JCO 2001). Practice guidelines issued by multidisciplinary expert panel recommended PMRT for patients with ≥4 LN+ and with T3 or Stage III tumors. Insufficient evidence to make recommendations for patients with 1–3 LN+.
- *ACR postmastectomy appropriateness criteria* (IJROBP 2009) PMRT indicated in patients with T3N1 and T4N1–2, and T1–2 disease with ≥ 4 positive nodes. Discuss risk and benefits of PMR for T1–2 patients with 1–3 positive nodes.

THREE CONTEMPORARY TRIALS USING SYSTEMIC THERAPY HAVE DEMONSTRATED DECREASED LRR (~20%) AND IMPROVED OS (~10%) WITH PMRT

Study	Patients	Randomization	Medial follow-up	Outcome	Comment
Danish 82b (New Engl J Med 1997)	1,708 Premenopausal patients status postmodified radical mastectomy	Adjuvant CMF chemo alone vs. chemo + RT	114 Months	Postmastectomy RT reduced LRF (32 vs. 9%), 10-year DFS (34 vs. 48%), and OS (45 vs. 54%) Improvement in LC and OS in all subsets regardless of tumor size or number of involved LN	Study criticized for inadequate LN dissection (mean of 7 LN). Internal mammary irradiation used
Danish 82c (Lancet 1999)	1,406 Postmenopausal patients status postmodified radical mastectomy	Adjuvant tamoxifen alone vs. tamoxifen + RT (48–50 Gy)	10 Years	RT improved LRF (35 vs. 8%), DFS (24 vs. 36%), and OS (36 vs. 45%). No survival benefit in N0 patients	Study criticized for inadequate LN dissection Internal mammary irradiation used
British-Columbia Trial (J Natl Cancer Inst 2005)	318 pLN+ Premenopausal patients status postmodified radical mastectomy	CMF chemo alone vs. chemo + RT	20 Years	RT reduced LRF (26→10%), and improved breast ca-specific survival (38→53%), and OS (37→47%)	Median 11 LN sampled

Meta-analyses and select nonrandomized studies PMRT

- EBCTCG RT (Early Breast Cancer Trialists' Collaborative Group 2005b). Metaanalysis of 78 randomized trials including 42,000 women. RT after BCS, and RT after mastectomy with axillary clearance in LN+ disease, produced significant absolute improvements in 5-year LR (17–19% benefit) and 15-year breast cancer mortality (5.4% benefit). RT produced similar proportional reductions in LR risk (~70% risk reduction) irrespective of age, grade, tumor size, ER status, or amount of LN involvement. Among patients treated with systemic therapy, the absolute benefits of RT on LR and breast cancer mortality, were 20% (at 5 years) and 5.9% (at 15 years), respectively. *Therefore, better local treatment adds to the effect of systemic therapy on LR, which can translate into a moderate breast cancer mortality benefit (4:1 ratio).* RT was associated with excess contralateral breast cancer, lung cancer, and mortality from heart disease. Yet, addition of RT improved 15-year OS by 5.3% after BCS and by 4.4% after mastectomy with axillary clearance for LN+ disease.
- Whelan et al. (2000). Metaanalysis of 18 contemporary postmastectomy trials (6,367 patients) demonstrated that the addition of postmastectomy RT reduced LRF by 75% and improved OS by 17%.
- ECOG, Recht et al. (1999). Retrospective review of 2,016 patients status postmastectomy and adjuvant CMF chemo without RT demonstrated that 10-year LRF was 13% for those with 1–3 LN+ compared to 29% for those with ≥4 LN+.
- Katz et al. (2000). Retrospective review of 1,031 patients treated with mastectomy and doxorubicin-based chemo without adjuvant RT. Ten-year LRF were 4, 10, 21, and 22% for patients with 0, 1–3, 4–9, or ≥10 LN involved, respectively. T stage, tumor size, and >2 mm ECE predictive for LRF.
- Taghian et al. (2004). Patterns of LRF reviewed for 5,758 patients enrolled on five NSABP trials; treated with mastectomy and adjuvant chemotherapy (± tam) with no PMRT. Ten-year LRF of 13.0, 24.4, and 31.9% for patients with 1–3, 4–9, and ≥10 +LN, and 14.9, 21.3, and 24.6%, and for patients with a tumor size of ≤2, 2.1–5.0, and >5.0 cm. Age, tumor size, premenopausal status, number of LN+, and number of dissected LN were significant predictors for LRF on multivariate analysis.
- CALGB 9741 (above) patients with 1–3+ LNs postmastectomy and no PMRT had 5-year LRR of 9.3% with AC and 5.2% with AC+T, as compared to 12.4% for patients with ≥4+ LN postmastectomy, no PMRT, and either chemo regiment.

V

LR management in the setting of neoadjuvant chemotherapy

- Accuracy of SLNBx is likely not reduced after neoadjuvant chemotherapy (Buchholz et al. 2008), thus it may be performed either pre or post neoadjuvant chemotherapy (at time of definitive surgery if post).
- BCT may be possible after neoadjuvant chemotherapy in properly selected patients.
  - Selection criteria for BCT after neoadjuvant chemotherapy remain to be defined
  - BCT contraindicated if residual skin ulceration, edema, chest wall fixation, or inflammatory breast cancer
- MRI to assess treatment response to neoadjuvant chemo appears promising.

- Chen et al. (2004). Retrospective review of 340 patients treated with neoadjuvant chemo + BCT demonstrated that acceptably low rates of LF (5% at 5 years) can be obtained when appropriate selection criteria are used.
- Huang et al. (2004). Retrospective review of 679 patients treated with neoadjuvant chemo + mastectomy with or without postmastectomy RT. At 10-year follow-up, addition of RT reduced LRF (11 vs. 22%) and improved breast ca-specific survival for patients with clinical T3 tumors or Stage III disease and for patients with ≥4 LN+.
- Huang et al. (2006) MD Anderson Prognostic Index for patients treated with neoadjuvant chemo and LRR risk based on local treatment (risk factors = cN2–3, LVI on bx or final pathology, multifocal residual disease, pathological tumor size >2 cm):

Number of risk factors	10-year LRR % with BCS +RT	10-year LRR % with MRM + RT	*p* Value
0–1	9	5	ns
2	28	12	0.28
3–4	61	19	0.009
All patients	12	9	ns

Isolated axillary disease with occult breast primary

Stage	Recommended treatment
TxN1–3	Workup: H&P, bilateral mammography, MRI of breast(s), PET–CT. Treatment: TM with ALND ± RT. Systemic therapy as indicated

LOCOREGIONAL RECURRENCE AND ISOLATED AXILLARY DISEASE

Stage	Recommended treatment
Isolated chest wall recurrence	■ Resection. Consider SLN bx. If no prior RT, post-op RT to chest wall and SCV. Adjuvant chemo, HT, and/or trastuzumab as indicated
Isolated axillary nodal recurrence	■ ALND + nodal RT if no prior RT, adjuvant chemo, HT and/or trastuzumab as indicated

RADIATION TECHNIQUES

- RT can usually begin within 2–4 weeks of surgery
- For patients receiving chemotherapy, RT begins 3–4 weeks after last cycle

V

- JCRT Sequencing (JCO 2005): 244 patients with Stage I/II breast ca status post lumpectomy randomized to adjuvant doxorubicin-based chemo followed by RT vs. adjuvant RT followed by four cycles of same chemo. With 11-year follow-up, there are no differences in OS, DM, time to any event, or site of first failure. For close margins (<1 mm), crude LR was 32% with chemo first vs. 4% with RT first; for + margins, crude LR was 20–23% in both arms.

INTACT BREAST

Simulation and field design

- Patients usually treated in supine position with customized immobilization device
- Bilateral arms abducted and externally rotated
- Wire all surgical scars
- Target volume is entire breast using tangential fields, and SCV fossa via third field as indicated (below)
- Mark estimated medial, lateral, cranial, and caudal field borders
  - Medial border at midsternum
  - Lateral border placed 2 cm beyond all palpable breast tissue (midaxillary line)
  - Inferior border is 2 cm from inframammary fold
  - Superior border is at head of clavicle or second intercostal space
  - Deep (intrathoracic) field border must be nondivergent and edges made coplanar

  - Use half-beam block techniques, or rotate gantry to make symmetric and align posterior edge of each tangent (gantry rotation angle = arctan ({0.5 × field width}/SAD) ~3° for 10 cm field
- Isocenter typically placed in the center of treatment field
- In general, 1–2 cm of underlying lung in the treatment field is acceptable
- For left-sided lesions, minimize the amount of heart in tangential fields
- CT-planning allows for more accurate dose distribution and is recommended
- Rarely need to treat completely dissected axilla (i.e., posterior axillary field) since axillary failure is uncommon
- Tangential RT usually covers a large percentage of the level I and II axillary nodes
- High tangent technique can be used to treat greater percentage of axilla if no axillary dissection performed
  - Top border placed within 2 cm of humeral head
  - Top of field should be 2–3 cm deep into lung
  - Best done with CT planning
- When using third field (SCV), attention to geometric match with tangential fields is essential
  - Half-beam block for caudal edge of supraclavicular field to eliminate divergence
  - Divergence of tangential fields superiorly can be eliminated with various techniques
    - Couch-kick away from tangents field: arctan ({0.5 × tangent field length})/SAD) but can adjust with multi-leaf collimators
    - Use of monoisocentric technique: SCV and tangents fields are half-beam blocked using same isocenter placed at edge of each respective field. Disadvantage: unable to collimate gantry for tangent fields, resulting in higher lung dose
  - Supraclavicular field is angled obliquely 10–15° laterally to keep off spinal cord
  - Inferior border of tangents field placed at inferior aspect of clavicular head
  - Superior border of supraclavicular field is above acromioclavicular joint, top of T1/first rib, short of flash
  - Medial border of supraclavicular field placed at the pedicles of vertebral bodies
  - Lateral border of supraclavicular field is coracoid process or lateral to humeral head

- Boost field is delivered with appositional field using electrons to tumor bed
- Each field should be treated on a daily basis, Monday through Friday
- Bolus should not be used

DOSE PRESCRIPTIONS

Conventional whole-breast tangents ± SCV

- 45–50 Gy at 1.8–2 Gy/fx to whole breast with tangential fields
- 45–50 Gy at 1.8–2 Gy/fx to supraclavicular fossa (when included)
- Boost irradiation with electrons to bring total tumor bed dose to 60–66 Gy (with 1–2 cm PTV expansion)
  - Electron energy is selected to allow the 85–90% isodose line to encompass target

V

Phase III boost trials

- EORTC Boost Trial (NEJM 2001, JCO 2007): 5,569 patients with Stage I/II breast ca status post lumpectomy (negative invasive margins, DCIS margins ignored) randomized to 50 Gy RT vs. 50 Gy + 16 Gy boost. At 10-year follow-up, boost decreased LF from 10.2 to 6.2% with largest benefit observed in patients ≤40 years (23.9→13%). All age groups benefited from boost, although benefit small if >60 year old. Boost had slightly increased rates of severe fibrosis (4.4 vs. 1.6%).
- Lyon Boost Trial (JCO 1997): 1,024 patients with early-stage breast ca status post lumpectomy (<3 cm tumor), ALND, and 50 Gy RT randomized to boost (10 Gy) vs. no boost. At median follow-up 3 years, addition of boost reduced LF (3.6 vs. 4.5%). No difference in self-assessed cosmetic response between two arms.

- At UCSF:
  - 1.8–2 Gy per fraction
  - DCIS and R-sided invasive disease receive 45–50 Gy whole-breast, L-sided invasive receives 45–50 Gy whole breast
  - SCV field receives 45–46 Gy or 50 Gy as indicated (below)
  - Tumor bed boosted to total of 60 Gy if negative margins, 64 Gy if close, and 66 Gy if + margins, on a case-by-case basis

- Boost not given if no residual disease was found on reexcision and ≥50 years old (Arthur et al. 2006)
  - 50 Gy whole-breast RT to both left and right-sided if no boost

Hypofractionation

- At UCSF, hypofractionation (42.5 Gy/2.66) is considered in right-sided disease (invasive), no chemotherapy, negative margins (>2 mm), no boost, ≥50 years old, ≤25 cm separation, and no SCV irradiation indicated and non-high grade.

- Whelan (IJROBP 2002; IJROBP 2008; NEJM 2010): 1,234 pN0 patients treated with BCS randomized to 50 Gy in 25 fxs vs. 42.5 Gy in 16 daily fxs, whole-breast RT. No boost. Large-breasted patients (>25 cm separation) not allowed. Only 11% of patients in each arm received chemotherapy, 25% <50 year old. No difference in 10-year LR (6.2 vs. 6.7%, respectively), DFS, OS, or good/excellent cosmetic outcome (70 vs. 71%).
- UK START A and B Trials (Bentzen et al. 2008a, b). Two phase III trials randomized 2,236 and 2,215 pT1–3 N0-1 patients to 50 Gy in 25 fxs vs. 41.6 Gy or 39 Gy in 13 fxs (START A) or 50 Gy in 25 fxs vs. 40 Gy in 15 fxs (START B), respectively. Twenty-one to twenty-three percent < 50 year old, 22–35% of patients had chemotherapy, 23–29% were LN+, 43–60% of post-BCS patients had boost, and 8–15% of patients had mastectomy. No difference in 5-year LRR. Photographic and patient-assessed late adverse effects were lower with 39 vs. 50 Gy and with 40 vs. 50 Gy. Estimated α/β of 4.6 Gy for tumor control and 3.4 Gy for late breast appearance change.
- RMH/GO3 (Owne Lancet Oncology 2006): 1,410 T1–3N01 patients randomized to 50 Gy in 25, 39 Gy in 13, or 42.9 Gy in 13 fractions. Thirty percent of patients <50 year old, 14% had chemotherapy, 75% had boost. Ten-year IBTR of 12.1, 14.8, and 9.6% (6.7–12.6) each arm, respectively (difference between 39 and 42.9 Gy groups: $p=0.027$). Estimated α/β of 4.0 Gy for tumor control.

Accelerated partial breast irradiation (APBI)

- APBI is considered investigational and is the subject of ongoing randomized clinical trials. Prescribed on protocol at UCSF.
- Techniques include intraoperative electron or X-rays, interstitial brachytherapy (HDR more common than LDR), balloon brachytherapy, or 3DCRT.
  - HDR/balloon brachytherapy dose: 3.4 Gy b.i.d. × 5 days
  - 3DCRT APBI dose: 3.85 Gy b.i.d. × 5 days

- RTOG 95-17 (Arthur et al. 2008; Vicini et al. 2003). Phase II multiinstitutional trial, 199 patients with Stage I–II breast ca (<3 cm, unifocal, invasive nonlobular, no ECE) treated with limited-field RT to region of tumor bed only (60% LDR, 45 Gy over 3.5–5 days, 40% HDR, 3.4 Gy b.i.d. × 10 fxs). Five-year in breast, regional, and contralateral failure rates of 3 and 6%, 5 and 0%, and 2 and 6%, with HDR and LDR, respectively.

- The American Society of Breast Surgeons' (ASBS) and the American Brachytherapy Society's patient selection criteria for APBI in lieu of whole breast RT:

	ASBS	**ABS**
Age (years)	≥45	≥50
Histology	IDCA or DCIS	Unifocal, IDCA
Tumor size	Total tumor size (invasive and DCIS) less than or equal to 3 cm	≤3 cm
Pathological margins	Negative microscopic surgical margins	Negative microscopic surgical margins
Lymph node status	Sentinel lymph node negative	Axillary node negative by level-I/II axillary dissection or sentinel node evaluation

ASBS: http://www.breastsurgeons.org/statements/APBI_statement_revised_100708.pdf

ABS: Arthur et al. (2003); http://www.americanbrachytherapy.org/resources/abs_breast_brachytherapy_taskgroup.pdf

ASTRO Consensus Statement for APBI		
"Suitable" patients meet all criteria	"Cautionary" patients meet any <u>one</u> criteria	"Unsuitable" patients meet any <u>one</u> of the following criteria
Age ≥ 60	Age 50–59	Age <50
T1	2.1–3 cm, T0 or T2	>3cm, T3-4
pN0	-	pN+ or no nodal surgery
ER+	ER-	
No LVI	Limited/focal LVSI	Extensive LVSI
Negative margins (>2mm)	Close margins (<2mm)	Positive margins
Unicentric and unifocal*	-#	Multicentric, microscopically multifocal >3cm in total size, or if clinically multifocal

ASTRO Consensus Statement for APBI		
"Suitable" patients meet all criteria	"Cautionary" patients meet any one criteria	"Unsuitable" patients meet any one of the following criteria
Not pure DCIS (associated LCIS and DCIS allowed)	Pure DCIS ≤3 cm	Pure DCIS > 3 cm
No EIC	EIC ≤3 cm	EIC >3 cm
Not ILCA	ILCA	-
BRCA1/2 mutation absent	-	BRCA1/2 mutation present
No neoadjuvant systemic tx	-	Received neoadjuvant systemic tx

* Microscopic multifocality allowed, provided the lesion is clinically unifocal and the total size of foci of multifocality and intervening normal parenchyma does not exceed 2 cm
# Microscopic multifocality allowed, provided the lesion is clinically unifocal and the total size of foci of multifocality and intervening normal parenchyma is between 2.1 and 3 cm
Adapted from: Smith BD, Arthur DW, Buchholz TA, et al. Accelerated partial breast irradiation consensus statement from the American Society for Radiation Oncology (ASTRO). *Int J Radiat Oncol Biol Phys.* Jul 15 2009;74(4):987–1001.

POSTMASTECTOMY

Simulation and field design

- Patient simulated in similar manner to early-stage disease.
- Target volume includes chest wall and supraclavicular fossa as indicated (below).
- Wire all surgical scars and drain sites.
- Entire mastectomy scar, flaps, surgical clips, and drain sites included in treatment field.
  - If outside of treatment field, drain site can be treated with local electron field 5 Gy × 2 fxs
- Attention to geometric match with SCV field to avoid junctional overdose.
- No boost is given to chest wall or scar with postmastectomy RT at UCSF, but it can be delivered using electrons in appositional field to chest wall and skin.
- Each field should be treated on a daily basis, Monday through Friday.

- TLD's are used at UCSF at assess skin dose.
- Five to ten millimeter bolus typically used every other day for duration of RT at UCSF.
  - Bolus thickness is dependent on photon beam energy
- Custom bolus provides improved dose distribution over the reconstructed breast (i.e., use of a form fitting Aquaplast cast and wax).
- RT is given to internal mammary nodes if clinically or pathologically positive, otherwise internal mammary node irradiation is controversial and at the discretion of the treating radiation oncologist (excellent reviews by Chen et al. 2008; Freedman et al. 2000).
  - Older Phase III randomized trials of IMLN dissection and irradiation showed no benefit (decreased 5-year OS with IMLN RT, NSABP 02)
  - Retrospective reports have reported no benefit with IMLN irradiation
  - CT treatment planning should be utilized in all cases where RT is delivered to the internal mammary lymph nodes
  - Internal mammary RT performed with matched electrons or with wide tangential field
- Posterior axillary boost (PAB) is controversial with no proven benefit, not routinely done at UCSF.

V

Dose prescriptions

- 50 Gy at 1.8–2 Gy/fx to chest wall using tangential fields.
- 45–50 Gy at 1.8–2 Gy/fx to supraclavicular fossa as indicated.
- Electron boost can be used to bring total scar dose to 60 Gy in high-risk patients.
  - Electron energy selected to allow the 85–90% isodose line to encompass target

Indications for nodal RT

- ≥4 involved axillary lymph nodes or inflammatory breast cancer are indications for SCV RT.
- Indications for SCV RT for 1–3 involved axillary lymph nodes less clear.
  - Consider SCV RT if ≥4 high risk features present (risk of SCV failure = 20% based on retrospective data): ECE, LVSI, less than 10 LN removed, ≥20% of dissected nodes +, largest + node >2 cm (Strom et al. 2005).
- SCV RT indications after good response to neoadjuvant chemotherapy are unclear.

- No axillary staging or no ALND in the case of +SLNB are relative indications for SCV RT.

DOSE LIMITATIONS

- Goal of treatment is to achieve homogeneous distribution throughout target volume.
- Careful attention must be paid to the amount of lung tissue and heart in treatment field.
- Wedging and weighting can achieve better dose distribution, although physical wedge increases scatter dose to contralateral breast (less so with virtual wedge or MLC).
- Field-within-field technique using static forward-planned IMRT often used to optimize dose distribution.
- At UCSF, ipsilateral lung V20 is limited to ≤10% with two-field tangents, and ≤20% with three-field (SCV) technique.
- Left ventricle and combined bilateral ventricle limits: V5≤10% and V25≤5%. Also record and attempt to minimize whole heart dose.
- Respiratory gating to minimize dose to lung and heart can be considered.
- ASTRO Consensus Statement dose constraints for 3DCRT APBI (*IJROBP 2009*): Contralateral breast Dmax≤3%, Ipsilateral lung V30%<15%, Contralateral lung V5%<15%, Heart V5%<5% for R-sided tumors and<40% for L-sided tumors

COMPLICATIONS

- Acute skin reaction, treated with:
  - Erythema alone: antifungal and hydrocortisol creams
  - Dry desquamation: moisturizing and vitamins A&D creams
  - Wet Desquamation: zinc Oxide and Bacitracin
- Late cosmetic impairment (edema, fibrosis, telangiectasia), including risk of breast reconstruction complications and/or cosmetic impairment.
- Upper extremity lymphedema: 1–5% risk with RT alone, 4–10% with SLNB, 10% risk with ALND, 12% risk with ALND+RT, and 16–20% risk with ALND + SCV/axillary RT.
- Uncommon: brachial plexopathy, pneumonitis, rib fracture.
- Risk of RT-induced cardiac toxicity can be minimized by modern techniques and cardiac risk modification (excellent review of cardiac risk: Harris 2008).

  - Fifty to seventy percent of patients treated with L-sided tangents exhibit perfusion defect on SPECT 3–6 years post-RT (Prosnitz et al. 2007).
  - Increased risk of cardiac toxicity with doxorubicin, trastuzumab, and aromatase inhibitors.
- Overall risk of second malignancies increased from ~4 to 5%, sarcoma ~0.5% risk in 20–30 years, lung cancer risk increased in smokers only, contralateral breast cancer risk increased from 15 to 16% with modern techniques, but may be higher in younger, positive family history, and BRCA1/2 patients.

FOLLOW-UP

- Monthly self-exam.
- H&P ever 3 months for 1–2 years, then every 6 months for 5 years, then annually.
- Bilateral breast mammograms annually. At UCSF, ipsilateral mammogram interval is 6 months for first 5 years.
- Cosmetic assessment.
- Median time to breast cancer recurrence is 5–7 years for women receiving adjuvant hormonal and/or chemotherapy, but is shorter for triple negative breast cancers (<3 years).

V

Acknowledgement We would like to thank the first edition authors of this chapter: Allen Chen, Alison Bevan, and Lawrence W. Margolis.

REFERENCES

Arthur DW, Cuttino LW, Neuschatz AC, et al. Tumor bed boost omission after negative re-excision in breast-conservation treatment. Ann Surg Oncol 2006;13(6):794-801.

Arthur D, Vicini F, Kuske RR, et al. Accelerated partial breast irradiation: an updated report from the American Brachytherapy Society. Brachytherapy 2003:2:124–130.

Arthur DW, Winter K, Kuske RR, et al. A Phase II trial of brachytherapy alone after lumpectomy for select breast cancer: tumor control and survival outcomes of RTOG 95-17. Int J Radiat Oncol Biol Phys 2008;72(2):467-473.

Bentzen SM, Agrawal RK, Aird EG, et al. The UK Standardisation of Breast Radiotherapy (START) Trial A of radiotherapy hypofractionation for treatment of early breast cancer: a randomised trial. Lancet Oncol 2008a;9(4):331-341.

Bentzen SM, Agrawal RK, Aird EG, et al. The UK Standardisation of Breast Radiotherapy (START) Trial B of radiotherapy hypofractionation for treatment of early breast cancer: a randomised trial. Lancet 2008;371(9618):1098-1107.

Bijker N, Meijnen P, Peterse JL, et al. Breast-conserving treatment with or without radiotherapy in ductal carcinoma-in-situ: ten-year results of European Organisation for Research and Treatment of Cancer randomized phase III trial 10853 a study by the EORTC Breast Cancer Cooperative Group and EORTC Radiotherapy Group. J Clin Oncol. Jul 20 2006;24(21):3381-3387.

Buchholz TA, Lehman CD, Harris JR, et al. Statement of the science concerning locoregional treatments after preoperative chemotherapy for breast cancer: a National Cancer Institute conference. J Clin Oncol 2008;26(5):791-797.

Chen AM, Meric-Bernstam F, Hunt KK, et al. Breast conservation after neoadjuvant chemotherapy: the M.D. Anderson Cancer Center experience. J Clin Oncol 2004;22:2303-2312.

Chen RC, Lin NU, Golshan M, Harris JR, Bellon JR. Internal mammary nodes in breast cancer: diagnosis and implications for patient management a systematic review. J Clin Oncol. Oct 20 2008;26(30):4981-4989.

Citron ML, Berry DA, Cirrincione C, et al. Randomized trial of dose-dense versus conventionally scheduled and sequential versus concurrent combination chemotherapy as postoperative adjuvant treatment of node-positive primary breast cancer: first report of Intergroup Trial C9741/Cancer and Leukemia Group B Trial 9741. J Clin Oncol 2003;21(8):1431-1439.

Demirci S, Nam J, Hubbs JL, Nguyen T, Marks LB. Radiation-induced cardiac toxicity after therapy for breast cancer: interaction between treatment era and follow-up duration. *Int J Radiat Oncol Biol Phys.* Mar 15 2009;73(4):980-987.

Early Breast Cancer Trialists' Collaborative Group. Effects of chemotherapy and hormonal therapy for early breast cancer on recurrence and 15-year survival: an overview o f the randomized trials. Lancet 2005;365:1687-1717.

Early Breast Cancer Trialists' Collaborative Group. Effects of radiotherapy and of differences in the extent of surgery for early breast cancer on local recurrence and 15-year survival: an overview of the randomized trials. Lancet 2005;366:2087-2106.

Fisher B, Bryant J, Dignam JJ, et al. Tamoxifen, radiation therapy, or both for prevention of ipsilateral breast tumor recurrence after lumpectomy in women with invasive breast cancers of one centimeter or less. J Clin Oncol 2002;20(20):4141-4149.

Fisher B, Bryant J, Dignam JL, et al. Tamoxifen, radiation therapy, or both for prevention of ipsilateral breast tumor recurrence after lumpectomy in women with invasive breast cancers of one centimeter or less. N Engl J Med 2002c;20:4141-4149.

Fisher B, Bryant J, Wolmark N, et al. Effect of preoperative chemotherapy on the outcome of women with operable breast cancer. J Clin Oncol 1998a;16:2672-2685.

Fisher B, Dignam J, Wolmark N, et al. Lumpectomy and radiation therapy for the treatment of intraductal breast cancer: findings from the national surgical adjuvant breast and bowel project B-17. J Clin Oncol 1998c;16:441-452.

Fisher B, Dignam J, Wolmark N, et al. Tamoxifen in treatment of intraductal breast cancer: national surgical adjuvant breast and bowel project B-24 randomized controlled trial. Lancet 1999;353:1993-2000.

Fisher B, Jeong JH, Bryant J, et al. Treatment of lymph-node-negative, oestrogen-receptor-positive breast cancer: long-term findings from National Surgical Adjuvant Breast and Bowel Project randomised clinical trials. Lancet 2004;364(9437):858-868.

Fisher B, Land S, Mamounas E, et al. Prevention of invasive breast cancer in women with ductal carcinoma in situ: an update of the national surgical adjuvant breast and bowel project experience. Semin Oncol 2001b;28:400-418.

Fisher ER, Land SR, Saad RS, et al. Pathologic variables predictive of breast events in patients with ductal carcinoma in situ. Am J Clin Pathol 2007;128(1):86-91.

Freedman GM, Fowble BL, Nicolaou N, et al. Should internal mammary lymph nodes in breast cancer be a target for the radiation oncologist? Int J Radiat Oncol Biol Phys. Mar 1 2000; 46(4): 805-814.

Fyles AW, McCready DR, Manchul LA, et al. Tamoxifen with or without breast irradiation in women 50 years of age or older with early stage breast cancer. N Engl J Med 2004;351:963-970.

Gnant M, Mlineritsch B, Schippinger W, et al. Endocrine therapy plus zoledronic acid in premenopausal breast cancer. N Engl J Med 2009;360(7):679-691.

Goodwin A, Parker S, Ghersi D, Wilcken N. Post-operative radiotherapy for ductal carcinoma in situ of the breast. Cochrane Database Syst Rev. 2009;(4):CD000563.

Goss PE, Ingle JN, Martino S, et al. A randomized trial of letrozole in postmenopausal women after five years of tamoxifen therapy for early stage breast cancer. N Engl J Med 2003;349:1793-1802.

Harris EE. Cardiac mortality and morbidity after breast cancer treatment. Cancer Control. Apr 2008;15(2):120-129.

Henderson IC, Berry DA, Demetri GD, et al. Improved outcomes from adding sequential Paclitaxel but not from escalating Doxorubicin dose in an adjuvant chemotherapy regimen for patients with node-positive primary breast cancer. J Clin Oncol. Mar 15 2003;21(6): 976-983.

Holli K, Hietanen P, Saaristo R, Huhtala H, Hakama M, Joensuu H. Radiotherapy after segmental resection of breast cancer with favorable prognostic features: 12-year follow-up results of a randomized trial. J Clin Oncol. Feb 20 2009;27(6):927-932.

Holmberg L, Garmo H, Granstrand B, et al. Absolute risk reductions for local recurrence after postoperative radiotherapy after sector resection for ductal carcinoma in situ of the breast. J Clin Oncol 2008;26(8):1247-1252.

Huang EH, Strom EA, Perkins GH, et al. Comparison of risk of local-regional recurrence after mastectomy or breast conservation therapy for patients treated with neoadjuvant chemotherapy and radiation stratified according to a prognostic index score. Int J Radiat Oncol Biol Phys 2006;66(2):352-357.

Huang EH, Tucker SL, Strom EA, et al. Postmastectomy radiation improves local-regional control and survival for selected patients with locally advanced breast cancer treated with neoadjuvant chemotherapy and mastectomy. J Clin Oncol 2004;22:4639-4647.

Hughes KS, Schnaper LA, Berry D, et al. Lumpectomy plus tamoxifen with or without irradiation in women 70 years of age or older with early breast cancer. N Engl J Med 2004;351:71-977.

Hughes LL, Wang M, Page DL, et al. Local excision alone without irradiation for ductal carcinoma in situ of the breast: a trial of the Eastern Cooperative Oncology Group. *J Clin Oncol.* Nov 10 2009;27(32):5319-5324.

Jones S, Holmes FA, O'Shaughnessy J, et al. Docetaxel With cyclophosphamide is associated with an overall survival benefit compared with doxorubicin and cyclophosphamide: 7-year follow-up of US Oncology Research Trial 9735. J Clin Oncol 2009;27:1177-1183.

Julien JP, Bijker N, Fentiman IS, et al. Radiotherapy in breast conserving treatment for ductal carcinoma in situ: first results of the EORTC randomized phase III trial 10853. Lancet 2000;353:528-533.

Katz A, Strom EA, Buchholz TA, et al. Locoregional recurrence patterns after mastectomy and doxorubicin-based chemotherapy: implications for postoperative irradiation. J Clin Oncol 2000;18:2817-2827.

Kim T, Giuliano AE, Lyman GH. Lymphatic mapping and sentinel lymph node biopsy in early-stage breast carcinoma: a metaanalysis. Cancer 2006;106(1):4-16.

Kuerer HM, Newman LA, Smith TL, et al. Clinical course of breast cancer patients with complete pathological primary tumor and axillary lymph node response to doxorubicin-based neoadjuvant chemotherapy. J Clin Oncol 1999;14:460-469.

Liljegren G, Holmberg L, Bergh J, et al. 10-Year results after sector resection with or without postoperative radiotherapy for stage I breast cancer: a randomized trial. J Clin Oncol 1999;17(8):2326-2333.

Louis-Sylvestre C, Clough K, Asselain B, et al. Axillary treatment in conservative management of operable breast cancer: dissection or radiotherapy? Results of a randomized study with 15 years of follow-up. J Clin Oncol 2004;22(1):97-101.

Mamounas EP, Bryant J, Lembersky B, et al. Paclitaxel after doxorubicin plus cyclophosphamide as adjuvant chemotherapy for node-positive breast cancer: results from NSABP B-28. J Clin Oncol 2005;23(16):3686-3696.

Mieog JS, van der Hage JA, van de Velde CJ. Neoadjuvant chemotherapy for operable breast cancer. Br J Surg 2007;94(10):1189-1200.

Paik S, Shak S, Tang G, et al. A multigene assay to predict recurrence of tamoxifen-treated, node-negative breast cancer. N Engl J Med. Dec 30 2004; 351(27): 2817-2826.

Paik S, Tang G, Shak S, et al. Gene expression and benefit of chemotherapy in women with node-negative, estrogen receptor-positive breast cancer. J Clin Oncol 2006;24(23):3726-3734.

Piccart-Gebhart MJ, Procter M, Leyland-Jones B, et al. Trastuzumab after adjuvant chemotherapy in HER2-postive breast cancer. N Engl J Med 2005;353:1659-1672.

Prosnitz RG, Hubbs JL, Evans ES, et al. Prospective assessment of radiotherapy-associated cardiac toxicity in breast cancer patients: analysis of data 3 to 6 years after treatment. Cancer 2007;110(8):1840-1850.

Rebbeck TR, Kauff ND, Domchek SM. Meta-analysis of risk reduction estimates associated with risk-reducing salpingo-oophorectomy in BRCA1 or BRCA2 mutation carriers. J Natl Cancer Inst 2009;101(2):80-87.

Recht A, Gray R, Davidson NE, et al. Locoregional failure 10 years after mastectomy and adjuvant chemotherapy with or without tamoxifen without irradiation: experience of the easten cooperative oncology group. J Clin Oncol 1999;17:1689-1700.

Romond EH, Perez EA, Bryant J, et al. Trastuzumab plus adjuvant chemotherapy for operable HER2-positive breast cancer. N Engl J Med 2005;353:1673-1684.

Sartor CI, Peterson BL, Woolf S, et al. Effect of addition of adjuvant paclitaxel on radiotherapy delivery and locoregional control of node-positive breast cancer: cancer and leukemia group B 9344. J Clin Oncol 2005;23(1):30-40.

Saslow D, Boetes C, Burke W, et al. American Cancer Society guidelines for breast screening with MRI as an adjunct to mammography. CA Cancer J Clin 2007;57(2):75-89.

Silverstein MJ. The University of Southern California/Van Nuys prognostic index for ductal carcinoma in situ of the breast. Am J Surg 2003;186:337-343.

Strom EA, Woodward WA, Katz A, et al. Clinical investigation: regional nodal failure patterns in breast cancer patients treated with mastectomy without radiotherapy. Int J Radiat Oncol Biol Phys 2005;63(5):1508-1513.

Taghian A, Jeong JH, Mamounas E, et al. Patterns of locoregional failure in patients with operable breast cancer treated by mastectomy and adjuvant chemotherapy with or without tamoxifen and without radiotherapy: results from five National Surgical Adjuvant Breast and Bowel Project randomized clinical trials. J Clin Oncol 2004;22(21):4247-4254.

The ATAC (Arimidex, Tamoxifen Alone or in Combination) Trialists Group. Anastrozole alone or in combination with tamoxifen versus tamoxifen alone for adjuvant treatment of postmenopausal women with early breast cancer: first results of the ATAC randomized trial. Lancet 2002;359:2131-2139.

Truong PT, Woodward WA, Thames HD, Ragaz J, Olivotto IA, Buchholz TA. The ratio of positive to excised nodes identifies high-risk subsets and reduces inter-institutional differences in locoregional recurrence risk estimates in breast cancer patients with 1-3 positive nodes: an analysis of prospective data from British Columbia and the M. D. Anderson Cancer Center. Int J Radiat Oncol Biol Phys 2007;68(1):59-65.

UK Coordinating Committee on Cancer Research. Radiotherapy and tamoxifen in women with completely excised ductal carcinoma in situ of the breast in the UK, Australia, and New Zealand: randomized controlled trial. Lancet 2003;362:95-102.

van der Vijver MJ, He YD, van't Veer LJ, et al. A gene-expression signature as a predictor of survival in breast cancer. New Engl J Med 2002;347(25):1999-2009.

Van Dongen JA, Voogd AC, Fentiman IS, Legrand C, et al. Long-term results of a randomized trial comparing breast-conserving therapy with mastectomy: European organization for research and treatment of cancer 10801 trial. J Natl Cancer Inst 2000;92:1143-1150.

Vicini FA, Kestin L, Chen P, et al. Limited-field radiation therapy in the management of early stage breast cancer. J Natl Cancer Inst 2003;95:1205-1211.

Vinh-Hung V, Verkooijen HM, Fioretta G, et al. Lymph node ratio as an alternative to pN staging in node-positive breast cancer. J Clin Oncol 2009;27(7):1062-1068.

Vogel VG, Costantino JP, Wickerham DL, et al. Effects of tamoxifen vs raloxifene on the risk of developing invasive breast cancer and other disease outcomes: the NSABP Study of Tamoxifen and Raloxifene (STAR) P-2 trial. Jama. Jun 21 2006;295(23):2727-2741.

Whelan TJ, Julian J, Wright J, et al. Does locoregional radiation therapy improve survival in breast cancer? A meta-analysis. J Clin Oncol 2000;18:1220-1229.

Whelan TJ, Pignol JP, Levine MN, et al. Long-term results of hypofractionated radiation therapy for breast cancer. *N Engl J Med.* Feb 11;362(6):513-520.

Wong JS, Kaelin CM, Troyan SL, et al. Prospective study of wide excision alone for ductal carcinoma in situ of the breast. J Clin Oncol 2006;24:1031-1036.

FURTHER READING

American Brachytherapy Society, 2007, http://www.americanbrachytherapy.org/resources/abs_breast_brachytherapy_taskgroup.pdf.

American College of Breast Surgeons, 2008, http://www.breastsurgeons.org/statements/APBI_statement_revised_100708.pdf.

Arriagada R, Le MG, Mouriesse H, et al. Long-term effect of internal mammary chain treatment. Results of a multivariate analysis of 1195 patients with operable breast cancer and positive axillary nodes. Radiother Oncol 1988;11:213-222.

Bartelink H, Horiot JC, Poortsmans P, et al. Recurrence rates after treatment of breast cancer with standard radiotherapy with or without additional radiation. N Engl J Med 2001;245:1378-1387.

Bellon JR, Come SE, Belman RS, et al. Sequencing of chemotherapy and radiation therapy in early-stage breast cancer: updated results of a prospective randomized trial. J Clin Oncol 2005;23:1934-1940.

Bijker N, Peterse JL, Duchateau L, et al. Risk factors for recurrence and metastases after breast-conserving therapy for ductal carcinoma in-situ: analysis of European organization for research and treatment cancer trial 10853. J Clin Oncol 2001;19:226-2271.

Boice JD, Harvey EB, Blettner M, et al. Cancer in the contralateral breast after radiotherapy for breast cancer. N Engl J Med 1992;326:781-785.

Bonadonna G, Valagussa P, Moliterni A, et al. Adjuvant cyclophosphamide, methotrexate, and fluorouracil in node-positive breast cancer: the results of 20 years of follow-up. N Engl J Med 1995;332:901-906.

Brito RA, Valero V, Buzdar AU, et al. Long-term results of combined-modality therapy for locally advanced breast cancer with ipsilateral supraclavicular metastases: the university of texas M.D. Anderson Cancer Center experience. J Clin Oncol 2001;19:628-633.

Buchholz TA, Tucker SL, Masullo L, et al. Predictors of local-regional recurrence after neoadjuvant chemotherapy and mastectomy without radiation. J Clin Oncol 2001;20:17-23.

Burstein HJ, Polyak K, Wong JS, et al. Ductal carcinoma in situ of the breast. N Engl J Med 2004;350:1430-1441.

Carlson RW, Allred DC, Anderson BO, et al. Breast cancer. Clinical practice guidelines in oncology. J Natl Compr Canc Netw 2009;7(2):122-192.

Chen AM, Obedian E, Haffty BG. Breast-conserving therapy in the setting of collagen vascular disease. Cancer J 2001;7:480-491.

Cole BF, Gelber RD, Gelber S, et al. Polychemotherapy for early breast cancer: an overview of the randomized clinical trials with quality-adjusted survival analysis. Lancet 2001;358:277-286.

Cuzick J, Stewart H, Rutqvist L, et al. Cause-specific mortality in long-term survivors of breast cancer who participated in trials of radiotherapy. J Clin Oncol 1994;12:447-453.

D'Orsi CJ. The American College of Radiology mammography lexicon: an initial attempt to standardize terminology. AJR Am J Roentgenol 1996;166(4):779-780.

Ellis MJ, Rigden CE. Initial versus sequential adjuvant aromatase inhibitor therapy: a review of the current data. Curr Med Res Opin. Dec 2006;22(12):2479-2487.

Esserman L, Kaplan E, Partridge S, et al. MRI phenotype is associated with response to doxorubicin and cyclophosphamide neoadjuvant chemotherapy in stage III breast cancer. Ann Surg Oncol 2001;8:549-559.

Fisher B, Anderson S, Bryant J, et al. Twenty-year follow-up of a randomized trial comparing total mastectomy, lumpectomy, and lumpectomy plus irradiation for the treatment of invasive breast cancer. N Engl J Med 2002a;347:1233-1241.

Fisher B, Cosantino J, Redmond C, et al. A randomized clinical trial evaluating tamoxifen in the treatment of patients with node-negative breast cancer who have estrogen-receptor positive tumors. N Engl J Med 1989;320:479-484.

Fisher B, Costantino JP, Wickerham DL, et al. Tamoxifen for prevention of breast cancer: report of the National Surgical Adjuvant Breast and Bowel Project P-1 Study. J Natl Cancer Inst 1998b;90:1371-1388.

Fisher B, Dignam J, Bryant J, et al. Five versus more than five years of tamoxifen for lymph node-negative breast cancer: updated findings from the national surgical adjuvant breast and bowel project B-14 randomized trial. J Natl Cancer Inst 2001a;93:684-690.

Fisher B, Dignam J, Wolmark N, et al. Tamoxifen and chemotherapy for lymph node-negative, estrogen receptor-positive breast cancer. J Natl Cancer Inst 1997;89:1673-1682.

Fisher B, Jeong JH, Anderson S, et al. Twenty-five year follow-up of a randomized trial comparing radical mastectomy, total mastectomy, and total mastectomy followed by irradiation. N Engl J Med 2002d;347:567-575.

Forrest AP, Stewart HJ, Everington D, et al. Randomized controlled trial of conservation therapy for breast cancer: 6-year analysis of the Scottish trial. Lancet 1996;348:708-713.

Fowble B, Gray R, Gilchrist K, et al. Identification of a subgroup of patients with breast cancer and histologically positive axillary lymph nodes receiving adjuvant chemotherapy who may benefit from postoperative radiotherapy. J Clin Oncol 1988;6:1107-1117.

Freedman GM, Anderson PR, Li T, Nicolaou N. Locoregional recurrence of triple-negative breast cancer after breast-conserving surgery and radiation. Cancer. Mar 1 2009;115(5):946-951.

Gage I, Schnitt SJ, Nixon AJ, et al. Pathologic margin involvement and the risk of recurrence in patients treated with breast-conserving therapy. Cancer 1996;78:1921-1928.

Galper S, Recht A, Silver B, et al. Factors associated with regional nodal failure in patients with early stage breast cancer with 0-3 positive axillary lymph nodes following tangential irradiation alone. Int J Radiat Oncol Biol Phys 1999;45:1157-1166.

Haffty BG, Fischer D, Rose M, et al. Prognostic factors for local recurrence in the conservatively treated breast cancer patient: a cautious interpretation of the data. J Clin Oncol 1991;9:997-1003.

Harris JR, Halpin-Murphy P, McNeese M, et al. Consensus statement on postmastectomy radiation therapy. Int J Radiat Oncol Biol Phys 1999;44:989-990.

Jaiyesimi IA, Buzdar AU, Hortobagyi GN, et al. Inflammatory breast cancer: a review. J Clin Oncol 1992;10:1014-1024.

Katz A, Buchholz TA, Strom EA, et al. Recursive partitioning analysis of locoregional recurrence following mastectomy and doxorubicin-based chemotherapy: implications for postoperative irradiation. Int J Radiat Oncol Biol Phys 2001;50:397-403.

Krag DN, Anderson SJ, Julian TB, et al. Technical outcomes of sentinel-lymph-node resection and conventional axillary-lymph-node dissection in patients with clinically node-negative breast cancer: results from the NSABP B-32 randomised phase III trial. Lancet Oncol. Oct 2007;8(10):881-888.

Krag D, Weaver D, Ashikaga A, et al. The sentinel node in breast cancer. N Engl J Med 1998;339:941-946.

Meric F, Buchholz TA, Mirza NQ, et al. Long-term complications associated with breast-conservation surgery and radiotherapy. Ann Surg Oncol 2002;9:543-549.

Morrow M, Strom EA, Bassett LW, et al. Standard for breast conservation therapy in the management of breast carcinoma. CA Cancer J Clin 2002;52:277-230.

NCCN practice guidelines. Screening for and evaluation of suspicious breast lesions. National Comprehensive Cancer Network. Oncology (Williston Park) 1998;12(11A):89-138.

Olson JE, Neuberg D, Pandya KJ, et al. The role of radiotherapy in the management of operable locally advanced breast carcinoma. Cancer 1997;79:1138-1149.

Overgaard M, Hansen PS, Overgaard J, et al. Postoperative radiotherapy in high-risk premenopausal women with breast cancer who receive adjuvant chemotherapy. N Engl J Med 1997;337:949-955.

Overgaard M, Jensen MB, Overgaard J, et al. Postoperative radiotherapy In high-risk postmenopausal breast cancer patients given adjuvant tamoxifen: Danish Breast Cancer Cooperative Group DBCG 82c randomized trial. Lancet 1999;353:1641-1648.

Park CC, Mitsumori M, Nixon A, et al. Outcome at 8 years after breast-conserving surgery and radiation therapy for invasive breast cancer: influence of margin status and systemic therapy on local recurrence. J Clin Oncol 2000;18:1668-1675.

Patel RR, Christensen ME, Hodge CW, Adkison JB, Das RK. Clinical outcome analysis in "high-risk" versus "low-risk" patients eligible for national surgical adjuvant breast and bowel B-39/radiation therapy oncology group 0413 trial: five-year results. Int J Radiat Oncol Biol Phys 2008;70(4):970-973.

Ragaz J, Jackson SM, Le N, et al. Adjuvant radiotherapy and chemotherapy in node-positive premenopausal women with breast cancer. N Engl J Med 1997;337:956-962.

Ragaz J, Olivotto I, Spinelli J, et al. Locoregional radiation therapy in patients with high-risk breast cancer receiving adjuvant chemotherapy: 20-year results of the British Columbia randomized trial. J Natl Cancer Inst 2005;97:116-126.

Rastogi P, Anderson SJ, Bear HD, et al. Preoperative chemotherapy: updates of National Surgical Adjuvant Breast and Bowel Project Protocols B-18 and B-27. J Clin Oncol. Feb 10 2008;26(5):778-785.

Recht A, Come SE, Henderson IC, et al. The sequencing of chemotherapy and radiation therapy after conservative surgery for early-stage breast cancer. N Engl J Med 1996;334:1356-1361.

Recht A, Edge SB, Solin LJ, et al. Postmastectomy radiotherapy: guidelines of the American society of clinical oncology. J Clin Oncol 2001;19:1539-1569.

Romestaing P, Lehingue Y, Carrie C, et al. Role of a 10-Gy boost in the conservative treatment of early breast cancer: results of a randomized trial. J Clin Oncol 1997;15:963-968.

Shapiro CL, Recht A. Side effects of adjuvant treatment of breast cancer. N Engl J Med 2001;344:1997-2008.

Silverstein MJ, Lagios MD, Groshen S, et al. The influence of margin width on local control of ductal carcinoma in situ of the breast. N Engl J Med 1999;340:1455-1461.

Singletary SE, McNeese MD, Hortobagyi GN, et al. Feasibility of breast-conservation surgery after induction chemotherapy for locally advanced breast carcinoma. Cancer 1992;69: 2849-2852.

Strom EA, McNeese MD. Postmastectomy irradiation: rationale for treatment field selection. Semin Radiat Oncol 1999;9:247-253.

Taylor ME, Haffty BG, Rabinovitch R, et al. ACR appropriateness criteria on postmastectomy radiotherapy expert panel on radiation oncology-breast. Int J Radiat Oncol Biol Phys 2009;73(4):997-1002.

Veronesi U, Cascinelli N, Mariani L, et al. Twenty-year follow-up of a randomized study comparing breast-conserving surgery with radical mastectomy for early stage breast cancer. N Engl J Med 2002;347:1227-1232.

Veronesi U, Luini A, Del Vecchio M, et al. Radiotherapy after breast-preserving surgery in women with localized cancer of the breast. N Engl J Med 1993;328:1587-1591.

Veronesi U, Marubini E, Marian L, et al. Radiotherapy after breast-conserving surgery in small breast carcinoma: long-term results of a randomized trial. Ann Oncol 2001;12:997-1003.

Veronesi U, Paganelli G, Viale G, et al. Sentinel-lymph-node biopsy as a staging procedure in breast cancer: update of a randomised controlled study. Lancet Oncol 2006;7(12):983-990.

Veronesi U, Paganelli G, Viale G, et al. Sentinel-lymph-node biopsy as a staging procedure in breast cancer: update of a randomised controlled study. Lancet Oncol. Dec 2006;7(12): 983-990.

Veronesi U, Saccozzi R, Del Vecchio M, et al. Comparing radical mastectomy with quadrantectomy, axillary dissection, and radiotherapy in patients with small cancers of the breast. N Engl J Med 1981;305:6-11.

Veronesi U, Salvadori, Luini A, et al. Breast conservation is a safe method in patients with small cancer of the breast: long-term results of three randomized trials on 1973 patients. Eur J Cancer 1995;31:1574-1599.

Veronesi U, Zucali R, Luini A. Local control and survival in early breast cancer: the Milan Trial. Int J Radiat Oncol Bio Phys 1986;12:717-720.

Whelan T, MacKenzie R, Julian J, et al. Randomized trial of breast irradiation schedules after lumpectomy for women with lymph node-negative breast cancer. J Natl Cancer Inst 2002;94(15):1143-1150.

Wong JS, Recht A, Beard CJ, et al. Treatment outcome after tangential radiation therapy without axillary dissection in patients with early-stage breast cancer and clinically negative axillary lymph nodes. Int J Radiat Oncol Biol Phys 1997;39:915-920.

PART VI
Digestive System

VI

Chapter 18
Esophageal Cancer

Charlotte Dai Kubicky, Hans T. Chung, and Marc B. Nash

PEARLS

- Esophageal cancer accounts for 5% of all GI cancers. There are 16,470 new cases and 14,280 deaths from esophageal cancer each year in the US. It is the sixth leading cause of death from cancer worldwide.
- Incidence increases with age, peaks at sixth to seventh decade.
- Male:female = 3.5:1.
- African-American males:White males = 5:1.
- Most common in China, Iran, South Africa, India, and the former Soviet Union.
- Risk factors: tobacco, EtOH, nitrosamines, Tylosis (congenital hyperkeratosis), Plummer Vinson syndrome, achalasia, GERD, and Barrett's esophagus.
- Four regions of the esophagus: Cervical = cricoid cartilage to thoracic inlet (15–18 cm from the incisor). Upper thoracic = thoracic inlet to tracheal bifurcation (18–24 cm). Midthoracic = tracheal bifurcation to just above the GE junction (24–32 cm). Lower thoracic = GE junction (32–40 cm).
- Barrett's esophagus: metaplasia of the esophageal epithelial lining. The squamous epithelium is replaced by columnar epithelium, with 0.5% annual rate of neoplastic transformation.
- Adenocarcinoma: rapid rise in incidence. Comprises 60–80% of all new cases compared to 10–15% 10 years ago. Predominately white men. Associated with Barrett's, GERD, and hiatal hernia. Locations: 75% in the distal esophagus and 25% in the upper and midesophagus.
- Squamous cell carcinoma: Associated with tobacco, alcohol, or prior history of H&N cancers. Locations: 50% midesophagus and 50% distal esophagus.

VI

WORKUP

- H&P: Dysphagia, odynophagia, cough, hoarseness (laryngeal nerve involvement), weight loss, use of EtOH, tobacco, nitrosamines, history of GERD. Examine for cervical or supraclavicular adenopathy.
- Labs: CBC, chemistries, LFTs.
- EGD: allow direct visualization and biopsy.
- EUS: assess the depth of penetration and LN involvement. Limited by the degree of obstruction.
- Barium swallow: can delineate proximal and distal margins.
- CT chest and abdomen: assess adenopathy and metastasis.
- PET scan: can detect up to 15–20% of metastases not seen on CT and EUS.
- Bronchoscopy: rule-out fistula in midesophageal lesions.
- Bone scan: recommended if elevated alkaline phosphatase or bone pain.
- Pulmonary function test: to evaluate whether medically operable and serve as baseline lung function for chemo-RT.
- Nutritional assessment.

STAGING: ESOPHAGEAL CANCER

Editors' note: All TNM stage and stage groups referred to elsewhere in this chapter reflect the 2002 AJCC staging nomenclature unless otherwise noted as the new system below was published after this chapter was written.

(AJCC 6TH ED., 2002)

Primary tumor (T)
TX: Primary tumor cannot be assessed
T0: No evidence of primary tumor
Tis: Carcinoma in situ
T1: Tumor invades lamina propria or submucosa
T2: Tumor invades muscularis propria
T3: Tumor invades adventitia
T4: Tumor invades adjacent structures

Regional lymph nodes (N)
NX: Regional lymph node metastasis cannot be assessed
N0: No regional lymph node metastasis
N1: Regional lymph node metastasis

Distant metastasis (M)
MX: Distant metastasis cannot be assessed
M0: No distant metastasis
M1: Distant metastasis
Tumors of the lower thoracic esophagus:
M1a: Metastasis in celiac lymph nodes
M1b: Other distant metastasis
Tumors of the midthoracic esophagus:
M1a: Not applicable
M1b: Nonregional lymph nodes and/or other distant metastasis
Tumors of the upper thoracic esophagus:
M1a: Metastasis in cervical nodes
M1b: Other distant metastasis

(AJCC 7TH ED., 2010)

Primary tumor (T)*
TX: Primary tumor cannot be assessed
T0: No evidence of primary tumor
Tis: High-grade dysplasia**
T1: Tumor invades lamina propria, muscularis mucosae, or submucosa
  T1a: Tumor invades lamina propria or muscularis mucosae
  T1b: Tumor invades submucosa
T2: Tumor invades muscularis propria
T3: Tumor invades adventitia
T4: Tumor invades adjacent structures
T4a: Resectable tumor invading pleura, pericardium, or diaphragm
T4b: Unresectable tumor invading other adjacent structures, such as aorta, vertebral body, trachea, etc.

*(1) At least maximal dimension of the tumor must be recorded and (2) multiple tumors require the T(m) suffix
**High-grade dysplasia includes all noninvasive neoplastic epithelia that was formerly called carcinoma in situ, a diagnosis that is no longer used for columnar mucosae anywhere in the gastrointestinal tract.

Regional lymph nodes (N)*
NX: Regional lymph nodes cannot be assessed
N0: No regional lymph node metastasis
N1: Metastasis in 1–2 regional lymph nodes
N2: Metastasis in 3–6 regional lymph nodes
N3: Metastasis in seven or more regional lymph nodes

continued

Stage grouping

0: TisN0M0
I : T1N0M0
IIA: T2N0M0, T3N0M0
IIB: T1N1M0, T2N1M0
III: T3N1M0, T4 Any N M0
IV: Any T, Any N, M1
IVA: Any T, Any N, M1a
IVB: Any T, Any N, M1b

*Number must be recorded for total number of regional nodes sampled and total number of reported nodes with metastasis

Distant metastasis (M)

M0: No distant metastasis
M1: Distant metastasis

Anatomic stage/prognostic groups

Squamous cell carcinoma (Fig. 18.1)*

Stage	T	N	M	Grade	Tumor location**
0:	Tis (HGD)	N0	M0	1, X	Any
IA:	T1	N0	M0	1, X	Any
IB:	T1	N0	M0	2–3	Any
	T2–3	N0	M0	1, X	Lower, X
IIA:	T2–3	N0	M0	1, X	Upper, middle
	T2–3	N0	M0	2–3	Lower, X
IIB:	T2–3	N0	M0	2–3	Upper, middle
	T1–2	N1	M0	Any	Any
IIIA:	T1–2	N2	M0	Any	Any
	T3	N1	M0	Any	Any
	T4a	N0	M0	Any	Any
IIIB:	T3	N2	M0	Any	Any
IIIC:	T4a	N1–2	M0	Any	Any
	T4b	Any	M0	Any	Any
	Any	N3	M0	Any	Any
IV:	Any	Any	M1	Any	Any

*Or mixed histology including a squamous component or NOS**Location of the primary cancer site is defined by the position of the upper (proximal) edge of the tumor in the esophagus.

Adenocarcinoma (Fig. 18.2)

Stage	T	N	M	Grade
0:	Tis (HGD)	N0	M0	1, X
IA:	T1	N0	M0	1–2, X
IB:	T1	N0	M0	3
	T2	N0	M0	1–2, X
IIA:	T2	N0	M0	3

continued

IIB:	T3	N0	M0	Any
	T1–2	N1	M0	Any
IIIA:	T1–2	N2	M0	Any
	T3	N1	M0	Any
	T4a	N0	M0	Any
IIIB:	T3	N2	M0	Any
IIIC:	T4a	N1–2	M0	Any
	T4b	Any	M0	Any
	Any	N3	M0	Any
IV:	Any	Any	M1	Any

Used with the permission from the American Joint Committee on Cancer (AJCC), Chicago, IL. The original source for this material is the AJCC Cancer Staging Manual, Seventh Edition (2010), published by Springer Science+Business Media.

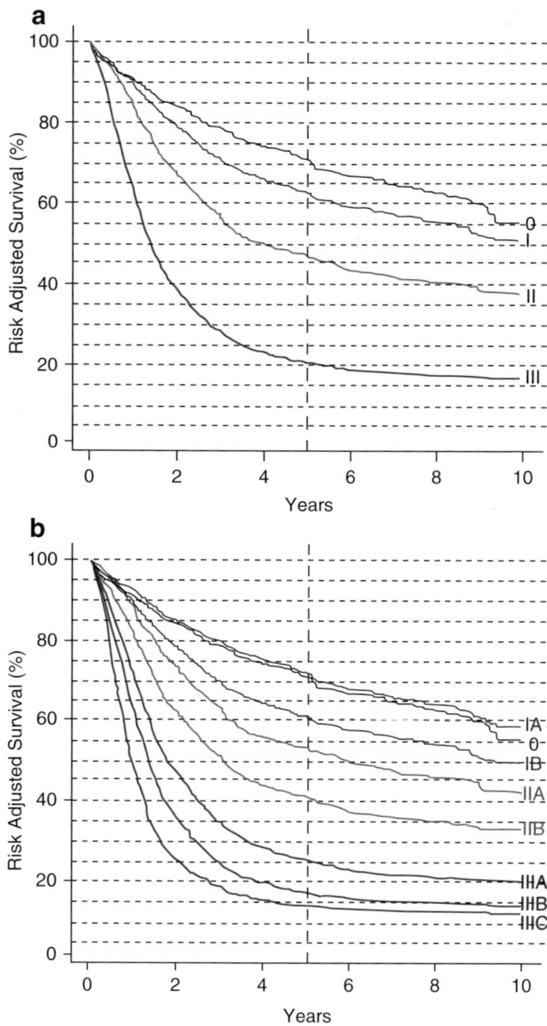

Fig. 18.1 (**a**) Survival after esophagectomy only for squamous cell carcinoma stratified by stage groupings, based on worldwide esophageal cancer collaboration (WECC) data. Condensed stage groupings. (**b**) Survival after esophagectomy only for squamous cell carcinoma stratified by stage groupings, based on worldwide esophageal cancer collaboration (WECC) data. Expanded stage groupings. (Used with permission from the American Joint Committee on Cancer (AJCC), Chicago, IL. The original source for this material is the AJCC Cancer Staging Manual, Seventh Edition (2010), published by Springer Science+Business Media)

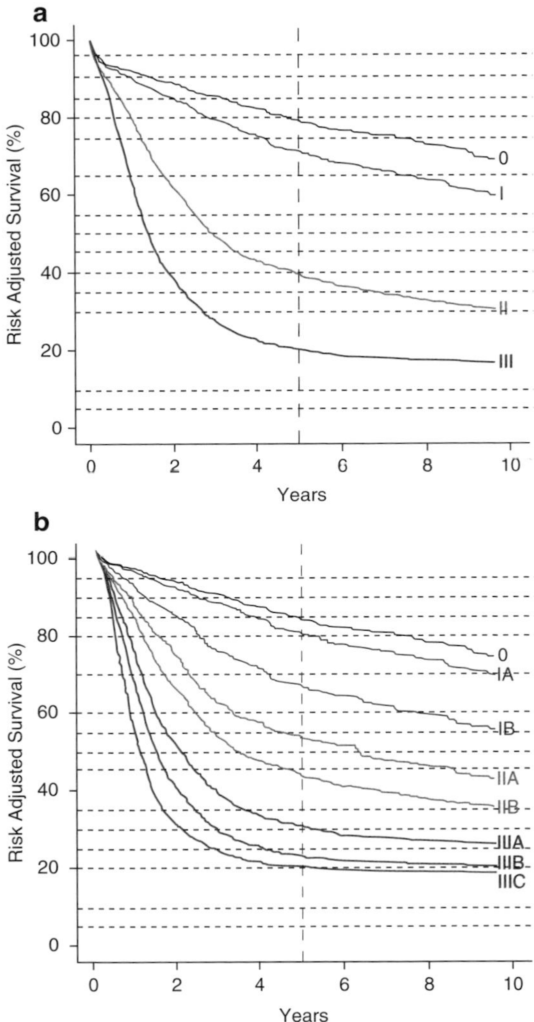

Fig. 18.2 (**a**) Survival after esophagectomy only for adenocarcinoma stratified by stage groupings, based on worldwide esophageal cancer collaboration (WECC) data. Condensed stage groupings. (**b**) Survival after esophagectomy only for adenocarcinoma stratifi ed by stage groupings, based on worldwide esophageal cancer collaboration (WECC) data. Expanded stage groupings. (Used with permission from the American Joint Committee on Cancer (AJCC), Chicago, IL. The original source for this material is the AJCC Cancer Staging Manual, Seventh Edition (2010), published by Springer Science+Business Media)

SURGICAL TECHNIQUES

- Transhiatal esophagectomy: for tumors anywhere in esophagus or gastric cardia. No thoracotomy. Blunt dissection of the thoracic esophagus. Left with cervical anastomosis. Limitations are lack of exposure of midesophagus and direct visualization and dissection of the subcarinal LN cannot be performed.
- Right thoracotomy (Ivor-Lewis procedure): good for exposure of mid to upper esophageal lesions. Left with thoracic or cervical anastomosis.
- Left thoracotomy: appropriate for lower third of esophagus and gastric cardia. Left with low-to-midthoracic anastomosis.
- Radical (en block) resection: for tumor anywhere in esophagus or gastric cardia. Left with cervical or thoracic anastomosis. Benefit is more extensive lymphadenectomy and potentially better survival, but increased operative risk.

TREATMENT RECOMMENDATIONS

2002 Stage	Recommended treatment
Stage I–III and IVA resectable* medically-fit	■ Pre-op chemo-RT (5-FU + cisplatin, 50 Gy) → surgery. Surgery preferred for adenocarcinoma regardless of response to chemo-RT. Three-year OS 20–30% (up to 50% if pCR). LF ~35% ■ Or, definitive chemo-RT (5-FU + cisplatin, 50 Gy). Chemo-RT is preferred for cervical esophagus lesions. Three-year OS 20–30%. LF ~45% ■ Or, surgery. Preferred upfront for noncervical T1N0 and young T2N0 patients with primaries of lower esophagus or gastroesophageal junction without high-risk features (poorly differentiated, LVSI). Perioperative chemo given for >T1N0 disease. Indications for post-op chemo-RT include: unfavorable T2N0, T3/4, LN+, and/or close/+ margin. Three-year OS 20–30%, LF ~40% *Resectable T4: involvement of pleura, pericardium or diaphragm only *Resectable stage IVA: resectable celiac nodes and no involvement of celiac artery, aorta, or other organs
Stage I–III inoperable	■ Definitive chemo-RT (5-FU + cisplatin, 50 Gy) (RTOG 85–01, RTOG 94–05, INT0123)

Stage IV palliative	■ Concurrent chemo-RT (5-FU + cisplatin, 50 Gy) or RT alone (e.g., 2.5 Gy × 14 fx) or chemo alone or best supportive care. RT palliates dysphagia in ~70% for average of ~6 months ■ Obstruction: stenting, laser, RT, chemo, or dilatation ■ Pain: medications ± RT ■ Bleeding: endoscopic therapy, surgery, or RT

STUDIES

SURGERY ALONE

- Three-year OS 6–35% (~20%). See control arms in Kelsen, Medical Research Council, and EORTC trials below.

RT ALONE

- Three-year OS 0%. See control arm in RTOG 85–01.

VI

PRE-OP AND POST-OP RT

- Five randomized trials of pre-op RT vs. surgery alone demonstrate no difference in LF and OS.
- Phase III data from outside the US demonstrate decreased LF, but no difference in OS or DM with post-op RT.

PRE-OP CHEMO

- *Metaanalysis* (Gebski et al. 2007). Ten randomized trials with 1,209 patients evaluating pre-op chemo-RT vs. surgery alone in resectable esophageal cancer. Conclusion was that concurrent pre-op chemo-RT improves OS in SCC and adenocarcinoma. Eight randomized studies with 1,724 patients evaluating chemo + surgey vs. surgery alone. Chemo alone improved survival in adenocarcinoma, but not SCC. Caveats: suboptimal RT, sequential chemo-RT included, older studies.
- *RTOG 8911/INT 133* (Kelsen et al. 1998; 2007). Phase III: 467 patients with resectable T1-2NxM0 SCC and adenocarcinoma randomized to surgery alone vs. pre-op chemo × 3c (cisplatin, 5-FU) → surgery. Pre-op chemo did not improve MS (16 vs. 15 months) or OS at 4 years (26 vs. 23%). 12% cCR and 2.5% pCR. No difference between histologies. Update 2007: only R0 resection resulted in significant long-term survival advantage. Five-year OS R0 32%, R1 5%.

- *Medical Research Council Oesophageal Cancer Working Group* (2002); (Allum et al. 2008). Phase III: 802 patients with resectable SCC and adenocarcinoma randomized to surgery alone vs. pre-op chemo × 2c (5-FU, cisplatin) → surgery. Nine percent of patients from each arm received pre-op RT. Pre-op chemo improved 5-year OS (17→23%) and complete resection rate (54 → 60%). Survival advantage was seen in adenocarcinoma (17 vs. 24%) and SCC (18 vs. 23%).

PERI-OP CHEMO

- *MAGIC trial* (Cunningham et al. 2006). Phase III: 503 patients, T1-3N0-1M0, with resectable adenocarcinoma of the stomach, GE junction, or lower esophagus randomized to perioperative chemo vs. surgery alone. Chemo was epirubicin, cisplatin, and 5-FU × 3 cycles pre-op and same regimen × three cycles post-op. Peri-op chemo improved 5-year OS 23 → 36% (HR 0.75).

PRE-OP CHEMO-RT

- See Gebski metaanalysis above.
- Walsh et al. (1996). Phase III: 113 patients, adenocarcinoma only, randomized to surgery alone vs. pre-op chemo-RT → surgery. RT was 40 Gy/15 fx. Chemo was 5-FU and cisplatin × 2c. Pre-op chemo-RT improved OS at 1 year (52 vs. 44%) and 3 years (32 vs. 6%) and MS (16 vs. 11 months). Twenty-five percent pCR rate in chemo-RT arm. Positive LN or mets at surgery: 42% Chemo-RT, 82% surgery alone. Caveats: small patient number, adenocarcinoma only, poor outcome of surgery alone arm, nonconventional fractionation, and short follow-up (only 11 months).
- *EORTC* (Bosset et al. 1997). Phase III: 282 patients, T1-3N0 and T1-2N1M0, SCC only, randomized to surgery alone vs. pre-op chemo-RT → surgery. Chemo was cisplatin × 2c. RT was 37 Gy/10 fx in two 1-week courses separated by 2 weeks. Surgery was one-stage en bloc esophagectomy and proximal gastrectomy. pCR 26%. No difference in OS and MS (18.6 months). Pre-op chemo-RT improved DFS ($p = 0.003$), had a higher rate of curative resection ($p = 0.017$), a lower rate of death from cancer ($p = 0.002$), and a higher rate of post-op death ($p = 0.012$). RT was split course, nonconventional fractionation, no 5-FU.
- Urba et al. (2001). Phase III: 100 patients, localized CA, 75% adenocarcinoma, 25% SCC randomized to pre-op chemo-RT

→ surgery vs. surgery alone. Chemo was cisplatin, vinblastine, and 5-FU. RT was 1.5 Gy b.i.d. to 45 Gy. Surgery was transhiatal esophagectomy. Pre-op chemo-RT significantly decreased LR (19 vs. 42%). Improved 3-year OS (30 vs. 15%) did not reach statistical significance ($p = 0.07$).

- Bates et al. (1996) Phase II: 35 patients, localized CA, 80% SCC, 20% adenocarcinoma treated with pre-op chemo-RT → surgery. Chemo was 5-FU + cisplatin. RT was 1.8/45 Gy. Surgery was Ivor-Lewis esophagectomy. pCR 51%, MS 25.8 months (all patients) with 36.8 months for pCR and 12.9 months for no pCR. Three-year DFS 43% (80% with CR, 13% with residual). Three-year OS 41% (61% with CR, 25% with residual). However, after chemo-RT, 41% of patients with negative repeat EGD still had residual tumor at surgery, indicating that preresection EGD alone is not reliable for detecting residual disease.
- Stahl et al. (2009) Phase III trial: 126 patients with locally advanced (uT3/4NxM0) but resectable adenocarcinoma of the lower esophagus or gastric cardia randomized to induction chemo (cisplatin, 5-FU, and leucovorin (PLF) × 2.5 cycles) + surgery vs. induction chemo (PLF × two cycles) + chemo-RT (30 Gy with cisplatin and etoposide) + surgery. Study prematurely closed but showed trend toward improved 3-year survival 47.4% in RT group vs. 27.7% in no RT group ($P = 0.07$). Chemo-RT group had increase in pCR (15.6 vs. 2%).
- *CALGB 9781* (Tepper et al. 2008). Phase III: 56 patients with resectable SCC and adenoCA (T1-3N1M0) randomized to surgery alone vs. concurrent chemo-RT (cisplatin, 5-FU × 2 cycles + 50.4 Gy in 28 fx)→ surgery. Trimodality therapy improved 5-year survival (16→ 39%), median survival (1.8→ 4.5 years), 40% pCR in patients with pre-op chemo-RT.
- Burmeister et al. (2005): 256 patients with T1-3N0-1 SCC or adenoCA (61%) randomized to pre-op concurrent chemo-RT vs. surgery alone. Chemo-RT = cisplatin and 5-FU with 35 Gy in 15 fx. No difference in 3-year DFS (~30–35%) or OS (~35%), but chemo-RT improved R0 resection rate (60 → 80%). Subgroup analysis showed SCC had improved DFS and OS with chemo-RT. No difference in patterns of failure. Thirteen percent of patients with pCR had 3-year OS 49%.

Definitive chemo-RT

- *RTOG 85-01* (Herskovic and Martz 1992; al-Sarraf M et al. 1997; Cooper et al. 1999). Phase III: 121 patients, T1-3N0-1M0, adenocarcinoma and SCC, randomized to RT alone vs. chemo-RT. Chemo was 5-FU and cisplatin on weeks 1, 5, 8, 11. RT alone arm was 50 + 14 Gy boost at 2 Gy/fx. Concurrent chemo-RT dose was 50 Gy. Interim analysis showed improved OS with chemo-RT. Additional 69 patients were treated according to the chemo-RT protocol and followed prospectively. Five-year OS for RT alone was 0%, for chemo-RT (randomized) 27% and for chemo-RT (nonrandomized) 14%. No differences in OS based on histology.

- *RTOG 94-05, INT0123* (Minsky 2002). Phase III: 236 patients, T1-4N0-1M0, SCC and adenocarcinoma, randomized to chemo-RT to 50 Gy vs. chemo-RT to 65 Gy. Chemo was 5-FU + cisplatin × 4c. Trial was stopped after an interim analysis. High-dose arm had higher treatment-related death (10 vs. 2%). Of the 11 deaths in high-dose arm, 7 occurred at ≤50.4 Gy. No differences in MS (13 vs. 18 months), 2-year OS (31 vs. 40%), or LRF (56 vs. 52%) between high-dose vs. low-dose arms.

Chemo-RT with and without surgery in high-risk patients

- Stahl et al. (2005, 2008). Phase III: 172 patients, T3-4N0-1M0, SCC, treated with chemo × 3c and then randomized to chemo-RT (2/40 Gy) → surgery (arm 1) vs. definitive chemo-RT (64–65 Gy, arm 2). Chemo was 5-FU, leucovorin, etoposide, and cisplatin when given alone, and cisplatin/etoposide when given with RT. RT in arm 2 was 2/50 + 1.5 Gy b.i.d./15 Gy boost (total 65 Gy) or 2/60 + 4 Gy HDR boost (total 64 Gy). Sixty-six percent of patients in arm 1 and 88% of patients in arm 2 completed treatment. pCR was 35% at surgery. No difference in MS (16 vs. 15 months) or 5-year/10-year OS (28/19 vs. 17/12%). Surgery improved 2-year freedom from local progression (64 vs. 41%), but definitive chemo-RT had less treatment-related mortality (13 vs. 4%) and preserved the esophagus. Patients with response to induction chemo had improved prognosis regardless of treatment group (3-year OS ~50%).
- *FFCD 9102* (Bedenne et al. 2007; Crehange et al. 2007): 259 patients with potentially resectable T3-4N0-1 SCC (90%) or adenoCA (10%) with ≥PR to chemo-RT (5-FU/cisplatin × 2c; concurrent RT (2/46 Gy or split-course 3/30 Gy)) randomized to surgery vs. three more cycles of 5-FU/cisplatin with RT boost during first cycle (2/20 Gy or split course 3/15 Gy). Two-third patients had split-course RT. Total RT doses were 2/66 or 3/45 Gy (split-course). *No difference* in 2-year OS (34–40%)

or MS (18–19 months). Worse QOL in post-op period and increased treatment-related mortality with surgery (1 → 9%). *Surgery reduced LF* (43 → 34%) and need for stents (32 → 5%). No change in DM. Split-course RT had worse local RFS (57 vs. 77%).

Brachytherapy

- *RTOG 9207 phaseI/II* (Gaspar et al. 2000): 49 patients T1-2N0-1M0, 92% SCC, 8% adenocarcinoma treated with concurrent chemo (5-FU, cisplatin) + RT (EBRT 50 Gy/25 fx + HDR 5 Gy × 3 or LDR 20 Gy × 1). Twenty-four percent Grade 4 toxicity, 12% fistula, 10% treatment-related deaths with MS 11 months. Three-year OS 29% and LF 63%. Brachytherapy not recommended due to high toxicity.

RTOG trials

- *RTOG 0246* (Swisher et al. 2007): Phase II study of resectable locoregionally advanced CA treated with induction chemo (5-FU, cisplatin, paclitaxel) → chemo-RT (50 Gy, 5-FU, cisplatin) → salvage surgery. Trial closed 3/17/2006. Preliminary results showed increased toxicity compared to historical controls, no significant improvement in outcomes, and study arm not suitable for phase III trial.
- *RTOG 0113*(Ajani et al. 2008): Randomized phase II study of inoperable localregional esophageal CA treated with 5-FU based vs. non-5-FU based induction chemo → chemo-RT. Trial closed 4/2005. Both arms associated with high morbidity (Grade 3 or 4). Study did not meet 1-year survival endpoint of ≥77.5% (5-FU based arm 1-year survival was 75.7%).
- *RTOG 0436*: Phase III trial evaluating the addition of cetuximab to paclitaxel, cisplatin, and RT for patients with esophageal cancer who are treated without surgery (50.4 Gy in 28 fractions). Trial activated 6/30/08.

VI

RADIATION TECHNIQUES

GENERAL PRINCIPLES

- Simulate patient supine with arms up so that lateral fiducials are possible.
- Immobilize with wing board or alpha cradle with arms above head.
- Use esophotrast to outline the esophagus and barium (2%, ReadiCat) to outline the stomach and small bowel.

FIELD DESIGN

- AP/PA fields deliver higher dose to the heart and lower dose to the lungs, whereas obliques and laterals deliver higher dose to the lungs and lower dose to the heart.
- At UCSF, we consider using a 3DCRT or IMRT plan throughout treatment, so that normal tissues such as the lungs receive a lower total integral dose. We generally weight AP/PA > obliques.
- Wedges and/or compensators may be needed.
- Tumors above the carina: treat SCV and mediastinal LN.
- GTV = primary lesion and involved LN; CTV = GTV + subclinical disease (regional LN and submucosal), 4 cm proximal/distal and 1 cm radial; PTV = CTV + 1–2 cm.
- Two options for field design:
  - SCV and primary tumor treated in one field. Consider AP 6 MV and PA 18 MV with off-cord boost to primary (after cord dose reaches 45 Gy). This technique might not be suitable if tumor volume includes excessive heart.
  - SCV field matched to primary tumor fields. Isocenter is placed at the matchline. SCV field is AP 6 MV to 50 Gy with half-beam block at clavicle and block placed over spinal cord. Primary tumor fields are beam split from above and use AP/PA and obliques. AP/PA fields are weighted » obliques and laterals.
- Tumors at or below the carina: treat mediastinal LN, and include celiac LN for lower 1/3 and gastroesophageal junction tumors.
  - Use a multifield technique including AP/PA and obliques or laterals. Weigh AP/PA » obliques and laterals.
- IMRT now being used more frequently, particularly cervical lesions; consider 4DCT and respiratory gating, especially for lower esophageal tumors.

DOSE PRESCRIPTIONS

- 1.8 Gy/fx to 50.4 Gy.
- If the stomach is in the field, consider reducing lower border to block stomach at 45 Gy if clinically possible.

DOSE LIMITATIONS

- Spinal cord D_{max} ≤45 Gy at 1.8 Gy/fx
- Lung: Limit 70% of both lungs <20 Gy
- Heart: Limit 50% of ventricles <25 Gy

COMPLICATIONS

- Acute side effects: esophagitis, weight loss, fatigue, and anorexia.
- Esophageal perforation may present with substernal chest pain, increased heart rate, fever and hemorrhage.
- Pneumonitis: subacute, occurs ~6 weeks after RT. Presents with cough, dyspnea, hypoxia, and fever. Depending on severity, treat with NSAIDs or steroids.
- Late strictures possible, half are due to LR. For benign strictures, dilation results in palliation in the majority of patients. For malignant strictures, dilation does not work as well.
- Pericarditis, coronary artery disease.
- With brachytherapy and/or EBRT, tumor involvement of the trachea can lead to fistula formation during RT (5–10%), secondary to tumor necrosis or natural progression of the disease.

FOLLOW-UP

- H&P every 4 months for 1 year, then every 6 months for 5 years, then annually thereafter. CBC, metabolic panel, CXR, endoscopy, CT chest, and PET should be considered when clinically indicated.
- For locally advanced esophageal cancers undergoing combined chemo-RT, metabolic response as determined by FDG-PET imaging before and after treatment is a strong predictor of OS (MS 6–7 months for non-PET responders vs. 16–23 months for PET responders) (Downey et al. 2003; Wieder et al. 2004).

VI

Acknowledgement We thank Richard M. Krieg, for his valuable advice in the preparation of this chapter.

REFERENCES

Ajani JA, Winter K, Komaki R, et al. Phase II randomized trial of two nonoperative regimens of induction chemotherapy followed by chemoradiation in patients with localized carcinome of the esophagus: RTOG 0113. *J Clin Oncol* 2008;26:551-4556.

al-Sarraf M, Martz K, Herskovic A, et al. Progress report of combined chemoradiotherapy versus radiotherapy alone in patients with esophageal cancer: an intergroup study. *J Clin Oncol* 1997;15:277-284.

Allum WH, Fogarty PJ, Stenning SP, et al. Long term results of the MRC OEO2 randomized trial of surgery with or without preoperative chemotherapy in resectable esophageal cancer. *Proc ASCO GI* 2008, abstr 9.

Bates BA, Detterbeck FC, Bernard SA, et al. Concurrent radiation therapy and chemotherapy followed by esophagectomy for localized esophageal carcinoma. *J Clin Oncol* 1996;14:156-163.

Bedenne L, Michel P, Bouché O, et al. Chemoradiation followed by surgery compared with chemoradiation alone in squamous cancer of the esophagus: FFCD 9102. J Clin Oncol. 2007 Apr 1;25(10):1160-1168.

Bosset JF, Gignoux M, Triboulet JP, et al. Chemoradiotherapy followed by surgery compared with surgery alone in squamous-cell cancer of the esophagus. *N Engl J Med* 1997;337:161-167.

Burmeister BH, Smithers BM, Gebski V, et al. Surgery alone versus chemoradiotherapy followed by surgery for resectable cancer of the oesophagus: a randomised controlled phase III trial. *Lancet Oncol* 2005;6:659-668.

Cooper JS, Guo MD, Herskovic A, et al. Chemoradiotherapy of locally advanced esophageal cancer: long-term follow-up of a prospective randomized trial (RTOG 85-01). Radiation Therapy Oncology Group. *JAMA* 1999;281:1623-1627.

Crehange G, Maingon P, Peignaux K, et al. Phase III trial of protracted compared with split-course chemoradiation for esophageal carcinoma: Federation Francophone de Cancerologie Digestive 9102. J Clin Oncol. 2007 Nov 1;25(31):4895-4901.

Cunningham D, Allum WH, Stenning SP, et al. Perioperative chemotherapy versus surgery alone for resectable gastroesophageal cancer. *N Eng J Med* 2006;355(1):11-20.

Downey RJ, Akhurst T, Ilson D, et al. Whole body 18FDG-PET and the response of esophageal cancer to induction therapy: results of a prospective trial. *J Clin Oncol* 2003;21:428-432.

Gaspar LE, Winter K, Kocha WI, et al. A phase I/II study of external beam radiation, brachytherapy, and concurrent chemotherapy for patients with localized carcinoma of the esophagus (Radiation Therapy Oncology Group Study 9207): final report. *Cancer* 2000;88:988-995.

Gebski V, Burmeister B, Smithers BM, et al. Survival benefits from neoadjuvant chemoradiotherapy or chemotherapy in oesophageal carcinoma: a meta-analysis. *Lancet Oncol* 2007;8(3):226-234.

Herskovic A, Martz K, al-Sarraf M, et al. Combined chemotherapy and radiotherapy compared with radiotherapy alone in patients with cancer of the esophagus. *N Engl J Med* 1992;326:1593-1598.

Kelsen DP, Ginsberg R, Pajak TF, et al. Chemotherapy followed by surgery compared with surgery alone for localized esophageal cancer. *N Engl J Med* 1998;339:1979-1984.

Kelson DP, Winter KA, Gunderson LL, et al. Long term results of RTOG Trial 8911 (USA Intergroup 113): a random assignment trial comparison of chemotherapy followed by surgery compared with surgery alone for esophageal cancer. *J Clin Oncol* 2007;25:3719-3725.

Medical Research Council Oesophageal Cancer Working Group. Surgical resection with or without preoperative chemotherapy in oesophageal cancer: a randomised controlled trial. *Lancet* 2002;359:1727-1733.

Minsky BD. Cancer of the Esophagus. In: Textbook of Radiation Oncology. 2nd ed. Philadelphia: Saunders; 2004. pp. 811-824.

Stahl M, Stuschke M, Lehmann N, et al. Chemoradiation with and without surgery in patients with locally advanced squamous cell carcinoma of the esophagus. *J Clin Oncol* 2005;23:2310-2317.

Stahl M, Wilke H, Lehmann M et al. Long-term results of a phase III study investigating chemoradiation with and without surgery in locally advanced squamous cell carcinoma (LA-SCC) of the esophagus. J Clin Oncol 26: 2008 ASCO abstract 4530.

Stahl M, Walz M, Stuschke M, et al. Phase III comparison of preoperative chemotherapy compared with chemoradiotherapy in patients with locally advanced adenocarcinoma of the esophagogastric junction. *J Clin Oncol* 2009;27:851-856.

Swisher S, Winters K, Komaki R, et al. A phase II study of a paclitaxel based chemoradiation regimen with selective surgical salvage for resectable locoregionally advanced esophageal cancer: initial reporting of RTOG 0246. *Int J Radiat Oncol Biol Phys* 2007;69(3):S106).

Tepper J, Krasna M, Niedzwiecki D, et al. Phase III trial of trimodality therapy with cisplatin, fluorouracil, radiotherapy, and surgery compared with surgey alone for esophageal cancer: CALGB 9781. *J Clin Oncol* 2008;26:1086-1092.

Urba SG, Orringer MB, Turrisi A, et al. Randomized trial of preoperative chemoradiation versus surgery alone in patients with locoregional esophageal carcinoma. J Clin Oncol. 2001 Jan 15;19(2):305-313.

Walsh TN, Noonan N, Hollywood D, et al. A comparison of multimodal therapy and surgery for esophageal adenocarcinoma. *N Engl J Med* 1996;335: 462-467.

Wieder HA, Brucher BL, Zimmermann F, et al. Time course of tumor metabolic activity during chemoradiotherapy of esophageal squamous cell carcinoma and response to treatment. *J Clin Oncol* 2004;22:900-908.

FURTHER READING

Czito BG, DiNittis AS, Willett CG. Esophageal Cancer. In: Halperin EC, Perez CA, Brady LW, et al., editors. Principles and Practice of Radiation Oncology. 5th ed: Lippincott Williams & Wilkins; 2007. pp. 1132-1153.

Enzinger PC, Mayer RJ. Esophageal cancer. *N Engl J Med* 2003;349:2241-2252.

Minsky BD, Pajak TF, Ginsberg RJ, et al. INT 0123 (Radiation Therapy Oncology Group 94-05) phase III trial of combined-modality therapy for esophageal cancer: high-dose versus standard-dose radiation therapy. *J Clin Oncol* 2002;20:1167-1174.

National Comprehensive Cancer Network. Clinical Practice Guidelines in Oncology: Esophageal Cancer. Available at: http://www.nccn.org/professionals/physician_gls/PDF/esophageal.pdf. Accessed on May 04, 2009.

Chapter 19
Gastric Cancer

Charlotte Dai Kubicky, Jennifer S. Yu, and Hans T. Chung

PEARLS

- 22,710 new cases and 11,780 deaths from gastric cancer each year in the US.
- Highest death rates are reported in Chile, Costa Rica, Japan, China, and the former Soviet Union.
- Median age of diagnosis is 65.
- Male:female = 1.5:1.
- Etiology and possible risk factors: low fruits and vegetables, high salts and nitrates, salted fish, smoked meats, *Helicobacter pylori*, hypochlorohydria, polyps, genetic alterations (p53 mutation, microsatellite instability, E-cadherin gene), previous radiation, gastrectomy, and pernicious anemia.
- Tumor location.
  - GE junction, cardia, and fundus 35% (diffuse subtype, incidence rising).
  - Body 25%.
  - Antrum and distal stomach 40% (intestinal subtype, incidence falling).
- Seven primary LN groups.
  - Perigastric LN along greater and lesser curvatures, gastroduodenal, paraaortics, celiac axis, porta-hepatic, suprapancreatic group, and splenic hilum. If GE junction, also distal paraesophageal.
- Histology: 90% adenocarcinoma. Others: sarcoma, GIST, carcinoid, small-cell, undifferentiated, MALT lymphoma, and leiomyosarcoma.
- Intestinal subtype: more commonly seen in patients >40 years, less aggressive.
- Diffuse subtype: affects younger patients, more aggressive.
- Borrmann's types:
  - I: polypoid
  - II: ulcerating
  - III: infiltrating and ulcerating

    - IV: infiltrating (linitis plastica)
    - Types I and II have better prognosis than III and IV
- Krukenberg tumor = ovarian met.
- Sister Mary Joseph node = periumbilical node.
- Virchow's node = left SCV.
- Irish's node = axillary lymphadenopathy.
- Blumer's shelf = metastatic tumor in the pelvic cul-de-sac, frequently palpable on rectal exam.

WORKUP

- H&P: dysphagia, indigestion, early satiety, loss of appetite, nausea, abdominal pain, weight loss, obstruction (pyloric lesion), anemia, hematemesis (10–15%), melena. Check for cervical, axillary, SCV, and periumbilical adenopathy.
- Laboratories: CBC, liver and renal function tests, CEA (elevated in one-third of cases), H. Pylori test.
- Upper endoscopy: allows direct visualization and biopsy.
- EUS: assesses the depth of penetration and LN involvement, but study is limited by the degree of obstruction.
- CT abdomen: assesses adenopathy and metastasis.
- CT or US of the pelvis in women in selected cases.
- Chest imaging, CT chest for gastroesophageal junction tumors to rule out mediastinal LN.
- PET scan: may be useful, not routinely done.
- Bone scan: recommended if elevated alkaline phosphatase or bone pain.
- Laparoscopy: performed prior to open laparotomy to assess extent of disease, peritoneal implants, and resectability. Should be performed if pre-op chemo-RT is being considered.
- Consider preradiation quantitative renal perfusion study to evaluate relative bilateral renal function, which may affect radiation planning and dose constraints.

STAGING: GASTRIC CANCER

Editors' note: All TNM stage and stage groups referred to elsewhere in this chapter reflect the 2002 AJCC staging nomenclature unless otherwise noted as the new system below was published after this chapter was written.

(AJCC 6TH ED., 2002)

Primary tumor (T)

TX: Primary tumor cannot be assessed
T0: No evidence of primary tumor
Tis: Carcinoma in situ: intraepithelial tumor without invasion of the lamina propria
T1: Tumor invades lamina propria or submucosa
T2: Tumor invades muscularis propria or subserosa*
- T2a: Tumor invades muscularis propria
- T2b: Tumor invades subserosa

T3: Tumor penetrates serosa (visceral peritoneum) without invasion of adjacent structures** and ***
T4: Tumor invades adjacent structures** and ***

**Note*: A tumor may penetrate the muscularis propria with extension into the gastrocolic or gastrohepatic ligaments, or into the greater or lesser omentum, without perforation of the visceral peritoneum covering these structures. In this case, the tumor is classified T2. If there is perforation of the visceral peritoneum covering the gastric ligaments or the omentum, the tumor should be classified T3.
**Note: The adjacent structures of the stomach include the spleen, transverse colon, liver, diaphragm, pancreas, abdominal wall, adrenal gland, kidney, small intestine, and retroperitoneum.

***Note: Intramural extension to the duodenum or esophagus is classified by the depth of the greatest invasion in any of these sites, including the stomach.

Regional lymph nodes (N)

NX: Regional lymph node(s) cannot be assessed
N0: No regional lymph node metastasis*

(AJCC 7TH ED., 2010)

Primary tumor (T)

TX: Primary tumor cannot be assessed
T0: No evidence of primary tumor
Tis: Carcinoma in situ: intraepithelial tumor without invasion of the lamina propria
T1: Tumor invades lamina propria, muscularis mucosae, or submucosa
- T1a: Tumor invades lamina propria or muscularis mucosae
- T1b: Tumor invades submucosa

T2: Tumor invades muscularis propria*
T3: Tumor penetrates subserosal connective tissue without invasion of visceral peritoneum or adjacent structures** and***
T4: Tumor invades serosa (visceral peritoneum) or adjacent structures** and ***
- T4a: Tumor invades serosa (visceral peritoneum)
- T4b: Tumor invades adjacent structures

*Note: A tumor may penetrate the muscularis propria with extension into the gastrocolic or gastrohepatic ligaments, or into the greater or lesser omentum, without perforation of the visceral peritoneum covering these structures. In this case, the tumor is classified T3. If there is perforation of the visceral peritoneum covering the gastric ligaments or the omentum, the tumor should be classified T4.

**The adjacent structures of the stomach include the spleen, transverse colon, liver, diaphragm, pancreas, abdominal wall, adrenal gland, kidney, small intestine, and retroperitoneum.
***Intramural extension to the duodenum or esophagus is classified by the depth of the greatest invasion in any of these sites, including the stomach.

continued

N1: Metastasis in 1–6 regional lymph nodes
N2: Metastasis in 7–15 regional lymph nodes
N3: Metastasis in more than 15 regional lymph nodes

Note: A designation of pN0 should be used if all examined lymph nodes are negative, regardless of the total number removed and examined.

Distant metastasis (M)
MX: Distant metastasis cannot be assessed
M0: No distant metastasis
M1: Distant metastasis

Stage grouping

0:	TisN0M0
IA:	T1N0M0
IB:	T1N1M0
	T2N0M0
II:	T1N2M0
	T2a/bN1M0
	T3N0M0
IIIA:	T2a/bN2M0
	T3N1M0
	T4N0M0
IIIB:	T3N2M0
IV:	T4N1–3M0
	T1–3N3M0
	Any T, any N, M1

Used with permission from the American Joint Committee on Cancer (AJCC), Chicago, IL. The original source for this material is the AJCC Cancer Staging Manual, Sixth Edition (2002), published by Springer Science+Business Media.

Regional lymph nodes (N)
NX: Regional lymph node(s) cannot be assessed
N0: No regional lymph node metastasis*
N1: Metastasis in 1–2 regional lymph nodes
N2: Metastasis in 3–6 regional lymph nodes
N3: Metastasis in seven or more regional lymph nodes
  N3a: Metastasis in 7–15 regional lymph nodes
  N3b: Metastasis in 16 or more regional lymph nodes

**Note*: A designation of pN0 should be used if all examined lymph nodes are negative, regardless of the total number removed and examined.

Distant metastasis (M)
M0: No distant metastasis
M1: Distant metastasis

Anatomic stage/prognostic groups

0:	Tis N0 M0
IA:	T1 N0 M0
IB:	T2 N0 M0
	T1 N1 M0
IIA:	T3 N0 M0
	T2 N1 M0
	T1 N2 M0
IIB:	T4a N0 M0
	T3 N1 M0
	T2 N2 M0
	T1 N3 M0
IIIA:	T4a N1 M0
	T3 N2 M0
	T2 N3 M0
IIIB:	T4b N0 M0
	T4b N1 M0
	T4a N2 M0
	T3 N3 M0
IIIC:	T4b N2 M0
	T4b N3 M0
	T4a N3 M0
IV:	Any T any N M1

continued

SURGERY

- General guidelines:
  - For distal (body and antrum): prefer subtotal gastrectomy.
  - For proximal (cardia): total or proximal gastrectomy.
  - Avoid splenectomy if possible.
  - Consider placing feeding jejunostomy-tube.
  - Aim for ≥5 cm proximal and distal margins whenever possible.
  - Remove minimum of 15 LNs.
- D1 dissection: removes involved proximal or distal or entire stomach, including the greater and lesser omental LN.
- D2 dissection: Also removes the omental bursa, the front leaf of the transverse mesocolon, and the corresponding arteries are completely cleared, including the portal, celiac, and splenic LN.
- Billroth I = end-to-end gastrojejunal anastomosis, gastric resection margin used for anastomosis.
- Billroth II = end-to-side gastrojejunal anastomosis, closure of the duodenal stump, and the lesser curvature of the stomach. Gastric resection margin is usually NOT used for anastomosis.
- Sites of LF after surgery:
  - Gastric bed ~50%, LN ~40%, anastomosis or stumps ~25%,

TREATMENT RECOMMENDATIONS

2002 Stage	Recommended treatment
T1N0	■ Surgery alone (partial or total gastrectomy with at least D1 LN dissection). Selected T1a patients may be candidates for endoscopic mucosal resection in experienced centers
T2–4 and/or LN+ resectable and operable	■ Surgery → post-op 5-FU/leucovorin (LV) × 1c → concurrent 5-FU/LV × 2c and RT (45 Gy) → 5-FU/LV × 2c (INT 0116). Surgery alone may be considered for selected pT2N0 patients with R0 resection and without high-risk features (poorly differentiated, high grade, LVSI, PNI, age <50 years) ■ Alternatively, pre-op ECF chemo (epirubicin, cisplatin, 5-FU) × 3c → surgery → post-op ECF chemo × 3c (MAGIC). ■ Post-op 5-FU based chemo-RT indicated in this setting for close or involved margin(s) or gross residual disease
T2–4 and/or LN+ unresectable or inoperable	■ Concurrent chemo-RT (5-FU and 45–50.4 Gy). ■ Alternatively, chemo alone (5-FU, cisplatin, oxaliplatin, taxane, or irinotecan-based) if patient not RT candidate. ■ Or, best supportive care for poor PS. RT alone may provide some palliation, but no survival benefit

continued

M1	■ Palliative chemo ± RT (5-FU + 45 Gy). Fifty to seventy-five percent patients experience improvement of symptoms such as gastric outlet obstruction, pain, bleeding, or biliary obstruction. Duration of palliation 4–18 months. Alternatively, palliative surgery or best supportive care.

STUDIES

EXTENT OF GASTRECTOMY

- *Gouzi* et al. 1989: Distal gastric CA randomized to subtotal vs. total gastretomy. Both arms had similar morbidity (33%), mortality (1.3 vs. 3.2%), and 5-year OS (48%).

EXTENT OF LYMPHADENECTOMY

- *Dutch trial* (*Bonenkamp et al.* 1999; *Hartgrink et al.* 2004): 711 patients with resectable gastric CA randomized to D1 vs. D2 lymph node dissection. D2 dissection led to a significantly higher rate of complications (43 vs. 25%, $p < 0.001$), more post-op deaths (10 vs. 4%, $p = 0.004$), and longer hospital stay (16 vs. 14 days). Similar 11-year OS (35 vs. 30%, $p = 0.53$) and rate of relapse.
- *MRC trial* (Cuschieri et al. 1999): 400 patients randomized to D1 vs. D2 lymph node dissection. D2 dissection led to a significantly increased postoperative morbidity (46 vs. 28%) and mortality (13 vs. 6.5%).
- *Italian Gastric Cancer Study Group* (Degiuli et al. 2004): 162 patients randomized to D1 or pancreas-sparing D2 dissection. No difference in morbidity (10.5 vs. 16.3%) and mortality (0 vs. 1.3%). Reported morbidity and mortality may be lower than that seen in MRC and Dutch trial because those studies included resection of the distal pancreas and spleen.
- *JCOG trial* (Sano et al. 2004, Sasako et al. 2008): 523 patients with resectable gastric CA randomized to standard D2 vs. D2 + paraaortic nodal dissection. No significant difference in 5-year OS (69.2 vs. 70.3% (D2 vs. D2 + PAND) or RFS. Overall morbidity was higher in the extended surgery group than the standard surgery group (28.1 vs. 20.9%; $p = 0.067$). There was no difference in the incidence of major complications including anastomotic leak, pancreatic fistula, abdominal abscess, and pneumonia.
- *Taiwanese trial* (Wu et al., 2006): 221 patients with resectable gastric adenocarcinoma randomized to D1 vs. D3 lymphadenectomy. Single institution with experienced surgeons. D3 dissection improved 5-year OS (54 → 60%) and DFS (58→63%). No pre-op or post-op chemo or RT.

PERI-OP CHEMO

- *MAGIC trial* (Cunningham et al. 2006): 503 patients with resectable adenocarcinoma of stomach (74%) GE junction, lower esophagus, randomized between surgery alone vs. ECF × three cycles preoperatively → surgery → ECF × three cycles. Similar rates of postoperative morbidity and mortality. Improved rates of downstaging, R0 resection, OS (36 vs. 23%, $p = 0.009$), PFS (HR 0.66, $p < 0.001$) in perioperative chemotherapy group. ECF (epirubicin, cisplatin, and continuous infusion 5-FU).
- *MAGIC-B* (phase III): Histologically confirmed, previously untreated stage IB–IV (M0) resectable disease of the stomach or GE junction randomized to pre-op ECX × 3c → surgery → ECX × 3c, or pre-op ECX-B → surgery → ECX-B × 3c. ECX (epirubicin, cisplatin, and capecitabine), B (bevacizumab).

PRE-OP CHEMO-RT

- Rule out peritoneal carcinomatosis by laparoscopic exam if considering pre-op chemoradiation.
- No phase III data.
- *RTOG 9904* (Ajani et al. 2006) *Phase II study*: 43 operable patients with localized gastric CA treated with pre-op chemo × 2c (5-FU, leucovorin, and cisplatin) → concurrent chemoradiation (45 Gy and infusional 5-FU and weekly paclitaxel) → surgery (with D2 dissection in 50% patients). Seventy-seven percent R0 resection rate, 26% pCR rate. For pCR, OS 82% at 1 year vs. 69% if <pCR. Patterns of failure: DM (30%) vs. tumor bed failure (19%) vs. nodal and regional failure (2%).

POST-OP CHEMO-RT

- *INT0116/SWOG 9008* (Macdonald et al. 2001, 2004, 2009): 556 patients with resected stage IB–IV M0 stomach and gastroesophageal junction tumors (20%) randomized to observation vs. post-op chemo × 1c → concurrent chemo × 2c + RT → chemo × 2c. Fifty-four percent had D0 dissection and 10% had D2 dissection. Chemo was 5-FU (425 mg/m²/day, reduced to 400 mg/m²/day with RT) + leucovorin (20 mg/m²/day) × 5 days. RT was 45 Gy/25 fx to tumor bed, regional nodes, and 2 cm proximal and distal margin. Forty-one percent Grade 3 and thirty percent Grade 4 toxicity in the chemo-RT arm. From 2004 abstract (Macdonald et al. 2004): median follow-up 7.4 years. Post-op chemo-RT improved MS (35 vs. 26 months, $p = 0.006$), DFS (30 vs. 19 months, $p < 0.001$), and 3-year OS (50 vs. 41%). No difference in DM.

From 2009 abstract (Macdonald et al. 2009): follow-up >10 years. Post-op chemo-RT improved DFS (HR = 1.51, $p < 0.001$) and OS (HR = 1.32, $p = 0.004$). All subsets of patients benefited from chemo-RT except diffuse histology. No increase in late toxicity. Criticism: extent of surgery suboptimal.

- *CALGB 80101* (phase III): Resected adenocarcinoma of stomach or GE junction randomized to adjuvant 5-FU/leucovorin → concurrent chemoradiation (45 Gy with infusional 5-FU) → 5-FU/leucovorin × 2c vs. adjuvant ECF → concurrent chemoradiation (45 Gy with infusional 5-FU) → ECF × 2c (result pending).
- *Dutch CRITICS* (phase III): Histologically confirmed, previously untreated stage IB–IV (M0) resectable disease of the stomach randomized to pre-op ECX × 3c → surgery → concurrent chemoradiation (45 Gy with cisplatin and capecitabine), or pre-op ECX × 3c → surgery → ECX × 3c, ECX (epirubicin, cisplatin, and capecitabine) (result pending).

VI

RADIATION TECHNIQUES

SIMULATION AND FIELD DESIGN

- Ensure adequate nutrition prior to radiation. Arrange for a nutrition consult. Recommend at least 1,500 Cal/day.
- Patient may require feeding tube (preferable if placed at the time of surgery).
- Patient instructed to fast for 3 h before simulation and all treatments.
- Simulate patient supine with arms up so that lateral fiducials are possible.
- Immobilize with wing board or alpha cradle with arms above head.
- Use pre-op CT, post-op CT, surgical clips, operative report, pathology report, and upper GI studies to guide target definition.
- Celiac axis is located at approximately T12–L1.
- Porta hepatis LN are covered by a field that extends 2 cm to the right of T11–L1.
- At UCSF, we use a 3DCRT or IMRT throughout the treatment to help reduce dose to normal tissues, such as small bowel, spinal cord, liver, and kidneys. Most 3DCRT plans include three to four fields.
- General target volume:
- Initial tumor bed: all patients. Exception is proximal T1–2aN0 patients with margin >5 cm.

- Remaining stomach: all patients. Exception is proximal T1–3N0 patients with margin >5 cm.
- Anastomotic site: all patients. Exception is proximal T1–2aN0 patients with margin >5 cm.
- Residual disease: all patients.
- Adjacent structures: see tables below.
- Regional LN (depends on location and TN stage; see tables below).
  - Perigastric LN: always. Exception: proximal T1–2aN0 patients with margins >5 cm and >10–15 LN resected.
  - Celiac and suprapancreatic LN: For T4, LN+, or T3N0 with <15 LN resected.
  - Porta-hepatic LN: for all T4 or LN+. Exception: proximal lesions with only 1–2 involved LN and >15 LN resected.
  - Splenic LN: for all T4 or LN+. Exception: distal lesions with only 1–2 involved LN and >15 LN resected.
  - Distal paraesophageal LN: for lesions with esophageal extension.
- The following are guidelines for target volume definition depending on the site of involvement (reprinted from Tepper and Gunderson (2002)).

GE JUNCTION TUMORS

Site/stage	Remaining stomach	Tumor bed**	Nodes
T2N0 with invasion of subserosa	Variable dependent on surgical-pathologic findings*	Medial left hemidiaphragm; adjacent body of pancreas	None or perigastric, periesophageal***
T3N0	Variable dependent on surgical-pathologic findings*	Medial left hemidiaphragm; adjacent body of pancreas	None or perigastric, periesophageal, mediastinal, or celiac***
T4N0	Preferable, but dependent on surgical-pathologic findings*	As for T3N0 plus site(s) of adherence with 3–5 cm margin	Nodes related to site(s) of adherence, ±perigastric, periesophageal, mediastinal, and celiac

continued

T1–2N+	Preferable	Not indicated for T1 As above for T2 into subserosa	Periesophageal, mediastinal, proximal perigastric, and celiac
T3–4N+	Preferable	As for T3–4N0	As for T1–2N+ and T4N0

*For tumors with wide (>5 cm) surgical margins confirmed pathologically, treatment of residual stomach is optional, especially if this would result in substantial increase in normal tissue morbidity.

**Use pre-op imaging (CT, barium swallow), surgical clips, and post-op imaging (CT, barium swallow).

***Optional node inclusion for T2–3N0 lesions if there has been an adequate surgical node dissection (D2 dissection) and at least 10–15 nodes have been examined pathologically.

Tolerance organ structures: heart, lung, spinal cord, and kidneys.

VI

CARDIA/PROXIMAL ONE-THIRD OF THE STOMACH TUMORS

Site/stage	Remaining stomach	Tumor bed**	Nodes
T2N0 with invasion of subserosa	Variable dependent on surgical-pathologic findings*	Medial left hemidiaphragm, adjacent body of pancreas (±tail)	None or perigastric
T3N0	Variable dependent on surgical-pathologic findings*	Medial left hemidiaphragm, adjacent body of pancreas (±tail)	None or perigastric, optional: periesophageal, and mediastinal, celiac****
T4N0	Variable dependent on surgical-pathologic findings*	As for T3N0, plus site(s) of adherence with 3–5 cm margin	Nodes related to site(s) of adherence, ±perigastric, periesophageal, mediastinal, and celiac
T1–2N+	Preferable	Not indicated for T1 As above for T2 into subserosa	Perigastric, celiac, splenic, suprapancreatic,

continued

			±periesophageal, mediastinal pancreaticoduodenal, and portahepatis***
T3–4N+	Preferable	As for T3–4N0	As for T1–2N+ and T4N0

*For tumors with wide (>5 cm) surgical margins confirmed pathologically, treatment of residual stomach is not necessary, especially if this would result in substantial increase in normal tissue morbidity.
**Use pre-op imaging (CT, barium swallow), surgical clips, and post-op imaging (CT, barium swallow).
***Pancreaticoduodenal and portahepatis nodes are at low risk if nodal positivity is minimal (i.e., 1–2 positive nodes with 10–15 nodes examined), and this region does not need to be irradiated. Periesophageal and mediastinal nodes are at risk if there is esophaphgeal extension.

****Optional nodes inclusion for T2–3N0 lesions if there has been an adequate surgical node dissection (D2 dissection) and at least 10–15 nodes have been examined pathologically.

Tolerance organ structures: kidneys, spinal cord, liver, heart, and lung.

BODY/MIDDLE ONE-THIRD OF THE STOMACH TUMORS

Site/stage	Remaining stomach	Tumor bed*	Nodes
T2N0 with invasion of subserosa – especially post wall	Yes	body of pancreas (±tail)	None or perigastric; optional: celiac, splenic, suprapancreatic, pancreaticoduodenal, and portahepatis**
T3N0	Yes	body of pancreas (±tail)	None or perigastric, optional: celiac, splenic, suprapancreatic, pancreaticoduodenal, and portahepatis**
T4N0	Yes	As for T3N0, plus site(s) of adherence with 3–5 cm margin	Nodes related to site(s) of adherence, ±perigastric, celiac, splenic,

continued

			suprapancreatic, pancreaticoduodenal, and portahepatis
T1–2N+	Yes	Not indicated for T1	perigastric, celiac, splenic, suprapancreatic, pancreaticoduodenal, and portahepatis
T3–4N+	Yes	As for T3–4N0	As for T1–2N+ and T4N0

*Use pre-op imaging (CT, barium swallow), surgical clips, and post-op imaging (CT, barium swallow).

**Optional nodes inclusion for T2–3N0 lesions if there has been an adequate surgical node dissection (D2 dissection) and at least10–15 nodes have been examined pathologically.

Tolerance organ structures: kidneys, spinal cord, liver.

VI

ANTRUM/PYLORUS/DISTAL ONE-THIRD OF THE STOMACH TUMORS

Site/stage	Remaining stomach	Tumor bed**	Nodes
T2N0 with invasion of subserosa	Variable dependent of surgical-pathologic findings*	Head of pancreas (±body), first and second part of the duodenum	None or perigastric; optional: pancreaticoduodenal, portahepatis, celiac, and suprapancreatic***
T3N0	Variable dependent of surgical-pathologic findings*	Head of pancreas (±body), first and second part of the duodenum	None or perigastric; optional: pancreaticoduodenal, portahepatis, celiac, and suprapancreatic***
T4N0	Preferable, but dependent on surgical-pathologic findings*	As for T3N0 plus site(s) of adherence with 3–5 cm margin	Nodes related to site(s) of adherence, ±perigastric, pancreaticoduodenal, portahepatis, celiac, and suprapancreatic

continued

T1–2N+	Preferable	Not indicated for T1	Perigastric, pancreaticoduodenal, portahepatis, celiac, suprapancreatic, and optional splenic hilum***
T3–4N+	Preferable	As for T3–4N0	As for T1–2N+ and T4N0

*For tumors with wide (>5 cm) surgical margins confirmed pathologically, treatment of residual stomach is optional if this would result in substantial increase in normal tissue morbidity.

**Use pre-op imaging (CT, barium swallow), surgical clips, and post-op imaging (CT, barium swallow).

***Optional node inclusion for T2–3N0 lesions if there has been an adequate surgical node dissection (D2 dissection) and at least 10–15 nodes have been examined pathologically.

Tolerance organ structures: kidneys, liver, and spinal cord.

DOSE PRESCRIPTIONS

- 1.8 Gy/fx to 45–50.4 Gy depending on margin status and presence/absence of residual disease.

DOSE LIMITATIONS

- Spinal cord D_{max} ≤45 Gy
- Heart: 50% of ventricles <25 Gy
- Liver: 70% of volume <30 Gy
- Kidneys: 70% of volume of each kidney <20 Gy

COMPLICATIONS

- Acute complications include nausea, anorexia, fatigue, and myelosuppression with chemo.
- Consider H2-blocker or proton pump inhibitor for ulcer prophylaxis.
- For severe nausea, recommend Ondansetron 8 mg 1 h before and 3 h after RT daily.
- Twenty-five percent of patients have persistent decrease in acid production for >1–5 years.
- Late complications: dyspepsia, radiation gastritis, and gastric ulcers.
- Gastric late effects are rare with 40–52 Gy. Incidence of late effects rises with higher doses.

FOLLOW-UP

- H&P every 4 months for first year, then every 6 months for 2 years, then annually thereafter. CBC, metabolic panel, endoscopies, CT as clinically indicated.
- Long-term parenteral vitamin B12 supplementation for all patients who undergo proximal or total gastrectomy.

Acknowledgement We thank Richard M. Krieg, MD, for his valuable advice in the preparation of this chapter.

REFERENCES

Ajani JA, Winter K, Okawara GS, et al. Phase II trial of preoperative chemoradiation in patients with localized gastric adenocarcinoma (RTOG9904): Quality of combined modality therapy and pathologic response. *J Clin Oncol* 2006;24:3953-3958.

Bonenkamp JJ, Hermans J, Sasako M, et al. Extended lymph-node dissection for gastric cancer. *N Engl J Med* 1999 Mar 25;340(12):908-914.

Cunningham D, Alum WH, Stenning SP, et al. Perioperative chemotherapy versus surgery alone for resectable gastroesophageal cancer. *N Engl J Med* 2006;355:11-20.

Cuschieri A, Weeden S, Fielding J, et al. Patient survival after D1 and D2 resections for gastric cancer: long-term results of the MRC randomized surgical trial. Surgical Co-operative Group. *Br J Cancer* 1999;79:1522-1530.

Degiuli M, Sasako M, Calgaro M, et al. Morbidity and mortality after D1 and D2 gastrectomy for cancer: interim analysis of the Italian Gastric Cancer Study Group (IGCSG) randomised surgical trial. *Eur J Surg Oncol* 2004;30:303-308.

Dutch CRITICS: http://clinicaltrials.gov/ct2/show/NCT00407186?term=critics+%26+gastric+cancer&rank=1Identifier NCT00407186. Assessed on February 19, 2010.

Gouzi JL, Huguier M, Fagniez PL et al. Total versus subtotal gastrectomy for adenocarcinoma of the gastric antrum. A French prospective controlled study. *Ann Surg* 1989 Feb;209(2): 162-166.

Hartgrink HH, van de Velde CJ, Putter H, et al. Extended lymph node dissection for gastric cancer: who may benefit? Final results of the randomized Dutch gastric cancer group trial. *J Clin Oncol* 2004;22:2069-2077.

Macdonald JS, Smalley SR, Benedetti J, et al. Chemoradiotherapy after surgery compared with surgery alone for adenocarcinoma of the stomach or gastroesophageal junction. *N Engl J Med* 2001;345:725-730.

Macdonald JS, Smalley SR, Benedetti J, et al. Postoperative combined radiation and chemotherapy improves disease-free survival (DFS) and overall survival (OS) in resected adenocarcinoma of the stomach and gastroesophageal junction: Update of the results of Intergroup Study INT-0116 (SWOG 9008). American Society of Clinical Oncology Gastrointestinal Cancers Symposium, Abstract no. 6, 2004.

Macdonald JS, Benedetti J, Smalley S, et al. Chemoradiation of resected gastric cancer: A 10-year follow-up of the phase III trial INT0116(SWOG 9008). 2009 American Society of Clinical Oncology Annual Meeting, Abstract no. 4515, 2009.

MAGIC-B: http://clinicaltrials.gov/ct2/show/NCT00450203?term=bevacizumab+%26+gastric&type=Intr&phase=2&rank=1. Identifier: NCT00450203.

National Comprehensive Cancer Network. Clinical Practice Guidelines in Oncology: Gastric Cancer. Available at: http://www.nccn.org/professionals/physician_gls/PDF/gastric.pdf. Accessed on May 29, 2009.

Sano T, Sasako M, Yamamoto S, et al. Gastric cancer surgery: morbidity and mortality results from a prospective randomized controlled trial comparing D2 and extended para-aortic lymphadenectomy – Japan Clinical Oncology Group study 9501. *J Clin Oncol* 2004;22: 2767-2773.

Sasako M, Sano T, et al. D2 lymphadenectomy alone or with para-aortic nodal dissection for gastric cancer – JCOG 9501. *N Engl J Med* 2008;359:453-462.

Tepper, JE, Gunderson, LL. Radiation treatment parameters in the adjuvant postoperative therapy of gastric cancer. *Semin Radiat Oncol* 2002;12:187-195.

Wu CW, Hsiung CA, Lo SS, et al. Nodal dissection for patients with gastric cancer: a randomised controlled trial. *Lancet Oncol* 2006 Apr;7(4):309-315.

VI

FURTHER READING

National Cancer Institute. Phase III randomized study of adjuvant chemoradiation after resection in patients with gastric or gastroesophageal adenocarcinoma. http://www.nci.nih.gov.

Soybel D, I, Zinner M, J. Stomach and Duodenum: Operative Procedures. In: Zinner M, J, Schwartz S, I, Ellis H, editors. Maingot's Abdominal Operations. 10th ed: Stamford: Appleton and Lange; 1997. pp. 1079-1127.

Willett CG, Gunderson LL. Stomach. In: Halperin EC, Perez CA, Brady LW, et al., editors. Principles and Practice of Radiation Oncology. 5th ed: Philadelphia: Lippincott Williams & Wilkins; 2007. pp. 1318-1335.

Chapter 20
Pancreatic Cancer

Jennifer S. Yu, Joy Coleman, and Jeanne Marie Quivey

PEARLS

- Fifth leading cause of cancer mortality, although only the ninth most common cancer.
- Found primarily in Western countries. Known risks include tobacco use, diets high in animal fat, ionizing radiation, chemotherapy, and exposure to 2-naphthylamine, benzene, and gasoline. Possible links between alcohol use, coffee use, chronic pancreatitis, and diabetes are less clear.
- Four parts: head (including uncinate process), neck, body, and tail. Two-third cancers present in the head.
- Most common presenting symptoms = jaundice (due to common bile duct obstruction), weight loss (due to malabsorption from pancreas exocrine dysfunction), diabetes (related to pancreas endocrine dysfunction), gastric outlet obstruction, and abdominal pain. Jaundice is most common in patients with lesions in the head. Patients with lesions arising in the body or tail typically present with midepigastric or back pain. May infrequently present with Trousseau's sign (migratory thrombophlebitis) or Courvoisier's sign (palpable gallbladder).
- Primary LN drainage includes the pancreaticoduodenal, suprapancreatic, pyloric, and pancreaticosplenic LN with the porta hepatic, infrapyloric, subpyloric, celiac, superior mesenteric, and paraaortic areas being involved in advanced disease.
- Most common type is of ductal origin. Cystadenocarcinomas, intraductal carcinomas, and solid and cystic papillary neoplasms (also known as *Hamoundi tumors*) have a more indolent course. Acinar cell cancers and giant cell tumors are aggressive and have poor survival. Five percent are tumors of the endocrine pancreas – these tumors are rare, slow growing, and have a long natural history.
- Seventy to hundred percent contain k-*ras* oncogene. TP53 mutation present in approximately 50%.

VI

- Peritoneal and liver mets are most common. Lung is most common location outside the abdomen.
- Postresection CA19-9 levels prognostic in patients treated with chemorad per RTOG 9704 (Berger et al. 2008).

WORKUP

- Main purpose of the workup is to determine resectability, establish a histologic diagnosis, reestablish biliary-tract outflow, and circumvent gastric outlet obstruction. Various diagnostic approaches exist.
- H&P, upper GI, CT scan, US, and ERCP, laparoscopy, or CT-guided biopsy.
- Laboratories: CBC, CEA, CA19-9, glucose, amylase, lipase, bilirubin, alkaline phosphatase, LDH, and LFTs.
- Endoscopy of the upper GI tract is extremely valuable with endobiliary stent placement. Endoscopic ultrasound can also be performed.

STAGING (AJCC 7TH ED., 2010): PANCREATIC CANCER

- The definition of TNM and anatomic stage/prognostic groupings has not changed from the sixth edition (2002) for exocrine pancreas.
- Pancreatic neuroendocrine tumors (including carcinoid tumors) are now staged by a single pancreatic staging system.

Primary tumor (T)
TX: Primary tumor cannot be assessed
T0: No evidence of primary tumor
Tis: Carcinoma in situ*
T1: Tumor limited to the pancreas, 2 cm or less in greatest dimension
T2: Tumor limited to the pancreas, more than 2 cm in greatest dimension
T3: Tumor extends beyond the pancreas but without involvement of the celiac axis or the superior mesenteric artery
T4: Tumor involves the celiac axis or the superior mesenteric artery (unresectable primary tumor)

*This also includes the "PanInIII" classification.

Regional lymph nodes (N)
NX: Regional lymph nodes cannot be assessed
N0: No regional lymph node metastasis
N1: Regional lymph node metastasis

Distant metastasis (M)
M0: No distant metastasis
M1: Distant metastasis

continued

Anatomic stage/prognostic groups

0: Tis N0 M0
IA: T1 N0 M0
IB: T2 N0 M0
IIA: T3 N0 M0
IIB: T1-T3 N1 M0
III: T4 Any N M0
IV: Any T Any N M1

- For practical purposes, tumors are generally classified as resectable (Stage I, II), unresectable (Stage III), and metastatic (Stage IV).
- Definition of resectability varies by institution, but generally includes no encasement (<180° involvement) of the celiac artery or superior mesenteric artery, and patency of portal vein and superior mesenteric vein. Splenic vein involvement does not necessarily mean a tumor is unresectable. Borderline resectable cases- tumor abutment (≤180 or ≤50%) of celiac artery or SMA circumference, or >180° or >50% common hepatic artery that is amenable to resection and repair, or SMV or portal vein occlusion amenable to resection and interposition grafting.
- Prognostic markers: surgical margins, nodal status, tumor grade.

VI

TREATMENT RECOMMENDATIONS

Stage	Recommended treatment

Resectable (10–15% of patients)	■ Pancreaticoduodenectomy. Mortality <5% when performed by experienced surgeons. Pylorus-preserving pancreaticoduodenectomy improves GI function and does not appear to compromise efficacy. Body/tail cancers (when resectable) should have a distal pancreatectomy with en bloc splenectomy
	■ Recommendations about adjuvant treatment are controversial. Options include
	  ■ Clinical trial
	  ■ Systemic gemcitabine followed by concurrent chemo-RT (5-FU based, 50.4 Gy)
	  ■ Chemotherapy alone (gemcitabine based)
	  ■ Due to post-op complications ~25% of patients do not receive intended post-op therapy
	■ *Open areas of investigation include*
	  ■ RT dose-escalation with IORT, radiosurgery, brachytherapy, proton therapy, IGRT

	■ Pre-op chemo-RT to decrease treatment toxicity, increase potential for negative margins, decrease risk of intraoperative tumor seeding, and ensure that operative complications do not cause omission of adjuvant therapy ■ Prophylactic hepatic irradiation in favorable patients due to the high incidence of liver metastasis. This has been tested and determined feasible by an RTOG study in patients with unresectable lesions which showed a 13% liver metastasis rate (lower than historic controls). Other RTOG trials pending. ■ Radiosensitizers, radioprotectants, and Yttrium-90 have also been studied
Borderline resectable	■ Staging laparoscopy. If negative, neoadjuvant therapy (concurrent 5-FU based chemo-RT ± systemic gemcitabine) followed by restaging and surgical resection if feasible.
Unresectable	■ Clinical trial preferred. Alternatively, definitive concurrent chemo-RT (5-FU based, 50–60 Gy) ± gemcitabine, or gemcitabine based chemotherapy alone. Multiinstitution cooperative ECOG and RTOG trials ongoing palliation with stents or surgical bypass
Metastatic	■ Palliation with stents, surgical bypass, chemo, RT, supportive care, or some combination of the above. Most randomized studies favor the use of gemcitabine over the use of 5-FU based chemo in the treatment of metastatic disease. Celiac nerve block is an effective palliative tool for local pain
Endocrine	■ Treatment surgical. Chemo for unresectable or metastatic disease. Effects of RT unknown, although anecdotal responses exist

STUDIES

RESECTABLE ADJUVANT TREATMENT

In favor of postoperative chemo-RT

- *GITSG 91-73* (Kalser and Ellenberg 1985): 43 patients with resectable pancreatic cancer were randomized to surgery followed by EBRT (40 Gy split course) with concurrent 5-FU vs. surgery alone. Adjuvant chemo-RT improved OS (2-year/5-year OS 43%/14% vs. 18%/5%).
  - Updated (GITSG 1987): additional 30 nonrandomized patients entered into adjuvant therapy group. Two-year OS 46%
  - Although touted by many as "the gold standard," few radiation oncologists currently use this split course regimen
- *Mayo Clinic* (Corsini 2008): retrospective review of 472 patients with R0 resection of T1-3N0-1M0 pancreatic cancer who

received adjuvant chemoradiation (50.4 Gy, 98% of patients received concurrent FU-based chemotherapy) or observation. Adjuvant chemoradiation cohort improved OS (MS 25.2 vs. 19.2 months, 2/5-year OS 50%/28 vs. 39%/17%).

- *Johns Hopkins* (Herman et al. 2008): review of 616 patients treated with pancreaticoduodenectomy. Patients who received adjuvant 5-FU based chemo-RT had improved MS (21 vs. 14 months), 2-year OS (44 vs. 32%), and 5-year OS (20 vs. 15%) compared to those who did not receive chemo-RT.
- *SEER* (Hazard et al. 2007): 3,008 patients receiving pre-op/post-op RT or surgery alone were reviewed. Patients (1,224) received RT. Majority of RT patients received post-op RT; only 23 patients got pre-op RT. Patients receiving RT (either pre or post-op) had improved survival (MS 17 vs. 12 months, 5-year OS 13 vs. 9.7%). RT improved OS in patients with direct extension of tumor beyond pancreas or positive regional nodes, but not T1-2N0M0. RT improved CSS in patients with positive regional nodes. No difference in OS between patients receiving pre-op or post-op RT. (Note that reanalysis of SEER database by Stessin showed improved OS in patients receiving pre-op RT. See Sect. "Neoadjuvant treatment").
- *Johns Hopkins-Mayo Clinic Collaborative Study* (Hsu 2009): retrospective OS was longer among patients receiving chemo-RT (50.4 Gy with concurrent 5-FU based chemo) vs. surgery alone (MS 21.1 vs. 15.5 months; 2/5-year OS 44.7%/22.3 vs. 34.6%/16.1%, $p<0.001$). Adjuvant chemo-RT also improved survival 33% when propensity score analysis used and stratified by age, margins, nodes, and T stage (RR = 0.57–0.75, $p<0.05$). Matched-pair analysis demonstrated OS was longer with chemo-RT vs. observation (MS 21.9 vs. 14.3 months; 2/5-year OS 45.5%/25.4 vs. 31.4%/12.2%, $p<0.001$).

VI

In favor of chemo

- *ESPAC-1* (Neoptolemos et al. 2001, 2004): 2 × 2 factorial design, 541 patients with resected pancreatic or periampullary carcinoma (only 289 of which were randomized). Arms were chemo-RT (40 Gy split course with 5-FU), adjuvant chemo alone (5-FU/leucovorin), both chemo-RT and chemo, or observation alone. Results contradictory when looking at randomized vs. nonrandomized patients in initial analysis. For all patients, chemo improved MS (19.7 vs. 14 months). For randomized patients only, chemo had no effect on MS (17.4 vs. 15.9 months). In final analysis (Neoptolemos et al. 2004) of the randomized patients, authors concluded that chemo was of benefit (5-year OS 21 vs. 8%), while chemo-RT was detrimental (5-year OS 10 vs. 20%).

- Criticisms: no RT quality assurance. Only 128 patients with RT details available, of whom only 90 patients got the prescribed dose of 40 Gy. Use of split-course RT. Progressive disease in 19% of patients precluded RT.

- *ESPAC metaanalysis* (Neoptolemos et al. 2009): 822 patients received either adjuvant 5-FU/folinic acid or observation after resection. Adjuvant 5-FU/FA improved MS (23.2 vs. 16.8 months).
- *CONKO-OO1* (Oettle et al. 2007): 368 patients with R0/R1 resection randomized to observation vs. gemcitabine × 6c. Adjuvant gemcitabine improved DFS (13.4 vs. 6.9 months, $p < 0.001$), but not OS (22 vs. 20 months, $p = 0.06$). Excluded patients with post-op CEA/CA19-9 levels ≥2.5 × upper limit of normal.
- *Metaanalysis* (Stocken et al. 2005): 875 patients with resected pancreatic cancer on six trials. Chemo improved MS (14→19 months) and 5-year OS (12→19%). No significant survival benefit for chemo-RT (MS 15.2–15.8 months). Subgroup analyses estimated that chemo-RT was more effective (and chemo less effective) for patients with positive resection margins.

In favor of observation

- *EORTC 40891* (Klinkenbijl et al. 1999; Smeenk et al. 2007): 218 patients with resectable pancreatic or periampullary cancer status postresection randomized to chemo-RT (40 Gy split course with 5-FU) vs. observation. Adjuvant treatment resulted in no significant difference in 10-year OS (18% overall, 8% pancreatic head group, 29% periampullary group) or PFS (median PFS 1.2 years in observation arm vs. 1.5 years in treatment arm). Criticisms: only 119 patients had pancreatic cancer, no maintenance therapy was given, and the study included patients with positive margins without stratification. No RT quality assurance.

Beyond adjuvant 5-FU chemo-RT

- *RTOG 97-04/SWOG/ECOG* (Regine et al. 2008): 451 patients with GTR of pancreatic cancer randomized to weekly gemcitabine vs. protracted venous infusion 5-FU for 3 weeks before and for 12 weeks after concurrent chemo-RT (5-FU, 50.4 Gy). Trend for improved MS (20.5 vs. 16.9 months) and 3-year OS (31 vs. 22%, $p = 0.09$) with gemcitabine. Patterns of failure similar in both arms: distant (71–77%) > local (23–28%) > regional (nodes associated with tumor site) 7–8%.

- *ACOSOG Z05031* (Picozzi 2008): multicenter phase II trial of 89 patients with R0/1 resection of pancreatic head carcinoma treated with 50.4 Gy RT with concurrent cisplatin, 5-FU, and alpha-interferon followed by additional 5-FU chemotherapy. Ninety-six percent of patients had grade 3+ toxicity, but no toxicity-related deaths were noted. MS is 27 months and 2-year OS is 55% after surgery. Local recurrence 46%, systemic recurrence 35%.

Ongoing trials

- ESPAC-3 (phase III): resected pancreatic adenocarcinoma randomized to adjuvant 5-FU vs. gemcitabine
- EORTC 40013 (phase II/III): resected pancreatic head adenocarcinoma randomized to gemcitabine vs. gemcitabine for 2c followed by gemcitabine and concomitant RT (50.4 Gy)

Neoadjuvant treatment

- No completed phase III studies.
- Krishnan et al. (2007): of 323 patients, 247 patients received neoadjuvant chemo-RT (30 Gy/10 fx or 50.4 Gy/28 fx with 5-FU, gemcitabine, or capecitabine), 27 patients received induction gemcitabine-based chemo → chemorad. RT encompassed regional nodes in 69% patients. Median follow-up 5.5 months. MS 8.5 months (chemo-RT group) vs. 11.9 months (induction chemo → chemo-RT group). No significant difference in patterns of failure between groups.
- Evans et al. (2008): phase II, 86 patients. Chemo-RT (30 Gy/10 fx and weekly gemcitabine × 7 weeks) → surgery. RT included pancreaticoduodenal, portahepatic, superior mesenteric, and celiac axis LN. All patients restaged after chemo-RT. Eighty-five percent patients went on to surgery. MS 22.7 months, 5-year OS 27%. Of patients who received surgery, MS 34 vs. 7 months for unresectable patients.
- *SEER* (Stessin et al. 2008): reanalysis of SEER database, 3,885 patients. Seventy patients (2%) pre-op RT, 1,478 patients (38%) post-op RT, 2,337 patients (60%) surgery alone. MS 23 months (pre-op RT), 17 months (post-op RT), 12 months (surgery alone).

VI

UNRESECTABLE

- *GITSG* (Moertel et al. 1981): 194 patients with unresectable pancreatic cancer randomized to split course EBRT (40 Gy) with concomitant bolus 5-FU vs. split course EBRT (60 Gy) with concomitant bolus 5-FU vs. EBRT (60 Gy) alone. Both concomitant chemo arms prolonged MS vs. EBRT alone (42.2, 40.3, and 22.9 weeks, respectively).

- *GERCOR* (Huguet et al. 2007): reviewed 181 patients with locally advanced disease treated with 5-FU or gemcitabine based chemo × 3 months without evidence of progression who then received either additional chemotherapy vs. chemo-RT (physician choice). Chemo-RT improved median PFS (7.4→10.8 months) and OS (11.7→15 months).
- *RTOG 9812* (Tyvin 2004): phase II study of 109 patients with unresectable pancreatic cancer treated with EBRT 50.4 Gy and weekly paclitaxel. All patients were restaged 6 weeks after completion of chemo-RT. If marked shrinkage, resection was attempted. MS 11.2 months with 1-year OS 43% and 2-year OS 13%. Forty percent grade III and 5% grade IV toxicity with 1 death due to treatment.
- Tempero et al. (2003): 92 patients with locally advanced and/or metastatic adenocarcinoma of the pancreas randomized to 2,200 mg/m^2 gemcitabine over 30 min or 1,500 mg/m^2 over 150 min on days 1, 8, and 15 of a 4-week cycle. Slow infusion resulted in increased median survival (5 vs. 8 months, $p = 0.031$) and decreased toxicity.
- Ko et al. (2007): phase II, 25 patients. Gemcitabine and cisplatin × 6c→chemo-RT (50.4 Gy/28 fx with capecitabine). Patients restaged during and after chemotherapy, and after chemo-RT. If progressed on chemo, then spared chemo-RT. Forty-eight patients completed treatment, 32% patients progressed during chemo. Well tolerated. Median time to progression 10.5 months, MS 13.5 months, and MS of patients completing treatment 17 months.
- Murphy et al. (2007): 74 patients with locally advanced pancreatic cancer treated with chemo-RT (36 Gy/15 fx) with full-dose gemcitabine (1,000 mg/m^2 on days 1, 8, and 15). PTV = GTV + 1 cm. Six-month OS 46%/13%, median OS 11.2 months.

RADIATION TECHNIQUES

SIMULATION AND FIELD DESIGN

- Treat tumor (or tumor bed) and nodal groups at risk using pre-op and post-op imaging studies as well as the findings at surgery. Three-dimensional planning is necessary to optimize dose distribution while minimizing dose to liver, kidneys, small bowel, and spinal cord.
- Sim supine, arms up, with oral contrast. Use gastrografin (proprietary name) oral contrast, not barium, if CT is planned within 2 days. Give renal contrast or use CT to identify kidneys.

- Pancreas lies at L1–L2. Celiac axis is at T12. SMA is at L1.
- Lesions at the pancreatic head: treat pancreaticoduodenal, suprapancreatic, and celiac nodes, porta hepatis, the entire duodenal loop, and the tumor with 2–3 cm margin on gross disease.
- Lesions in the body/tail: treat pancreaticoduodenal, portal hepatic, lateral suprapancreatic nodes, the nodes of the splenic hilum, and the gross tumor with 2–3 cm margin. Porta hepatis and duodenal bed do not need to be covered.
- In general, patients are treated with a three or four field design – AP (50–80% of dose), two laterals or slightly off-axis superior/inferior obliques (20% of dose), plus or minus a posterior field. High energy photon fields (e.g., 18 MV) are useful particularly for the lateral/oblique fields.
- In general, for tumors of the pancreatic head treated with AP/PA fields: superior border = T10/T11; inferior border = L3/4; left border = 2 cm to the left of the edge of the vertebral body or 2 cm from the tumor; right border = pre-op location of the duodenum. On the laterals, anterior margin = 1.5–2 cm beyond the gross disease (being sure to include the duodenum); posterior margin = blocks the cord but covers 1.5–2 cm of the vertebral body.
- 4DCT or fluoroscopy is useful at the time of simulation to evaluate organ movement during respiration, which can have an impact on the position of the target volume and the kidneys. Some groups use respiratory gating, and abdominal compression to limit organ motion and decrease field size.
- Conedown to gross tumor (or preoperative tumor extent) + 2 cm margin at 45 Gy.
- For unresectable/palliative cases, consider using smaller field sizes, particularly if giving concurrent chemo-RT: GTV = primary tumor excluding draining LN, CTV = GTV ± 0.5 cm, PTV = CTV ± 0.5 cm.

VI

DOSE PRESCRIPTIONS

- Treat to 45 Gy at 1.8 Gy/fx followed by conedown to 50.4 Gy. In definitive chemo-RT setting, consider boosting to 54–59.4 Gy if feasible, respecting normal tissue tolerance.
- Multiple dose-escalation studies with hyperfractionation, brachytherapy, IORT, radiosurgery, hypofractionation, and other methods are under investigation.

DOSE LIMITATIONS

- Doses up to 50 Gy are tolerated by small volumes of stomach and intestine. Most common late effects are mucosal ulceration and bleeding. Perforation is rare.

- Limit the equivalent of at least one kidney to <20 Gy.
- Limit the whole liver to <20 Gy and 70% of liver to <30 Gy to prevent radiation hepatitis. Small volumes of liver can be treated to high doses.

COMPLICATIONS

- Critical normal tissues include liver, small bowel, stomach, cord, and kidney.
- Because the pancreas is a gland with both exocrine and endocrine secretions, both can decrease acutely or chronically following treatment. Adequate monitoring for diabetes is integral to treatment as is supplementation with pancreatic enzymes if exocrine insufficiency is suspected (pancrealipase with each meal).
- Acute – nausea and vomiting (use antiemetics, proton pump inhibitor, or H2 blocker). Diarrhea less common. If jaundice develops during RT or following treatment, ascending cholangitis must be considered as a potential etiology.
- Late – possible side effects include ulceration, stricture formation, obstruction, and (less commonly) perforation of GI tract. Side effects to cord, kidney, liver should not occur if normal tissue tolerances are followed.

FOLLOW-UP

- H&P, laboratories, and abdominal CT every 2 months to evaluate for disease recurrence/progression.

REFERENCES

Ann Surg Oncol. 2010 (epub ahead of print so no page numbers yet)

Berger AC, Garcia M, Jr, Hoffman JP, et al. Postresection CA 19-9 predicts overall survival in patients with pancreatic cancer treated with adjuvant chemoradiation: a prospective validation by RTOG 9704. JCO 2008;26(36):5918-5922.

Corsini MM, Miller RC, Haddock MG, et al. Adjuvant radiotherapy and chemotherapy for pancratic carcinoma: The Mayo Clinic experience (1975-2005). J Clinical Oncology 2008; 21:3511-3516.

Evans DB, Varadhachary GR, Crane CH, et al. Preoperative gemcitabine-based chemoradiation for patients with resectable adenocarcinoma of the pancreatic head. JCO 2008;26(21):3496-3502.

GITSG, Further evidence of effective adjuvant combined radiation and chemotherapy following curative resection of pancreatic cancer. Gastrointestinal Tumor Study Group. Cancer 1987;59(12):2006-2010.

Hazard L, Tward JD, Szabo A, et al. Radiation therapy is associated with improved survival in patients with pancreatic adenocarcinoma: results of a study from the surveillance, epidemiology, and end results (SEER) registry data. Cancer 2007;11(10):2191-2201.

Herman JM, Swartz MJ, Hsu CC, et al. Analysis of fluorouracil-based adjuvant chemotherapy and radiation after pancreaticoduodenectomy for ductal adenocarcinoma of the pancreas: results of a large, prospectively collected database at the Johns Hopkins Hospital. J Clin Oncol 2008;26(21):3503-3510.

Hsu CC, Herman JM, Corsini MM, et al. Adjuvant chemoradiation for pancreatic adenocarcinoma: The Johns Hopkins Hospital-Mayo Clinic collaborative study.

Huguet F, Andre T, Hammel P, et al. Impact of chemoradiotherapy after disease control with chemotherapy in locally-advanced pancreatic adenocarcinoma in GERCOR Phase II and III studies. J Clin Oncol 2007;25:326-331.

Kalser M, Ellenberg S. Pancreatic cancer. Adjuvant combined radiation and chemotherapy following curative resection. Arch Surg 1985;120(8):899-903. Erratum in: Arch Surg 1986;121(9):1045.

Klinkenbijl JH, Jeekel J, Sahmoud T, et al. Adjuvant radiotherapy and 5-fluorouracil after curative resection of cancer of the pancreas and periampullary region: phase III trial of the EORTC gastrointestinal tract cancer cooperative group. Ann Surg 1999;230(6):776-782; discussion 782-784.

Ko AH, Quivey JM, Venook AP, et al. A phase II study of fixed-dose rate gemcitabine plus low-dose cisplatin followed by consolidative chemoradiation for locally advanced pancreatic cancer. Int J Radiat Oncol Biol Phys 2007:68(3):809-816.

Krishnan S, Rana V, Janjan NA, et al. Induction chemotherapy selects patients with locally advanced, unresectable pancreatic cancer for optimal benefit from consolidative chemoradiation therapy. Cancer 2007;110(1):47-55.

Moertel CG, Frytak S, Hahn RG, et al. Therapy of locally unresectable pancreatic carcinoma: a randomized comparison of high dose (6000 rads) radiation alone, moderate dose radiation (4000 rads + 5-fluorouracil), and high dose radiation + 5-fluorouracil: The Gastrointestinal Tumor Study Group. Cancer 1981;48(8):1705-1710.

Murphy JD, Adusumilli S, Griffith KA, et al. Full dose gemcitabine and concurrent radiotherapy for unresectable pancreatic cancer. Int J Radiat Oncol Biol Phys 2007;68:801-808.

Neoptolemos JP, Dunn JA, Stocken DD, et al. Adjuvant chemoradiotherapy and chemotherapy in resectable pancreatic cancer: a randomised controlled trial. Lancet 2001;358(9293): 1576-1585.

Neoptolemos JP, Stocken DD, Friess H, et al. MW; European Study Group for Pancreatic Cancer. A randomized trial of chemoradiotherapy and chemotherapy after resection of pancreatic cancer. N Engl J Med 2004;350(12):1200-1210. Erratum in: N Engl J Med 2004; 351(7):726.

Neoptolemos JP, Stocken DD, Smith CT, et al. Adjuvant 5-fluourouracil and folinic acid vs observation for pancreatic cancer: composite data from the ESPAC-1 and -3(v1) trials. Br J Cancer 2009;100:246-250.

Oettle H, Post S, Neuhaus P, et al. Adjuvant chemotherapy with gemcitabine vs observation in patients undergoing curative-intent resection of pancreatic cancer (CONKO-001). JAMA 2007;297(3):267-276.

Picozzi VJ, Abrams RA, Traverso LW, et al. ACOSOG Z05031: Initial report of a multicenter, phase II trial of a novel chemoradiation protocol using cistplatin, 5-FU, and alpha-interferon as adjuvant therapy for resected pancreatic cancer. ASCO 2008 Gastrointestical Cancers Symposium, abstract 125.

Regine WF, Winter KA, Abrams RA, et al. Flurorouracil vs gemcitabine chemotherapy before and after fluorouracil-based chemoradiation following resection of pancreatic adenocarcinoma. JAMA 2008;299(9):1019-1026.

Smeenk HG, van Eijck CHJ, Hop WC, et al. Long-term survival and metastatic pattern of pancreatic and periampullary cancer after adjuvant chemoradiation or observation: long-term results of the EORTC trial 40891. Ann Surg 2007;246(5):734-740.

Stessin AM, Meyer JE, and Sherr DL. Neoadjuvant radiation is associated with improved survival in patients with resectable pancreatic cancer: an analysis of data from the surveillance, epidemiology, and end results (SEER) registry. Int J Radiat Oncol Biol Phys 2008;72(4): 1128-1133.

Stocken DD, Buchler MW, Dervenis C, et al. Meta-analysis of randomised adjuvant therapy trials for pancreatic cancer. Br J Cancer 2005;25:92(8):1372-1381.

Tempero M, Plunkett W, Ruiz Van Haperen V, et al. Randomized phase II comparison of dose-intense gemcitabine: thirty-minute infusion and fixed dose rate infusion in patients with pancreatic adenocarcinoma. J Clin Oncol 2003;21(18):3402-3408.

Tyvin R, Harris J, Abrams R, et al. Phase II study of external irradiation and weekly paclitaxel for nonmetastatic, unresectable pancreatic cancer: RTOG-98-12. Am J Clin Oncol 2004; 27:51-56.

VI

FURTHER READING

Abrams R. Primary Malignancies of the Pancreas, Periampullary Region and Hepatobiliary Tract – Considerations for the Radiation Oncologist (no. 310). Presented at the American Society of Therapeutic Radiology and Oncology Annual Meeting, San Francisco, CA; 2001.

American Society of Therapeutic Radiology and Oncology. Active Protocols. http://www.rtog.org/members/protocols/97-04/97-04.pdfandhttp://www.rtog.org/members/protocols/98-12/98-12.pdf. Accessed February, 2005.

Crane CH, Evans DB, Wolff RA, Abbruzzese JL, Pisters PWT, Janjan NA. The Pancreas. In: Cox JD, Ang KK, editors. Radiation oncology: rationale, technique, results. 8th ed. St. Louis: Mosby; 2003. pp. 465-480.

Lillis-Hearne P. Cancer of the Pancreas. In: Leibel SA, Phillips TL, editors. Textbook of Radiation Oncology. 2nd ed. Philadelphia: Saunders; 2004. pp. 837-856.

NCCN Physician Guidelines. Available at http://www.nccn.org/professionals/physician_gls/PDF/pancreatic.pdf. Accessed May 7, 2009.

Nukui Y, Picozzi VJ, Traverso LW. Interferon-based adjuvant chemoradiation therapy improves survival after pancreaticoduodenectomy for pancreatic adenocarcinoma. Am J Surg 2000;179:367-371.

Talamonti MS, Small W Jr, Mulcahy MF, et al. A multi-institutional phase ii trial of preoperative full-dose gemcitabine and concurrent radiation for patients with potentially resectable pancreatic carcinoma. Ann of Surg Oncol 2005;13(2):150-158.

Chapter 21
Hepatobiliary Cancer

Chien Peter Chen, Kim Huang, and Mack Roach III

GENERAL PEARLS

- ~22,000 cases and 17,000 deaths per year in the U.S.
- Frequency: hepatocellular carcinoma (most common) > gallbladder cancer > extrahepatic cholangiocarcinoma > intrahepatic cholangiocarcinoma (least common).

LIVER (HEPATOCELLULAR)

VI

PEARLS

- 100–250× more common in patients with chronic Hepatitis B.
- 3–4× more common in men.
- Cirrhosis, Hepatitis C, and aflatoxin B exposure are also risk factors.
- Prevention: Hepatitis B vaccine.
- Screening tools frequently used in high-risk patients: serum alpha-fetoprotein, liver ultrasound.

WORKUP

- Labs: CBC, LFTs, chemistries, coagulation panel, serum AFP (10–15% false negative), Hepatitis B/C panels.
- Abdominal CT scan (special contrast protocol).
- FNA can be performed but is not always needed.

STAGING: HAPATOCELLULAR

Editors' note: All TNM stage and stage groups referred to elsewhere in this chapter reflect the 2002 AJCC staging nomenclature unless otherwise noted as the new system below was published after this chapter was written.

(AJCC 6TH ED., 2002)

Primary tumor (T)

TX: Primary tumor cannot be assessed
T0: No evidence of primary tumor
T1: Solitary tumor without vascular invasion
T2: Solitary tumor with vascular invasion or multiple tumors not more than 5 cm
T3: Multiple tumors more than 5 cm or tumor involving a major branch of the portal or hepatic vein(s)
T4: Tumor(s) with direct invasion of adjacent organs other than the gallbladder or with perforation of visceral peritoneum

Regional lymph nodes (N)

NX: Regional lymph nodes cannot be assessed
N0: No regional lymph node metastasis
N1: Regional lymph node metastasis

Distant metastasis (M)

MX: Distant metastasis cannot be assessed
M0: No distant metastasis
M1: Distant metastasis

Stage grouping		**~5-year OS by stage**
I:	T1N0M0	I: 50–60%
II:	T2N0M0	II: 30–40%
IIIA:	T3N0M0	III: 10–20%
IIIB:	T4N0M0	
IIIC:	Any T, N1, M0	
IV:	Any T, Any N, M1	IV: <10%

(AJCC 7TH ED., 2010)

Primary tumor (T)

TX: Primary tumor cannot be assessed
T0: No evidence of primary tumor
T1: Solitary tumor without vascular invasion
T2: Solitary tumor with vascular invasion or multiple tumors not more than 5 cm
T3a: Multiple tumors more than 5 cm
T3b: Single tumor or multiple tumors of any size involving a major branch of the portal vein or hepatic vein
T4: Tumor(s) with direct invasion of adjacent organs other than the gallbladder or with perforation of visceral peritoneum

Regional lymph nodes (N)

NX: Regional lymph nodes cannot be assessed
N0: No regional lymph node metastasis
N1: Regional lymph node metastasis

Distant metastasis (M)

M0: No distant metastasis
M1: Distant metastasis

Anatomic stage/prognostic groups

I: T1 N0 M0
II: T2 N0 M0
IIIA: T3a N0 M0
IIIB: T3b N0 M0
IIIC: T4 N0 M0
IVA: Any T N1 M0
IVB: Any T Any N M1

continued

VI

TREATMENT RECOMMENDATIONS

Presentation	Recommended treatment
Resectable	■ Partial hepatectomy
Unresectable, medically inoperable	■ Liver transplant ■ Ablation (radiofrequency, cryotherapy, alcohol) ■ chemoembolization ■ Conformal RT ■ RT with concurrent chemotherapy ■ SBRT ■ Chemotherapy alone ■ Supportive care

SURGERY

- Partial hepatectomy is a treatment of choice if tumor can be resected with negative margins and patient has enough functional reserve to tolerate procedure.
  - Five-year overall survival ~35–40%
- Total hepatectomy with liver transplant is an option for patients with advanced cirrhosis and tumors smaller than 5 cm without vascular invasion.
  - Five-year overall survival as high as ~70% in selected patients
- Local failure is common.
- Role of adjuvant and neoadjuvant therapy unclear.

ABLATIVE PROCEDURES/OTHER INTERVENTIONS

- Radiofrequency ablation best for deep tumors with a diameter of 3 cm or less.
- Cyroablation can treat tumors up to 6 cm in size but requires laparotomy.
- Alcohol injection is commonly used because it is inexpensive but is limited to small tumors and may require several injections to be effective.
- Cryoablation and alcohol injection no longer used in the US.
- Chemoembolization and intrahepatic artery chemotherapy have response rates of 40–50% but may not improve survival.
- Systemic chemotherapy not useful, response rates <20%, no survival benefit, what about sorafinib?
- Antiviral therapy for patients with chronic hepatitis.

RADIATION THERAPY

- *EBRT definitive*
  - Option for unresectable tumors.

- Use local field for each lesion.
- High doses may improve survival, use conformal techniques, SBRT.
- Consider addition of concurrent FUDR hepatic arterial chemotherapy.

- *EBRT palliative*
  - Whole liver.
  - Consider for patients with multiple small lesions and liver related symptoms who are not candidates for other therapies.
- ^{131}I Lipiodol
  - Intraarterial injection.
  - May decrease recurrences and improve overall survival.
- *Yttrium microspheres*

STUDIES

VI

- Borgelt et al. (1981): Whole liver RT can relieve symptoms of abdominal pain, nausea, vomiting, fever, night sweats, ascites, anorexia, abdominal distention, weakness, fatigue.
- Russell et al. (1993): RTOG whole liver fractionation paper. patients treated with 1.5 b.i.d with dose escalation 27 Gy → 30 Gy → 33 Gy. No liver injury at 27 and 30 Gy. 5/51 patients had toxicity at 33 Gy. Authors suggest that 21 Gy may be insufficient radiation dose.
- Dawson et al. (2000): University of Michigan method for treating with high dose 3DCRT. Sixty-eight percent response rate. Survival improved with tumor doses of 70 Gy or higher.
- Dawson et al. (2002): Liver tolerance histograms. No radiation induced liver disease (RILD) with mean liver dose <31 Gy. Whole organ TD_{50} for mets 45.8 Gy, for primary hepatobiliary 39.8 Gy.
- Mornex et al. (2006): Prospective phase II trial including 25 patients with small-size HCC (1 nodule ≤5 cm or 2 nodules ≤3 cm) received 66 Gy in 2 Gy/fraction 3DCRT. CR achieved in 80% and PR in 12%. Stable disease in 8%. Grade 4 toxicities occurred only in Child-Pugh B patients.
- Seong et al. (2007): Retrospective analysis of 305 patients undergoing radiotherapy for HCC. Median survival was 11 months. The 1-, 2-, and 5-year OS were 45%, 24%, and 6%, respectively.
- Tse et al. (2008): 41 patients (31 with HCC and 10 with intrahepatic cholangiocarcinoma) completed six-fraction SBRT. Median dose was 36 Gy. Median survival of HCC was 11.7 months.
- Lau et al. (2008): 43 patients underwent curative resection for HCC and randomly assigned to one 1,850 MBq dose of

^{131}I-lipiodol or no adjuvant therapy. The 5-, 7-, and 10-year DFS in treatment and control groups were 62% vs. 32% ($p = 0.04$), 52% vs. 32% ($p = 0.02$), and 48% vs. 27% ($p = 0.09$), respectively. The 5-, 7-, and 10-year OS in treatment and control groups were 67% vs. 36% ($p = 0.04$), 67% vs. 32% ($p = 0.02$), and 52% and 27% ($p = 0.09$), respectively. DFS and OS difference became statistically insignificant at 8 year.

- Zeng et al. (2004): Retrospective analysis of 203 patients with unresectable hepatocellular carcinoma received transcetheter arterial chemoembolization (TACE) or combination therapy with external beam radiotherapy. OS for radiotherapy and non-radiotherapy groups for 1, 2, and 3 years were 72% vs. 60%, 42 vs. 26%, and 24% vs. 11%, respectively.
- Abou-Alfa et al. (2006): Phase II study including 137 patients with inoperable HCC, Child-Pugh A or B, no prior systemic treatment received oral sorafenib. Median OS 9.2 months.
- Llovet et al. (2008): Phase III, multicenter RCT including 602 patients with advanced HCC randomized to either sorafenib or placebo. Median OS was 10.7 months vs. 7.9 months ($p < 0.001$) for treatment vs. placebo. One-year OS 44% vs. 33% ($p = 0.009$).

RADIATION TECHNIQUES

SIMULATION AND FIELD DESIGN

- Supine with arms above head (out of field).
- Use wingboard to immobilize arms and alpha cradle to stabilize torso.
- Whole Liver (palliation only).
  - AP/PA, chose borders based on CT scan
  - 3DCRT reasonable because permits generation of kidney and lung DVHs
- Partial Liver (definitive option).
  - 3D treatment planning
  - Give contrast with planning CT scan to visualize tumor
  - CTV = gross tumor + 1 cm in all directions
  - PTV = CTV + 0.5 cm for setup error + 0.3–3 cm for organ motion error secondary to breathing (determined using fluoroscopy)
  - Stereotactic radiosurgery investigational

DOSE PRESCRIPTIONS

- Whole liver: 21 Gy/7 fx.
- Partial liver: determined individually.

- Prescribe dose that gives 10% risk of RILD based on NTCP model.
- Limit isocenter dose to 90 Gy even if risk of RILD is less than 10%.
- 1.5 Gy BID with at least 6 h between fractions.

DOSE LIMITATIONS

- Whole liver
  - TD 5/5: 30 Gy/15 fx
  - TD 50/5: 42 Gy/21fx
- 2/3 of liver TD 5/5: 50.4 Gy/28 fx
- 1/3 of liver TD 5/5: 68.4 Gy/38 fx

COMPLICATIONS

- Refer to Dawson paper (above) to estimate risk of RILD.
- RILD occurs 2–8 weeks after treatment.
- Signs/symptoms include fatigue, RUQ pain, ascites, hepatomegaly.
- Alkaline phosphatase and transaminase levels are frequently markedly elevated while bilirubin levels remain near normal.

VI

FOLLOW-UP

- Office visit, CT scan, and labs (LFTs, AFP) every 3 months for 2 years, then every 6 months.

GALLBLADDER

PEARLS

- Chronic gallbladder inflammation (usually from gallstones) increases risk of development of gallbladder cancer.
- Generally considered to have poor prognosis, frequently advanced stage at presentation.
- Usually undiagnosed before cholecystectomy.
- Can be found incidentally after simple cholecystectomy for benign etiology.

WORKUP

- Labs: CBC, LFTs, chemistries, coagulation panel, serum CEA, CA 19–9.
- Right upper quadrant US and/or abdominal CT scan and/or MRI.
- ERCP or percutaneous needle biopsy for diagnosis.

STAGING: GALLBLADDER

Editors' note: All TNM stage and stage groups referred to elsewhere in this chapter reflect the 2002 AJCC staging nomenclature unless otherwise noted as the new system below was published after this chapter was written.

(AJCC 6TH ED., 2002)

Primary tumor (T)

TX: Primary tumor cannot be assessed
T0: No evidence of primary tumor
Tis: Carcinoma in situ
T1: Tumor invades lamina propria or muscle layer
  T1a: Tumor invades lamina propria
  T1b: Tumor invades muscle layer
T2: Tumor invades perimuscular connective tissue; no extension beyond serosa or into liver
T3: Tumor perforates the serosa (visceral peritoneum) and/or directly invades the liver and/or another adjacent organ or structure, such as the stomach, duodenum, colon, or pancreas, omentum or extrahepatic bile ducts
T4: Tumor invades main portal vein or hepatic artery or invades multiple extrahepatic organs or structures

Regional lymph nodes (N)

NX: Regional lymph nodes cannot be assessed
N0: No regional lymph node metastasis
N1: Regional lymph node metastasis

Distant metastasis (M)

MX: Distant metastasis cannot be assessed
M0: No distant metastasis
M1: Distant metastasis

(AJCC 7TH ED., 2010)

Primary tumor (T)

TX: Primary tumor cannot be assessed
T0: No evidence of primary tumor
Tis: Carcinoma in situ
T1: Tumor invades lamina propria or muscular layer
  T1a: Tumor invades lamina propria
  T1b: Tumor invades muscular layer
T2: Tumor invades perimuscular connective tissue; no extension beyond serosa or into liver
T3: Tumor perforates the serosa (visceral peritoneum) and/or directly invades the liver and/or another adjacent organ or structure, such as the stomach, duodenum, colon, pancreas, omentum, or extrahepatic bile ducts
T4: Tumor invades main portal vein or hepatic artery or invades two or more extrahepatic organs or structures

Regional lymph nodes (N)

NX: Regional lymph nodes cannot be assessed
N0: No regional lymph node metastasis
N1: Metastases to nodes along the cystic duct, common bile duct, hepatic artery, and/or portal vein
N2: Metastases to periaortic, pericaval, superior mesenteric artery, and/or celiac artery lymph nodes

Distant metastasis (M)

M0: No distant metastasis
M1: Distant metastasis

continued

Stage grouping

Stage	
0:	TisN0M0
IA:	T1N0M0
IB:	T2N0M0
IIA:	T3N0M0
IIB:	T1N1M0, T2N1M0, T3N1M0
III:	T4, Any N, M0
IV:	Any T, Any N, M1

Used with the permission from the American Joint Committee on Cancer (AJCC), Chicago, IL. The original source for this material is the AJCC Cancer Staging Manual, Sixth Edition (2002), published by Springer Science+Business Media.

Anatomic stage/prognostic groups

Stage	
0:	Tis N0 M0
I:	T1 N0 M0
II:	T2 N0 M0
IIIA:	T3 N0 M0
IIIB:	T1-3 N1 M0
IVA:	T4 N0-1 M0
IVB:	Any T N2 M0
	Any T Any N M1

Used with the permission from the American Joint Committee on Cancer (AJCC), Chicago, IL. The original source for this material is the AJCC Cancer Staging Manual, Seventh Edition (2010), published by Springer Science+Business Media.

VI

TREATMENT RECOMMENDATIONS

Presentation	Recommended treatment
Incidental finding on cholecystectomy pathology, T1a	■ Cholecystectomy is adequate surgery. ■ No adjuvant therapy
Incidental finding on cholecystectomy pathology, T1b or more advanced	■ Additional resection with lymphadenectomy ■ Adjuvant treatment with RT and concurrent 5FU based chemo
Mass on imaging or jaundice, resectable	■ Surgery with lymphadenectomy ■ Adjuvant treatment with RT and concurrent 5FU based chemo
Mass on imaging or jaundice, unresectable	■ Biliary decompression if needed ■ RT with concurrent 5FU based chemo ■ Gemcitabine or 5FU based chemo alone ■ Supportive care

SURGERY

- Cholecystectomy possible in ~30% of patients.
- Radical cholecystectomy with partial hepatectomy for node negative patients with invasion of perimuscular connective tissue.
- Palliation.

ADJUVANT THERAPY

- Role of EBRT and chemo-RT unclear, but generally recommended for residual disease after surgery.

STUDIES

- Cubertafond et al. (1999): Review of surgical data for 724 patients. Five-year survival: Tis 93%, T1 18%, T2 10%. No 3-year survivors with T3/4 cancer.
- North et al. (1998): Review of surgical data for 162 patients. Median survival: complete resection 67 months, microscopic residual disease 9 months, gross residual disease 4 months. Some patients received chemo and/or RT.
- Mojica et al. (2007): Retrospective analysis of 3,187 cases of gallbladder cancer in SEER registry. Adjuvant RT was used in 17% of cases. Median survival for patients receiving adjuvant RT was 14 months compared to 8 months ($p \leq 0.001$) for those not receiving RT. Survival benefit only for those with regional spread and tumors infiltrating liver.

- Duffy et al. (2008): Retrospective analysis of 435 patients with gallbladder cancer. Median OS was 10 months with median survival of stage Ia-III of 12.9 months and stage IV of 6 months. Of those who received curative resections (123 patients), 20% received adjuvant therapy. Median survival for those who received adjuvant therapy was 23.4 months, but was not statistically significant.
- Czito et al. (2005): Retrospective analysis of 22 patients with primary and nonmetastatic gallbladder cancer treated with surgical resection followed by concurrent radiotherapy (median dose 45 Gy) and 5FU chemotherapy. Five-year LRC, DFS, and OS were 59%, 33%, and 37%, respectively. Median survival was 1.9 year.
- *SEER* (Wang 2008): 4,180 patients with resected gallbladder cancer, 18% received adjuvant RT. Adjuvant RT improved MS for ≥T2N+ disease from 8 to 15 months. Some patients with ≥T2N0 disease may benefit, but to a smaller degree. Nomogram derived in paper.

RADIATION TECHNIQUES

SIMULATION AND FIELD DESIGN

- Supine with arms above head (out of field).
- Use wingboard to immobilize arms and alpha cradle to stabilize torso.
- CT scan for treatment planning.
- Cover tumor bed and local regional lymph nodes including portahepatis, pericholechal, celiac, and pancreaticoduodenal.

DOSE PRESCRIPTION

- 45 Gy/25 fx followed by boost to reduced fields.

DOSE LIMITATIONS

- Small bowel <45–50.4 Gy/25–28 fx
- Spinal cord <45 Gy/25 fx
- Liver (see previous sections, use NTCP model)
- Kidney 1/3 ≤ 20 Gy

COMPLICATIONS

- RILD
- Small bowel obstruction
- Fistula formation

FOLLOW-UP

- See liver section above

BILE DUCT

PEARLS

- Divided into intrahepatic (IHCC) and extrahepatic (EHCC) cholangiocarcinoma.
- Klatskin (hilar) tumor is located at birufication of common hepatic duct and is classified as extrahepatic.
- History of primary sclerosing cholangitis gives 10% lifetime risk of developing cholangiocarcinoma.
- Chronic inflammation from tape worm infection increases risk of developing cholangiocarcinma.
- Cholecystectomy decreases risk of cholangiocarcinoma.
- ~55% of patients are lymph node positive at diagnosis.

WORKUP

- Labs: CBC, LFTs, chemistries, coagulation panel, CA 19–9, CEA, Hepatitis B/C.
- Right upper quadrant US and/or abdominal CT scan and/or MRI.
- ERCP with biopsy.

STAGING: INTRAHEPATIC BILE DUCT

Editors' note: All TNM stage and stage groups referred to elsewhere in this chapter reflect the 2002 AJCC staging nomenclature unless otherwise noted as the new system below was published after this chapter was written.

(AJCC 6TH ED., 2002)

Primary tumor (T)

TX: Primary tumor cannot be assessed
T0: No evidence of primary tumor
Tis: Carcinoma in situ
T1: Tumor confined to bile duct histologically
T2: Tumor invades beyond wall of bile duct
T3: Tumor invades the liver, gallbladder, pancreas, and/or unilateral branches of the portal vein (right or left) or hepatic artery (right or left)
T4: Tumor invades any of the following: main portal vein or its branches bilaterally, common hepatic artery, or other adjacent structures, such as the colon, stomach, duodenum, or abdominal wall

Regional lymph nodes (N)

NX: Regional lymph nodes cannot be assessed
N0: No regional lymph node metastasis
N1: Regional lymph node metastasis

Distant metastasis (M)

MX: Distant metastasis cannot be assessed
M0: No distant metastasis
M1: Distant metastasis

Stage grouping

0: TisN0M0
IA: T1N0M0
IB: T2N0M0
IIA: T3N0M0
IIB: T1N1M0, T2N1M0, T3N1M0

(AJCC 7TH ED., 2010)

Primary tumor (T)

TX: Primary tumor cannot be assessed
T0: No evidence of primary tumor
Tis: Carcinoma in situ (intraductal tumor)
T1: Solitary tumor without vascular invasion
T2a: Solitary tumor with vascular invasion
T2b: Multiple tumors, with or without vascular invasion
T3: Tumor perforating the visceral peritoneum or involving the local extra hepatic structures by direct invasion
T4: Tumor with periductal invasion

Regional lymph nodes (N)

NX: Regional lymph nodes cannot be assessed
N0: No regional lymph node metastasis
N1: Regional lymph node metastasis present

Distant metastasis (M)

M0: No distant metastasis
M1: Distant metastasis present

Anatomic stage/prognostic groups

0: Tis N0 M0
I: T1 N0 M0
II: T2 N0 M0
III: T3 N0 M0
IVA: T4 N0 M0
Any T N1 M0
IVB: Any T any N M1

continued

III: T4, any N, M0
IV: Any T, any N, M1

Used with the permission from the American Joint Committee on Cancer (AJCC), Chicago, IL. The original source for this material is the AJCC Cancer Staging Manual, Sixth Edition (2002), published by Springer Science+Business Media.

Used with the permission from the American Joint Committee on Cancer (AJCC), Chicago, IL. The original source for this material is the AJCC Cancer Staging Manual, Seventh Edition (2010), published by Springer Science+Business Media.

STAGING (AJCC 7TH ED., 2010): PERIHILAR BILE DUCT

Editors' note: All TNM stage and stage groups referred to elsewhere in this chapter reflect the 2002 AJCC staging nomenclature unless otherwise noted as the new system below was published after this chapter was written.

Primary tumor (T)

TX: Primary tumor cannot be assessed
T0: No evidence of primary tumor
Tis: Carcinoma in situ
T1: Tumor confined to the bile duct, with extension up to the muscle layer or fibrous tissue
T2a: Tumor invades beyond the wall of the bile duct to surrounding adipose tissue
T2b: Tumor invades adjacent hepatic parenchyma
T3: Tumor invades unilateral branches of the portal vein or hepatic artery
T4: Tumor invades main portal vein or its branches bilaterally; or the common hepatic artery; or the second-order biliary radicals bilaterally; or unilateral second-order biliary radicals with contralateral portal vein or hepatic artery involvement

Regional lymph nodes (N)

NX: Regional lymph nodes cannot be assessed
N0: No regional lymph node metastasis
N1: Regional lymph node metastasis (including nodes along the cystic duct, common bile duct, hepatic artery, and portal vein)
N2: Metastasis to periaortic, pericaval, superior mesenteric artery, and/or celiac artery lymph nodes

Distant metastasis (M)

M0: No distant metastasis
M1: Distant metastasis

Anatomic stage/prognostic groups

0: Tis N0 M0
I: T1 N0 M0
II: T2a-b N0 M0
IIIA: T3 N0 M0
IIIB: T1-3 N1 M0
IVA: T4 N0-1
IVB: Any T N2 M0
Any T any N M1

STAGING (AJCC 7TH ED., 2010): DISTAL BILE DUCT

Editors' note: All TNM stage and stage groups referred to elsewhere in this chapter reflect the 2002 AJCC staging nomenclature unless otherwise noted as the new system below was published after this chapter was written.

Primary tumor (T)

TX: Primary tumor cannot be assessed
T0: No evidence of primary tumor
Tis: Carcinoma in situ
T1: Tumor confined to the bile duct histologically
T2: Tumor invades beyond the wall of the bile duct

continued

T3: Tumor invades the gallbladder, pancreas, duodenum, or other adjacent organs without involvement of the celiac axis, or the superior mesenteric artery
T4: Tumor involves the celiac axis, or the superior mesenteric artery

Regional lymph nodes (N)
NX: Regional lymph nodes cannot be assessed
N0: No regional lymph node metastasis
N1: Regional lymph node metastasis

Distant metastasis (M)
M0: No distant metastasis
M1: Distant metastasis

Anatomic stage/prognostic groups
0: Tis N0 M0
IA: T1 N0 M0
IB: T2 N0 M0
IIA: T3 N0 M0
IIB: T1-T3 N1 M0
III: T4 Any N M0
IV: Any T any N M1

Used with the permission of the American Joint Committee on Cancer (AJCC), Chicago, IL. The original source for this material is the AJCC Cancer Staging Manual, Seventh Edition (2010), published by Springer Science+Business Media.

STAGING (AJCC 7TH ED., 2010): AMPULLA OF VATER

Primary Tumor (T)
TX: Primary tumor cannot be assessed
T0: No evidence of primary tumor
Tis: Carcinoma in situ
T1: Tumor limited to ampulla of Vater or sphincter of Oddi
T2: Tumor invades duodenal wall
T3: Tumor invades pancreas
T4: Tumor invades peripancreatic soft tissues or other adjacent organs or structures other than pancreas

Regional Lymph Nodes (N)
NX: Regional lymph nodes cannot be assessed
N0: No regional lymph node metastasis
N1: Regional lymph node metastasis

Distant Metastasis (M)
M0: No distant metastasis
M1: Distant metastasis

Anatomic Stage/Prognostic Groups
0: Tis N0 M0
IA: T1 N0 M0
IB: T2 N0 M0
IIA: T3 N0 M0
IIB: T1-T3 N1 M0
III: T4 Any N M0
IV: Any T Any N M1

Used with the permission of the American Joint Committee on Cancer (AJCC), Chicago, Illinois. The original source for this material is the AJCC Cancer Staging Manual, Seventh Edition (2010) published by Springer Science+Business Media.

TREATMENT RECOMMENDATIONS

Presentation	Recommended treatment
Intrahepatic cholangiocarcinoma	
Resectable No residual disease	■ Surgery followed by observation
Resectable Residual disease (MS 10–20 months; 5-year OS 20–35%)	■ Surgical resection, repeat resection if possible ■ Ablative procedure ■ RT with concurrent 5FU based chemo ■ Consider SBRT ■ Gemcitabine based chemo alone
Unresectable (MS 7 months; 5-year OS 0%)	■ Ablative procedure ■ RT with concurrent 5FU based chemo ■ Consider SBRT ■ 5FU or gemcitabine based chemo alone ■ Supportive care
Extrahepatic cholangiocarcinoma	
Resectable No residual disease (MS 20–25 months; 5-year OS 30%)	■ Surgery followed by observation
Resectable Residual disease (MS 13 months)	■ Surgery followed RT with concurrent 5FU based chemo
Unresectable (MS 6–12 months)	■ RT with concurrent 5FU based chemo (consider brachytherapy boost) ■ RT with concurrent 5FU based chemo followed by transplant ■ 5FU or gemcitabine based chemo alone ■ Supportive care

VI

SURGERY

- Complete surgical resection is the most effective treatment.
- Surgical procedure depends on tumor location and extent of disease.
  - Partial hepatectomy or lobectomy for intrahepatic tumors.
  - Roux-en-y hepaticojejunostomy for hilar tumors.
  - Pancreaticoduodenectomy for distal lesions.
  - Liver transplant.
- Palliative Options - biliary enteric bypass, percutaneous transhepatic biliary drainage, stents.

ADJUVANT THERAPY

- Not studied prospective.
- Adjuvant RT and chemotherapy may improve overall survival.

STUDIES

- Todoroki et al. (2000): 63 patients. Treatment: surgical resection. RT given to 28/47 with microscopic disease and 13/14 with gross residual disease. 5-year OS with RT 32 months vs. surgery alone 13.5 months. RT group OS: IORT+EBRT 39%, IORT alone 17%, EBRT alone 0%. LRC with RT 79% vs. with surgery alone 31.2%. IORT dose recommendations - 20 Gy, 8 MeV electrons, 6 cm cone.
- Schoenthaler et al. (1994): UCSF experience. 129 patients, retrospective, extrahepatic ducts only. Treatment: 62 patients surgery alone, 45 patients surgery + conventional RT (46 Gy median), 22 patients surgery + charged particles (60 GyE median). MS: 6.5 months with surgery, 11 months with surgery + EBRT, 14 months with surgery + particles, 7 months with gross residual disease, 19 months with microscopic residual disease, and 39 months with negative margins.
- Alden and Mohiuddin (1994): Unresectable disease. Higher RT doses improve survival. MS: 44 Gy = 4.5 months, 45–54 Gy = 18 months, >54 Gy = 24 months. Recommended dose is 45 Gy EBRT with a 25-Gy intraluminal brachytherapy boost.
- Crane et al. (2002): 52 patients, locally advanced, unresectable treated with RT + chemo (73% of patients, PVI 5FU). Median time to local progression: 9 months after 30 Gy, 11 months after 36–50.4 Gy, 15 months after 54–85 Gy (p = ns). MS 10 months. Grade 3 toxicity similar in all groups.
- Borghero et al. (2008): Retrospective analysis of 65 patients with extrahepatic bile duct adenocarcinoma treated with curative-intent resection (S). For those with high-risk of local regional recurrence (42 patients), adjuvant chemoradiation (S-CRT) was implemented. Five-year OS and LRR for S- vs. S-CRT groups were 36% vs. 42% and 38% vs. 37%, respectively.
- Nelson et al. (2009): Retrospective analysis of 45 patients underwent resection followed by concurrent chemoradiation. Thirty-three patients underwent adjuvant radiotherapy and 12 neoadjuvant radiotherapy. Five-year OS, DFS, LRC were 33%, 37%, and 78%, respectively. Median survival was 34 months. Patients treated neoadjuvantly showed a trend toward longer 5-year OS (53% vs. 23%) but was not statistically significant.

RADIATION TECHNIQUES

SIMULATION AND FIELD DESIGN

- Supine with arms above head (out of field).
- Use wingboard to immobilize arms and alpha cradle to stabilize torso.
- CT scan for treatment planning.
- Cover tumor bed, porta hepatis, celiac axis + 1.5 cm margins.
- Consider extending field 3–5 cm into liver to cover additional intrahepatic bile duct length for margin.
- Add additional margins as needed to account for organ motion secondary to breathing, determined using fluoroscopy or perform 4D CT to define ITV.

DOSE PRESCRIPTION

- 45 Gy/25 fx to large field described above.
- Additional boost dose should be given. Options include: EBRT with conedown to tumor bed to 60 Gy total; ^{192}Ir intraluminal brachytherapy (20–25 Gy); IORT at time of surgery.

DOSE LIMITATIONS

- See liver and gallbladder sections.

COMPLICATIONS

- RILD rare, as much of the liver can be excluded from the field.
- Cholangitis after brachytherapy.
- Small bowel damage (ulcer, bleeding, obstruction).

FOLLOW-UP

- See liver section above.

REFERENCES

Abou-Alfa GK, Schwartz L, Ricci S, et al. Phase II Study of Sorafenib in Patients with Advanced Hepatocellular Carcinoma. J Clin Oncol 2006;24: 4293-4300.

Alden ME, Mohiuddin M. The Impact of Radiation Dose in Combined External Beam and Intraluminal Ir-192 Brachytherapy for Bile Duct Cancer. Int J Radiat Oncol Biol Phys 1994;28:945-951.

Borgelt BB, Gelber R, Brady LW, et al. The Palliation of Hepatic Metastases: Results of the Radiation Therapy Oncology Group Pilot Study. Int J Radiat Oncol Biol Phys 1981;7: 587-591.

Borghero Y, Crane CH, Szklaruk J, et al. Extrahepatic Bile Duct Adenocarcinoma: Patients at High-Risk for Local Recurrence Treated with Surgery and Adjuvant Chemoradiation Have an Equivalent Overall Survival to Patients with Standard-Risk Treated with Surgery Alone. Ann Surg Oncol 2008;15: 3147-3156.

Crane CH, MacDonald KO, Vauthey JN, et al. Limitations of Conventional Doses of Chemoradiaion for Unresectable Biliary Cancer. Int J Radiat Oncol Biol Phys 2002;53:969-974.

Cubertafond P, Mathonnet M, Gainant A, et al. Radical Surgery For Gallbladder Cancer. Results of the French Surgical Association Survey. Hepatogastroenerology 1999;46:1567-1571.

Czito BG, Hurwitz HI, Clough RW, et al. Adjuvant External-Beam Radiotherapy with Concurrent Chemotherapy After Resection of Primary Gallbladder Carcinoma: A 23-Year Experience. Int J Radiat Oncol Biol Phys 2005;62: 1030-1034.

Dawson LA, McGinn CJ, Normolle D, et al. Escalated Focal Liver Radiation and Concurrent Hepatic Artery Flourodeoxyuridine for Unresectable Intrahepatic Malignancies. J Clin Oncol 2000;18:2210-2218.

Dawson LA, Normolle D, Balter JM, et al. Analysis of Radiation-Induced Liver Disease Using the Lyman NTCP Model. Int J Radiat Oncol Biol Phys 2002;53:810-821.

Duffy A, Capanu M, Abou-Alfa GK, et al. Gallbladder Cancer (GBC): 10-Year Experience at Memorial Sloan Kettering Cancer Centre (MSKCC). J Surg Oncol 2008; 98:485-489.

Lau WY, Lai EC, Leung TW, et al. Adjuvant Intra-arterial Iodine-131 Labeled Lipiodol for Resectable Hepatocellular Carcinoma: A Prospective Randomized Trial – Update on 5-Year and 10-Year Survival. Ann Surg 2008;247:43-48.

Llovet JM, Ricci S, Mazzaferro V, et al. Sorafenib in Advanced Hepatocellular Carcinoma. N Engl J Med 2008;359:378-390.

Mojica P, Smith D, and Ellenhorn J. Adjuvant Radiation Therapy is Associated with Improved Survival for Gallbladder Carcinoma with Regional Metastatic Disease. J Surg Oncol 2007;96:8-13.

Mornex F, Girarda N, Beziat C, et al. Feasibility and efficacy of high-dose three-dimensional radiotherapy in cirrhotic patients with small-size hepatocellular carcinoma non-eligible for curative therapies – mature results of the French phase II RTF-1 trial. Int J Radiat Oncol Biol Phys 2006;66:1152-8.

National Comprehensive Cancer Network. Clinical Practice Guidelines in Oncology: Hepatobiliary Cancers. Available at: http://www.nccn.org/professionals/physician_gls/PDF/hepatobiliary.pdf. Accessed on May 11, 2009.

Nelson JW, Ghafoori AP, Willett CG, et al. Concurrent Chemoradiotherapy in Resected Extrahepatic Cholangiocarcinoma. Int J Radiat Oncol Biol Phys 2009;73:148-153.

North JH, Pack MS, Hong C, et al. Prognostic Factors for Adenocarcinoma of the Gallbladder: An analysis of 162 Cases. Am Surg 1998;64:437-440.

Russell AH, Clyde C, Wasserman TH, et al. Accelerated Hyperfractionated Hepatic Irradiation in the Management of Patients with Liver Metastases: Results of the RTOG Dose Escalating Protocol. Int J Radiat Oncol Biol Phys 1993;27:117-123.

Seong J, Shim SJ, Lee IJ, et al. Evaluation of the prognostic value of Okuda, Cancer of the Liver Italian Program, and Japan Integrated Staging systems for hepatocellular carcinoma patients undergoing radiotherapy. Int J Radiat Oncol Biol Phys 2007;67:1037-1042.

Schoenthaler R, Phillips TL, Efrid JT, et al. Carcinoma of the Extrahepatic Bile Ducts, the University of California at San Francisco Experience. Annals of Surgery 1994;219:267-274.

Tse RV, Kim JJ, Hawkins M, et al. Phase I Study of Individualized Stereotactic Body Radiotherapy for Hepatocellular Carcinoma and Intrahepatic Cholangenic Sarcoma. J Clin Oncol 2008;Epub Jan 2.

Todoroki T, Ohara K, Kawamoto T, et al. Benefits of Adjuvant Radiotherapy After Radical Resection of Locally Advanced Main Hepatic Duct Carcinoma. Int J Radiat Oncol Biol Phys 2000;46:581-587.

Wang SJ, Fuller CD, Kim JS, et al. Prediction model for estimating the survival benefit of adjuvant radiotherapy for gallbladder cancer. J Clin Oncol 2008; 26: 2116-2117.

Zeng ZC, Tang ZY, Fan J, et al. A comparison of chemoembolization combination with and without radiotherapy for unresectable hepatocellular carcinoma. Cancer J 2004;10:307-316.

FURTHER READING

Bartlet DL, Di Bisceglie AM, Dawson LA. Cancer of the Liver. In: DeVita VT, Lawrence TS, Rosenberg SA, editors. Cancer, Principles and Practice of Oncology. 8th ed. Philadelphia: Lippincott Willaims & Wilkins, 2008. 1129-1156.

Ben-Josef E, Lawrence TS. Hepatobiliary Tumors. In: Gunderson LL, Tepper JE, editors. Clinical Radiation Oncology. 2nd ed. Philadelphia: Churchill Livingstone; 2007. 1083-1100.

Cheng SH, Huang AT. Liver and Hepatobiliary Tract. In: Halperin EC, Perez CA, Brady LW, et al, editors. Principles and Practice of Radiation Oncology. 5th ed. Philadelphia: Lippincott Williams & Wilkins; 2008. 1349-1365.

Fritz P, Brambs HJ, Schraube P, et al. Combined External Beam Radiotherapy and Intraluminal High Dose Rate Brachytherapy on Bile Duct Carcinomas. Int J Radiat Oncol Biol Phys 1994;29:855-861.

Greene FL, American Joint Committee on Cancer, American Cancer Society. AJCC Cancer Staging Manual. 6th ed. New York: Springer-Verlag; 2002.

Morganti AG, Trodella L, Valentini V, et al. Combined Modality Treatment in Unresectable Extrahepatic Biliary Carcinoma. Int J Radiat Oncol Biol Phys 2000;46:913-919.

Stevens, KR. The Liver and Biliary System. In: Cox JD, Ang KK, editors. Radiation Oncology: Rationale, Technique, Results. 8th ed. St. Louis: Mosby; 2003. 481-496.

Urego M, Flickinger JC, Carr BI. Radiotherapy and Multimodality Management of Cholangiocarcinoma. Int J Radiat Oncol Biol Phys 1999;44:121-126.

Wagman R, Schoenthaler R. Cancer of the Liver, Bile Duct, and Gallbladder. In: Leibel SA, Phillips TL, editors. Textbook of Radiation Oncology. 2nd ed. Philadelphia: Saunders; 2004. 857-884.

Chapter 22
Colorectal Cancer

Marc B. Nash, Hans T. Chung, and Kavita K. Mishra

VI

PEARLS

- Third most frequently diagnosed cancer in the US men and women.
- 108,070 new cases of colon cancer and 40,740 new cases of rectal cancer in the US in 2008. Combined mortality for colorectal cancer 49,960 in 2008.
- Rectum begins at the rectosigmoid junction at level of S3 vertebra. It is divided into three ~5 cm segments by transverse folds: upper, mid, lower rectum. Cancer of rectum is defined as those straddling or inferior to the peritoneal reflection.
- Rectal nodal drainage: superior half rectum drains to pararectal, sacral, sigmoidal, inferior mesenteric; inferior half rectum drains to internal iliacs; lower rectum and tumors extending to anal canal may drain to superficial inguinal nodes.
- Rectal metastases travel along portal drainage to liver via superior rectal vein, as well as systemic drainage to lung via middle and inferior rectal veins.
- Colon nodal drainage: left colon to inferior mesenteric; right colon to superior mesenteric. Periaortic nodes at risk if cancer invades retroperitoneum. External iliac nodes at risk if cancer invades adjacent pelvic organs.
- Hematochezia most common presentation in rectal and lower sigmoid CA; abdominal pain common with colon CA.

SCREENING

- Average risk persons (age ≥ 50 years, asymptomatic, no FH): colonoscopy q10 year (preferred) or FOBT q1 year + flexible sigmoidoscopy q5 year or double-contrast barium enema q5 year.
- Inflammatory bowel disease: colonoscopy q1–2 years, initiate 8 years after symptom onset if pancolitis or 15 years after symptom onset if L-sided colitis.

- Family Hx (non-FAP/HNPCC): colonoscopy q1–5 years, initiate at age 40 years or 10 years prior to earliest cancer diagnosis in family.
- Familial adenosis polyposis (lifetime cancer risk ~100% by age 50): APC gene testing, early screening, colectomy, or procto-colectomy after onset of polyposis.
- Hereditary nonpolyposis colorectal cancer: colonoscopy q1–2 years, initiate at age 20–25 or 10 years younger than earliest cancer diagnosis in family.

WORKUP

- H&P including DRE and complete pelvic exam in women. Note size, location, ulceration, mobile vs. tethered vs. fixed, and sphincter function on rectal exam.
- Labs including CBC, LFTs, CEA.
- Complete colonoscopy with endoscopic biopsy, pathology review.
- Endorectal US to assess tumor extension and nodal status.
- CT chest/abdomen/pelvis. Consider pelvic MRI.
- ~20% of patients may be over or understaged clinically (Guillem 2008; Sauer et al. 2004).

STAGING: COLORECTAL CANCER

Editors' note: All TNM stage and stage groups referred to elsewhere in this chapter reflect the 2002 AJCC staging nomenclature unless otherwise noted as the new system below was published after this chapter was written.

(AJCC 6TH ED., 2002)

Primary tumor (T)

TX: Primary tumor cannot be assessed
T0: No evidence of primary tumor
Tis: Carcinoma in situ: intraepithelial or invasion of lamina propria
T1: Tumor invades submucosa
T2: Tumor invades muscularis propria
T3: Tumor invades through the muscularis propria into the subserosa, or into nonperitonealized pericolic or perirectal tissues
T4: Tumor directly invades other organs or structures, and/or perforates visceral peritoneum

Regional lymph nodes (N)

NX: Regional lymph nodes cannot be assessed
N0: No regional lymph node metastasis
N1: Metastasis in 1–3 regional lymph nodes
N2: Metastasis in four or more regional lymph nodes

Metastases (M)

MX: Distant metastasis cannot be assessed
M0: No distant metastasis
M1: Distant metastasis

Stage grouping		Dukes	Modified Aster-Coller	~5-year OS	
0:	TisN0M0	–	–		
I:	T1N0M0	A	A	I:	80–95%
	T2N0M0	A	B1		
IIA:	T3N0M0	B	B2	II:	50–90%
IIB:	T4N0M0	B	B3		

(AJCC 7TH ED., 2010)

Primary tumor (T)

TX: Primary tumor cannot be assessed
T0: No evidence of primary tumor
Tis: Carcinoma in situ: intraepithelial or invasion of lamina propria*
T1: Tumor invades submucosa
T2: Tumor invades muscularis propria
T3: Tumor invades through the muscularis propria into pericolorectal tissues
T4a: Tumor penetrates to the surface of the visceral peritoneum**
T4b: Tumor directly invades or is adherent to other organs or structures**,***

**Note*: Tis includes cancer cells confined within the glandular basement membrane (intraepithelial) or mucosal lamina propria (intramucosal) with no extension through the muscularis mucosae into the submucosa.
**Note: Direct invasion in T4 includes invasion of other organs or other segments of the colorectum as a result of direct extension through the serosa, as confirmed on microscopic examination (for example, invasion of the sigmoid colon by a carcinoma of the cecum) or, for cancers in a retroperitoneal or subperitoneal location, direct invasion of other organs or structures by virtue of extension beyond the muscularis propria (i.e., respectively, a tumor on the posterior wall of the descending colon invading the left kidney or lateral abdominal wall; or a mid or distal rectal cancer with invasion of prostate, seminal vesicles, cervix, or vagina).
****Note*: Tumor that is adherent to other organs or structures, grossly, is classified cT4b. However, if no tumor is present in the adhesion, microscopically, the classification should be pT1-4a depending on the anatomical depth of wall invasion. The V and L classifications should be used to identify the presence or absence of vascular or lymphatic invasion, whereas the PN site-specific factor should be used for perineural invasion.

continued

VI

IIIA:	T1-2N1M0	C	C1	III:	30–60%
IIIB:	T3-4N1M0	C	C2/C3		
IIIC:	Any T, N2, M0	C	C1/C2/C3		
IV:	Any T, any N, M1		D	IV:	<5%

Used with the permission from the American Joint Committee on Cancer (AJCC), Chicago, IL. The original source for this material is the AJCC Cancer Staging Manual, Sixth Edition (2002), published by Springer Science+Business Media.

Regional lymph nodes (N)

NX: Regional lymph nodes cannot be assessed
N0: No regional lymph node metastasis
N1: Metastasis in 1–3 regional lymph nodes
- N1a: Metastasis in one regional lymph node
- N1b: Metastasis in 2–3 regional lymph nodes
- N1c: Tumor deposit(s) in the subserosa, mesentery, or nonperitonealized pericolic or perirectal tissues without regional nodal metastasis

N2: Metastasis in four or more regional lymph nodes
- N2a: Metastasis in 4–6 regional lymph nodes
- N2b: Metastasis in seven or more regional lymph nodes

Note: A satellite peritumoral nodule in the pericolorectal adipose tissue of a primary carcinoma without histologic evidence of residual lymph node in the nodule may represent
discontinuous spread, venous invasion with extravascular spread (V1/2), or a totally replaced lymph node (N1/2).

Replaced nodes should be counted separately as positive nodes in the N category, whereas discontinuous spread or venous invasion should be classified and counted in the Site-Specific Factor category Tumor Deposits (TD).

Distant metastasis (M)

M0: No distant metastasis
M1: Distant metastasis
- M1a: Metastasis confined to one organ or site (e.g., liver, lung, ovary, nonregional node)
- M1b: Metastases in more than one organ/site or the peritoneum

Anatomic stage/prognostic groups

Stage	T	N	M	Dukes*	MAC*
0:	Tis	N0	M0	–	–
I:	T1	N0	M0	A	A
	T2	N0	M0	A	B1
IIA:	T3	N0	M0	B	B2

continued

IIB:	T4a	N0	M0	B	B2
IIC:	T4b	N0	M0	B	B3
IIIA:	T1–T2	N1/N1c	M0	C	C1
	T1	N2a	M0	C	C1
IIIB:	T3–T4a	N1/N1c	M0	C	C2
	T2–T3	N2a	M0	C	C1/C2
	T1–T2	N2b	M0	C	C1
IIIC:	T4a	N2a	M0	C	C2
	T3–T4a	N2b	M0	C	C2
	T4b	N1–N2	M0	C	C3
IVA:	Any T	Any N	M1a	–	–
IVB:	Any T	Any N	M1b	–	–

Note: cTNM is the clinical classification, pTNM is the pathologic classificationThe *y* prefix is used for those cancers that are classified after neoadjuvant pretreatment (e.g., ypTNM). Patients who have a complete pathologic response are ypT0N0cM0 that may be similar to Stage Group 0 or I. The *r* prefix is to be used for those cancers that have recurred after a disease-free interval (rTNM).
*Dukes B is a composite of better (T3 N0 M0) and worse (T4 N0 M0) prognostic groups, as is Dukes C (any TN1 M0 and any T N2 M0). MAC is the modified Astler-Coller classification.

VI

TREATMENT RECOMMENDATIONS

2002 Stage	Rectal cancer	~5-year LF/OS
I	▪ TME with APR (low lesions) or LAR (midupper lesions). If pT1-2N0, no adjuvant treatment ▪ Consider local excision for favorable tumors (<3 cm size, <30% circumference, within 8 cm of anal verge, well-moderately differentiated; margin >3 mm, no LVSI/PNI). Following local excision, favorable T1 lesions may be observed, while T2 lesions should receive adjuvant 5-FU/RT	<5% LF 90% OS
II and III (locally resectable)	▪ Pre-op 5-FU/RT → LAR/APR → adjuvant 5-FU-based therapy* × 3 cycles (preferred) ▪ If patient treated with surgery initially, then pt should receive adjuvant 5-FU × 2 cycles → concurrent chemoRT → 5-FU × 2 cycles	T3N0 and T1-2N1: 5–10% LF 80% OS T4N0 and T3N1: 10–15% LF 60% OS T4N1 and T3/4N2: 15–20% LF 40% OS
III (T4/ locally unresectable)	▪ If obstructed, may need diverting colostomy or stent placed prior to definitive treatment. 5-FU/RT → resection if possible. Consider IORT for microscopic disease (after 50 Gy EBRT, give IORT 12.5–15 Gy to 90% IDL) or brachytherapy for macroscopic disease → adjuvant 5-FU-based therapy*	
IV	▪ Individualized options, including combination 5-FU-based chemo alone, or chemo ± resection ± RT	
Recurrent	▪ Individualized options. If no prior RT, then consider chemoRT, followed by surgery ± IORT or brachytherapy. If prior RT, then chemo → surgery ± IORT or brachytherapy as appropriate	

*Consider post-op 5-FU ± leucovorin vs. FOLFOX (infusional 5-FU/leucovorin/oxaliplatin) vs. FOLFIRI (infusional 5-FU/leucovorin/irinotecan).

Stage	**Colon cancer****
I	Colectomy + LND
IIA	Colectomy + LND. For adverse pathologic features, consider adjuvant chemo
IIB	Colectomy + LND. Consider adjuvant chemo
III	Colectomy + LND adjuvant chemo
IV	Consider resection and neoadjuvant/ adjuvant chemo

**No clear OS/LC benefit with RT in colon CA. May consider post-op RT in setting of node-negative disease if close/+ margins and tumor bed can be clearly identified.

STUDIES

RECTAL

PRE-OP RT VS. SURGERY ALONE

- *Dutch Colorectal Cancer Group* (Kapiteijn et al. 2001, ASCO 2002; Peeters 2007): 1,861 patients with resectable rectal CA randomized to pre-op RT (25 Gy/5 fx) and surgery vs. surgery alone (TME surgery). Pre-op RT improved 2-year LR (2% vs. 8%) and 5-year LR (6% vs. 12%). No difference in survival. At 5 year, RT increased fecal incontinence (62 vs. 33%), pad wearing, bleeding (11 vs. 3%), and mucous discharge.
- *Swedish Rectal Cancer Trial* (Pahlman et al. 1997; Folkesson et al. 2005): 1,168 patients with resectable rectal CA randomized to pre-op RT (25 Gy/5 fx) and surgery vs. surgery alone (non-TME surgery). Pre-op RT improved 5-year LR (11% vs. 27%) and 5-year OS (58% vs. 48%). Thirteen-year OS was 38% vs. 30%.

PRE-OP VS. POST-OP CHEMORT

- *German Rectal Cancer Study Group* (Sauer et al. 2004): 823 patients with T3/4 or N+ rectal CA randomized to pre-op vs. post-op chemoRT. Both arms had 50.4 Gy with concurrent 5-FU; post-op arm had additional 5.4 Gy boost. Pre-op chemoRT improved 5-year LR rate (6% vs. 13%); increased rate of sphincter saving procedures (39% vs. 19%); and decreased grade 3–4 acute and late toxicity and late anastomotic strictures. Twenty-five percent of pre-op group compared to 40% post-op had positive LN, and there was pCR in 8% of pre-op group. In post-op arm, 18% of initially eligible patients were overstaged and excluded due to finding of pT1-2N0 disease at time of surgery. No difference in survival.

- *MRC CR07/NCIC-CTG C016* (Sebag-Montefiore et al. 2009): Phase III. 1,350 patients with resectable rectal CA randomized to short-course pre-op RT (25 Gy/5fx) + surgery vs. surgery + selective post-op chemoRT (45 Gy and 5-FU) restricted to patients with involvement of the circumferential resection margin. Reduction in LR for pre-op RT vs. selective post-op chemoRT (4.4% vs. 10.6%). No difference in OS. Quirke et al. (2009): 1,156 patients evaluated in terms of plane of surgery achieved and the involvement of the circumferential resection margin. Plane of surgery classified as good (mesorectal), intermediate (intramesorectal), and poor (muscularis propria plane). Three-year LRR 4% (mesorectal), 7% (intramesorectal), and 13% (muscularis propria group). Patients in short-course RT group with resection in mesorectal plane had 3-year LRR 1%. All pt groups with pre-op short-course RT had decreased local recurrence.

PRE-OP CHEMORT VS. PRE-OP RT

- Pre-op chemoRT appears to increase pCR (~5→15%) and LC (~80–85%→90%), but not sphincter saving surgery (~50%) or OS (~65%) compared with pre-op RT alone.
- *French FFCD 9203* (Gerard 2006): 733 eligible patients with T3-4N0 resectable adenoca rectum randomized to pre-op RT (1.8/45 Gy) vs. pre-op concurrent RT + bolus 5FU and LV d1-5 weeks 1 and 5. All patients had adjuvant 4c of FU-LV chemo. Pre-op chemoRT increased pCR (4→11%) and LC (83→92%), but also grade 3–4 toxicity (3→15%). No difference in sphincter saving surgery (52%), EFS, or OS (67%).
- *EORTC 22921* (Bosset et al. 2006; JCO 2007): 1,011 patients with resectable rectal CA randomized to pre-op RT, pre-op chemoRT, pre-op RT + post-op chemo, or pre-op chemoRT + post-op chemo. RT consisted of 45 Gy and chemo consisted of 5-FU and leucovorin (pre-op chemo × 2 cycles, post-op chemo × 4cycles). No difference in 5-year OS between pre-op and post-op chemo groups (64.8% vs. 65.8%). Five-year LRR improved for chemoRT groups (8.7, 9.6, and 7.6%) compared to RT alone group (17.1%), and chemoRT increased the pCR rate (5→14%).
- *Polish Colorectal Study Group* (Bujko et al. 2006): Phase III trial. 312 patients with T3/4 resectable rectal CA randomized to pre-op RT (25 Gy/5fx) + surgery vs. pre-op chemoRT (50.4 Gy with bolus 5-FU and leucovorin) + surgery. Early radiation toxicity was higher in the chemoRT group (18.2% vs. 3.2%). Neoadjuvant chemoRT did not increase OS, LC, or late toxicity

compared to short-course RT alone, although there was increased downstaging with chemoRT.

POST-OP CHEMO, RT, AND/OR CHEMORT

- Post-op RT increases LC, while chemo increases LC and OS; PVI 5-FU during RT improves OS vs. bolus 5-FU.
- *GITSG 7175* (Thomas and Lindblad, 1988): 227 patients with stage B2-C rectal CA randomized postoperatively to no adjuvant therapy vs. chemo alone vs. RT alone vs. concurrent chemoRT. ChemoRT arm improved 5-year DFS and OS over control.
- *Intergroup/NCCTG* (O'Connell et al. 1994): 660 patients with stage II or III rectal CA randomized to postoperative bolus 5-FU vs. PVI 5-FU during post-op pelvic RT. Chemo given ± semustine. PVI 5-FU improved 4-year OS (70% vs. 60%) and relapse-free rate (63% vs. 53%). No benefit with semustine.
- *Intergroup 0114* (Tepper et al. 2002; JCO 2001): 1,695 patients with T3/4 or N+ rectal CA randomized to postoperative bolus 5-FU vs. 5-FU and leucovorin vs. 5-FU and levamisole vs. 5-FU, leucovorin, and levamisole. All received concurrent pelvic RT 50.4–54 Gy. No difference in 7-year OS (~56%) and DFS (~50%) between 4 chemo arms. Number of LN examined was associated with OS for N0 patients. Recommend minimum 14 LN should be examined.
- *NSABP R-01* (JNCI 1988): 555 patients with B-C (II-III) rectal cancer treated with surgery alone vs. post-op RT (46–47 Gy) vs. post-op chemo (5-FU, semustine, vincristine). RT improved LF (25→16%), while chemo improved DFS (30→42%) and OS (43→53%) vs. observation.
- *NCCTG 79-47-51* (NEJM 1991): 204 patients with T3/4 or LN+ (B2-C) randomized to post-op RT (45–50.4 Gy) vs. chemoRT (bolus 5-FU concurrent). ChemoRT improved LF (25→14%), DM, DFS, and OS (48→58%) vs. RT alone.
- *NSABP R-02* (JNCI 2000): 694 patients with Dukes' B-C (II-III) treated with surgery→post-op chemo (5-FU/LV vs. MOF) + concurrent RT. Post-op RT reduced 5-year LF (14→8%), but there was no difference in DFS or OS.
- *Pooled-analysis* (Gunderson et al. 2004): Pooled rectal analysis of 3,791 patients on NCCTG trials, Int 0144, NSABP RO1, and RO2. Increasing T and N stage negatively impacted survival, but N stage alone does not determine survival. For intermediate-risk patients, post-op chemo appeared to improve OS after surgery (to ~85%), similar to post-op chemoRT. For moderately high-risk and high-risk patients, DFS, OS, and LF tended to be better with chemoRT than with chemo alone.

VI

Risk group	~5-year OS	~DFS	~LR	~DM
Low T1-2N0	90%	90%	<5%	10%
Intermediate T1-2N1, T3N0	80% (75–85%) with S+C+-RT	75% (65–80%)	5–10%	15–20%
Moderately high T1-2N2, T3N1, T4N0	60% (40–80%)	55% (45–60%)	10–20% C only >15% CRT 10–15%	30–35%
High T3N2, T4N+	40% (25–60%)	30–35%	15–20% C only >20% CRT <20%	>40%

LOCAL EXCISION

- Rationale for local excision is to avoid APR for lesions <8 cm from verge, but not to avoid LAR which still allows sphincter sparing.
- If high-grade, LVSI, signet ring cells, or ≥T2, local failure is >15% and incidence of involved mesorectal and/or pelvic LN is 10–20%, so do not use WLE alone.
- *RTOG 89-02* (Russell et al. 2000): 65 patients in phase II trial of sphincter-sparing local excision for low-lying rectal tumors ≤4 cm, ≤40% circumference, mobile, N0 status. 51 higher-risk patients also received post-op chemoRT. RT dose 45–50 Gy with boost to total 50–65 Gy. Five-year OS 78%, 11 patients failed. LRF correlated with T stage (T1 4%, T2 16%, T3 23%) and percentage of rectal circumference involved. DM correlated with T stage.
- *MDACC* (Bonnen 2004): Reviewed 26 patients with T3 rectal cancer who refused APR after pre-op chemoRT and were treated with WLE. Fifty-four percent had pCR, 35% had micro residual dz, and 12% had gross residual dz. Only 2/26 (6%) pelvic failures.

COLON

- *INT0130 Trial* (2004): 222 patients with resected T3N1-N2 or T4 colon CA randomized to chemo vs. chemoRT. RT given as 45 Gy/25 fx ± 5.4 boost to tumor bed. No difference in survival or local recurrence.
- Andre et al. (2004): 2,246 patients with stage II or III colon CA randomized to postoperative 5-FU/leucovorin vs. 5-FU/leucovorin/oxaliplatin. Oxaliplatin improved 3-year DFS (78% vs. 73%).

- Twelves eta l. (2005): 1,987 patients with resected stage III colon CA randomized to oral capecitabine vs. bolus 5FU/LV. Capecitabine had at least equivalent DFS, with improved RFS with fewer adverse events.
- Moertel et al. (1990): 1,296 patients with resected colon cancer, which either was locally invasive (Stage B2–3) or had regional nodal involvement (Stage C), were randomized to observation vs. treatment for one year with levamisole and fluorouracil. Overall death rate was reduced by 33% in chemo treatment arm.

RADIATION TECHNIQUES

RECTAL CANCER

SIMULATION AND FIELD DESIGN

- Prone position; radiopaque markers include anal, vaginal, rectal, perineal skin; wire perineal scar if present; small bowel contrast, ensure bladder full.
- Rectal field designed to cover tumor with margin, presacral, and internal iliac nodes (if T4, external iliac nodes also).
- *Whole Pelvis* (PA field) borders: Superior = L5-S1; inferior = 3 cm below initial tumor volume or inferior obturator foramen, whichever most inferior; lateral = 1.5 cm outside pelvic inlet.
- *Whole Pelvis* (Lateral fields) borders: Posterior = behind bony sacrum; anterior = posterior pubic symphysis if T3 vs. anterior pubic symphysis if T4. Corner blocks as needed.
- Avoid flashing posterior skin, unless s/p APR, and then include perineal scar in all fields.
- *Tumor bed boost* borders: tumor + 2–3 cm margin superior/inferior/anterior; posterior border includes sacral hollow. Corner blocks used to protect small bowel.
- *For rectal cancers extending inferior to dentate lone:* inguinal nodes are at risk and IMRT is used in this situation to decrease dose to the genitalia (Fig. 22.1).
- IORT: consider for close/+ microscopic margins, especially for T4 or recurrent CA.
- Brachytherapy: consider for macroscopic residual after pre-op chemoRT and resection.
- Chemo: Concurrent PVI 5-FU-based therapy with RT given as 5-FU 225 mg/m^2 over 24 h 7 days/week during RT. Use of oral 5-FU is becoming common.

VI

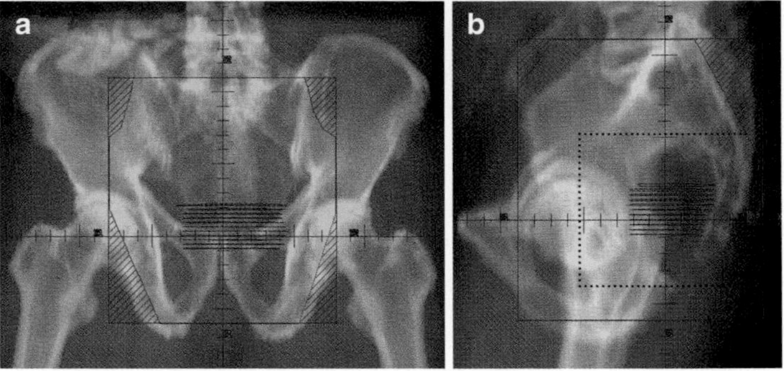

Fig. 22.1 (**a**) PA and (**b**) lateral DRRs of fields used to treat a T3N0 rectal primary. The lateral boost field is indicated by the black dotted line. *Note*: radiopaque markers not shown

DOSE PRESCRIPTIONS

- Whole Pelvis: 3 field with PA + opposed laterals; use lateral wedges as appropriate. 45 Gy (1.8 Gy × 25 fx) then boost. Use high energy photon beams for lateral fields. Choose appropriate energy photon beam for PA field based on the depth of sacral hollow.
- Boost: opposed laterals only; 5.4 Gy (1.8 Gy × 3 fx), to total dose 50.4 Gy. Consider second boost to 54 Gy if all small bowel is out of field.
- If no planned surgical intervention, definitive RT dose is 45 Gy to whole pelvis, then tumor boost including primary and sacral hollow to 50.4 Gy as above. Then second boost to primary tumor, off small bowel, with additional 9–59.4 Gy.

DOSE LIMITATIONS (AT STANDARD FRACTIONATION)

- Small bowel 45–50 Gy
- Femoral head and neck 42 Gy
- Bladder 65 Gy
- Rectum 60 Gy

RADIATION TECHNIQUES: COLON CANCER

- No clear evidence of survival benefit with RT. However, RT may be useful in the setting of node-negative disease with close/+ microscopic margins at the primary site, where a target can be clearly demarcated. If RT is included in treatment regimen,

field should include margin around tumor bed based on pre-op imaging and/or surgical clips.
- Dose 45–50 Gy in 25–28 fx.

COMPLICATIONS

- Potential side effects include diarrhea, dysuria, fatigue, skin irritation, and hematologic toxicity. Long term GI complications include change in bowel habits, rectal urgency, diarrhea, anastomotic stricture, small bowel obstruction.
- Check weekly CBC and skin reaction on treatment.

FOLLOW-UP

- H+P, CEA every 3 months × 2 years, then every 6 months × 5 years.
- Consider CT scan if high risk of recurrence approximately every 4–6 months. Recurrence commonly occurs within 2 years after initial therapy. However, late failures even beyond 5 years have been noted after local excision.
- Colonoscopy in 1 year, then every 2–3 years if negative.

Acknowledgement We thank Richard M. Krieg, M.D., for his valuable advice in the preparation of this chapter.

REFERENCES

Andre T, Boni C, Mounedii-Boudiaf L, et al. Oxaliplatin, fluorouracil, and leucovorin as adjuvant treatment for colon cancer. N Engl J Med 2004;350:2343-2351.

Add Collette L, Bosset JF, den Dulk M et al. Patients with curative resection of cT3-4 rectal cancer after preoperative radiotherapy or radiochemotherapy: does anybody benefit from adjuvant fluorouracil-based chemotherapy? A trial of the European Organisation for Research and Treatment of Cancer Radiation Oncology Group. J Clin Oncol. 2007 Oct 1;25(28):4379-4386.

Add Fisher B, Wolmark N, Rockette H et al. Postoperative adjuvant chemotherapy or radiation therapy for rectal cancer: results from NSABP protocol R-01. J Natl Cancer Inst. 1988 Mar 2;80(1):21-29.

Add Tepper JE, O'Connell MJ, Niedzwiecki D et al. Impact of number of nodes retrieved on outcome in patients with rectal cancer. J Clin Oncol. 2001 Jan 1;19(1):157-163.

Bonnen M, Crane C, Vauthey JN, et al. Long-term results using local excision after preoperative chemoradiation among selected T3 rectal cancer patients. IJROBP 2004;60(4):1098-1105.

Bosset J, Collette L, Calais G, et al. Chemotherapy with preoperative radiotherapy in rectal cancer. N Engl J Med 2006;355:1114-1123.

Bujko K, Nowacki MP, Nasierowska-Guttmejer A, et al. Long-term results of a randomized trial comparing preoperative short-course radiotherapy with preoperative conventionally fractionated chemoradiation for rectal cancer. Br J Surg 2006;93:1215-1223.

Folkesson J, Birgisson H, Pahlman L, et al. Sweedish Rectal Cancer Trial: long lasting benefits from radiotherapy on survival and local recurrence rate. J Clin Oncol 2005;23:5644-5650.

Gérard JP, Conroy T, Bonnetain F et al. Preoperative radiotherapy with or without concurrent fluorouracil and leucovorin in T3-4 rectal cancers: results of FFCD 9203. J Clin Oncol. 2006 Oct 1;24(28):4620-4625.

Guillem JG, Diaz-Gonzalez JA, MInsky BD, et al. cT3N0 rectal cancer: potential overtreatment with preoperative chemoradiotherapy is warranted. J Clin Oncol 2008;26(3):368-373.

Gunderson LL, Sargent DJ, Tepper JE, et al. Impact of T and N stage and treatment on survival and relapse in adjuvant rectal cancer: a pooled analysis. J Clin Oncol 2004;22:1785-1796.

Kapiteijn E, Marijnen CAM, Nagtegaal ID, et al. Preoperative radiotherapy combined with total mesorectal excision for resectable rectal cancer. N Engl J Med 2001;345:638-646.

Krook JE, Moertel CG, Gunderson LL, et al. Effective surgical adjuvant therapy for high-risk rectal carcinoma. N Engl J Med. 1991;324(11):709-715.

Moertel CG, Fleming TR, Macdonald JS, et al. Levamisole and fluorouracil for adjuvant therapy of resected colon carcinoma. N Engl J Med 1990;322:352-358.

NSABP R-02 reference: Wolmark N, Wieand HS, Hyams DM et al. Randomized trial of postoperative adjuvant chemotherapy with or without radiotherapy for carcinoma of the rectum: National Surgical Adjuvant Breast and Bowel Project Protocol R-02. J Natl Cancer Inst. 2000 Mar 1;92(5):388-396.

O'Connell MJ, Martenson JA, Wieand HS, et al. Improving adjuvant therapy for rectal cancer by combining protracted-infusion fluorouracil with radiation therapy after curative surgery. N Engl J Med 1994;331:502-507.

Pahlman L, Glimelius B, et al. Improved survival with preoperative radiotherapy in resectable rectal cancer: Swedish Rectal Cancer Trial. N Engl J Med 1997;336:980-987.

Peeters KC, Marijnen CA, Nagtegaal ID et al. The TME trial after a median follow-up of 6 years: increased local control but no survival benefit in irradiated patients with resectable rectal carcinoma. Ann Surg. 2007 Nov;246(5):693-701.

Quirke P, Steele R, Monson J, et al. Effect of the plane of surgery achieved on local recurrence in patients with operable rectal cancer: a prospective study using data from the MRC CR07 and NCIC-CTG C016 randomized clinical trial. Lancet 2009;373:821-828.

Russell AH, Harris J, Rosenberg PJ, et al. Anal sphincter conservation for patients with adenocarcinoma of the distal rectum: long term results of Radiation Therapy Oncology Group Protocol 89-02. Int J Radiat Oncol Biol Phys 2000;46:313-322.

Sauer R, Becker H, Hohenberger W, et al. Preoperative versus postoperative chemoradiotherapy for rectal cancer. N Engl J Med 2004;351:1731-1740.

Sebag-Montefiore D, Stephens R, Monson J, et al. Preoperative radiotherapy versus selective postoperative chemoradiotherapy in patients with rectal cancer (MRC CR07 and NCIC-CTG C016): a multicentre, randomized trial. Lancet 2009;373:811-820.

Tepper JE, O'Connell M, Niedzwiecki D, et al. Adjuvant therapy in rectal cancer: analysis of stage, sex, and local control–final report of Intergroup 0114. J Clin Oncol 2002;20:1744-1750.

Thomas PR, Lindblad AS. Adjuvant postoperative radiotherapy and chemotherapy in rectal carcinoma: a review of the Gastrointestinal Tumor Study Group experience. Radiother Oncol 1988;13:245-252.

Twelves C, Wong A, Nowacki MP, et al. Capecitabine as adjuvant treatment for stage III colon cancer. N Engl J Med 2005;352:2696-2704.

FURTHER READING

Janjan NA, Delclos ME, Ballo MT, et al. The Colon and Rectum. In: Cox JD, Ang KK, editors. Radiation oncology: rationale, technique, results. 8th ed. St. Louis: Mosby; 2003. pp. 497-536.

Martenson Jr JA, Willet CG, Sargent DJ, et al. Phase III study of adjuvant chemotherapy and radiation therapy compared with chemotherapy alone in the surgical adjuvant treatment of colon cancer: results of Intergroup protocol 0130. J Clin Oncol 2004;22:3277-3283.

Minsky BD. Cancer of the Colon. In: Leibel SA, Phillips TL, editors. Textbook of radiation oncology. 2nd ed. Philadelphia: Saunders; 2004. pp. 885-895.

Minsky BD. Cancer of the Rectum. In: Leibel SA, Phillips TL, editors. Textbook of radiation oncology. 2nd ed. Philadelphia: Saunders; 2004. pp. 897-912.

Mohiuddin M, Willett CG. Colon and Rectum. In: Halperin EC, Perez CA, Brady LW, et al., editors. Principles and practice of radiation oncology. 5th ed. Philadelphia: Lippincott Williams & Wilkins; 2008. pp. 1366-1382.

National Comprehensive Cancer Network. Clinical Practice Guidelines in Oncology: Colon Cancer. Available at:http://www.nccn.org/professionals/physician_gls/PDF/colon.pdf. Accessed on May 24, 2009.

National Comprehensive Cancer Network. Clinical Practice Guidelines in Oncology: Rectal Cancer. Available at:http://www.nccn.org/professionals/physician_gls/PDF/rectal.pdf. Accessed on May 24, 2009.

Tepper JE, O'Connell MJ, Petroni GR, et al. Adjuvant postoperative fluorouracil-modulated chemotherapy combined with pelvic radiation therapy for rectal cancer: initial results of Intergroup 0114. J Clin Oncol 1997;15:2030-2039.

Chapter 23
Anal Cancer

Amy Gillis, Hans T. Chung, and Gautam Prasad

PEARLS

- 5,070 new cases in 2008 with increasing incidence over the last three decades.
- Majority are SCC (75–80%); others are adenocarcinoma or melanoma.
- *HPV*: strongly associated with SCC and may be requisite for disease formation. High-grade intraepithelial lesions are precursors. In particular HPV-16, 18 as in cervical cancer.
- *AIDS* is associated with anal cancer, likely through an association with immunodeficiency in the setting of HPV coinfection. Increased risk if CD4 < 200.
- *Additional Risk Factors*: >10 sexual partners, history of anal warts, history of anal intercourse < age 30 or with multiple partners, history of STDs.
- *Anatomy*: anal canal is 3–4 cm long. Extends from anal verge to the anorectal ring. The dentate line lies within the anal canal and divides it by histology. Proximal to the dentate line is colorectal mucosa, distal to it is nonkeratinizing squamous epithelium. The dentate line contains transitional mucosa. Anal margin is 5 cm ring of skin around the anus. Use CT to measure depth of inguinal nodes using the femoral vessels as a surrogate: large variations exist (Koh et al. 1993).
- *Anal margin tumors*: may behave like skin cancers, and can be treated as skin cancer as long as there is no involvement of the anal sphincter, tumor <2 cm, moderately or well-differentiated.
- *Adenocarcinoma*: higher local and distant recurrence rates with chemo-RT compared to SCC. Use 5-FU chemo-RT pre-op followed by APR (Papagikos et al. 2003).
- *Lymph node drainage*: superiorly (above dentate line) along hemorrhoidal vessels to perirectal and internal iliac nodes; inferior canal (below dentate line) and anal verge to inguinal nodes.
- *Presentation*: bleeding, anal discomfort, pruritis, rectal urgency.

VI

WORKUP

- H&P. Include inguinal LN evaluation. Note anal sphincter tone, pain, bleeding, HIV risk factors, inflammatory bowel disease, prior RT. For women, a comprehensive gynecologic exam should be performed. Note anal sphincter function by tone on DRE and whether prone/supine, clock location, distance from verge, cicumferential involvement, size, superior extent.
- Labs: CBC, HIV test if any risk factors. CD4 counts if HIV-positive.
- Proctoscopy with biopsy.
- May biopsy inguinal nodes if clinically suspicious. Only FNA, avoid open biopsy.
- CXR or Chest CT. CT abdomen and pelvis or MRI.
- PET/CT recommended to evaluate extent of disease including lymph nodes and/or distant metastases (Cotter et al. 2006; Trautmann and Zuger, 2005). PET/CT can also be used as baseline to gauge posttreatment response (Schwarz et al. 2008).
- Transanal ultrasound (considered optional, but may be helpful to visualize perirectal nodes)

STAGING (AJCC 7TH ED., 2010): ANAL CANAL

- The definitions of TNM and the stage groupings for this chapter have not changed from the AJCC 6th Ed., 2002.

Primary tumor (T)
TX: Primary tumor cannot be assessed
T0: No evidence of primary tumor
Tis: Carcinoma in situ (Bowen's disease, high-grade squamous intraepithelial lesion (HSIL), anal intraepithelial neoplasia II–III (AIN II–III)
T1: Tumor 2 cm or less in greatest dimension
T2: Tumor more than 2 cm, but not more than 5 cm in greatest dimension
T3: Tumor more than 5 cm in greatest dimension
T4: Tumor of any size invades adjacent organ(s), e.g., vagina, urethra, bladder*

**Note*: Direct invasion of the rectal wall, perirectal skin, subcutaneous tissue, or the sphincter muscle(s) is not classified as T4.

Regional lymph nodes (N)
NX: Regional lymph nodes cannot be assessed
N0: No regional lymph node metastasis
N1: Metastasis in perirectal lymph node(s)
N2: Metastasis in unilateral internal iliac and/or inguinal lymph node(s)
N3: Metastasis in perirectal and inguinal lymph nodes and/or bilateral internal iliac and/or inguinal lymph nodes

Distant metastasis (M)
M0: No distant metastasis
M1: Distant metastasis

Anatomic stage/prognostic groups
0: Tis N0 M0
I: T1 N0 M0

continued

II:	T2 N0 M0
	T3 N0 M0
IIIA:	T1-T3 N1 M0
	T4 N0 M0
IIIB:	T4 N1 M0
	Any T N2 M0
	Any T N3 M0
IV:	Any T Any N M1

Used with the permission from the American Joint Committee on Cancer (AJCC), Chicago, IL. The original source for this material is the AJCC Cancer Staging Manual, Seventh Edition (2010), published by Springer Science+Business Media.

TREATMENT RECOMMENDATIONS

Situation	Recommended Treatment

T1, small, well-differentiated	■ Local excision (Boman, Cancer 1984; Greenall et al. 1985)
	  ■ Consider only if small, <2 cm, well-differentiated and superficially invasive, negative margins on excision
	  ■ Not to be used if sphincter involved or if >40% of circumference (would cause loss of continence, so use chemo-RT)
	  ■ Consider only in very compliant patients as close follow-up is needed. Better if anal dysplasia clinic available for close follow-up
	  ■ With proper selection, local control >90%
	■ Radiotherapy alone (Martenson and Gunderson 1993)
	  ■ Final dose to primary of 65 Gy with 45 Gy prophylaxis to LN

T1-2N0 status post excision, close or involved margins	■ May consider abbreviated concurrent chemo-RT (Hatfield et al. 2008)
	  ■ ~5% local failures after 42 month follow-up in 21 patients
	  ■ Used 30 Gy with one cycle of mitomycin + 5-FU
	■ At UCSF with positive microscopic margins, we use ~45 Gy final dose (36 Gy to primary and elective LN with 9 Gy boost to primary) and two cycles of mitomycin + 5-FU

I–III with intact sphincter	■ Concurrent chemo-RT with 5-FU/mitomycin C ■ CR7 ~50–90% depending on stage
IV	■ Individualized treatment depending on case
Salvage, or if prior pelvic RT	■ APR with colostomy – salvage rate after chemo-RT failure is ~50%

continued

VI

Anal margin tumors	■ Wide local excision with ≥1 cm margin. Well-differentiated T1N0 can be observed with close follow-up. All others get definitive chemo-RT to primary with elective inguinal LN RT for T2-4 and poorly differentiated tumors. Include pelvic LN if involvement of anal canal above dentate line. Alternative is post-op RT or chemo-RT with inguinal management as above. Dose 45 Gy elective, 60 Gy to gross disease

TRIALS

CHEMO-RT VS. RT

- *UKCCCRi* (1996): 585 patients. RT: 45 Gy + boost (15 Gy EBRT or 25 Gy brachy) ± 5-FU+mitomycin. Six week break in RT. Chemo-RT improved 3-year LC (59 vs. 36%), but no significant change in 3-year OS (65 vs. 58%). Poorer results with RT alone may be due to mandatory 6 week break.
- *EORTC* (Bartelink et al. 1997): 110 patients. T3-4N0-3 or T1-2N1-3. RT (45 Gy + 15–20 Gy boost) + concurrent chemo (bolus 5-FU+mitomycin) vs. RT alone. Six week break in RT, prior to boost. Chemo-RT improved CR rate (80 vs. 54%), 5-year LC (68 vs. 50%), colostomy-free survival (72 vs. 40%), and PFS (61 vs. 43%). No difference in OS (57 vs. 52%). Poorer results with RT alone may again be due to mandatory 6 week break.
- *RTOG 87-04* (Flam et al. 1996): 291 patients. 45 Gy + 5FU ±mitomycin. If no CR at 6 weeks, gave 9 Gy boost + 5-FU/cisplatin. 5-FU given bolus × 4 day starting d1, d29 (1,000 mg/m^2/day). Mitomycin given as 10 mg/m^2 bolus d1, d29. Mitomycin improved CR rate (92 vs. 85%) and decreased 4-year colostomy rate (9 vs. 22%). No difference in 4-year OS (75 vs. 70%).
- *RTOG 92-08* (John et al. 1996): dose escalation, phase II. 5-FU+ mitomycin+ 59.6 Gy. Two week break included. Closed early. Colostomy rate at 2 years: 30%. Higher colostomy rate may be due to 2 week break.

ROLE OF CISPLATIN

- *ACT II* (James et al. 2009): 940 patients with anal cancer [stage T1–T2 (50%), T3–T4 (43%); LN-(62%), LN+ (30%)] treated with 5-FU (1,000 mg/m^2/day on d1-4 and 29–32) and RT (50.4 Gy in 28 fx), randomized to either concurrent MMC (12 mg/m^2, d1) or cisplatin (60 mg/m^2 on d1 and 29), and also randomized to maintenance therapy (2c of cisplatin/5-FU weeks 11 and 14) 4 weeks after chemo-RT or no maintenance therapy. There was no difference in CR rate (94–95%). MMC patients had more acute grade 3/4 hematological toxicities (25 vs. 13%). Preliminary analysis shows no significant difference in RFS ($p = 0.42$) or OS ($p = 0.19$) for the maintenance comparison. The authors conclude that 5-FU, MMC with RT remains the standard of care.

- Based on the above results of those of RTOG 98-11 (see below), most believe that 5-FU/MMC chemotherapy remains the standard of care.

NEOADJUVANT CHEMO

- *RTOG 98-11* (Ajani et al. 2008): 644 patients. Neoadjuvant cisplatin + 5-FU × 2 followed by concurrent cisplatin + 5-FU × 2 and 45–59 Gy vs. concurrent 5-FU + mitomycin and 45–59 Gy. No significant difference in 5-year OS (70 vs. 75%) or 5-year DFS (54 vs. 60%). Cumulative colostomy rate less for mitomycin arm (10%) than cisplatin arm (19%).
- *CALGB 9281* (Meropol et al. 2008): 45 patients. Neoadjuvant chemo trial for poor prognosis anal carcinoma (T3/T4 and/or N2/N3), phase II. Neoadjuvant cisplatin + 5-FU × 2 followed by concurrent mitomycin + 5-FU × 2 and 45 Gy followed by possible single cycle of cisplatin + 5-FU and 9 Gy boost. Two week break included. Four-year data: OS 68%, DFS 61, 23% colostomy rate.
- No proven advantage to neoadjuvant chemo exists, but it may be used in cases of abscess or fistula.

INFUSIONAL 5-FU VS. CAPECITABINE

- Phase II data exist with substitution of infusional 5-FU with oral capecitabine concurrently with mitomycin and RT in anal cancer with overall low toxicity (Glynne-Jones et al. 2008).
- Phase III data needed.

HIV

- Hoffman et al. (1999): seventeen HIV+ patients. Nine had CD4 ≥ 200: no hospitalization or colostomy. Eight had CD4 < 200: 4 hospitalized, 4 colostomies.

BRACHYTHERAPY

- Higher complication rates. Not frequently used in North America due to the risk of necrosis. Six percent complication requiring surgery (Ng 1988). Rates of necrosis in the range of 7–15% (Sandhu et al. 1998; Gerard et al. 1998).

IMRT

- Salama et al. (2007): retrospective analysis of 53 patients treated at three institutions with concurrent IMRT and 5-FU-MMC (in most cases). Eighteen months OS 93%, colostomy-free survival 84%, pCR 93%. No grade 4+ skin/GI toxicity. Thiry-eight percent had grade 3 skin toxicity and 15% grade 3 GI toxicity. Compares favorably with results of RTOG 98-11.
- Milano et al. (2005): retrospective analysis of 17 patients treated at single institution with concurrent IMRT and 5-FU-MMC (in most cases). Two-year OS 91%, colostomy-free survival 82%. No grade 3+ nonhematologic toxicity.

POSTTREATMENT BIOPSY

- Cummings et al. (1991): no benefit to routine rebiopsy at 6 weeks postchemo-RT. Continued regression of tumor for up to 12 months, mean time to regression 3 months.
- Follow patients clinically. Biopsy for clinically suspicious lesions.

SALVAGE APR

- Ellenhorn et al. (1994): retrospective review of 38 patients treated with RT + 5-FU + mitomycin. Overall, 5-year OS was 44% when salvage APR used for chemo-RT failure.

RADIATION TECHNIQUES

GENERAL POINTS

- No randomized data of chemo-RT vs. surgery alone, but chemo-RT produces better survival with sphincter preservation as compared to historical controls.
- Chemotherapy is concurrent 5-FU/mitomycin.
- Plan to treat inguinal nodes.
- Minimize breaks (try to keep under 2 weeks).
- HIV+ patients with CD4 < 200.

  - Smaller field: superior border of initial pelvic field is usually the bottom of SI joints.
  - Increased morbidity (Hoffman et al. 1999).
  - Final tumor dose may need to be decreased to 50 Gy.
  - A second cycle of MMC is often withheld and 5-FU may be dose reduced.
- IMRT is currently used in most cases at UCSF.

SIMULATION AND PLANNING

- Simulate patient supine with alpha cradle to immobilize legs
- Anal marker to mark anal verge
- Wire perianal area
- Wire inguinal node regions
- If possible, treat with full bladder to minimize small bowel toxicity and use small bowel contrast 90 min prior to simulation

CONVENTIONAL PLANNING (RTOG 98-11 TECHNIQUE)

- Targets: primary tumor, grossly enlarged LN, internal/external iliac LN, inguinal LN.
- Initial large field (all patients) treated AP/PA, energy 18 MV AP, 6 MV PA, dose 30.6 Gy at 1.8 Gy/fx.
  - Borders: superior = L5/S1. Inferior = 2.5 cm margin on anus and tumor. AP field includes lateral inguinal nodes. PA field = 2 cm lateral to greater sciatic notch (not including lateral inguinal LN).
  - Supplementary RT delivered to inguinal nodes with anterior electron fields matched with exit of PA field.
- Reduced field #1 (all patients) drops AP/PA superior border to inferior border of sacroiliac joints and is treated 14.4 Gy at 1.8 Gy/fx (total 45). If N0, field reduced off inguinal nodes after 36 Gy.
- Reduced field #2 (for T3–T4, LN+, and T2 lesions with residual disease after 45 Gy).
  - Boost original tumor plus 2–2.5 cm margin 10–14 Gy at 2 Gy/fz(total 55–59 Gy) using either a multifield technique or laterals or a direct photon or electron perineal field.
  - Involved pelvic LN should be included if small bowel can be avoided. Involved inguinal LN also boosted with 2–2.5 cm margin 10–14 Gy at 2 Gy/fx (total 55–59 Gy) with electrons.

UCSF IMRT PLANNING (MOST CASES AT UCSF CURRENTLY)

- Use bolus on palpable groin nodes. If not palpable, no bolus needed.
- Plan with 2–4 mm of inguinal skin sparing as appropriate.
- Targets: primary tumor, grossly enlarged LN, internal/external iliac LN, inguinal LN.
- CTV margins.
  - Primary tumor: 3 cm around gross disease in anal area and include perirectal nodes along with anal canal.
  - LN: 1.5–2 cm around gross disease.
- Uses sequential plans, cumulative dose to primary tumor is 55.8 Gy.
- PTV and dose prescriptions.
  - For N0 patients.
    - PTV1 = Anal area, inguinal LN, and pelvic LN extending from L5/S1 down to 3 cm below tumor (always include anal verge). Dose 36 Gy at 1.8 Gy/fx.
    - PTV2 = Primary tumor. 19.8 Gy at 1.8 Gy/fx (total 55.8 Gy).
  - For N+ patients, LN ≤ 1.5 cm:
    - PTV1 = same as N0
    - PTV2 = Primary tumor and LN ≤ 1.5 cm. 9 Gy at 1.8 Gy/fx (total 45 Gy)
    - PTV3 = Primary tumor. 10.8 Gy at 1.8 Gy/fx (total 55.8 Gy)
  - For N+ patients, LN > 1.5 cm:
    - PTV1 = same as N0
    - PTV2 = Primary tumor and LN > 1.5 cm. 19.8 Gy at 1.8 Gy/fx (total 55.8 Gy)
- Patients are generally treated with 7-field IMRT plan: 2 AO, 2 laterals, 2 PO, and 1 PA.
- Beams are 18 MV, except for anterior obliques which are 6 MV. However, if disease extends to the anal verge or margin, use 6 MV for PA and PO fields.

RTOG IMRT TECHNIQUE (BASED ON RTOG 05-29)

- RTOG has published an anorectal contouring atlas (Myerson et al. 2008; see Fig. 23.1)
- Uses dose-painting (all PTVs treated simultaneously), rather than shrinking-field IMRT (as at UCSF)
- For T2N0
  - PTVA (primary tumor): 50.4 Gy in 28 fx of 1.8 Gy
  - PTV42 (all nodal regions receives): 42 Gy in 28 fx of 1.5 Gy

- For T3-4N0
  - PTVA: 54 Gy in 30 fx of 1.8
  - PTV45: 45 Gy in 30 fx of 1.5 Gy
- For N+:
  - PTVA: 54 Gy in 30 fx of 1.8 Gy
  - PTV45 (uninvolved LN): 45 Gy in 30 fx of 1.5 Gy
  - PTV50 (LN≤3 cm): 50.4 Gy in 30 fx of 1.68 Gy
  - PTV54 (LN>3 cm): 54 Gy in 30 fx of 1.8 Gy
- For further details, see http://www.rtog.org/members/protocols/0529/0529.pdf (Figs. 23.1a–c and 23.2)

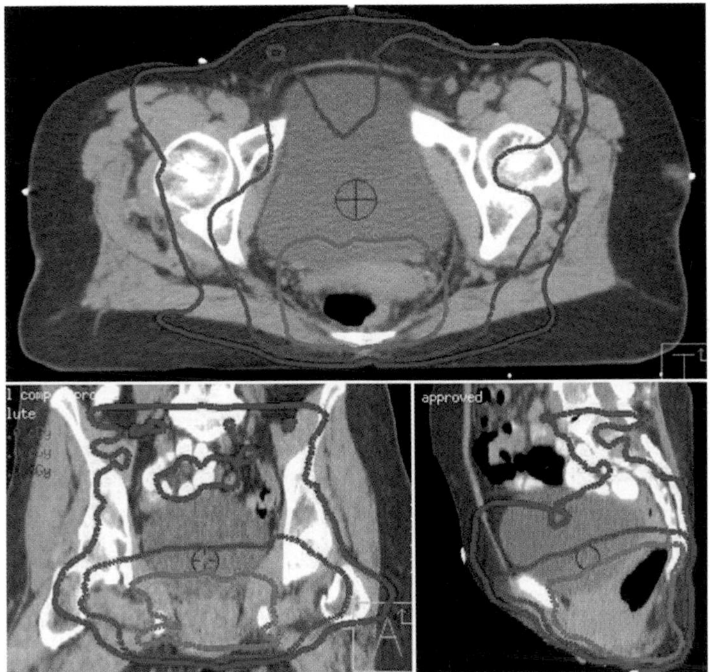

Fig. 23.1 A 71-year-old woman treated with UCSF IMRT technique for cT2N1M0 (stage IIIA) anal carcinoma. Isodose lines: 36 Gy (*pink*), 45 Gy (*brown*), and 55 Gy (*aqua*). PTV1 was treated to 36 Gy at 1.8 Gy/fx at the 93% IDL, PTV2 to 45 Gy cumulative (9 Gy boost at 1.8 Gy/fx) at the 90% IDL, and PTV3 to 55.8 Gy cumulative (10.8 Gy second boost at 1.8 Gy/fx) at the 90% IDL. Note that PTV2 is directed primarily to the left due to the presence of an FDG-avid lymph node

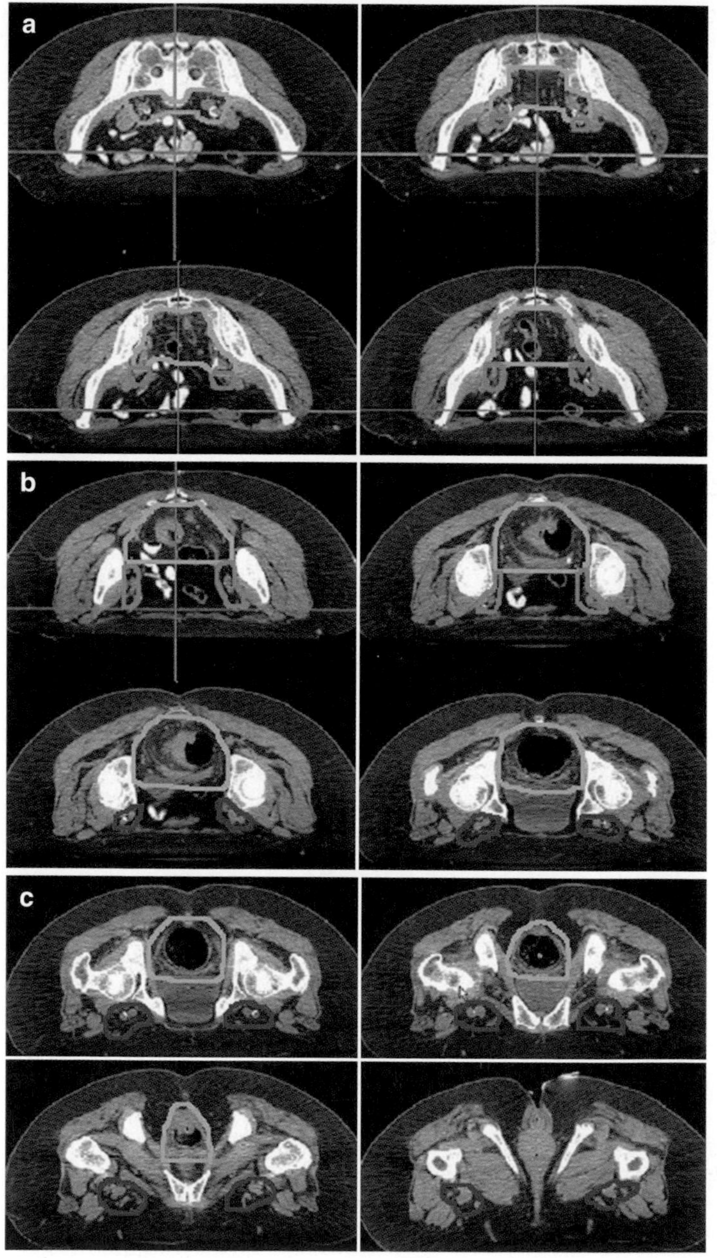
a
b
c

DOSE LIMITATIONS

- Small bowel: 45–50 Gy max point dose; V30 < 200 cc
- Vulva/Penis: 25 Gy max point dose; V20 < 50%
- Femoral Neck: 45 Gy
- Additional dose constraints are listed in RTOG protocol 0529 referenced above

COMPLICATIONS

- Acute complications: skin reaction/desquamation, leukopenia, thrombocytopenia, proctitis, diarrhea, cystitis.
- Subacute and late complications include chronic diarrhea, rectal urgency, sterility, impotence, vaginal dryness, vaginal fibrosis/stenosis (use vaginal dilator status post XRT to help avoid), and possibly decreased testosterone.

FOLLOW-UP

- H&P and anal exam every 6 weeks until CR, then every 3 months for first year, every 4 months for second year, every 6 months for third year, then annually.
- Consider PET/CT ~2 months after treatment as persistently abnormal FDG uptake correlated with poor 2-year CSS (39%, Schwarz et al. 2008).
- For T3–T4 or inguinal LN+: consider annual CXR and pelvic CT for 3 years.
- On exam if mass increases in size, or new clinical symptoms develop (pain, bleeding, incontinence) → biopsy. If + → salvage APR.
- If tumor decreasing in size, continue to follow. Median time to regression ~3 months, but may take 12 months.
- Most recurrences occur within 2 years. Most are at primary site.
- Anal pap, if available, is useful for follow-up.
- Consider vaginal dilator in women who are treated and do not regularly engage in intercourse to help prevent stenosis/narrowing.
- Male patients may notice decrease in ejaculate; testosterone levels may be checked for sexual difficulties.

Fig. 23.2 RTOG consensus contours for elective clinical target coverage for anorectal cancer. *Yellow* = CTVA (perirectal, presacral, internal iliac), *blue* = CTVB (external iliac), *red* = CTVC (inguinal). Upper pelvis; mid-pelvis; lower pelvis. (Reprinted with the permission from Elsevier. Adapted from Myerson et al. 2008)

Acknowledgement We thank Richard M. Krieg for his valuable advice in the preparation of this chapter.

REFERENCES

Ajani JA, Winter KA, Gunderson LL, et al. Fluorouracil, mitomycin, and radiotherapy vs fluorouracil, cisplatin, and radiotherapy for carcinoma of the anal canal: a Randomized Controlled Trial. *JAMA* 2008;299(16):1914-1921.

Bartelink H, Roelofsen F, et al. Concomitant radiotherapy and chemotherapy is superior to radiotherapy alone in the treatment of locally advanced anal cancer: results of a phase iii randomized trial of the European Organization for Research and Treatment of Cancer Radiotherapy and Gastrointestinal Cooperative Groups. *J Clin Oncol* 1997;15:2040-2049.

Cotter SE, Grigsby PW, Siegel BA, et al. FDG-PET/CT in the evaluation of anal carcinoma. *Int J Radiat Oncol Biol Phys* 2006;65:720-725.

Cummings BJ, Keane TJ, O'Sullivan B, et al. Epidermoid anal cancer: treatment by radiation alone or by radiation and 5-fluorouracil with and without mitomycin-c. *Int J Radiat Oncol Biol Phys* 1991;21(5):1115-1125.

Ellenhorn JDI, Enker WE, Quan SH. Salvage abdominoperineal resection following combined chemotherapy and radiotherapy for epidermoid carcinoma of the anus. *Ann Surg Oncol* 1994;1:105-110.

Flam M, Madhu J, et al. Role of mitomycin in combination with fluorouracil and radiotherapy, and of salvage chemoradiation in the definitive nonsurgical treatment of epidermoid carcinoma of the anal canal: results of a Phase III Randomized Intergroup Study. *J Clin Oncol* 1996;14:2527-2539.

Gerard JP, Ayzac L, et al. Treatment of anal canal carcinoma with high dose radiation therapy and concomitant fluorouracil-cisplatinum. Long-term results in 95 patients. *Radiother Oncol* 1998;46(3):249-256.

Glynne-Jones R, Meadows H, Wan S, et al. Extra – a multicenter phase ii study of chemoradiation using a 5 day per week oral regimen of capecitabine and intravenous mitomycin c in anal cancer. *Int J Radiat Oncol Biol Phys* 2008;72(1):119-126.

Greenall MJ, Quan HQ, Decosse JJ. Epidermoid cancer of the anus. *Br J Surg* 1985;72:S97.

Hatfield P, Cooper R, Sebag-Montefiore D. involved-field, low-dose chemoradiotherapy for early-stage anal carcinoma. *Int J Radiat Oncol Biol Phys* 2008;70(2):419-424.

Hoffman R, Welton ML, et al. The significance of pretreatment CD4 count on the outcome and treatment tolerance of HIV-positive patients with anal cancer. *Int J Radiat Oncol Biol Phys* 1999;44:127-131.

James R, Wan S, Glynne-Jones D, et al. A randomized trial of chemoradiation using mitomycin or cisplatin, with or without maintenance cisplatin/5FU in squamous cell carcinoma of the anus (ACT II). Abstract LBA4009. Presented at ASCO annual meeting, May 30, 2009.

John M, Pajak T, et al. Dose escalation in chemoradiation for anal cancer: preliminary results of RTOG 92-08. *Cancer J Sci Am* 1996;2(4):205.

Koh WJ, Chiu M, Stelzer KJ, et al. Femoral vessel depth and the implications for groin node radiation. *Int J Radiat Oncol Biol Phys* 1993;27:969-974.

Martenson JA, Gunderson LL. External radiation therapy without chemotherapy in the management of anal cancer. *Cancer* 1993;71(5):1736-1740.

Meropol NJ, Niedzwiecki D, Shank B, et al. Induction therapy for poor-prognosis anal canal carcinoma: a Phase II Study of the Cancer and Leukemia Group B (CALGB 9281). *J Clin Oncol* 2008;26(19):3229-3234.

Milano MT, Jani AB, Farrey KJ, et al. Intensity-modulated radiation therapy (IMRT) in the treatment of anal cancer: toxicity and clinical outcome. *Int J Radiat Biol Phys* 2005;63:354-361.

Myerson RJ, et al. Elective clinical target volumes for conformal therapy in anorectal cancer: an Radiation Therapy Oncology Group consensus panel contouring atlas. *Int J Radiat Oncol Biol Phys* 2008;74:824-830.

Ng Y, Ying Kin NY, Pigneux J, et al. Our experience of conservative treatment of anal cancal carcinoma combining external irradiation and interstitial implants. *Int J Radiat Oncol Biol Phys* 1988;14:253-259.

Papagikos M, Crane CH, et al. Chemoradiation for adenocarcinoma of the anus. *Int J Radiat Oncol Biol Phys* 2003;55:669-678.

Salama JK, Mell LK, Schomas DA, et al. Concurrent chemotherapy and intensity-modulated radiation therapy for anal canal cancer patients: a multicenter experience. *J Clin Oncol* 2007;29:4851-4856.

Sandhu APS, Symonds RP, et al. Interstitial Iridium-192 implantation combined with external radiotherapy in anal cancer: ten years experience. *Int J Radiat Oncol Biol Phys* 1998;40: 575-581.

Schwarz JK, Siegel BA, Dehdashti F, et al. Tumor response and survival predicted by post-therapy FDG-PET/CT in anal cancer. *Int J Radiat Oncol Biol Phys* 2008;71(1):180-186.

Trautmann TG, Zuger JH. Positron emission tomography for pretreatment staging and post-treatment evaluation in cancer of the anal canal. *Mol Imaging Biol* 2005;7:309-313.

UKCCCR Anal Cancer Trial Working Party. Epidermoid anal cancer: results from the UKCCCR randomized trial of radiotherapy alone versus radiotherapy, 5-fluorouracil, and mitomycin. *Lancet* 1996;348:1049-1054.

FURTHER READING

Boman BM, Moertel CG, et al. Carcinoma of the anal canal. A clinical and pathological study of 188 cases. Cancer 1984;54:114-125.

Janjan NA, Ballo MT et al. The Anal Region. In: Cox JD, Ang KK, editors. Radiation oncology: rationale, technique, results. 8th ed. St. Louis: Mosby; 2003. 537-556.

Jemal A, Siegel R, Ward E, et al. Cancer statistics, 2008. *CA Cancer J Clin* 2008;52(2):71-96.

Minsky BD. Cancer of the Anal Canal. In: Leibel SA, Phillips TL, editors. Textbook of radiation oncology. 2nd ed. Philadelphia: Saunders; 2004. 913-922.

Papillon J, Montbarbon JF. Epidermoid carcinoma of the anal canal. A Series of 276 cases. *Dis Colon Rectum* 1987;30:324-333.

Peiffert D, Bey P, Pernot M, et al. Conservative treatment by irradiation of epidermoid carcinomas of the anal margin. *Int J Radiat Oncol Biol Phys* 1997;39:57-66.

PART VII

Genitourinary Sites

VII

STAGING: RENAL CELL CARCINOMA

Editors' note: All TNM stage and stage groups referred to elsewhere in this chapter reflect the 2002 AJCC staging nomenclature unless otherwise noted as the new system below was published after this chapter was written.

(AJCC 6TH ED., 2002)

Primary tumor (T)

TX: Primary tumor cannot be assessed
T0: No evidence of primary tumor
T1: Tumor 7 cm or less in greatest dimension, limited to the kidney
  T1a: Tumor 4 cm or less in greatest dimension, limited to the kidney
  T1b: Tumor more than 4 cm but not more than 7 cm in greatest dimension, limited to the kidney
T2: Tumor more than 7 cm, limited to the kidney
T3: Tumor extends into major veins or invades adrenal gland or perirenal and/or renal sinus fat, but not beyond Gerota's fascia
  T3a: Tumor directly invades adrenal gland or perirenal and/or renal sinus fat, but not beyond Gerota's fascia
  T3b: Tumor grossly extends into the renal vein or its segmental (muscle-containing) branches, or vena cava below the diaphragm
  T3c: Tumor grossly extends into vena cava above diaphragm or invades the wall of the vena cava
T4: Tumor invades beyond Gerota's fascia

Regional lymph nodes* (N)

NX: Regional lymph nodes cannot be assessed
N0: No regional lymph node metastasis
N1: Metastases in a single regional lymph node
N2: Metastasis in more than one regional lymph node

*Laterality does not affect the N classification

Regional lymph nodes: Renal hilar, paracaval, aortic (paraaortic, periaortic, lateral aortic), Retroperitoneal NOS.

Note: If a lymph node dissection is performed, pathologic evaluation would ordinarily include at least eight nodes.

(AJCC 7TH ED., 2010)

Primary tumor (T)

TX: Primary tumor cannot be assessed
T0: No evidence of primary tumor
T1: Tumor 7 cm or less in greatest dimension, limited to the kidney
  T1a: Tumor 4 cm or less in greatest dimension, limited to the kidney
  T1b: Tumor more than 4 cm, but not more than 7 cm in greatest dimension limited to the kidney
T2: Tumor more than 7 cm in greatest dimension, limited to the kidney
  T2a: Tumor more than 7 cm, but less than or equal to 10 cm in greatest dimension, limited to the kidney
  T2b: Tumor more than 10 cm, limited to the kidney
T3: Tumor extends into major veins or perinephric tissues, but not into the ipsilateral adrenal gland and not beyond Gerota's fascia
  T3a: Tumor grossly extends into the renal vein or its segmental (muscle-containing) branches, or tumor invades perirenal and/or renal sinus fat, but not beyond Gerota's fascia
  T3b: Tumor grossly extends into the vena cava below the diaphragm
  T3c: Tumor grossly extends into the vena cava above the diaphragm or invades the wall of the venacava
T4: Tumor invades beyond Gerota's fascia (including contiguous extension into the ipsilateral adrenal gland)

Regional lymph nodes (N)

NX: Regional lymph nodes cannot be assessed
N0: No regional lymph node metastasis
N1: Metastasis in regional lymph node(s)

continued

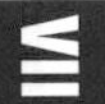

Distant metastasis (M)

MX: Distant metastasis cannot be assessed
M0: No distant metastasis
M1: Distant metastasis

Stage grouping

0: TisN0M0
I : T1N0M0
II: T2N0M0
III: T3N0M0, T1-3N1M0
IV: T4N0-1M0, AnyTN2M0 Any M1

~5-Years OS by stage

I: ~85–90%
II: ~65–85%
III: ~40–60%
IV: ~30% if only 1 metastatic site <10% if >1 metastatic site

Used with the permission from the American Joint Committee on Cancer (AJCC), Chicago, IL. The original source for this material is the AJCC Cancer Staging Manual, Sixth Edition (2002), published by Springer Science+Business Media.

Distant metastasis (M)

M0: No distant metastasis
M1: Distant metastasis

Anatomic stage/prognostic groups

I: T1 N0 M0
II: T2 N0 M0
III: T1 or T2 N1 M0
T3 N0 or N1 M0
IV: T4 Any N M0
Any T Any N M1

Used with the permission from the American Joint Committee on Cancer (AJCC), Chicago, IL. The original source for this material is the AJCC Cancer Staging Manual, Seventh Edition (2010), published by Springer Science+Business Media.

TREATMENT RECOMMENDATIONS

2002 Stage	Recommended treatment

I–III	■ Nephrectomy
	  ■ Open radical nephrectomy, but laparoscopic gaining popularity. Nephron sparing surgery via partial nephrectomy, if possible (open or laparoscopic)
	  ■ Possible to spare adrenal gland in ~75% cases
	■ No role for adjuvant chemo/immunotherapy
	■ No widely accepted role for neoadjuvant or adjuvant radiotherapy. Retrospective data suggest possible utility in select cases:
	  ■ Positive surgical margins
	  ■ Locally advanced disease with perinephric fat invasion and adrenal invasion (IVC/renal vein extension alone does not increase local recurrence significantly)
	  ■ LN+
	  ■ Unresectable (pre-op RT)

IV	■ *Cytoreductive nephrectomy*: improved survival with nephrectomy followed by interferon alpha vs. interferon alpha alone (Flanigan et al. 2001)
	■ *Systemic therapy*
	  ■ Immunotherapy (IL-2, interferon alpha, or combination)
	    ■ High dose IL-2 only FDA approved treatment for Stage IV RCC
	  ■ Biologic agents show promise in recent trials
	    ■ Bevacizumab
	    ■ Sorafenib or sunitinib
	    ■ Temsirolimus
	Consider chemo (gemcitabine ± 5-FU or capecitabine)
	  ■ Focal palliation of metastases
	    ■ RT alone
	    ■ Metastasectomy
	    ■ Combination of both

TRIALS

RADIOTHERAPY

- Two prospective randomized European trials (Rotterdam trial, Sweden trial) showed no benefit to preoperative radiotherapy in terms of OS or PFS.
- Two prospective randomized trials (Fugitt, Cancer, 1973; Kjaer et al. 1987) showed no benefit to postoperative radiotherapy, yet these trials did not select a patient population that was likely to benefit from adjuvant RT. LR in radical nephrectomy series is

~5%. These excellent results are driven mainly by completely resected stage I/II tumors. However, with incomplete resection or +LN, LR rises dramatically to ~20–30%, suggesting a role for adjuvant RT in these patients. The following two studies retrospectively analyze patients at high risk for local recurrence and support a role for adjuvant RT in select patients.

- Kao et al. (1994): Retrospective study of 12 consecutive patients with locally advanced RCC (perinephric invasion or +margins) who received adjuvant RT 41–63 Gy (1.8–2 Gyfx) – 100% 5-year LC, with 5-year actuarial DFS 75% compared with 30% in 12 consecutive patients of similar stage treated with surgery alone.
- Stein et al. (1992): Retrospective study of 147 patients treated with post-op RT (median 46 Gy) vs. observation. In the T3N0 patients, LR was 10% vs. 37% favoring adjuvant RT. Also, 3/19 recurrences at the scar.

SYSTEMIC THERAPY

- *Escudier/AVOREN* (Escudier et al. 2007b): randomized, phase III trial; 649 patients with untreated metastatic RCC given interferon-alfa with either bevacizumab vs. placebo. PFS 10.2 vs. 5.4 months (HR 0.63, $p = 0.0001$).
- *Escudier/TARGET* (Escudier et al. 2007a): randomized, phase III trial; 903 patients with treatment-resistant RCC given sorafenib vs. placebo. PFS 5.5 vs. 2.8 months (HR 0.44; $p < 0.01$) favoring sorafenib. Toxicity higher in sorafenib arm.
- Motzer et al. (2007): randomized, phase III trial; 750 patients with untreated, metastatic RCC given sunitinib vs. interferon-alfa. PFS 11 vs. 5 months (HR 0.42; $p < 0.001$), RR 31 vs. 6% ($p < 0.001$), favoring sunitinib.

RADIATION TECHNIQUES

SIMULATION AND FIELD DESIGN

Primary site

- Supine, arms-up to allow visualization of lateral isocenter marks, immobilize with wing-board or alpha cradle, wire scar, planning CT scan.
- *Volume*: nephrectomy bed (involved kidney if pre-op), lymph-node drainage sites, surgical clips; scar failures reported [Stein], so if not possible to include scar in treatment volume, treat it with electrons to full dose. SRS currently under active study.

Metastatic site (non-CNS)

- Proper immobilization depending on site; planning CT if 3DCRT needed to spare normal tissue
- *Volume:* focal treatment of metastasis with 2–3 cm margin
- See Chap. 40 for management of CNS metastases

DOSE PRESCRIPTIONS

- Pre-op: 40–50 Gy (1.8–2 Gy/fx)
- Post-op: 45–50 Gy with 10–15 Gy boost to micro/gross disease; total 50–60 Gy
- Metastases: 45–50 Gy in 3–4.5 weeks

DOSE LIMITATIONS

- Contralateral kidney: limit to ≤20 Gy in 2–3 weeks
- Liver: limit to <30% receiving >36–40 Gy
- Spinal cord: <45 Gy
- Small bowel: <40 Gy

FOLLOW-UP (NCCN 2009 RECOMMENDATIONS)

VII

- *Stage I–III*: every 6 months × 2 years, then every 1 year × 5 years – H&P, CXR, Labs with LDH; CT chest/abdomen/pelvis at 4–6 months then as indicated.

REFERENCES

Escudier B, Eisen T, Stadler WM, et al. TARGET study group. Sorafenib in advanced clear cell renal-cell carcinoma. NEJM 2007;356:125–134.

Escudier B, Pluzanska A, Koralewski P. AVOREN trial investigator. Bevacizumab plus interferon alfa-2a for treatment of metastatic renal cell carcinoma: a randomized, double-blind phase III trial. Lancet 2007;370:2103–2111.

Flanigan RC, Salmon SE, Blumenstein BA, et al. Nephrectomy followed by interferon alfa-2b compared with interferon alfa-2b alone for metastatic renal-cell cancer. N Engl J Med 2001;345(23):1655–1659.

Fugitt RB, Wu GS, Martinelli LC. An evaluation of postoperative radiotherapy in hypernephroma treatment - a clinical trial. Cancer 1973;32(6):1332-1334.

Kao GD, Malkowicz SB, Whittington R, et al. Locall advanced renal cell carcinoma: low complication rate and efficacy of postnephrectomy planned with CT. Radiology 1994;193(3):725–730.

Kjaer M, Frederiksen PL, Engelholm SA. Postoperative radiotherapy in stage II and III renal adenocarcinoma. A randomized trial by the Copenhagen Renal Cancer Study Group. Int J Radiat Oncol Biol Phys 1987;13(4):665–672.

Motzer RJ, Hudson TE, Tomczak P, et al. Sunitinib versus interferon alfa in metastatic renal cell carcinoma. NEJM 2007;356:115–124.

National Comprehensive Cancer Network. Clinical Practice Guidelines in Oncology: Kidney Cancer. Available at: http://www.nccn.org/professionals/physician_gls/PDF/kidney.pdf. Accessed on May 1, 2009.

Stein M, Kuten A, Halpern J, et al. The value of postoperative irradiation in renal cell cancer. Radiother Oncol 1992;24(1):41–44.

FURTHER READING

Finney R. The value of radiotherapy in the treatment of hypernephroma – a clinical trial. Br J Urol 1973;45(3):258–269.

Greene FL; American Joint Committee on Cancer, American Cancer Society. AJCC Cancer Staging Manual. 6th ed. New York: Springer; 2002.

Juusela H, Malmio K, Alfthan O, et al. Preoperative irradiation in the treatment of renal adenocarcinoma. Scand J Urol Nephrol 1977;11:277–281.

Michalski JM. Kidney, Renal Pelvis, and Ureter. In: Halperin EC, Perez CA, Brady LW, et al., editors. Principles and Practice of Radiation Oncology. 5th ed. Philadelphia: Lippincott Williams & Wilkins; 2008. pp. 1397–1411.

Redman BG, Kawachi M, Hurwitz M. Urothelial and kidney cancers. In: Pazdur R, Coia L, Hoskins W., Wagman L, editors. Cancer Management: A Multidisciplinary Approach. 8th ed. New York: CMP Healthcare Media; 2004. pp. 403–418.

Schefter T, Rabinovitch R. Cancer of the Kidney In: Leibel SA, Phiilips TL, editors. Textbook of Radiation Oncology. 2nd ed. Philadelphia: Saunders; 2004. pp. 923–938.

van der Werf-Messing B, van der Heul RO, Ledeboer RC. Renal cell carcinoma trial. Strahlentherapie (Sonderb) 1981;76:169–715.

Chapter 25
Bladder Cancer

William Foster, Brian Lee, and Joycelyn L. Speight

PEARLS

- Risk factors: smoking, napthylamines, dyes, cytoxan exposure. Chronic irritation, i.e., bladder stones, chronic indwelling foley catheter
- Primary lymphatic drainage: hypogastric, obturator, iliac (internal and external), perivesical, sacral, presacral
- Secondary lymphatic drainage: common iliac
- Tumors tend to be multifocal in nature
- Transitional cell carcinoma (TCC) constitutes 93% of cases in the U.S.; TCC with squamous or glandular features behaves like pure TCC
- Squamous cell carcinoma (SCC) constitutes 5% of cases (primary histology seen in Egypt due to Schistosoma infections)
- Adenocarcinoma uncommon 1–2% (most often in dome of bladder; urachal remnant)
- Most common sites = trigone (inferiorly below ureterovesical junctions), lateral and posterior walls, and bladder neck
- Common presenting symptoms: hematuria (gross or microscopic; 75% of cases), irritative voiding (25–30%), pelvic pain, obstructive uropathy, hydronephrosis
- At presentation, 75% of cases are Ta, Tis, or T1
- Probability of lymph node (LN) involvement (~20% overall): pT1 5%, pT2-T3a 30%, pT3b 64%, pT4 50% (Skinner et al.)
- Incidence of distant metastases (DM) at diagnosis ~8–10%; lung, bone, liver

WORKUP

- H&P; Labs: CBC, BUN, Cr, alkaline phosphatase, UA
- Urine cytology: identifies 50–80% of poorly differentiated CA, but only 20% of well-differentiated CA
- Cystoscopy with bladder mapping and EUA

- TURBT with random biopsies of normal appearing mucosa to exclude CIS. If trigone involved, biopsy prostatic urethra
- CT A/P with contrast including imaging of upper urinary tracts; historically, IVP used
- Chest X-ray (CXR) and/or CT chest if stage ≥T2; bone scan if symptomatic or alkaline phosphatase elevated
- Pre-op MRI valuable to evaluate depth of invasion, staging

STAGING: BLADDER CANCER

Editors' note: All TNM stage and stage groups referred to elsewhere in this chapter reflect the 2002 AJCC staging nomenclature unless otherwise noted as the new system below was published after this chapter was written.

(AJCC 6TH ED., 2002)

Primary tumor (T)
TX: Primary tumor cannot be assessed
T0: No evidence of primary tumor
Ta: Noninvasive papillary carcinoma
Tis: Carcinoma in situ
T1: Tumor invades subepithelial connective tissue
T2: Tumor invades muscle
  pT2a: Tumor invades superficial muscle (inner half)
  pT2b: Tumor invades deep muscle (outer half)
T3a: Perivesical tumor, microscopic
T3b: Perivesical tumor, macroscopic
T4a: Tumor invades prostate, uterus, vagina
T4b: Invades pelvic wall, abdominal wall

Regional lymph nodes (N)
N1: Metastasis in single lymph node, 2 cm or less in greatest dimension
N2: Metastasis in single lymph node, more than 2 cm but not more than 5 cm in greatest dimension; or multiple lymph nodes, not more than 5 cm in greatest dimension
N3: Metastasis in a lymph node, more than 5 cm in greatest dimension

Metastases (M)
MX: Distant metastasis cannot be assessed
M0: No distant metastasis
M1: Distant metastases

Stage grouping
0a: TaN0M0
0is: TisN0M0

(AJCC 7TH ED., 2010)

Primary tumor (T)
TX: Primary tumor cannot be assessed
T0: No evidence of primary tumor
Ta: Noninvasive papillary carcinoma
Tis: Carcinoma in situ: "flat tumor"
T1: Tumor invades subepithelial connective tissue
T2: Tumor invades muscularis propria
  pT2a: Tumor invades superficial muscularis propria (inner half)
  pT2b: Tumor invades deep muscularis propria (outer half)
T3: Tumor invades perivesical tissue
  pT3a: Microscopically
  pT3b: Macroscopically (extravesical mass)
T4: Tumor invades any of the following: prostatic stroma, seminal vesicles, uterus, vagina, pelvic wall, abdominal wall
  T4a: Tumor invades prostatic stroma, uterus, vagina
  T4b: Tumor invades pelvic wall, abdominal wall

Regional lymph nodes (N)
Regional lymph nodes include both primary and secondary drainage regions. All other nodes above the aortic bifurcation are considered distant lymph nodes.

NX: Lymph nodes cannot be assessed
N0: No lymph node metastasis
N1: Single regional lymph node metastasis in the true pelvis (hypogastric, obturator, external iliac, or presacral lymph node)
N2: Multiple regional lymph node metastasis in the true pelvis (hypogastric, obturator, external iliac, or presacral lymph node metastasis)
N3: Lymph node metastasis to the common iliac lymph nodes

continued

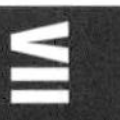

I: T1N0M0
II: T2aN0M0
T2bN0M0
III: T3aN0M0
T3bN0M0
T4aN0M0
IV: T4bN0M0
Any T N1 M0
Any T N2 M0
Any T N3 M0
Any T Any N M1

Survival (5-year OS)
Ta: 95%
T1 (G3): 50–80%
T2: Cystectomy/cystoprostatectomy = 77% (pT2N0 USC series), bladder preservation = 60%
T3-T4N0: Cystectomy/cystoprostatectomy = 47% (pT3-4N0 USC series), bladder preservation = 40–50%

pN+: Cystectomy/cystoprostatectomy = 31% (pN+ USC series)
M1: Untreated median survival <6 months; 13 months with chemotherapy

Distant metastasis (M)
M0: No distant metastasis
M1: Distant metastasis

Anatomic stage/prognostic groups
0a: Ta N0 M0
0is: Tis N0 M0
I: T1 N0 M0
II: T2a N0 M0
T2b N0 M0
III: T3a N0 M0
T3b N0 M0
T4a N0 M0
IV: T4b N0 M0
Any T N1-3 M0
Any T Any N M1

TREATMENT RECOMMENDATIONS

2002 Stage	Recommended treatment
Nonmuscle invasive (Ta, Tis, T1)	■ TURBT alone: 70% local recurrence (15–30% invasive) ■ Indications for adjuvant treatment: persistent abnormal or equivocal urine cytology, multifocal, grade II/III, Tis/CIS, T1, or subtotal resection ■ Multicolor fluorescence in situ hybridization has been shown to be useful in predicting recurrences in patients with negative or equivocal cytology (Whitson et al. BJU Int 2009) ■ TURBT + BCG × 6 weeks (alternative intravesical chemotherapies (IVC): mitomycin C, gemcitabine, doxorubicin) ■ Disease persistence 6 months status post IVC → use another agent with BCG × 3 weeks q6 months × 2 years ■ Disease persistence >1 year or multiple recurrences → radical cystectomy (10-year DFS = 80–90%; DSS = 75–80%) ■ Or, consider Bladder preservation with chemo-RT for previously untreated T1G3, 5/10-year PFS 87%/71%; 5/10-year DSS – 80%/71%; progression to T2 = 29%; bladder preservation 80% (Weiss et al. 2006)
Muscle invasive (T2–T4)	■ Treatment options: (i) Radical cystectomy/cystoprostatectomy and reconstruction, (ii) partial cystectomy*, (iii) bladder preservation with chemo-RT, (iv) radical RT (poor surgery/chemo candidate) *Small tumors in the dome without CIS may be treated with partial cystectomy ■ "Optimum" bladder preservation candidate: unifocal T2-T4, <5 cm, no hydronephrosis/hydroureter, good bladder function, and visibly complete TURBT ■ Consider bladder preservation as suitable alternative for all appropriate patients ■ In general, 5-year OS = 50–60%; greater than 50% of patients have intact functioning bladder. Sixty percent of patients with CR to chemo-RT remain free of any recurrence including superficial. Fifty percent of relapses are superficial ■ Multifocal T2-T3a, T3b-T4, presence of Tis, hydroureter/hydronephrosis, subtotal resection is generally treated with neoadjuvant chemo and cystectomy vs. radical cystectomy ± RT ■ T3b-T4: consider pre-op chemo; cystectomy + LN dissection + adjuvant chemo

continued

VII

Local recurrence (LR)	■ Status post TURBT + IVC: cystectomy/cystoprostatectomy or may consider chemo-RT ■ Status post cystectomy/cystoprostatectomy: chemo (usually platinum-based) + RT to 40–45 Gy to true pelvis, 50–54 Gy to sidewall if clinical recurrence, 60–64 Gy to LR ■ Status post chemo-RT: 20% of patients with CR to chemo-RT develop superficial LR → treat with TURBT + intravesical therapy ■ Ten to twenty percent of patients with CR to chemo-RT develop invasive LR → treat with radical cystectomy/cystoprostatectomy

Treatment	**Description**

Radical cystectomy	■ En bloc removal of bladder, perivesical tissue, urethra, and prostate, seminal vesicles or uterus, fallopian tubes, ovaries, and anterior vaginal wall
	■ Local recurrence after cystectomy = 5–10% for pT2-T3a, but 30–50% with T3b-T4
	■ USC series (Stein et al. 2001): 30% relapses, 85% in the first 3 years, distant > local (2–3:1)
	■ If (+) margins, post-op chemo, or post-op RT and concurrent platinum-based chemotherapy. Problem with post-op RT = 20–40% GI complications
	■ Pre-op RT not routinely used, but may be considered for cT3b lesions (Cole et al. 1995)
	■ Neoadjuvant chemo before cystectomy provides 5% OS advantage @ 5 years based on metaanalysis
	■ Patients may have either an incontinent or a continent urinary diversion
	■ In an incontinent diversion, the ureters are attached to an ileal loop conduit to the skin surface. Requires bag to collect urine
	■ Continent urinary diversions provide ~80% continence rates
	   ■ Cutaneous diversion: ureters drain into a bowel segment that is reconstructed into a pouch that is connected to skin via stoma that does not allow continuous urine drainage. Needs to be catheterized periodically. Used when urethra or bladder neck is nonfunctional or involved by tumor
	   ■ Othotopic neobladder: intestinal detubularized segment anastomosed to intact urethra, allows volitional voiding

Bladder preservation	■ Maximal TURBT → induction chemo-RT to 40–45 Gy → second look cystoscopy with multiple biopsies and urine cytology (if surgical candidate; ~70–80% of

continued

patients have CR). If residual tumor ≥T1, salvage cystectomy. If CR, consolidation chemo-RT boost to primary (total dose 60–65 Gy)

- Follow-up cystoscopy with biopsy and cytology (4–6 weeks) → adjuvant chemo
- Persistence of superficial disease → consider BCG (IVC) vs. radical cystectomy
- Presence of invasive disease → salvage cystectomy

STUDIES

- No randomized trials have been completed comparing radical cystectomy vs. bladder preservation.
- *USC surgical series* (Stein et al. 2001): radical cystectomy in the treatment of invasive bladder cancer: long-term results in 1,054 patients. Median FU 10.2 years. All patients: 5(10)-OS 60% (43%), 5(10)-RFS 68% (66%). Organ confined disease: 5(10)-OS 78% (56%), 5(10)-RFS 85% (82%). Extravesical disease (pT3-pT4): 5(10)-OS 47% (27%), 5(10)-RFS 58% (55%).
- *MD Anderson retrospective analysis* of pre-op RT + radical cystectomy (RC) vs. RC alone (Cole et al. 1995): 50 Gy/25 fractions to pelvis associated with improved 5-year LC 91 vs. 72% SS. Nonsignificant improvements in DFS, OS, and freedom from DM. Benefits seen in T3b patients.
- *NCIC* (Coppin et al. 1996): 99 patients T2-4. RT alone or pre-op RT ± concurrent cisplatin × 3. Concurrent chemo decreased LRF, but no change OS.
- *RTOG* 8512, (Tester et al. 1993): 42 patients T2-T4N0-2. Phase II = WP 2/40 Gy + cisplatin × 2. Restage 2 weeks after with cystoscopy, biopsy, EUA, CT. If CR, 2/24 Gy with third cycle cisplatin. No CR = cystectomy. Follow-up = cystoscopy q3 months. *Results*: 67% CR. Five-year OS = 52%. All LC = 42%. Invasive only LC = 50%. Five-year LF = 25%.
- *RTOG* 8802, (Tester et al. 1996): 91 patients. Phase II neoadjuvant MCV (methotrexate, cisplatin, vinblastine), RT + cisplatin same as RTOG 8512. *Results*: 75% CR, 5-year OS 62%.
- *RTOG* 8903, (Shipley et al. 1998): 123 patients T2-4aNx status post maximal TURBT. Phase III. Randomized to [neoadjuvant MCV × 2c concurrent cisplatin × 2c + WP 1.8/39.6 Gy] vs. [same but no MCV]. Both restaged 4 weeks later with cystoscopy, biopsy, EUA, cytology. If CR, 1.8/25.2 Gy boost (total dose = 64.8 Gy) + cisplatin × 1c. Stopped early due to MCV toxicity (14% died). *Results*: no significant change in CR, OS, or DMFS.

VII

- *RTOG* 9506, (Kaufman et al. 2000): 34 patients T2-T4aNx without hydronephrosis. Phase II = TURBT → WP 3 Gy (b.i.d.)/24 Gy + concurrent 5-FU + cisplatin. Restage 4 weeks later. If CR, 2.5 Gy (b.i.d.)/20 Gy + concurrent 5-FU + cisplatin. No CR = cystectomy. *Results*: 67% CR. 3-year OS 83%, with intact bladder = 66%. Twenty percent grade 3/4 toxicity. In follow-up, 45% superficial recurrence.
- *MGH*, (Shipley et al. 2002): RTOG 8903 style technique. 190 patients, 6.7-year follow-up. Results: only 35% needed cystectomy (including salvage for recurrence). Five-year OS 54% (T2 = 62%, T3-4a = 47%). Five-year DSS 63% (T2 = 74%, T3-4a = 53%). Five-year DSS with intact bladder 46% (T2 57%, T3-4a 35%). Hydronephrosis not significant.
- *RTOG* 9706, (Hagan et al. 2003): 52 patients T2-T4aN0. TURBT → within 6 weeks, WP 1.8 Gy qAM + bladder 1.6 Gy qPM × 13 days (=WP 21.6 Gy, bladder 40.8 Gy) + concurrent cisplatin. Restage at 4 weeks with biopsy and cytology. If CR, b.i.d. RT × 8 days (total WP 45.6, bladder 64.8) + concurrent cisplatin. If no CR, cystectomy. All got MCV × 3. *Results*: similar to 8903 but more toxic. Seventy-five percent CR. Three-year OS 61%, with intact bladder 48%. Only 45% of patients completed MCV × 3. Three-year LRF = 27%, DM = 29%.
- *RTOG 9906*, (Kaufman et al. 2008): 80 patients T2-T4aNx without hydronephrosis. Phase I–II TURBT → induction CTI weeks 1–3 (b.i.d. XRT × 13 days + paclitaxel + cisplatin) → Restage week 7. If pT0, Ta or Tis → Consolidation weeks 8–9 (b.i.d. XRT × 8 days + Paclitaxel + Cisplatin). If ≥T1, Radical Cystectomy (week 9). All patients had four cycles of adjuvant chemo (Gemcitabin + Cisplatin). *Results:* CR 81%, 3-OS 67% (with bladder 59%), 5-OS 56% (with bladder 47%), 4% G3 bladder toxicity at 5 years. Five-year LR 29%, 5-year DM 31%.
- *Metaanalysis of neoadjuvant chemo trials*. (Lancet 2003): neoadjuvant multiagent cisplatin based chemo gives 5% OS @ 5 years. No data to support single agent cisplatin.
- Weiss et al. (2006). Bladder preserving protocol in T1 high-risk lesions, without prior BCG therapy. One hundred and forty-one patients (81 T1G3). Results: CR 88% (89%), 5-year PFS 81% (87%), 10-year PFS 70% (71%), 5-year DSS 82% (80%), 10-year DSS 73% (71%); >80% bladder preservation.
- Harland et al. (2007): 210 patients with T1G3 disease: group 1 (unifocal disease, no Tis) randomized to RT alone (no chemotherapy) vs. observation after TURBT, and group 2 (multifocal disease and/or Tis) randomized to IVC vs. RT after TURBT.

Median follow-up = 44 months. *Results:* no difference in time to progression or in OS, 5-year PFS 66% (control) vs. 49% (RT). However, poorer than expected results (compared to Erlangen series: 5-year PFS = 83%) may be due to lack of concurrent sensitizing chemotherapy.

RADIATION TECHNIQUES

SIMULATION AND FIELD DESIGN

- Simulate patient supine with immobilization and bladder emptied by patients
- Need CT scan (preferably with contrast) and highly recommend consulting bladder map from TURBT for planning
- Alternatively, double-contrast cystogram = introduce via Foley typically 25–30 mL radiopaque contrast + 10–15 mL air. May need more contrast to equal PVR volume
- For non-3D simulation: to identify anterior rectal wall, instill 50 cc rectal barium (for lateral sim films) administered *after* AP field film
- Use of fiducials and IGRT may allow decrease in PTV expansion
- Volumes
  - GTV: macroscopic tumor visible on CT/MRI/cystoscopy
  - CTV_{pelvis}: GTV + whole bladder + lymph Nodes (obturator, external + internal iliacs), proximal urethra, prostate + prostatic urethra in men
  - PTV: (not described in RTOG protocols) CTV + 1.5–2 and 2–3 cm superiorly (can probably be reduced to 1 cm and 1.5–2 cm superiorly with the use of fiducials + IGRT)
- Field design (RTOG protocol)
  - Whole pelvis AP/PA borders = S2–S3, lower pole of obturator foramen, widest bony pelvis margin + 1.5–2 cm. Block medial border of femoral heads
  - Whole pelvis lateral borders = 2 cm beyond CTV_{pelvis}, same inferior and superior borders as for APPA field. Block rectum, small bowel
- Treat with empty bladder
- Boost volumes = entire bladder or partial bladder. CTV = GTV + 0.5 cm. PTV = CTV + 1.5 cm
- Use of IMRT controversial. If used, strongly consider IGRT

DOSE PRESCRIPTIONS

- Bladder preservation: treat bladder and nodal drainage to 40–45 Gy with concurrent chemo; if CR on postinduction cystoscopy, boost to a total dose of 60–65 Gy.

VII

- LR status post cystectomy → cisplatin + RT to 45–50 Gy to pelvic nodes, 60–64 Gy to gross local recurrence.

DOSE LIMITATIONS

- Whole bladder 50 Gy = 5–10% late grade 3–4 effects
- Whole bladder 60 Gy = 10–40% late grade 3–4 effects
- More than 1/3 bladder: 60 Gy = 5–10% late effects; 70 Gy = 20%
- Urethra: max dose <70 Gy associated with <5% risk of stricture
- Small bowel: TD 5/5 1/3: 50 Gy, 3/3 40 Gy

COMPLICATIONS

- Chemo-RT trials = 0–13% late sequelae
- Urinary tract infection; treat with antibiotic
- Irritative urinary symptoms/bladder spasm. Use terazosin or tamsulosin
- Acute dysuria. Treat with ibuprofen or pyridium
- Seventy-five percent of late bladder symptoms present within 3 years = frequency, dysuria, intermittent hematuria. Seventy percent will resolve within 2–3 years
- Urethral stricture: 5–10%
- Five to fifteen percent late bowel complications
- Quality of life (QoL) after bladder preservation therapy remains good; Urodymanic studies and patient reported QoL posttreatment (median = 6.3 years) showed >75% patient retained normal bladder function and >85% reported no bothersome urinary side effects. Bowel symptoms were reported by 22% (Zietman et al. 2003

FOLLOW-UP

- Follow-up with urine cytology and cystoscopy every 3 months × 1 year, every 6 months × 2 year, then annually. CT abdomen and pelvis q 1–2 year.

REFERENCES

Advanced Bladder Cancer Meta-Analysis Collaboration. Neoadjuvant chemotherapy in invasive bladder cancer: a systematic review and meta-analysis. Lacet 2003;361:1927-1934.

Cole CJ, Pollack A, Gunar K, et al. Local control of muscle-invasive bladder cancer: Preoperative radiotherapy and cystectomy versus cystectomy alone. Int J Radiat Oncol Biol Phys 1995;32(2):331-340.

Coppin CM, Gospodarowicz MK, James K, et al. Improved local control of invasive bladder cancer by concurrent cisplatin and preoperative or definitive radiation. The National Cancer Institute of Canada Clinical Trials Group. J Clin Oncol 1996;14:2901-2907.

Hagan MP, Winter KA, Kaufman DS, et al. RTOG 97-06: initial report of a phase I-II trial of selective bladder conservation using TURBT, twice-daily accelerated irradiation sensitized with cisplatin, and adjuvant MCV combination chemotherapy. Int J Radiat Oncol Biol Phys 2003;57:665-672.

Harland SJ, Kynaston H, Grigor K, et al. A Randomized trial of radical radiotherapy for the management of pT1G3 NXM0 transitional cell carcinoma of the bladder. J Urol 2007;178:807-813.

Kaufman DS, Winter KA, Shipley WU, et al. The initial results in muscle-invading bladder cancer of RTOG 95-06: phase I/II trial of transurethral surgery plus radiation therapy with concurrent cisplatin and 5-fluorouracil followed by selective bladder preservation or cystectomy depending on the initial response. Oncologist 2000;5:471-476.

Kaufman DS, Winter KA, Shipley WU, et al. Phase I-II RTOG Study (99-06) of patients with muscle-invasive bladder cancer undergoing transurethral surgery, paclitaxel, cisplatin, and twice-daily radiotherapy followed by selective bladder preservation or radical cystectomy and adjuvant chemotherapy. Urology 2009;73(4):833-837.

Shipley WU, Winter KA, Kaufman DS, et al. Phase III trial of neoadjuvant chemotherapy in patients with invasive bladder cancer treated with selective bladder preservation by combined radiation therapy and chemotherapy: initial results of Radiation Therapy Oncology Group 89-03. J Clin Oncol 1998;16:3576-3583.

Shipley WU, Kaufman DS, Zehr E, et al. Selective bladder preservation by combined modality protocol treatment: long-term outcomes of 190 patients with invasive bladder cancer. Urology 2002;60:62-67; discussion 67-68.

Stein JP, Lieskovsky G, Skinner DG, et al. Radical cystectomy in the treatment of invasive bladder cancer: long-term results in 1,054 patients. JCO 2001;19(3):666-675.

Tester W, Porter A, Asbell S, et al. Combined modality program with possible organ preservation for invasive bladder carcinoma: results of RTOG protocol 85-12. Int J Radiat Oncol Biol Phys 1993;25:783-790.

Tester W, Caplan R, Heaney J, et al. Neoadjuvant combined modality program with selective organ preservation for invasive bladder cancer: results of Radiation Therapy Oncology Group phase II trial 8802. J Clin Oncol 1996;14:119-126.

Weiss C, Wolze C, Rodel C, et al. Radiochemotherapy after transurethral resection for high-risk T1 bladder cancer: an alternative to intravesical therapy or early cystectomy? JCO 2006;24(15):2318-2324.

ZIetman AL, Sacco D, Skowronski U, et al. Organ conservation in invasive bladder cancer by transurethral resection, chemotherapy and radiation: results of a urodynamic and quality of life study on long-term survivors. J Urol 2003;170:1772-1776.

FURTHER READING

Milosevic MF, Gospodarowicz MK. The Urinary Bladder. In: Cox JD, Ang KK, editors. Radiation Oncology: Rationale, Technique, Results. 8th ed. St. Louis: Mosby; 2003. pp. 575-602.

National Comprehensive Cancer Network. Clinical Practice Guidelines in Oncology: Bladder Cancer v.2.2008. Available at: http://www.nccn.org/professionals/physician_gls/PDF/bladder.pdf

Petrovich Z, Stein JP, Jozsef G, Formenti SC. Bladder. In: Perez CA, Brady LW, Halperin ED, editors. Principles and Practice of Radiation Oncology. 5th ed. Philadelphia: Lippincott Williams & Wilkins; 2008. pp. 1412-1438.

Skinner DG, Tift JP, Kaufman JJ. High dose, short course preoperative radiation therapy and immediate single stage radical cystectomy with pelvic node dissection in the management of bladder cancer. J Urol 1982;127(4):671-674.

Whitson J, Berry A, Carroll P, et al. A multicolour fluorescence in situ hybridization test predicts recurrence in patients with high-risk superficial bladder tumours undergoing intravesical therapy. BJU Int 2009;104(3):336-339.

Zelefsky MJ, Small EJ. Cancer of the Bladder. In Leibel SA, Phillips TL, editors. Textbook of Radiation Oncology. 2nd ed. Philadelphia: Saunders; 2004. pp. 939-957.

Chapter 26
Prostate Cancer

Siavash Jabbari, Eric K. Hansen, and Mack Roach III

PEARLS

- Prostate cancer is the #1 noncutaneous cancer in men (~186,320 estimated cases in the US in 2008), and is the #2 cause of cancer mortality (~28,660 deaths in 2008) after lung cancer (~90,810 deaths).
- The median age at diagnosis is 70, but with increased screening, more younger men are being diagnosed.
- Due to its long natural history, many men may not benefit from treatment if their life expectancy is short (<5–10 years) and if they have early-stage, low-grade disease.
- Prostate gland consists of the peripheral zone (70% of glandular prostate and site of nearly all cancers), the central zone (25% of the glandular prostate), the transition zone (surrounding the urethra and the site of BPH), and the anterior fibromuscular stroma.
- Approximately 50–80% of tumors involve the prostate apex, and ~85% of patients have multifocal disease in the prostate.
- At the apex, the capsule is not well-defined and true ECE is difficult to recognize.
- ECE is most common at the posterior lateral portion of the prostate (associated with regions penetrated by nerves).
- More than 95% of prostate cancers are adenocarcinomas.
- Routine screening not recommended by the American Cancer Society, but when done should begin with PSA and digital exam at age 50 if life expectancy is >10 years. It is recommended that discussion should take place starting at age 45 for men at high risk of developing prostate cancer. This includes African-American men and men who have a first-degree relative (father, brother, or son) diagnosed with prostate cancer at an early age (younger than age 65). This discussion should take place at age 40 (the age at which the American Urological Association (AUA) recommends screening) for men at even higher risk

(those with several first-degree relatives who had prostate cancer at an early age).

- Two Randomized Trials studying the impact of screening on survival have been completed to date with conflicting results, the PLCO trial (Prostate, Lung, Colorectal, and Ovarian; USA), a negative study (Andriole et al. 2009) and the ERSPC trial (European Randomized Study of Screening for Prostate Cancer), a positive study (Schroder et al. 2009).

Study	Number of patients	Follow-up (years)	~Age (Estimated. median)	Cases detected in screened vs. control	Control group screened	Reduction in mortality
Multicenter (USA)	76,000	7	60–64	1.17 @ 10 years	52% at sixth year	NS
Multi-country (European)	182,000	9	60	1.7 @ 9 years	Very low	20%

Comment: As above, the European study was larger, has longer follow-up, and less contamination of the observation (nonscreened) arm. Consequently, this study appears to be better powered and implemented to answer the question of screening. In addition, patients treated in the U.S. were prescreened, while the European study included index cases diagnosed at the time of recruitment.

- Risk of finding prostate cancer on biopsy is related to PSA level:
  - Approximately 5–25% for PSA<4 (Thompson et al. 2004).
  - Up to ~50–67% for PSA >10.
  - Upper range of normal PSA is ~(age/10)-1.
  - For PSA <4, rule-of-thumb: risk of Gleason score (GS) 7–10 prostate cancer is 2× the PSA level.
- LN drainage is primarily to the internal iliac, obturator, external iliac, and presacral nodes, but disease also may spread to perirectal, common iliac, and paraaortic nodes.
  - Standard prostatectomy LN dissection samples only obturator and external iliac nodes.
  - More extensive LN dissection increases chance of involved LN. Forty to sixty percent of involved LN are located in the

internal iliac and presacral chains (outside standard LN dissection).

- GS represents the sum (2–10) of the major and minor glandular patterns [ranging from slight disorganization (1) to anaplastic (5)].
- Most frequently used prognostic factors are GS, clinical stage, pretreatment PSA.
- Additional prognostic factors:
  - Percentage of biopsy cores positive (>50% behaves more aggressively).
  - Perineural invasion.
  - Gleason 7 with tertiary component (>10%) Gleason 5 have biochemical recurrence-free survival similar to Gleason 8–10 (Patel 2007).
  - PSA velocity >2 ng/mL in the year before radical prostatectomy (RP) or EBRT suggested as prognostic for increased risk of death from prostate cancer (D'Amico et al. 2004a, 2005), but the value of pretreatment PSA kinetics (PSA velocity and doubling time) as independent predictors of outcome questioned in a recent systematic review (Vickers et al. 2009).

VII

WORKUP

- H&P (including American Urology Association (AUA) symptom scores, baseline erectile function, bony pain, and DRE).
- Labs include PSA, testosterone, CBC, and LFTs.
- TRUS-guided biopsy is used for pathologic diagnosis (>8 separate cores is recommended, and the highest GS is used).
- Upgrading of biopsy GS from ≤6 to ≥7 or from 7 to >7 occurs in ~25–30% of patients who subsequently undergo prostatectomy even with >10 biopsy cores (Chun 2006).
- Downgrading of GS uncommon.
- Note prostate volume and whether pubic arch interference is present if considering brachytherapy.
- Bone scan and pelvic CT or MRI are usually ordered for T3–T4, GS ≥8, PSA ≥20, or symptoms.
- MR spectroscopy shows decreased citrate and increased choline with prostate cancer, but its role in routine management remains controversial.
- Prostascint (an In-111 labeled monoclonal Ab) has limited sensitivity (60–70%), but may be useful for staging high-risk disease, nodes, and/or sites of recurrence.

STAGING: PROSTATE CANCER

Editors' note: All TNM stage and stage groups referred to elsewhere in this chapter reflect the 2002 AJCC staging nomenclature unless otherwise noted as the new system below was published after this chapter was written.

(AJCC 6TH ED., 2002)

Primary tumor (T) – clinical

TX: Primary tumor cannot be assessed
T0: No evidence of primary tumor
T1: Clinically inapparent tumor neither palpable nor visible on imaging
- T1a: Tumor incidental histologic finding in 5% or less of tissue resected
- T1b: Tumor incidental histologic finding in more than 5% of tissue resected
- T1c: Tumor identified by needle biopsy (e.g., because of elevated PSA)

T2: Tumor confined within the prostate
- T2a: Tumor involves 1/2 of one lobe or less
- T2b: Tumor involves more than 1/2 of one lobe, but not both lobes
- T2c: Tumor involves both lobes

T3: Tumor extends through prostate capsule
- T3a: Extracapsular extension (unilateral or bilateral)
- T3b: Tumor invades seminal vesicle(s)

T4: Tumor is fixed or invades adjacent structures other than seminal vesicles: bladder neck, external sphincter, rectum, levator muscles, and/or pelvic wall

Regional lymph nodes (N)

NX: Regional lymph nodes were not assessed
N0: No regional lymph node metastasis
N1: Regional lymph node metastasis

Metastases (M)

MX: Distant metastasis cannot be assessed (not evaluated by any modality)
M0: No distant metastasis
M1: Distant metastasis
M1a: Nonregional lymph node(s)
M1b: Bone(s)
M1c: Other site(s) with or without bone disease

(AJCC 7TH ED., 2010)

Primary tumor (T) – clinical

TX: Primary tumor cannot be assessed
T0: No evidence of primary tumor
T1: Clinically inapparent tumor neither palpable nor visible by imaging
- T1a: Tumor incidental histologic finding in 5% or less of tissue resected
- T1b: Tumor incidental histologic finding in more than 5% of tissue resected
- T1c: Tumor identified by needle biopsy (e.g., because of elevated PSA)

T2: Tumor confined within prostate*
- T2a: Tumor involves one-half of one lobe or less
- T2b: Tumor involves more than one-half of one lobe, but not both lobes
- T2c: Tumor involves both lobes

T3: Tumor extends through the prostate capsule**
- T3a: Extracapsular extension (unilateral or bilateral)
- T3b: Tumor invades seminal vesicle(s)

T4: Tumor is fixed or invades adjacent structures other than seminal vesicles such as external sphincter, rectum, bladder, levator muscles, and/or pelvic wall

**Note*: Tumor found in one or both lobes by needle biopsy, but not palpable or reliably visible by imaging, is classified as T1c.
***Note*: Invasion into the prostatic apex or into (but not beyond) the prostatic capsule is classified not as T3 but as T2

Pathologic (pT)*

pT2: Organ confined
- pT2a: Unilateral, one-half of one side or less

continued

Grade
GX: Grade cannot be assessed
G1: Well-differentiated (slight anaplasia, Gleason 2–4)
G2: Moderately-differentiated (moderate anaplasia, Gleason 5–6)
G3–4: Poorly-differentiated/ undifferentiated (marked anaplasia, Gleason 7–10)

Stage grouping
I: T1aN0M0 G1
II: T1aN0M0 G2–4, T1-2N0M0 any G
III: T3N0M0 any G
IV: T4N0M0; any TN1M0; any T any N M1

Used with the permission from the American Joint Committee on Cancer (AJCC), Chicago, IL. The original source for this material is the AJCC Cancer Staging Manual, Sixth Edition (2002), published by Springer Science+Business Media

pT2b: Unilateral, involving more than one-half of side but not both sides
pT2c: Bilateral disease
pT3: Extraprostatic extension
pT3a: Extraprostatic extension or microscopic invasion of bladder neck**
pT3b: Seminal vesicle invasion
pT4: Invasion of rectum, levator muscles, and /or pelvic wall
**Note*: There is no pathologic T1 classification
***Note*: Positive surgical margin should be indicated by an R1 descriptor (residual microscopic disease)

Regional lymph nodes (N)
Clinical
NX: Regional lymph nodes were not assessed
N0: No regional lymph node metastasis
N1: Metastasis in regional lymph node(s)

Pathologic
pNX: Regional nodes not sampled
pN0: No positive regional nodes
pN1: Metastases in regional node(s)

Distant metastasis (M)*
M0: No distant metastasis
M1: Distant metastasis
M1a: Nonregional lymph node(s)
M1b: Bone(s)
M1c: Other site(s) with or without bone disease

**Note*: When more than one site of metastasis is present, the most advanced category is used. pM1c is most advanced.

Anatomic stage/prognostic groups*

Group	T	N	M	PSA	Gleason
I	T1a – c	N0	M0	PSA < 10	Gleason ≤6
IIA:	T2a	N0	M0	PSA < 10	Gleason ≤6
IIB:	T1 – 2a	N0	M0	PSA X	Gleason X

continued

VII

III:	T1a – c	N0	M0	PSA < 20	Gleason 7
IV:	T1a – c	N0	M0	PSA ≥10 < 20	Gleason ≤6
	T2a	N0	M0	PSA < 20	Gleason ≤7
	T2b	N0	M0	PSA < 20	Gleason ≤7
	T2b	N0	M0	PSA X	Gleason X
	T2c	N0	M0	Any PSA	Any gleason
	T1 – 2	N0	M0	PSA ≥ 20	Any gleason
	T1 – 2	N0	M0	Any PSA	Gleason ≥8
	T3a – b	N0	M0	Any PSA	Any gleason
	T4	N0	M0	Any PSA	Any gleason
	Any T	N1	M0	Any PSA	Any gleason
	Any T	Any N	M1	Any PSA	Any gleason

*When either PSA or Gleason is not available, grouping should be determined by T stage and/or either PSA or Gleason as available.

RISK CLASSIFICATION SCHEMES

NCCN risk categories	**~5–10-Year bPFS/CSS**
Low: T1-2a and GS ≤6 and PSA <10	80–90%/>95%
Intermediate: T2b–T2c and/or GS 7 and/or PSA 10–20	70–85%/75–90%
High: T3a or GS 8-10 or PSA >20 (very high T3b-T4)	30–60%/60–80%
(Also consider PSA kinetics, % involved biopsy cores)	
RTOG metaanalysis risk groups – predict DSS and OS	**10-Year DSS**
I: T1-2 and GS ≤6 (Low)	86%
II: T1-2 and GS 7, or T3 or N1 with GS ≤6 (intermediate)	75%
III: T1-2 and GS 8-10, or T3 or N1 with GS 7 (high)	62%
IV: T3 or N1 with GS 8-10 (very high)	34%

Partin nomograms predict pathologic stage (organ confined, ECE, seminal vesicle invasion, or LN involvement) based on T stage, GS, and pretreatment PSA

Brignanti nomograms (using extended LN dissection) show higher rates and support importance of obtaining larger # of LN (e.g., 28 to detect 90%) to improve chance of detecting involvement

Roach formulas estimate pathologic stage based on original Partin data

ECE = 3/2 × PSA + 10 × (GS-3)

Seminal vesicle involvement = PSA + 10 × (GS-6)

LN involvement = 2/3 × PSA + 10 × (GS-6)

Kattan nomograms are computerized and predict primarily PSA recurrence, but some also predict PFS as well as prostate cancer specific mortality after RP, 3DCRT, or brachytherapy. (Online access: http://www.nomograms.org)

VII

TREATMENT RECOMMENDATIONS

Stage	Recommended treatment	5–10-Year bPFS	5–10-Year CSS
Low-risk	■ For life expectancy <10 years, active surveillance or definitive RT (3DCRT/IMRT with IGRT, or brachytherapy) ■ For life expectancy ≥10 years, RT, RP ± pelvic LN dissection, or active surveillance. Consider adjuvant RT if +margin(s) after RP	75–90%	>95%

continued

Intermediate-risk	■ For life expectancy <10 years, active surveillance, RT ± short-term androgen deprivation therapy(ADT), or RP ■ For life expectancy ≥10 years, RT + short-term ADT (4–6 month), high-dose RT alone, or RP ± pelvic LN dissection ■ RT is 3DCRT/IMRT with IGRT ± brachytherapy boost. Brachytherapy monotherapy considered for select GS seven patients. Consider whole pelvic RT, especially if multiple adverse features. Adjuvant RT ± short-term ADT indicated for +margin(s) or pT3 disease	50–85%	85–90%
High-risk	■ RT (3DCRT/IMRT with IGRT ± brachytherapy boost) with neoadjuvant, concurrent, and adjuvant ADT (2–3 years). Four to six-month ADT considered for select patients with single adverse feature with GS 6–7. Whole pelvic RT indicated. Consider RP with pelvic LN dissection only for select patients with low-volume disease and no fixation. Adjuvant RT ± short-term ADT indicated for +margin(s) or pT3 disease	T1-2: 60% T3/N+: 20%	T1-2: 80–85% N+: 60%
Node+	■ Life long or long-term ADT (≥2 years) alone or combined with RT (3DCRT/IMRT with IGRT ± brachytherapy boost; sometimes preferred over ADT alone when limited nodal disease)	10-year OS 35–60% 5-year PFS 20–50%	
Metastatic	■ Long-term ADT (≥2 years) ± palliative RT ± bisphosphonates. For hormone-refractory disease, docetaxel and prednisone	Median survival for androgen-independent disease is ~18 months	
Adjuvant or salvage RT after RP	■ Adjuvant RT indicated if persistent local disease on imaging or biopsy, or pT3 disease or +margin(s).	*Adjuvant RT* 5-year bPFS ~75% 5–10-year LF 5–8%	

continued

	■ Best candidates for salvage RT for rising PSA after RP: pretreatment low-risk disease with PSA velocity <2 ng/mL in year before diagnosis; pathologic GS ≤7, +margin(s), negative LN, and no SVI; time to ■ PSA failure >3 years after RP, and ■ low PSA at time of salvage <1 ng/mL. Short-term ADT considered for patients with high-risk features	*Salvage RT* See Trock and Stephenson nomograms
Residual disease or recurrence after RT	■ If metastatic or not a candidate for local therapy, ADT or observation. If +biopsy and no evidence (or low-risk) of metastases, surgery, salvage brachytherapy, or cryotherapy considered. Salvage RP provides 5-year PSA control in up to 85, 55, and 30% of patients with pre-op PSA <4, 4–10, and >10, respectively. However, high risk of morbidity, including incontinence (~50–70%), erectile dysfunction, and bladder neck contracture or stricture (~15–30%)	

VII

STUDIES

ACTIVE SURVEILLANCE

- Active surveillance generally consists of DRE and PSA every 3–6 months with routine repeat biopsy in 1–2 years to rule-out Gleason grade progression.
- Active surveillance avoids side effects of therapy that may be unnecessary.
- Disadvantages of active surveillance include:
  - Chance of missed opportunity for cure.
  - Risk of progression and/or metastases
  - Subsequent treatment may be more intense with increased risk of side effects.
  - Increased anxiety.
  - Uncertain long-term natural history of prostate cancer.

- Life expectancy can be estimated using the Social Security Administration tables, available at: http://www.ssa.gov.
  - Life expectancy can then be adjusted using the clinicians assessment of overall health:
    - Best quartile of health – add 50%.
    - Worst quartile of health - subtract 50%.
    - Middle two quartiles of health - no adjustment.
- *Swedish trial* (Bill-Axelson et al. 2002, 2005, 2008): Randomized 695 patients with T1b-T2 to WW vs. RP. With median follow-up 10.8 years, RP reduced 12-year death from prostate cancer (20→14%) and DM (26→19%), but no longer a difference in OS ($p > 0.09$). Patients with ECE had 14× risk of prostate cancer death vs. those without ECE. On subgroup analysis, men younger than 65 years at diagnosis had significant improvements with RP, while there was no discernable difference among those above 65 years.
- *SEER* (Wong et al. 2006): Compared ~32,000 treated patients age 65–80 with T1–2 GS 2–7 vs. ~12,000 patients observed. Treatment group had 31% lower mortality (HR 0.69). Benefits for specific subgroups: age 75–80 years 27% benefit, PSA era diagnosis 38% benefit, no comorbidities 29% benefit, cT1–T2a GS 2–4 21% benefit.
- Klotz et al. (2004): Phase II study of 299 patients with low-risk or intermediate risk disease (if >70 years) treated with active surveillance with delayed intervention for PSA DT ≤2 years or grade progression on rebiopsy. Eight-year DSS and OS were 99 and 85%, respectively.

ANDROGEN DEPRIVATION THERAPY ALONE OR WITH RT

- *Scandinavian SPCG-7* (Widmark 2008): 875 patients with locally advanced nonmetastatic disease with PSA <70 (78% T3, 19% T2; median PSA 16) randomized to 3 month combined androgen blockade followed by continuous flutamide ± RT. RT was 50 Gy to P+SV and 20 Gy boost to P. Addition of RT improved 10-year prostate cancer specific mortality (24→12%; including 16% benefit for T2 patients), overall mortality (39→30%), and PSA recurrence (75→26%). QOL was only slightly worse with RT, including urinary stricture (0→2%), urinary urgency (8→14%), moderate to severe urinary leakage (3→7%), and ED (81→89%).
- *EORTC 30891* (Studer et al. 2006): 985 patients with T0-4N0-2 who refused or were not eligible for local treatment randomized to immediate vs. deferred androgen ablation (orchiectomy or LHRH analog). Immediate AA improved OS (42→48%), but not prostate

cancer specific survival or symptom-free survival. In deferred arm, median time to start of androgen ablation was 7 years. Causes of death: prostate CA ~36%, cardiovascular disease ~34%.

- *Medicare analysis* (Lu-Yao et al. 2008): >19,000 men >66 years with T1–2 disease followed conservatively or treated with primary ADT (PADT). PADT reduced 10-year PCSS by 2% with no OS difference. Exception was 5% improvement in PCSS for poorly differentiated cancer.

RADICAL PROSTATECTOMY (RP)

- Retropubic approach allows bilateral pelvic lymph node dissection to precede prostatectomy in patients with LN risk. Perineal approach associated with better exposure of urethral stump and reduced risk of involved apical margin, but increased risk of rectal damage.
- A pelvic LN dissection frequently excluded in patients with <7% probability of LN metastases by nomograms.
- High volume surgeons in high volume centers generally provide better outcomes.
- Results with laparoscopic and robot-assisted RP in experience hands are comparable to open approaches.
- Recovery of erectile function is directly related to the degree of preservation of the cavernous nerves.
- Numerous studies of 3-month neoadjuvant HT before RP vs. RP alone demonstrate decreased margin positivity and tumor volume, but no change in bPFS.
- *Outcome for GS 7* patients (Tollefson 2006): ~1,600 patients at Mayo Clinic had RP for GS 7. GS 3+4 vs 4+3: 10-year bRFS (48 vs. 38%), DM (8 vs. 15%), and CSS (97 vs. 93%).
- *Outcome for GS 8–10* patients (Lau 2002): 407 patients at Mayo Clinic with GS 8–10 who had RP. Twenty-six percent pT2, 48% pT3, 27% LN+. Ten-year CSS 85%, OS 67%, b/cPFS 36%. Among pT2 patients, 10-year CSS 96%.
- *Occult LN* (Pagliarulo et al. 2006): 274 patients with pT3 with bilateral LND. Occult +LN found by immunohistochemistry in 13% of pN0 patients by H&E. Occult LN+ patients had similar recurrence and survival to pN+ patients.

RADIATION DOSE ESCALATION

- Six randomized trials show 10–20% improvements in bPFS with dose escalation, but no OS benefit.

Study	Patients	Doses	Med follow-up	Benefit	Late toxicity
MDACC, (Kuban et al. 2008; Pollack et al. 2000)	301 patients T1-3N0 No ADT	70 vs. 78 Gy to isocenter (initial four-field box to 46 Gy)	8.7 years	8-year Biochemical clinical freedom from failure. Low-risk: 63→88%; intermediate-risk: 65→94%; high-risk: 26→63% only if PSA>10, No OS difference	Gr≥2 GI toxicity: 13→26% ($p = 0.013$) (16 vs. 46% when <25% vs. >25% rectum received >70 Gy). Gr≥2 GU toxicity: 8→13% ($p >$ ns)
Zietman et al. 2005; correction Zietman 2008)	393 patients T1b-T2b and PSA <15 58% low, 33% intermediate-risk. No ADT	70.2 vs. 79.2 Gy with proton boost after 50.4 Gy photon to P&SV	5.5 years	5-year bFFS:Low risk: 84→98% Intermediate-risk: 79→91% No OS diff	No difference in Gr≥3 GU/GI toxicity
Netherlands, (Peeters 2006; Al-Mamgani et al. 2008)	664 patients T1b-T4N0 PSA<60 18% low, 28% intermediate, 54% high-risk, 10% STADT, 11% LTADT	68 vs. 78 Gy to PTV (prostate ± SV)	70 months	7-year bFFS: 45→56%, greatest risk reduction for intermediate-risk and high-risk, but not low-risk. No OS diff	Gr≥2 GI Toxicity: 25→35%. No difference in GU toxicity

continued

MRC RT01, (Dearnaley et al. 2007)	843 patients T1b-T3N0, PSA <50 25% low, 30% intermediate, 45% high. 3–6-month nADT	64 vs. 74 Gy–Prostate + SV	63 months	5-year bPFS: 60→71%, benefit in all risk groups. No OS diff	G≥2 GI toxicity 24→33%. G≫2 GU toxicity 8–11%
GETUG (Beckendorf 2008)	306 patients pN0 if Partin risk >10%. No ADT	70 vs. 80 Gy	59 months	5-year PSA failure 31→24%, benefit most if PSA >15	
Sathya et al. (2005)	104 patients T2-3N0 40% intermediate, 60% high No ADT	66 Gy EBRT vs. 40 Gy EBRT to P&SV with 35 Gy Ir-192 implant		bFFS: 29→61% No OS diff	

VII

HYPOFRACTIONATION

- Kupelian et al. (2007): 770 patients treated with 70 Gy at 2.5 Gy/fx in 5 weeks. Low 34%, intermediate 28%, and high-risk 38%. Sixty percent got HT. Five-year bRFS for low 94%, intermediate 83%, and high-risk 72%. Late grade 2–4 rectal toxicity 4.5%, late grade 2–3 urinary toxicity 5.2%.
- Yeoh et al. (2006): 217 T1-2N0 patients randomized to 55 Gy at 2.75-Gy/fx vs. 2/64 Gy. Worse acute GI and GU toxicity with hypofractionation, but no difference in bF or OS.
- Pollack (2006): Randomized 100 intermediate (65%) and high (35%) risk patients to 76 Gy/38 fx vs. 70.2 Gy/26 fx to P+proximal SV for intermediate and P+SV+LN for high-risk patients. Slight increase in acute GI toxicity for first month with hypofractionation, predicted by V65 Gy.

RT + SHORT-TERM HT (STHT)

- Randomized trials of STHT vs. no HT demonstrate that 3–6-month HT improves bPFS by 15–25% and CSS by 3–8% vs. no HT. A 10–15% OS benefit was only seen in the D'Amico and RTOG 8610 (GS 6 patients only).

Study	Patients	Arms	Benefit	Toxicity
RTOG 8610, (Pilepich et al. 2001; Roach 2008)	456 patients Palpable T2-4	44 WP → 66–70 Gy ± 4-month ADT (2 months neo-adjuvant and 2 months con-current)	10-year CSS: 64→77% DM: 47→35% OS trend for all patients: 34→43% ($p = 0.12$) 8-year OS for GS2-6 subset: 52→70% ($p < 0.05$)	No difference in fatal cardiac events. RTOG 8531, 8610, 9202 (Lawton 2007). 2,922 patients. Compared to RT alone, RT + STHT reduced late grade 3+ GU (9→5% cystitis, hematuria), GI (4→1% proctitis, rectal bleeding), and other (2→1%; osteoporosis, fistula) toxicity
D'Amico et al. 2004b, 2008	206 patients T1-2b plus G7-10 or PSA 10–40 (or lower PSA or GS if ECE or SVI on MRI) 80% intermediate-risk, 15% G8-10	45 Gy to P&SV → boost P to 70 Gy±6-month ADT (2 month before, during, and after)	8-year OS: 61→74% for all patients, mainly those with no or minimal comorbidities 5-year: bF: 45→21% CSS: 94→100% FF salvage HT: 57→82%	Unplanned retrospective pooled analysis D'amico, TTROG, and Crook randomized trials (JCO 2007). Men ≥65 years who received 6-month ADT had shorter time to fatal MIs (cumulative incidence ~7%) compared to men who did not receive AST (5–6%) and men <65 (2%). There was no difference in time to fatal MI between 3 vs. 6–8 month AST for men >65 (5%). However, the data from

continued

VII

TTROG, (Denham et al. 2005)	818 patients T2b-T4 Median PSA 15 ~15% intermediate, 85% high-risk	66 Gy to prostate and SV 0 vs. 3 vs. 6 months nADT (starting 2 and 5 months before RT, respectively)	Compared to no ADT, 3- and 6-month nADT improved: 5-year LF: 28 vs. 17 vs. 12% bFFS: 38 vs. 52 vs. 56% DFS: 32 vs. 49 vs. 52% Freedom from salvage tx: 63 vs. 68 vs. 78% 6 months vs. no nADT further improved DM and PCSS 6 vs. 3-month nADT further increased freedom from salvage tx	other large phase III Trials (RTOG 8610, 8531, 9202 and EORTC) do not support an association with ADT and the risk of MI
Crook et al. 2004, 2009	378 patients T1c-T4 ~25% low, 45% intermediate, 30% high-risk	66–67 Gy to prostate (+WP 45–46 Gy if risk of LN >15%) 3 vs. 8-month nADT	No difference in 5-year FFF or OS. For high-risk patients only, DFS improved in the 8-month arm (71% vs. 42%, $p = 0.01$)	

continued

Lavadiere 2004	481 patients T2-3N0 Median PSA>12 70% inter-mediate risk	64 Gy to prostate-only in 2 trials:**1**: 0 vs. 3-month nADT vs. 10-month n&cADT. **2**: 5-month n&cADT vs. 10-month ncaADT	7-year bPFS: 42→67% with 3–10-month HT vs. no HT. No diff in bPFS with 5 vs. 10-month ADT in second study	
RTOG 9413, (Roach et al. 2003; Lawton 2007)	1,323 patients Risk LN >15% Median PSA 23 66% T2c-T4 73% G7-10 Only 23% T1c-T2a	70.2 Gy (50.4 Gy to WP if on WP arms) 4 arms: whole pelvis (WP) vs. prostate-only (PO) RT and neoadjuvant and concurrent HT (ncHT) vs. adjuvant HT (aHT)	Initial results: WP + ncHT improved progression free survival (PFS) (61%) vs. the other 3 arms (45–49%). With 6.6-year follow-up, WP+ncHT had better PFS vs. PO+ncHT ($p = 0.034$) and WP+aHT ($p = 0.02$), but not PO+aHT ($p = 0.75$). WP+aHT had trend for worse OS vs. other arms. Cause specific survival: at 10 years, WP+ncHT, PO+aHT, WP+aHT, and PO+ncHT = 90, 85, 80, and 80%, respectively ($p > 0.43$).	No diff in acute grade 3 toxicity, but WP+NHT had slightly higher late grade 3 GI toxicity (5 vs. 1–2%)

VII

- RTOG 9408 (ASTRO 2009 late breaking abstract, not published by ASTRO). Randomized 1979 T1b-T2b pts to 66.6 Gy +/- 4 mo nCHT. HT improved 8 yr OS for intermediate-risk pts (66→72%) with trend for high-risk pts (58→66%) and no difference for low-risk pts (73 vs 76%). No increase in deaths from intercurrent disease with HT.

RT + LONG-TERM HT

- For high-risk patients, HT for ≥2–3 years improves OS by ~10–15%, CSS by ~5%, and DFS by ~20–30% vs. no HT or 4–6-month HT.

Study	Patients	Arms	Benefit	Toxicity
RTOG 8531, (Pilepich et al. 1997; JCO 2005; IJROBP 2005; ASCO 2007; JCO 2009)	945 patients cT3, pT3, or LN+	65–70 Gy (50 Gy WP) ± indefinite goserelin starting the last week of RT	10-year OS for all patients: 39→49% On subset analysis, OS benefit only for G7–10 DSS: 78→84% DM: 39→24%	No difference in 9-year cardiac mortality with ADT *Pooled results of RTOG 8531, 8610*, 9202 (Lawton 2007). RT + LTHT reduced late GU toxicity (9→6%), but not GI (3%) or other (1%)
EORTC 22863 (Bolla et al. 2002; ASTRO 2008)	415 patients T3-4 or T1-2 G≥7 (only 34 of these patients) Median PSA >20	70 Gy (50 Gy WP) ±3-year goserelin starting on first day of RT	10-year OS: 40–>58% CSS: 69→89%	No difference in 10-year cardiac mortality (8–11%)
RTOG 9202 (JCO 2003; JCO 2008)	1,554 patients T2c-T4 PSA <150 Median PSA 20	65–70 Gy (44–45 Gy WP) + 4-month ncHT ±2-year goserelin	10-year OS: 52→54% overall, p = ns, but GS 8–10: 32→45% CSS: 84→89% DM: 23→15% bF: 68→52% LF: 22→12%	No difference in long-term CV mortality. Traditional cardiac risk factors, including age, prevalent CVD, and diabetes, were significantly associated with greater cardio-vascular mortality (Efstathiou 2008)

continued

VII

EORTC 22961 (Bolla et al. 2009)	970 patients T2c-T4N0/+ or T1c-2bN+ Median PSA 18	70 Gy (50 Gy WP) 6-month vs. 3-year HT	3-year HT improved 5-year overall mortality: 19 vs. 15.2% Prostate cancer mortality: 4.7 vs. 3.2% Clinical progression: 39.5 vs. 25% Biochemical progression: 52 vs. 29.4% No difference in fatal cardiac events (3–4%) More hot flushes, decreased sexual function with 3-year HT

SELECTED STUDIES ON FIELD SIZE

- Whole pelvic RT used in all high-risk trials, controversial for intermediate-risk patients, and not indicated for low-risk patients.
- Whole Pelvic RT defined with L5-S1 superior border vs. mini-pelvic field at bottom of SI joints.
- *RTOG 9413 field size* (Roach 2006): Compared results for ncHT arms for WP vs. mini-pelvic (largest PO fields) vs. smallest PO fields. WP improved 7-year PFS (40%) vs. mini-pelvis (35%) or PO RT (27%). No difference in late GU toxicity, but small increase in late grade 3+ GI toxicity (1→4%) with WP.
- *GETUG-01* (Pommier 2007): 444 patients with T1b-T3N0M0 randomized to 66–70 Gy to prostate ± 46 Gy to pelvis (top border S1/S2): 4–8-month NCHT allowed for "high-risk" patients (≥T3, GS ≥7, or PSA ≥3x normal). Approximately 55% of patients had LN risk <15% using Roach formula. Median PSA 12, ~25% T3, and ~10% GS 8–10. With 42-month follow-up, pelvic RT did not improve OS or PFS regardless of LN risk group, although risk of LN was the most significant prognostic factor on multivariate analysis. Pelvic RT slightly increased acute mild GI toxicity (p=ns) and late GI grade 2+ toxicity (p=ns), but not acute or late urinary toxicity. No difference in QOL. Criticism: WPRT superior border only extended to S1/S2.
- *Yale* (Aizer et al. 2009): Retrospective review of 277 consecutive patients with ≥15% risk of LN involvement treated with prostate-only (75.5%) or whole pelvic RT (24.5%) and median RT dose 75.6 Gy. Despite higher T stage, GS, and pretreatment PSA at baseline, WPRT group had improved 4-year bDFS (69.4 vs. 86.3%). Predictors of bDFS were pretreatment PSA, GS, use of HT, and use of WPRT. WPRT increased acute GI, but not acute GU or late toxicity.
- *UCSF* (Seaward et al. 1998): Retrospective review. High-risk patients ($n=201$) who received WPRT had improved freedom from PSA failure vs. PO-RT (median PFS = 34 vs. 21 month). Multivariate analysis revealed type of RT as most significant predictor of outcome.
- *University of Michigan* (Pan et al. 2002): Retrospective review of 1,832 patients treated with 3D-CRT divided into three categories of LN involvement: low, 0–5%; intermediate, >5–15%; and

VII

high, >15% (Partin Tables). Multivariate analysis demonstrated significant benefit for entire population treated with WPRT, with benefit most pronounced among intermediate-risk group (2-year bNED 90 vs. 81%).

- *Fox Chase* (Jacob et al. 2005): Retrospective review of 460 patients with LN risk ≥15% or T2c GS 6–10 PSA <100 treated with 3DCRT (74–82 Gy) with whole pelvic (65%), partial pelvic (16%), or prostate-only (10%) fields. Sixteen percent received STAD. RT dose was the major determinant of PSA control and field size and STAD were not associated. Criticism: WP fields only extended superiorly to the inferior SI joints.
- *Stanford* (Spiotto 2007): See below under adjuvant/salvage.
- Da Pozzo et al. (2009): See below under node+.

CHEMO WITH RT

- RTOG 9902 (Rosenthal et al. 2009): 397 patients with GS ≥7 and PSA 20–100 or T2, GS ≥8, PSA <100 randomized to RT + 2-year 4-month HT ± paclitaxel, estramustine, and etoposide chemotherapy. Terminated early due to increased toxicity. Chemo increased GI and heme toxicity including two deaths from neutropenic infection and three cases of AML or myelodysplasia.

LDR BRACHYTHERAPY

- Multiinstitutional review (Zelefsky 2007): 2,693 patients with T1–2 treated with brachy monotherapy (68% I-125, 32% Pd-103): 8-year PSA RFS: 93% if D90 ≥130 Gy vs. 76% if <130 Gy; 92% if PSA nadir <0.5, 86% if PSA nadir 0.5 to <1, 79% if PSA nadir 1 to <2, 67% if PSA nadir >2.
- Multiinstitutional review (Stone 2009): 1,078 patients with Gleason 7–10 treated with LDR brachy ± supplemental EBRT (58%) and/or STADT (62%): 5-year bFFF was 80% for all. On subset, BED predicted 5-year bFFF: BED <200 (76%), BED 200–220: 84%, BED >220: 88%.

HDR BRACHYTHERAPY

- Galalae et al. (2004): Reviewed 611 patients on three studies treated with EBRT (45–50 Gy to prostate, seminal vesicles, and pelvic LN) with a HDR boost of 2–4 fractions during EBRT. Included 177 patients treated with short-course N&CHT. Five-year bPFS / CSS for low-risk (≤T2a and GS ≤6 and PSA ≤10) = 96/100%, intermediate-risk (one factor: ≥T2b or GS ≥7 or PSA ≥10) = 88/99%, and high-risk (≥2 intermediate risk factors) = 69/95%. Predictors of failure were risk group, stage, PSA, and GS. Short-course N&CHT did not improve outcome. Five-year OS for all groups was 85–88%.

COMPARISON OF MODALITIES

- Kupelian et al. (2004): Compared 2,991 consecutive patients treated at Cleveland Clinic and Memorial Sloan Kettering with RP, EBRT <72 Gy, EBRT >72 Gy, permanent seed implant (PPI), and combined PPI + EBRT. Patients treated with RP were younger and had more favorable tumor characteristics. ≤6-month neoadjuvant HT was used in 21% of patients (mainly the RT groups). bPFS was defined as PSA >0.2 for RP or 3 consecutive rises for all others. The 5-year bPFS was: RP 81%, EBRT <72Gy 51%, EBRT >72Gy 81%, PPI 83%, PPI+EBRT 77%. Only EBRT <72 Gy was worse. Pretreatment PSA, GS, and year of therapy predicted bPFS, but T stage and HT did not.
- D'Amico et al. (1998): Reviewed 1,872 patients treated at University of PA or the Joint Center in Boston with RP, EBRT, or LDR implant ± neoadjuvant HT. Using old ASTRO PSA failure definition and D'Amico risk groups, there was no difference in bPFS for low-risk patients. For intermediate-risk patients, there was no difference between RP, EBRT, implant + neoadjuvant HT. For high-risk patients, implants (± NHT) had lower bPFS than RP or EBRT.
- Eade et al. (2008): 374 low-risk patients treated at Fox Chase with IMRT and IGRT to 74–78 Gy or with I-125 implant to 145 Gy. patients treated with IMRT were more likely to be older and have worse baseline urinary function. IMRT had lower 3-year rates of grade 2+ GI toxicity (2.4 vs. 7.7%) and GU toxicity (3.5 vs. 19.2%).

VII

- Beyer and Brachman (2000): Reviewed >2,200 patients with T1–2 disease treated with either EBRT ($n > 1{,}527$) or PPI ($n > 695$) at a single institution. There was no difference in 5-year FFS for T1 or T2 disease with GS <7 and PSA <10. For patients with GS 8–10 or PSA >10 to <20, EBRT provided improved FFS.
- Jabbari (2009): Comparison of 249 low/intermediate-risk patients treated with LDR brachytherapy ± EBRT ± ADT at UCSF and University of Michigan, and the high-dose (79.2 Gy) arm of the Zietman proton boost PIII trial. bNED at 5 and 7 years with LDR brachy is 92 and 86%, and equivalent to 3DCRT and proton boost. No change in results when censoring ADT patients. Lower PSA nadirs achieved with LDR brachytherapy as compared to 3DCRT or proton boost.
- Grills et al. (2004): Review of 65 consecutive patients treated with HDR monotherapy (Ir-192, 9.5 Gy b.i.d. × 2 day) and 84 patients treated with LDR monotherapy (Pd-103, 120 Gy) at William Beaumont Hospital. The majority had T1c-T2a, GS ≤6, and PSA <10; 36% received neoadjuvant HT. Three-year biochemical control (ASTRO definition) was 98% for HDR and 97% for LDR. HDR was associated with reduced acute grade 1–3 dysuria, urinary frequency/urgency, and rectal pain, as well as late urinary frequency/urgency and impotence.

ADJUVANT AND SALVAGE RT AFTER RP

- PSA failure occurs in 15–40% of patients after RP.
- Patients with rising PSA after RP have up to 60% probability of developing DM and 20% risk of prostate CA mortality within 10 years if left untreated.
- Median time from PSA failure to DM is ~8 years, but only ~3 years for high GS or short PSA doubling time <3 month. Median time from DM to death is ~5 years (Pound 1999; Freedland 2005).

ADJUVANT RADIOTHERAPY TRIALS

Study	Patients	Arms	Benefits of adjuvant RT	Toxicity
SWOG 8794 (Thompson 2009; Swanson 2007)	431 patients pN0M0 s/p RP with ECE, +margin, or SVI	Observation (~1/3 ultimately got RT) vs. 60–64 Gy	15-year OS: 37→47% 15-year DMFS: 38→46% 10-year bF: 77→55% 10-year LF 22→8% ADT at 12 years: 50→39% Risk of DM or death greater in RT patients with detectable PSA vs. those treated with an undetectable PSA	QOL study in 217 patients (JCO 2008): increased urinary frequency and bowel dysfunction in RT grp, although bowel difference disappeared by 2 years. No difference in erectile dysfunction. Global health related QOL initially worse in RT group, but improved over time and favored RT group in the long-term due to prevention of disease progression and ADT use
EORTC 22911 (Van der Kwast 2007; Bolla 2005)	1,005 patients pN0 with ECE, +margin, or SVI	Observation (~1/2 ultimately got RT) vs. 60 Gy	5-year OS: no diff (~93%) bPFS:53→74% cPFS: 77→85%) LRF: 15→5% +Margin status strongest predictor of benefit	No significant difference in 2–4% grade 3+ toxicity
German ARO 96-02 (Wiegel 2007; Wiegel et al. 2009)	385 patients pT3 or + margins	Observation vs. 60 Gy	bNED: 54→72% for patients with undetectable post-op PSA	1% grade 1–2 rectal toxicity, 2% grade 1–2 genitourinary toxicity. 0.3% late grade 3 toxicity

VII

SALVAGE RADIOTHERAPY

- Stephenson et al. (2007): Retrospective review 1,540 patients with PSA ≥0.2 followed by another higher value or single PSA ≥0.5 after RP. All treated with salvage RT (median 64 Gy). Overall 6-year bPFS (PSA >0.2 higher than nadir after RT) was 32%; 48% for pre-RT PSA ≤0.5, 40% for 0.5–1, 28% for 1–1.5, and 18% for >1.5. bPFS 41% for patients with GS8–10 and PSADT <10 month if initiated with pre-RT PSA ≤0.5. Predictors of poor outcome were higher pre-RT PSA, GS 8–10, PSADT <10 month, -margins, ADT, and LN+ (Fig. 26.1).
- Trock et al. (2008): Retrospective review of 635 men status post-RP for T1–2 with PSA >0.2 with no further tx (63%) vs. salvage RT (25%) or salvage RT and HT (12%): 10-year PCSS was 62, 86, and 82%, respectively. On multivariate analysis, salvage RT reduced risk of death by >65%. Strongest predictor of improved PCSS was PSA-DT <6 month. For PSA-DT >6 month, salvage RT only improved PCSS for subgroup of patients with +margins and G8–10. Salvage RT improved PCSS only if given sooner than 2 years after recurrence. Salvage RT benefit for patients with rapid PSADT and high GS suggests prevalence of local recurrence may be higher than previously thought. Study underpowered to determine if salvage RT benefits men whose PSA never became undetectable. PCSS similar for men with salvage RT ± HT, despite HT patients having worse prognostic factors, suggesting possible benefit of HT. Salvage RT improved OS for pT3 patients up to 98% (Fig. 26.2).
- Beyer (2003) reviewed the literature on salvage brachytherapy after EBRT and noted that 5-year freedom from second relapse after salvage brachytherapy is ~50% overall, but with careful selection may be as high as 83%. Patients most likely to benefit include those with histologically confirmed local recurrence, no evidence of distant disease, adequate urinary function, >5–10-year life expectancy, >2-year disease-free interval after EBRT, PSADT >6–9 month, GS ≤6, and PSA <10 at time of recurrence).

ROLE OF HT WITH SALVAGE OR ADJUVANT RT

- King (2004): Retrospective analysis of 122 patients treated with salvage RT ± HT. Addition of HT improved 5-year bNED 31→57% and OS 87→100%. For GS ≤7 5-year bNED 38→58% and OS 98–100%. For GS ≥8 bNED 17→65% and OS 54→100%.
- Cheung (2005): Retrospective analysis of 101 patients treated with salvage RT ± HT. HT provided benefit for all patients

Pre-RT PSA
≤ 2.0
> 2.0
4-year PFP (CI)
52% (49–56)
980 patients
4-year PFP (CI)
19% (15–24)
346 patients
Gleason score
4–7
8–10
4-year PFP (CI)
58% (54–62)
689 patients
4-year PFP (CI)
27% (19–35)
151 patients
Surgical margins
Positive
Negative
4-year PFP (CI)
61% (55–67)
360 patients
4-year PFP (CI)
55% (49–61)
314 patients
Surgical margins
Positive
Negative
4-year PFP (CI)
33% (22–43)
151 patients
4-year PFP (CI)
18% (7–29)
63 patients
PSADT
> 10
≤ 10
4-year PFP (CI)
69% (59–79)
110 patients
4-year PFP (CI)
57% (49–66)
196 patients
PSADT
> 10
≤ 10
4-year PFP (CI)
61% (50–72)
96 patients
4-year PFP (CI)
48% (40–56)
175 patients
PSADT
> 10
≤ 10
4-year PFP (CI)
5C% (16–86)
14 patients
4-year PFP (CI)
30% (17–44)
50 patients

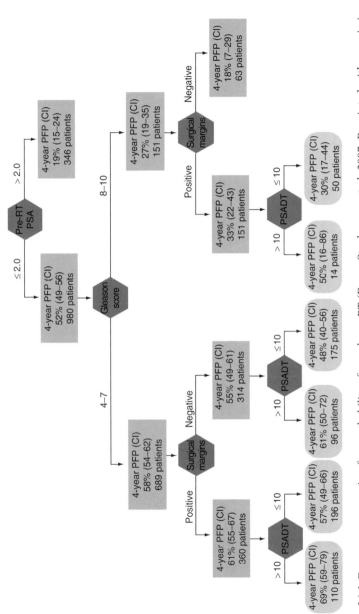

Fig. 26.1 Four-year progression free probability after salvage RT (From: Stephenson et al. 2007. Reprinted with permission. Copyright 2008 American Society of Clinical Oncology. All rights reserved)

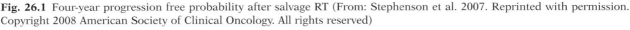

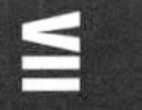

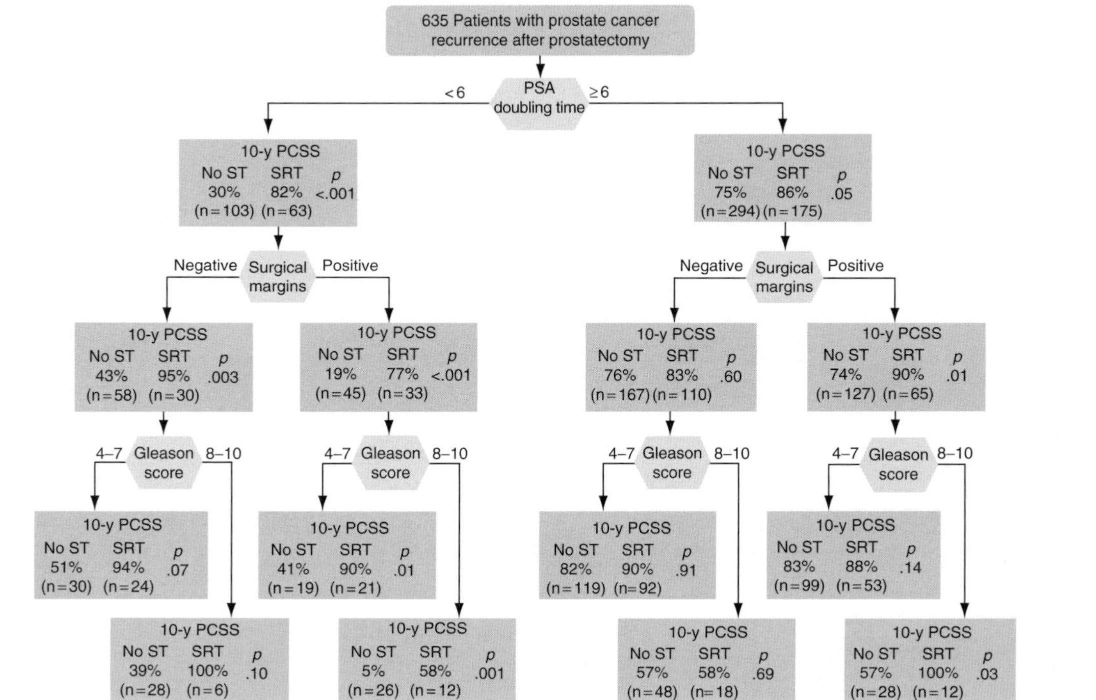

Fig. 26.2 Ten-year PCSS rates following recurrence in men who received no salvage therapy (ST) vs. salvage radiotherapy (SRT; with or without hormonal therapy) (From: Trock et al. 2008. Copyright (2008) American Medical Association. All rights reserved)

except those with +margin and PSA <0.5 (favorable): 5-year bPFS for favorable patients ~80→100% p = ns, ~60→80% for unfavorable patients (p = 0.03).

- Spiotto (2007): 160 patients treated with adjuvant or salvage RT. Sixty-three percent of 114 patients with high-risk features (GS ≥8, pPSA ≥20, SVI, ECE, or +LN) received WPRT, while remaining received prostate bed only RT. Among high-risk patients (>20% risk of LN = pT3, LN+, pPSA >20, G8–10), WPRT improved 5-year bRFS vs. PO RT (21→47%), but there was no difference for lower-risk patients. Benefit only seen for patients given ADT concurrently (bRFS 18→53%), despite worse prognostic features among WPRT group. Also, the addition of ADT to WPRT improved bRFS vs. WPRT alone (35→53%).
- *RTOG 85-31* (Corn 1999): 139 post-op patients had ECE or SVI. 71 got RT+HT and 68 got RT alone. RT+HT improved 5-year bPFS (42→65%).

NODE+ DISEASE

- No proven OS benefit by the addition of local treatment to ADT.
- No randomized trial of long-term LHRH vs. LHRH + RT yet published, but trial of long-term antiandrogen after initial combined ADT showed OS advantage with the addition of RT (Widmark et al. 2009).
- Messing et al. (1999); Messing (2006): 98 LN+ patients who had a RP and pelvic lymphadenectomy were randomized to immediate goserelin or bilateral orchiectomy vs. observation. At 12-year, immediate ADT improved MS (11.3→13.9 years) and MPFS (2.4–4.1→13.9 years). All but three patients died of prostate cancer in observation arm.
- *RTOG 8531* (JCO 2005): 173 patients had biopsy pN+ and randomized to RT vs. RT + goserelin indefinitely. Addition of LTHT improved OS (5 year 50→72%, 9 year 38→62%), bPFS (5 year 33→54%, 9 year 4→10%), and DM (48→33%).
- Zagars et al. (2001): Retrospective 255 pN+ patients were treated with early androgen ablation alone or with 70 Gy EBRT to the prostate. Adding EBRT improved 10-year OS (46→67%) and freedom from relapse or rising PSA (25→80%).
- Da Pozzo et al. (2009): Retrospective review of 250 consecutive pLN+ patients treated with HT alone (48%) or HT and RT (52%). Seventy-four percent of patients received pelvic and prostate bed RT. Median dose 66.6 Gy. 5/8-year bRFS 72/61%, CSS 89/83%. In multivariate analysis, adjuvant RT and # of

VII

positive LN predicted bRFS and CSS. Patients treated with aHT alone had 2.6× risk of prostate cancer mortality vs. HT and RT after accounting for other predictors.

METASTATIC DISEASE

- Prognosis is best approximated by the absolute level of PSA, the PSA doubling time, initial stage, and, most importantly, tumor grade.
- Earlier ADT may be better than delayed ADT, although the definitions of early are controversial.
- Patients with an elevated PSA (>50 ng/mL) and/or a shorter PSA doubling time (or a rapid PSA velocity) and an otherwise long life expectancy should consider early ADT.
- Treatment should begin immediately in the presence of tumor-related symptoms or overt metastases.
- Earlier ADT will delay the appearance of symptoms and of metastases, but it is not clear whether it will prolong survival.
  - *MRC* (The Medical Research Council Prostate Cancer Working Party Investigators Group 1997): 934 patients with T2–4 or asymptomatic M1 disease were randomized to immediate androgen ablation (AA) (LHRH analog or orchiectomy) vs. deferred AA. Early treatment decreased local and metastatic disease progression, and increased OS and CSS (mostly among M0 patients).
- LHRH agonist (medical castration) and bilateral orchiectomy (surgical castration) appear to be equally effective. Combined androgen blockade (medical or surgical castration combined with an antiandrogen) provides no proven benefit over castration alone in patients with metastatic disease.
- Antiandrogen therapy should precede or be coadministered with LHRH agonist and be continued in combination for at least 7–14 days to reduce risk of developing symptoms associated with the flare in testosterone with initial LHRH agonist alone.
- Antiandrogen monotherapy appears to be less effective than medical or surgical castration and should not be recommended.
- Intermittent ADT may reduce side effects without altering survival compared to continuous ADT, but the long-term efficacy remains unproven.
  - Miller (2007): 335 patients with node+ or metastatic prostate CA randomized to goserelin and bicalutamide intermittent vs. continuous. No difference in time to progression or death

or incidence of adverse events. Patients on intermittent experienced >40% off-treatment periods.

- Patients who do not achieve adequate suppression of serum testosterone (less than 50 ng/mL) with medical or surgical castration can be considered for additional hormonal manipulations (with estrogen, antiandrogens, or steroids), although the clinical benefit is not clear.
- Give supplemental calcium (1,200 mg daily) and vitamin D3 (800–1,000 IU daily) and consider bisphosphonate therapy.
- For men with androgen-independent disease, every 3-week docetaxel and prednisone is the preferred first-line chemotherapy treatment based on two randomized trials that demonstrated ~3-month survival benefit with docetaxel based therapy vs. mitoxantrone / prednisone (SWOG 99-16, NEJM 2004; Tannock et al. 2004).

RADIATION TECHNIQUES

EBRT

- At UCSF, patients are treated supine with alpha cradle or "knee sponge" to consistently align thighs.
- Alternatively, patients may be treated prone with thermoplastic shell immobilization. A randomized trial by Bayley et al. (2004), however, noted that there was significantly less prostate motion in the supine position and that prone position resulted in increased dose to critical structures.
- Patients are instructed to have a full bladder and empty rectum (following an enema) for simulation.
- At UCSF, a daily electronic portal imaging device (EPID) is used to monitor prostate position. Gold marker seeds are placed in the base and apex of the prostate 7–10 day prior to simulation. If EPIDs are unavailable, transabdominal US-based daily imaging may be used.
- If gold seeds are not placed, retrograde urethrography is used in conjunction with CT for identifying the inferior border of the prostate. The prostate apex is assumed to be 1–1.5 cm superior to the point at which the dye narrows. Retrograde urethrography is particularly useful in the post-op setting.
- Planning is CT-based. The prostate appears larger inferiorly and posteriorly on noncontrast CT images compared to TRUS or MRI.
- Indications for seminal vesicle irradiation include + biopsy, + TRUS, + MRI, or calculated risk >15% (using the Roach formula).

- Indications for whole pelvic RT at UCSF include involved LN, seminal vesicle involvement, a calculated risk of lymph node involvement >15% (using the Roach formula), patients with T3 GS 6 disease, and patients with high intermediate risk (>50% + biopsies) or high-risk disease.
- For traditional whole pelvic RT, initial field borders are: superior = L5/S1; inferior = 0.5–1 cm below the area where the dye narrows on the urethrogram (or 1–1.5 cm below in the post-op setting); lateral = 1.5 cm lateral to the bony margin of the true pelvis. On the AP/PA fields, corners are blocked to decrease dose to the femoral heads, bowel, and bone marrow. On the lateral fields, the anterior border is anterior to the pubic synthesis. The posterior border splits the sacrum to S2/3 and a beam's eye view is generated with CT contours of the rectum present in order to draw the rectal bloc excluding the posterior rectum. "Mini-pelvic" fields are not recommended.
- For the conedown on the prostate + seminal vesicles or the prostate alone, nonuniform field edge margins of 0.5–1.5 cm are used in order to account for set-up error, movement error, and beam penumbra.
- With daily EPID imaging, the margins are reduced to 0.5–1 cm.
- Weekly port films are obtained throughout treatment.
- Alternatively, IMRT may be used for both whole pelvic and boost portions of treatment. With whole pelvic IMRT, careful review of lymph node mapping is recommended (Shih et al. 2005; Taylor et al. 2005; Chao and Lin 2002).
- RTOG GU Consensus on pelvic LN CTV volumes (Lawton et al. 2008; Lawton et al. 2009):
  - Commence contouring the pelvic CTV LN volumes at the L5/S1 interspace (the level of the distal common iliac and proximal presacral lymph nodes).
  - Place a 7-mm margin around the iliac vessels connecting the external and internal iliac contours on each slice, carving out bowel, bladder, and bone.
  - Contour presacral lymph nodes (subaortic only) S1 through S3, posterior border being the anterior sacrum, and anterior border approximately 10 mm anterior to the anterior sacral bone carving out bowel, bladder, and bone.
  - Stop external iliac CTV lymph node contours at the top of the femoral heads (bony landmark for the inguinal ligament).
  - Stop contours of the obturator CTV lymph nodes at the top of the public (Figs. 26.3 and 26.4).

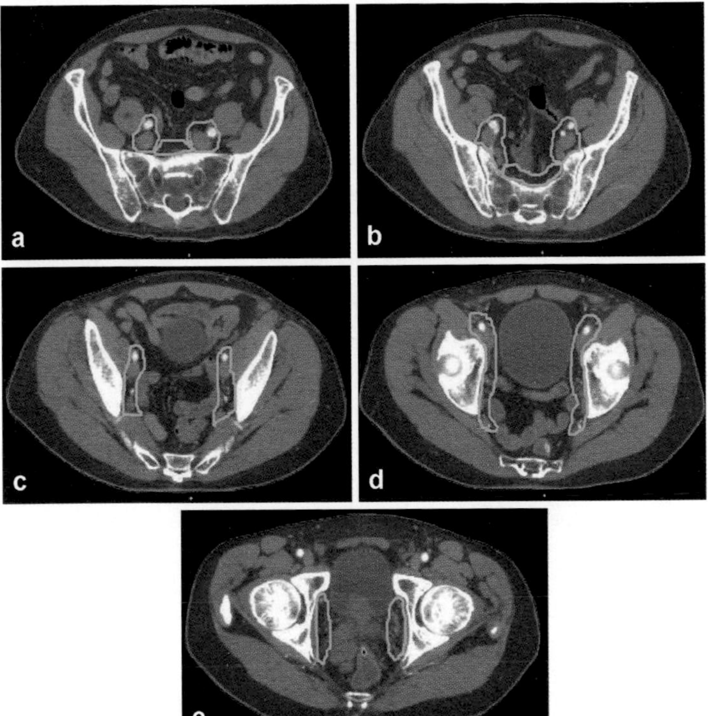

Fig. 26.3 Representative pelvic LN CTV contours: (**a**) Common iliac and presacral (L5/S1). (**b**) External iliac, internal iliac, and presacral (S1–S3). (**c**) External and internal Iliac (below S3). (**d**) End of external iliac (at top of femoral head, bony landmark for the inguinal ligament). (**e**) Obturator (above the top of the pubic symphysis) (Reprinted with permission from Elsevier. Adapted from: Lawton et al. 2009)

- In the postoperative setting, the CTV is based on preoperative imaging, histopathologic size of the prostate, tumor extent, surgical margins, and input from the Urologist.
  - Inferior border: top of penile bulb or 1.5 cm below urethral beak or 8 mm below vesicourethral anastamosis.
  - Anterior border: posterior edge of pubic symphysis including entire bladder neck until above symphysis, then off bladder.
  - Posterior border: to anterior aspect of rectum and mesorectal fascia.

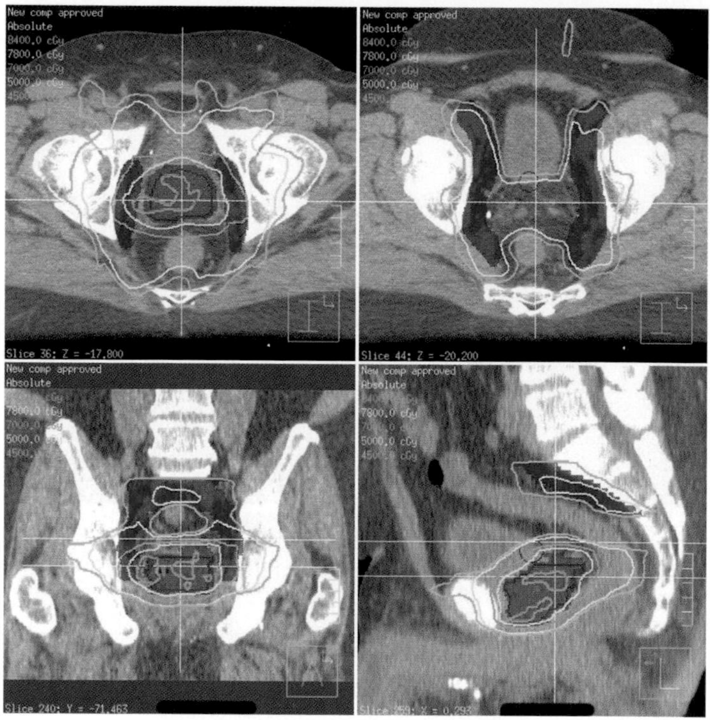

Fig. 26.4 Representative definitive UCSF IMRT plan for a man with cT2b, Gleason 4+5 PSA 17.2 adenocarcinoma of the prostate. Purple colorwash: prostate and SV PTV, blue colorwash: lymph node PTV

- Lateral borders: to medial edge of obturator internus muscles.
- Superior border: just above pubic symphysis anteriorly and including surgical clips or 5 mm above inferior border of vas deferens.
- PTV expansion: 0.6–1.5 cm (Fig. 26.5).

EBRT DOSE

- Prophylactic dose to the pelvic LN is 1.8 Gy/fx to 45 Gy. Involved LN receive 54–56 Gy or higher with IMRT.
- Prophylactic dose to the seminal vesicles is 54 Gy. Documented seminal vesicle disease receives full-dose.
- Conedown boosts using 3DCRT or IMRT cover the prostate to 74–78 Gy. The minimum central axis dose is 78 Gy.

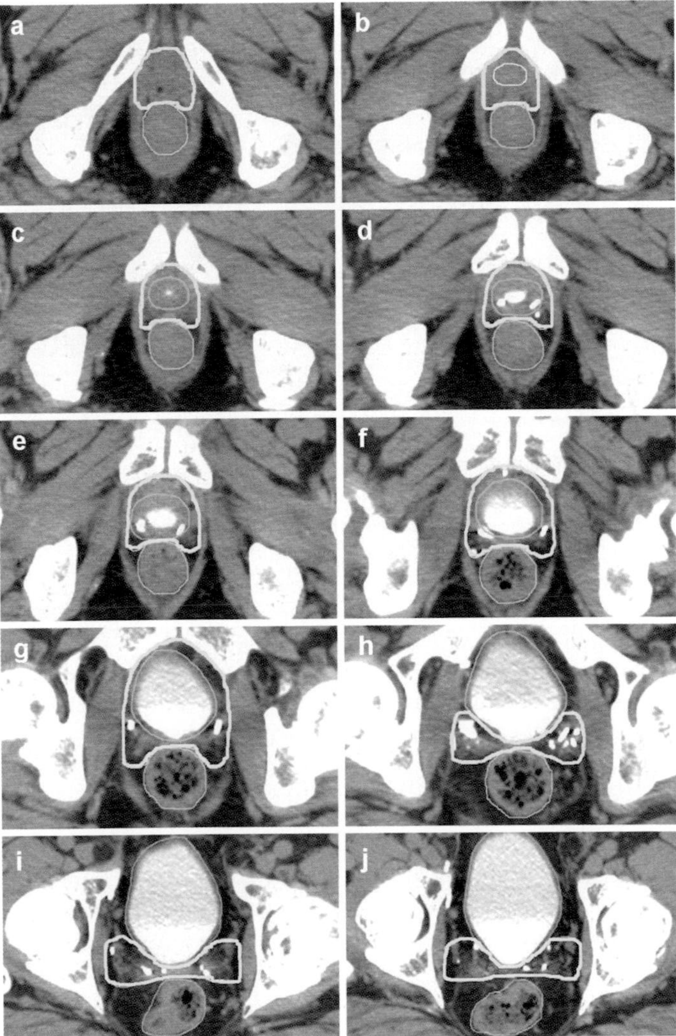

Fig. 26.5 Representative postoperative prostate bed CTV, *yellow*; vesicourethral anastomosis, *white*; rectum, *blue*; bladder, *green*; vas deferens, *red*. (**a–c**) Delayed scan following IV contrast so as to ascertain the most inferior slice where urine is last visible (**c**). The anastomosis is one slice below this (**b**), and the most inferior CTV slice 5 mm lower (**a**). (**d–g**) The anterior border of the inferior CTV lies behind the symphisis pubis. (**h–j**) The most superior slice of the CTV (**j**) encompasses the last slice where the vas deferens is visible and all nonvascular surgical clips (Reprinted with permission by Elsevier. Adapted from: Sidhom et al. 2008)

- In the postoperative setting, the prostate bed is typically treated to 64.8–66.6 Gy at 1.8-Gy per fraction, but may be boosted higher if local residual disease is documented.

EXAMPLE EBRT DOSE CONSTRAINTS

- Bladder
  - V75 <25%, V70 <35%, V65 <25–50%, V55 <50%, V40 <50%.
- Rectum
  - V75 <15%, V70 <20–25%, V65 <17%, V60 <40%, V50 <50%, V40 <35–40%.
- Femoral heads: V50 <5%
- Small bowel: V52 0%
- Penile bulb: Mean dose <52.5 Gy

LDR BRACHYTHERAPY

- ABS monotherapy indications: T1c-T2a, GS <7, PSA ≤10.
- ABS indications for supplemental EBRT: ≥T2c, GS≥7, PSA >10 (any 1 factor).
- Contraindications include metastases, gross seminal vesicle involvement, and large T3 disease that cannot be easily implanted due to geometrical impediments.
- Patients unlikely to cope well with a temporary exacerbation of obstructive symptoms may be better served with EBRT or RP (e.g., significant pretreatment urinary obstructive symptoms, such as AUA score >15. Other relative contraindications are prostate size (>50 cm^3) related to pubic arch interference, prostatitis, and median lobe hypertrophy.
- Implants are typically preplanned from TRUS images of the prostate taken in the lithotomy position at 5-mm intervals from the base through the apex ≤7 days before the implant.
  - The patient is set up with the midgland symmetrically in center of template grid (6 cm R/L × 5.5 cm A/P). Fluid in bladder helps define base. Rectal wall aligned to row 1. Pubic arch interference is then ruled out. The base is referred to as 0.0 retraction and is set on axial and sagittal views. A Foley catheter is then inserted into bulbomembranous urethra and 2 mL water is inserted into the balloon to occlude the urethra. Aerated K-Y jelly is then inserted slowly into urethra to improve visualization. Images of the prostate are then captured into the treatment planning system. At least one extra slice above and below prostate is captured.

- Recently, intraoperative planning based on intraoperative TRUS image capture has been used.
- The goal of treatment planning is to cover the prostate with a 3–5-mm margin to cover potential ECE.
- For the procedure, pre-op bowel preparation is necessary and spinal, epidural, or general anesthesia is generally used, but local anesthesia is used at some centers.
- In the OR, a catheter or aerated gel is used to visualize the urethra. TRUS frequencies of 5–7 MHz are used. The TRUS is supported on an adjustable 0.5 cm stepping unit mounted to the table. If using a preplan, match the intra-op images to the pre-op images using the seminal vesicles and the base of the gland. Needles are inserted through the template holes until they are viewed in the desired plane. Rotating the needle allows two distinct lines to be seen, corresponding to the bevel. Seeds are deposited from preloaded needles or the Mick applicator. Seeds may be single or suture-mounted. An extended lithotomy position may help reduce pubic arch interference.
- Typically, the patient is discharged after he is able to urinate. Prescriptions are generally provided for Flomax, NSAIDs, and Cipro ×3 day. Patients are cautioned to avoid constipation in postimplant periord.

LDR DOSE

- Brachytherapy monotherapy doses: I-125 144 Gy; Pd-103 125 Gy.
- After 40–50 Gy EBRT: I-125 110 Gy; Pd-103 90 Gy.
- I-125: source activity 0.2–0.9 mCi, half-life 60 day, photon energy 28 KeV.
- Pd-103: source activity 1.1–2.5 mCi, half-life 17 day, photon energy 21 KeV.
- Review isodose overlays to determine significance of under and overdosed regions.
- Dosimetric goals.
  - V100 is the percent of the prostate volume covered by 100% of the prescription dose.
  - D90 is the % prescription dose that covers 90% of the prostate volume.
  - Prostate: V100 >95–99%, D90 >90–100%, V150 <70%, V200 <20%.
  - Urethra: D30% <130%, Dmax <150%, V100 <60%.
  - Rectum: D0.1 mL <200 Gy, D2mL <100%, RV100% <1 mL.

HDR BRACHYTHERAPY

- Generally, HDR implants are performed less frequently than LDR implants.
- HDR after-loading catheters are inserted under TRUS guidance and secured into position. A CT scan captures the catheter position into the treatment planning system. Each catheter is sequentially loaded with Ir-192 by computer-driven stepping motors. The treatment planning software determines the optimal loading and duration of the source in a given position in order to accomplish a desired dose distribution.
- Temporary implants are usually administered using multiple fractionated treatments delivered over 1–3 out-patient or in-patient visits.

HDR DOSE

- After EBRT, HDR is given as 9.5 Gy × 2 fractions in one implant.
- As monotherapy, HDR dose is 9.5 Gy b.i.d. × 2 day or 10.5 Gy × 3 fractions with one implant.
- Goals:
  - Prostate: V100 ≥ 90–96%, V150 < 40%, D90 > 90%.
  - Rectum and Bladder: V75 < 1 mL.
- Urethra: V120 < 0.8 mL.

GYNECOMASTIA DUE TO ANTIANDROGENS

- EBRT 4 Gy × 3 with 9 MeV e– reduces risk of gynecomastia by 70%.

COMPLICATIONS

Acute EBRT complications	**Incidence**	**Time of onset (week)**	**Management**
Dysuria, urgency, frequency, nocturia	Most	2	NSAID, alpha-blockers, pyridium
Urinary retention	Rare	>1	Catheter
Diarrhea	25–75%	2	Diet, antidiarrheals,
Rectal irritation, pain, bleeding	<10–20%	2–6	sitz baths, rectal steroids
Fatigue	Most	>3	Reassurance

- Late EBRT complications.
  - Urinary stricture <4%, unless prior TURP or prostatectomy 4–9% risk of stricture or stress incontinence.
  - Rectal bleeding <5–10% (technique/volume/dose related).
- In a metaanalysis (Robinson et al. 2002), posttreatment impotence rates were:
  - Brachtherapy alone 24%.
  - Brachtherapy + EBRT 40%.
  - EBRT alone 45%.
  - Nerve-sparing RP 66%.
  - Nonnerve sparing RP 75%.
  - Cryosurgery 87%.
- Decreased volume of ejaculate is seen with both EBRT and brachytherapy.
- Perioperative brachytherapy complications include pain, dysuria, urinary retention, hematuria, and urinary frequency.
  - Obstructive symptoms occur in ~10% of patients and tend to resolve 6–12 month after the implant. Retention usually resolves in 1–3 day. Urinary retention risk is related to preimplant AUA score.
    - AUA <10: 2–9%.
    - AUA 11–20: 10–20%.
    - AUA >20: 25 30%.
  - Urinary incontinence, urethral stricture or necrosis, hematuria: <1–3%.
  - Rectal injury is technique related and occurs in about 1–5% of patients.
- Complications of hormone therapy include hot flashes, impotence, liver dysfunction (due to antiandrogen), anemia, and osteoporosis.
  - Testosterone returns ~6–8 month after 1-month LHRH injection, 10–14 month after 3-month injection.
  - If nonmetastatic on ADT, annual zolendronate 4 mg IV ×1 and daily Ca 500 mg and Vit D 400 IU can maintain bone mineral density for 1 year (JCO 2007).
  - For metastatic patients, or patients with osteoporosis (T score <2.5), zolendronate 4 mg IV q3 weeks decreases skeletal complications.
- Prostatectomy.
  - Prostate cancer outcomes study (Penson 2005): ~1,300 men treated with RP in a population based cohort. Five-year outcomes.

VII

  - Urinary symptoms: Only 35% had complete urinary control, 51% had occasional leakage, 11% had frequent urinary leakage, and 3% no urinary control.
  - Sexual dysfunction: Only 28% had erections sufficient for intercourse.
- Second cancers (SEER, Tward 2008): Reviewed >92,000 RP patients, >9,000 EB+brachytherapy patients, and >10,000 brachytherapy patients and found no statistically elevated risk of developing any overall or particular "in-field" malignancy.

FOLLOW-UP

- H&P with DRE and PSA every 6 month for 5 years and then annually. In the first 1–3 years after definitive RT, PSA may be ordered more frequently (e.g., every 3–6 month).
- The definition of PSA failure following surgery is controversial and values ≥0.2, ≥0.3, and ≥0.4 ng/mL have been used.
- New AUA standard is PSA ≥0.2 ng/mL on two measurements (J Urol 2007).
- The 1996 ASTRO definition of PSA failure following EBRT is three consecutive PSA rises, with the time of failure backdated to the midpoint between the PSA nadir and the first rising PSA, or any rise great enough to provoke initiation of salvage therapy; a minimum follow-up of 2 years was recommended for presentation or publication of data.
- The "Phoenix Definition" (current ASTRO/RTOG definition) of PSA failure after EBRT, with or without short-term HT, is defined as a rise by ≥2 ng/mL above the nadir PSA (defined as the lowest PSA achieved), with the date of failure "at call" and not backdated. Patients who undergo salvage therapy (e.g., with HT, RP, brachytherapy, or cryosurgery) are declared failures at the time of + biopsy or salvage therapy administration (whichever comes first). Alternatively, for patients treated with EBRT alone, a modified stricter version of the ASTRO definition may continue to be used. For presentations and publications, the stated date of control should be listed as 2 years short of the median follow-up.
- The PSA nadir after RP is ~3 weeks, after EBRT ~2–3 years (but can be up to 4–5 years), and after brachytherapy ~3–4 years.
- PSA "bounce" consists of transient PSA rises (usually <2 ng/mL) after RT with a subsequent fall in the value. After brachytherapy, ~20% of patients have a bounce , and ~90% occur within 3 years with median duration 14 month. The median time to bounce

after EBRT is ~9–12 month and ~10–20% of patients have a bounce. Risk factors for PSA bounce after brachytherapy include age <65, higher implant dose, sexual activity, and larger prostate volume. PSA bounce after brachytherapy or EBRT does not predict PSA failure.

REFERENCES

Aizer AA, Yu JB, McKeon AM, et al. Whole pelvic radiotherapy versus prostate only radiotherapy in the management of locally advanced or aggressive prostate adenocarcinoma. Int J Radiat Oncol Biol Phys. 2009;75(5):1344-1349.

Al-Mamgani A, van Putten WL, Heemsbergen WD, et al. Update of Dutch multicenter dose-escalation trial of radiotherapy for localized prostate cancer. Int J Radiat Oncol Biol Phys 2008;72(4):980-988.

Bayley AJ, Catton CN, Haycocks T, et al. A randomized trial of supine vs. prone positioning in patients undergoing escalated dose conformal radiotherapy for prostate cancer. Radiother Oncol 2004;70:37-44.

Beyer DC, Brachman DG. Failure free survival following brachytherapy alone for prostate cancer: comparison with external beam radiotherapy. Radiother Oncol 2000;57:263-267.

Beyer DC. Brachytherapy for recurrent prostate cancer after radiation therapy. Semin Radiat Oncol 2003;13:158-165.

Bill-Axelson A, Holmberg L, Filen F, et al. Radical prostatectomy versus watchful waiting in localized prostate cancer: the Scandinavian prostate cancer group-4 randomized trial. J Natl Cancer Inst 2008;100(16):1144-1154.

Bill-Axelson A, Holmberg L, Ruutu M, et al. Radical prostatectomy versus watchful waiting in early prostate cancer. N Engl J Med 12 2005;352(19):1977-1984.

Bill-Axelson A, Holmberg L, Ruutu M, et al. Radical prostatectomy versus watchful waiting in early prostate cancer. N Engl J Med 2005;352:1977-1984.

Black PC, Basen-Engquist K, Wang X, et al. A randomized prospective trial evaluating testosterone, haemoglobin kinetics and quality of life, during and after 12 months of androgen deprivation after prostatectomy: results from the Postoperative Adjuvant Androgen Deprivation trial. BJU Int 2007;100(1):63-69.

Bolla M, Collette L, Blank L, et al. Long-term results with immediate androgen suppression and external irradiation in patients with locally advanced prostate cancer (an EORTC study): a phase III randomised trial. Lancet 2002;360:103-106.

Bolla M, de Reijke TM, Van Tienhoven G, et al. Duration of androgen suppression in the treatment of prostate cancer. NEJM 2009;360:2516-2527.

Chao KS, Lin M. Lymphangiogram-assisted lymph node target delineation for patients with gynecologic malignancies. Int J Radiat Oncol Biol Phys 2002;54:1147-1152.

Cheung MR, Tucker SL, Dong L, et al. Investigation of bladder dose and volume factors influencing late urinary toxicity after external beam radiotherapy for prostate cancer. Int J Radiat Oncol Biol Phys 2007;67(4):1059-1065.

Cheung R, Kamat AM, de Crevoisier R, et al. Outcome of salvage radiotherapy for biochemical failure after radical prostatectomy with or without hormonal therapy. Int J Radiat Oncol Biol Phys 2005;63(1):134-140.

Chun FK, Briganti A, Shariat SF, et al. Significant upgrading affects a third of men diagnosed with prostate cancer: predictive nomogram and internal validation. BJU Int 2006;98(2):329-334.

Corn BW, Winter K, Pilepich MV. Does androgen suppression enhance the efficacy of postoperative irradiation? A secondary analysis of RTOG 85-31. Radiation Therapy Oncology Group. Urology 1999;54(3):495-502.

Crook J, Ludgate C, Malone S, et al. Final report of multicenter Canadian Phase III randomized trial of 3 versus 8 months of neoadjuvant androgen deprivation therapy before conventional-dose radiotherapy for clinically localized prostate cancer. Int J Radiat Oncol Biol Phys 2009;73(2):327-333.

D'Amico AV, Chen MH, Roehl KA, et al. Preoperative PSA velocity and the risk of death from prostate cancer after radical prostatectomy. N Engl J Med 2004a;351:125-135.

D'Amico AV, Manola J, Loffredo M, et al. 6-month androgen suppression plus radiation therapy vs radiation therapy alone for patients with clinically localized prostate cancer: a randomized controlled trial. JAMA 2004b;292:821-827.

D'Amico AV, Renshaw AA, Sussman B, et al. Pretreatment PSA velocity and risk of death from prostate cancer following external beam radiation therapy. JAMA 2005;294:440-447.

VII

D'Amico AV, Whittington R, Malkowicz SB, et al. Biochemical outcome after radical prostatectomy, external beam radiation therapy, or interstitial radiation therapy for clinically localized prostate cancer. JAMA 1998;280:969-974.

D'Amico AV, Chen MH, Renshaw AA, Loffredo B, Kantoff PW. Risk of prostate cancer recurrence in men treated with radiation alone or in conjunction with combined or less than combined androgen suppression therapy. J Clin Oncol 2008;26(18):2979-2983.

D'Amico AV, Chen MH, Renshaw AA, Loffredo M, Kantoff PW. Androgen suppression and radiation vs radiation alone for prostate cancer: a randomized trial. JAMA 2008;299(3):289-295.

Da Pozzo LF, Cozzarini C, Briganti A, et al. Long-term follow-up of patients with prostate cancer and nodal metastases treated by pelvic lymphadenectomy and radical prostatectomy: the positive impact of adjuvant radiotherapy. Eur Urol. 2009;55(5):1003-1011.

Dearnaley DP, Sydes MR, Graham JD, et al. Escalated-dose versus standard-dose conformal radiotherapy in prostate cancer: first results from the MRC RT01 randomised controlled trial. Lancet Oncol 2007;8(6):475-487.

Eade TN, Horwitz EM, et al. A comparison of acute and chronic toxicity for men with low-risk prostate cancer treated with intensity-modulated radiation therapy or (125)I permanent implant. Int J Radiat Oncol Biol Phys 2008;71(2):338-345.

Efstathiou JA, Bae K, Shipley WU, et al. Cardiovascular mortality and duration of androgen deprivation for locally advanced prostate cancer: analysis of RTOG 92-02. Eur Urol 2008;54(4):816-823.

Freedland SJ, Humphreys EB, Mangold LA, et al. Risk of prostate cancer-specific mortality following biochemical recurrence after radical prostatectomy. JAMA 2005;294(4):433-439.

Galalae RM, Martinez A, Mate T, et al. Long-term outcome by risk factors using conformal high-dose-rate brachytherapy (HDR-BT) boost with or without neoadjuvant androgen suppression for localized prostate cancer. Int J Radiat Oncol Biol Phys 2004;58:1048-1055.

Grills IS, Martinez AA, Hollander M, et al. High dose rate brachytherapy as prostate cancer monotherapy reduces toxicity compared to low dose rate palladium seeds. J Urol 2004;171:1098-1104

Immediate versus deferred treatment for advanced prostatic cancer: initial results of the Medical Research Council Trial. The Medical Research Council Prostate Cancer Working Party Investigators Group. Br J Urol 1997;79:235-246.

Jabbari S, Weinberg VK, Shinohara K, et al. Equivalent biochemical control and improved prostate-specific antigen nadir after permanent prostate seed implant brachytherapy versus high-dose three-dimensional conformal radiotherapy and high-dose conformal proton beam radiotherapy boost. Int J Radiat Oncol Biol Phys 76(1):36-42.

Jacob R, Hanlon AL, Horwitz EM, et al. Role of prostate dose escalation in patients with greater than 15% risk of pelvic lymph node involvement. Int J Radiat Oncol Biol Phys 2005;61(3):695-701

King CR, Presti JC, Jr., Gill H, Brooks J, Hancock SL. Radiotherapy after radical prostatectomy: does transient androgen suppression improve outcomes? Int J Radiat Oncol Biol Phys 2004;59(2):341-347.

Klotz L. Active surveillance with selective delayed intervention: using natural history to guide treatment in good risk prostate cancer. J Urol 2004;172:S48-50; discussion S50-S41.

Kuban DA, Tucker SL, Dong L, et al. Long-term results of the M. D. Anderson randomized dose-escalation trial for prostate cancer. Int J Radiat Oncol Biol Phys 2008;70(1):67-74.

Kupelian PA, Potters L, Khuntia D, et al. Radical prostatectomy, external beam radiotherapy <72 Gy, external beam radiotherapy > or =72 Gy, permanent seed implantation, or combined seeds/external beam radiotherapy for stage T1-T2 prostate cancer. Int J Radiat Oncol Biol Phys 2004;58:25-33.

Kupelian PA, Willoughby TR, Reddy CA, Klein EA, Mahadevan A. Hypofractionated intensity-modulated radiotherapy (70 Gy at 2.5 Gy per fraction) for localized prostate cancer: Cleveland Clinic experience. Int J Radiat Oncol Biol Phys 2007;68(5):1424-1430.

Lau WK, Bergstralh EJ, Blute ML, Slezak JM, Zincke H. Radical prostatectomy for pathological Gleason 8 or greater prostate cancer: influence of concomitant pathological variables. J Urol 2002;167(1):117-122.

Laverdiere J, Gomez JL, Cusan L, et al. Beneficial effect of combination hormonal therapy administered prior and following external beam radiation therapy in localized prostate cancer. Int J Radiat Oncol Biol Phys 1997;37(2):247-252.

Lawton CA, Bae K, Pilepich M, Hanks G, Shipley W. Long-term treatment sequelae after external beam irradiation with or without hormonal manipulation for adenocarcinoma of the prostate: analysis of radiation therapy oncology group studies 85-31, 86-10, and 92-02. Int J Radiat Oncol Biol Phys 2008;70(2):437-441.

Lawton CA, DeSilvio M, Roach M III, et al. An update of the phase III trial comparing whole pelvic to prostate only radiotherapy and neoadjuvant to adjuvant total androgen suppression: updated analysis of RTOG 94-13, with emphasis on unexpected hormone/radiation interactions. Int J Radiat Oncol Biol Phys 2007;69(3):646-655.

Lawton CA, Michalski J, El-Naqa I, et al. RTOG GU radiation oncology specialists reach consensus on pelvic lymph node volumes for high-risk prostate cancer. Int J Radiat Oncol Biol Phys 2009;74(2):383-387.

Lu-Yao GL, Albertsen PC, Moore DF, et al. Survival following primary androgen deprivation therapy among men with localized prostate cancer. JAMA 2008;300(2):173-181.

Messing EM, Manola J, Sarosdy M, et al. Immediate hormonal therapy compared with observation after radical prostatectomy and pelvic lymphadenectomy in men with node-positive prostate cancer. N Engl J Med 1999;341:1781-1788.

Messing EM, Manola J, Yao J, et al. Immediate versus deferred androgen deprivation treatment in patients with node-positive prostate cancer after radical prostatectomy and pelvic lymphadenectomy. Lancet Oncol 2006;7(6):472-479.

Miller J, Smith A, Kouba E, Wallen E, Pruthi RS. Prospective evaluation of short-term impact and recovery of health related quality of life in men undergoing robotic assisted laparoscopic radical prostatectomy versus open radical prostatectomy. J Urol 2007;178(3 Pt 1): 854-858; discussion 859.

Ng LG, Yip S, Tan PH, Yuen J, Lau W, Cheng C. Improved detection rate of prostate cancer using the 10-core biopsy strategy in Singapore. Asian J Surg 2002;25(3):238-243.

Pagliarulo V, Hawes D, Brands FH, et al. Detection of occult lymph node metastases in locally advanced node-negative prostate cancer. J Clin Oncol 2006;24(18):2735-2742.

Pan CC, Kim KY, Taylor JM, et al. Influence of 3D-CRT pelvic irradiation on outcome in prostate cancer treated with external beam radiotherapy. Int J Radiat Oncol Biol Phys 2002;53(5):139-1145

Patel AA, Chen MH, Renshaw AA, D'Amico AV. PSA failure following definitive treatment of prostate cancer having biopsy Gleason score 7 with tertiary grade 5. JAMA 2007;298(13):1533-1538.

Peeters ST, Heemsbergen WD, Koper PC, et al. Dose-response in radiotherapy for localized prostate cancer: results of the Dutch multicenter randomized phase III trial comparing 68 Gy of radiotherapy with 78 Gy. J Clin Oncol 2006;24(13):1990-1996.

Penson DF, McLerran D, Feng Z, et al. 5-year urinary and sexual outcomes after radical prostatectomy: results from the prostate cancer outcomes study. J Urol 2005;173(5):1701-1705.

Penson DF. An update on randomized clinical trials in localized and locoregional prostate cancer. Urol Oncol 2005;23(4):280-288.

Pilepich MV, Caplan R, Byhardt RW, et al. Phase III trial of androgen suppression using goserelin in unfavorable-prognosis carcinoma of the prostate treated with definitive radiotherapy: report of Radiation Therapy Oncology Group Protocol 85-31. J Clin Oncol 1997;15:1013-1021.

Pilepich MV, Winter K, John MJ, et al. Phase III radiation therapy oncology group (RTOG) trial 86-10 of androgen deprivation adjuvant to definitive radiotherapy in locally advanced carcinoma of the prostate. Int J Radiat Oncol Biol Phys 2001;50:1243-1252.

Pollack A, Hanlon AL, Horwitz EM, et al. Dosimetry and preliminary acute toxicity in the first 100 men treated for prostate cancer on a randomized hypofractionation dose escalation trial. Int J Radiat Oncol Biol Phys 2006;64(2):518-526.

Pollack A, Zagars GK, Smith LG, et al. Preliminary results of a randomized radiotherapy dose-escalation study comparing 70 Gy with 78 Gy for prostate cancer. J Clin Oncol 2000;18: 3904-3911.

Pommier P, Chabaud S, Lagrange JL, et al. Is there a role for pelvic irradiation in localized prostate adenocarcinoma? Preliminary results of GETUG-01. J Clin Oncol 2007;25(34):5366-5373.

Pound CR, Partin AW, Eisenberger MA, Chan DW, Pearson JD, Walsh PC. Natural history of progression after PSA elevation following radical prostatectomy. JAMA 1999;281(17):1591-1597.

Roach M III, DeSilvio M, Valicenti R, et al. Whole-pelvis, "mini-pelvis," or prostate-only external beam radiotherapy after neoadjuvant and concurrent hormonal therapy in patients treated in the Radiation Therapy Oncology Group 9413 trial. Int J Radiat Oncol Biol Phys 2006; 66(3):647-653.

Roach M III. Targeting pelvic lymph nodes in men with intermediate- and high-risk prostate cancer, and confusion about the results of the randomized trials. J Clin Oncol 1 2008;26(22):3816-3817; author reply 3817-3818.

Robinson JW, Moritz S, Fung T. Meta-analysis of rates of erectile function after treatment of localized prostate carcinoma. Int J Radiat Oncol Biol Phys 2002;54:1063-1068.

Rosenthal SA, Bae K, Pienta KJ, et al. Phase III multi-institutional trial of adjuvant chemotherapy with paclitaxel, estramustine, and oral etoposide combined with long-term androgen suppression therapy and radiotherapy versus long-term androgen suppression plus radiotherapy alone for high-risk prostate cancer: preliminary toxicity analysis of RTOG 99-02. Int J Radiat Oncol Biol Phys 2009;73(3):672-678.

Sandler HM, DeSilvio M, Pienta K, et al. Preliminary analysis of RTOG 9902: increased toxicity observed with the use of adjuvant chemotherapy. Proceedings of the American Society for Therapeutic Radiology and Oncology 47th Annual Meeting. 10 January 2005, Int J Radiat Oncol Biol Phys 2005;63(Suppl 1):S123.

Sathya JR, Davis IR, Julian JA, et al. Randomized trial comparing iridium implant plus external-beam radiation therapy with external-beam radiation therapy alone in node-negative locally advanced cancer of the prostate. J Clin Oncol 2005;23:1192-1199.

Seaward SA, Weinberg V, Lewis P, et al. Improved freedom from PSA failure with whole pelvic irradiation for high-risk prostate cancer. Int J Radiat Oncol Biol Phys 1998;42(5):1055-1062

Shih HA, Harisinghani M, Zietman AL, et al. Mapping of nodal disease in locally advanced prostate cancer: Rethinking the clinical target volume for pelvic nodal irradiation based on vascular rather than bony anatomy. Int J Radiat Oncol Biol Phys 2005;63:1262-1269.

Sidhom MA, et al. Post-prostatectomy radiation therapy: consensus guidelines of the Australian and New Zealand Radiation Oncology Genito-Urinary Group. Radiother Oncol 2008;88(1):10-19.

Spiotto MT, Hancock SL, King CR. Radiotherapy after prostatectomy: improved biochemical relapse-free survival with whole pelvic compared with prostate bed only for high-risk patients. Int J Radiat Oncol Biol Phys 2007;69(1):54-61.

Stephenson AJ, Scardino PT, et al. Predicting outcome of salvage radiation therapy for recurrent prostate cancer after radical prostatectomy. J Clin Oncol 2007;25:2035-2041.

Stone NN, Stock RG, Cesaretti JA, Unger P. Local control following permanent prostate brachytherapy: effect of high biologically effective dose on biopsy results and oncologic outcomes. Int J Radiat Oncol Biol Phys 76(2):355-360.

Studer UE, Whelan P, Albrecht W, et al. Immediate or deferred androgen deprivation for patients with prostate cancer not suitable for local treatment with curative intent: European Organisation for Research and Treatment of Cancer (EORTC) Trial 30891. J Clin Oncol 2006;24(12):1868-1876.

Swanson GP, Riggs MW, Herman M. Long-term outcome for lymph node-positive prostate cancer. Prostate Cancer Prostatic Dis 2008;11(2):198-202.

Tannock IF, de Wit R, Berry WR, et al. Docetaxel plus prednisone or mitoxantrone plus prednisone for advanced prostate cancer. N Engl J Med 2004;351:1502-1512.

Taylor A, Rockall AG, Rezneck RH, Powell ME. Mapping pelvic lymph nodes: guidelines for delineation in intensity-modulated radiotherapy. Int J Radiat Oncol Biol Phys 2005;63:1604-1612.

Thompson IM, Pauler DK, Goodman PJ, et al. Prevalence of prostate cancer among men with a prostate-specific antigen level < or =4.0 ng per milliliter. N Engl J Med 2004;350:2239-2246.

Thompson IM, Tangen CM, Paradelo J, et al. Adjuvant radiotherapy for pathological T3N0M0 prostate cancer significantly reduces risk of metastases and improves survival: long-term followup of a randomized clinical trial. J Urol 2009;181(3):956-962.

Tollefson MK, Leibovich BC, Slezak JM, Zincke H, Blute ML. Long-term prognostic significance of primary Gleason pattern in patients with Gleason score 7 prostate cancer: impact on prostate cancer specific survival. J Urol 2006;175(2):547-551.

Trock BJ, Han M, et al. Prostate cancer–specific survival following salvage radiotherapy vs observation in men with biochemical recurrence after radical prostatectomy. JAMA 2008;299(23):2760-2769

Tward JD, Lee CM, Pappas LM, Szabo A, Gaffney DK, Shrieve DC. Survival of men with clinically localized prostate cancer treated with prostatectomy, brachytherapy, or no definitive treatment: impact of age at diagnosis. Cancer 2006;107(10):2392-2400.

Van der Kwast TH, Bolla M, Van Poppel H, et al. Identification of patients with prostate cancer who benefit from immediate postoperative radiotherapy: EORTC 22911. J Clin Oncol 2007;25(27):4178-4186.

Vickers AJ, Savage C, O'Brien MF, Lilja H. Systematic review of pretreatment prostate-specific antigen velocity and doubling time as predictors for prostate cancer. J Clin Oncol 2009;27(3): 398-403.

Widmark A, Klepp O, Solberg A, et al. Endocrine treatment, with or without radiotherapy, in locally advanced prostate cancer (SPCG-7/SFUO-3): an open randomised phase III trial. Lancet 2009;373(9660):301-308.

Wiegel T, Bottke D, Steiner U, et al. Phase III postoperative adjuvant radiotherapy after radical prostatectomy compared with radical prostatectomy alone in pT3 prostate cancer with postoperative undetectable prostate-specific antigen: ARO 96-02/AUO AP 09/95. J Clin Oncol 2009;27(18):2924-2930.

Wong YN, Mitra N, Hudes G, et al. Survival associated with treatment vs observation of localized prostate cancer in elderly men. JAMA 2006;296(22):2683-2693.

Yeoh EE, Holloway RH, Fraser RJ, et al. Hypofractionated versus conventionally fractionated radiation therapy for prostate carcinoma: updated results of a phase III randomized trial. Int J Radiat Oncol Biol Phys 2006;66(4):1072-1083.

Zagars GK, Pollack A, von Eschenbach AC. Addition of radiation therapy to androgen ablation improves outcome for subclinically node-positive prostate cancer. Urology 2001;58:233-239.

Zelefsky MJ, Kuban DA, Levy LB, et al. Multi-institutional analysis of long-term outcome for stages T1-T2 prostate cancer treated with permanent seed implantation. Int J Radiat Oncol Biol Phys 2007;67(2):327-333.

Zelefsky MJ, Yamada Y, Cohen GN, et al. Five-year outcome of intraoperative conformal permanent I-125 interstitial implantation for patients with clinically localized prostate cancer. Int J Radiat Oncol Biol Phys 2007;67(1):65-70.

Zietman AL, DeSilvio M, Slater JD, et al. Comparison of conventional-dose vs high-dose conformal radiation therapy in clinically localized adenocarcinoma of the prostate. JAMA 2005;294:1233-1239.

Zietman AL. Correction: inaccurate analysis and results in a study of radiation therapy in adenocarcinoma of the prostate. JAMA 2008;299(8):898-899.

FURTHER READINGS

Andriole GL, Grubb RL 3rd, Buys SS, et al. Mortality Results from a Randomized Prostate-Cancer Screening Trial. N Engl J Med. 2009;360(13):1310-1319.

Cagiannos I, Karakiewicz P, Eastham JA, et al. A preoperative nomogram identifying decreased risk of positive pelvic lymph nodes in patients with prostate cancer. J Urol 2003;170:1798-1803.

Chung T, Speight J, Roach M 3rd. Intermediate and high-risk prostate cancer. In: Perez CA, Brady LW, Halperin EC, et al., editors. Principles and practice of radiation oncology. 5th ed. Philadelphia: Lippincott Williams & Wilkins; 2008. pp. 1483-1502.

Crook J, Ludgate C, Malone S, et al. Report of a multicenter Canadian phase III randomized trial of 3 months vs. 8 months neoadjuvant androgen deprivation before standard-dose radiotherapy for clinically localized prostate cancer. Int J Radiat Oncol Biol Phys 2004;60:15-23.

Bolla M, Van Poppel H, Collette L, et al. Postoperative radiotherapy after radical prostatectomy: a randomised controlled trial (EORTC 22911). Lancet 2005;366:572-578.

Bolla M, van Poppel H, Collette L, et al. Postoperative radiotherapy after radical prostatectomy: a randomised controlled trial (EORTC trial 22911). Lancet 13-19 2005;366(9485):572-578.

D'Amico AV, Denham JW, Crook J, et al. Influence of androgen suppression therapy for prostate cancer on the frequency and timing of fatal myocardial infarctions. J Clin Oncol 2007;25(17):2420-2425.

D'Amico AV, Keshaviah A, Manola J, et al. Clinical utility of the percentage of positive prostate biopsies in predicting prostate cancer-specific and overall survival after radiotherapy for patients with localized prostate cancer. Int J Radiat Oncol Biol Phys 2002;53:581-587.

D'Amico AV, Renshaw AA, Cote K, et al. Impact of the percentage of positive prostate cores on prostate cancer-specific mortality for patients with low or favorable intermediate-risk disease. J Clin Oncol 2004c;22:3726-3732.

D'Amico AV, Whittington R, Malkowicz SB, et al. Clinical utility of the percentage of positive prostate biopsies in defining biochemical outcome after radical prostatectomy for patients with clinically localized prostate cancer. J Clin Oncol 2000;18:1164-1172.

Denham JW, Steigler A, Lamb DS, et al. Short-term androgen deprivation and radiotherapy for locally advanced prostate cancer: results from the Trans-Tasman Radiation Oncology Group 96.01 randomised controlled trial. Lancet Oncol 2005;6:841-850.

Efstathiou JA, Bae K, Shipley WU, et al. Cardiovascular mortality after androgen deprivation therapy for locally advanced prostate cancer: RTOG 85-31. J Clin Oncol 2009;27(1):92-99.

Gleason DF, Mellinger GT. Prediction of prognosis for prostatic adenocarcinoma by combined histological grading and clinical staging. J Urol 1974;111:58-64.

Gottschalk AR, Roach M 3rd. The use of hormonal therapy with radiotherapy for prostate cancer: analysis of prospective randomised trials. Br J Cancer 2004;90:950-954.

Greene FL. American Joint Committee on Cancer. American Cancer Society. AJCC cancer staging manual. 6th ed. New York: Springer; 2002.

Grimm PD, Blasko JC, Sylvester JE, et al. 10-year biochemical (prostate-specific antigen) control of prostate cancer with (125)I brachytherapy. Int J Radiat Oncol Biol Phys 2001;51:31-40.

Grossfeld GD, Latini DM, Lubeck DP, et al. Predicting disease recurrence in intermediate and high-risk patients undergoing radical prostatectomy using percent positive biopsies: results from CaPSURE. Urology 2002;59:560-565.

Hanks GE, Lu J, Machtay M, et al. RTOG protocol 92-02: a phase III trial of the use of long term androgen supression following neoadjuvant hormonal cytoreduction and radiotherapy in locally advanced carcinoma of the prostate. Int J Radiat Oncol Biol Phys 2000;48 (3 Suppl 1):112.

Hanks GE, Pajak TF, Porter A, et al. Phase III trial of long-term adjuvant androgen deprivation after neoadjuvant hormonal cytoreduction and radiotherapy in locally-advanced carcinoma of the prostate: The Radiation Therapy Oncology Group Protocol 92-02. J Clin Oncol 2003;21:3972-3978.

Holmberg L, Bill-Axelson A, Helgesen F, et al. A randomized trial comparing radical prostatectomy with watchful waiting in early prostate cancer. N Engl J Med 2002;347(11):781-789.

Jemal A, Siegel R, Ward E, et al. Cancer statistics, 2006. CA Cancer J Clin 2006;56:106-130.

Kattan MW, Karpeh MS, Mazumdar M, et al. Postoperative nomogram for disease-specific survival after an R0 resection for gastric carcinoma. J Clin Oncol 2003;21:3647-3650.

Kattan MW, Zelefsky MJ, Kupelian PA, et al. Pretreatment nomogram that predicts 5-year probability of metastasis following three-dimensional conformal radiation therapy for localized prostate cancer. J Clin Oncol 2003;21:4568-4571.

Klein EA, Thompson IM, Lippman SM, et al. SELECT: the next prostate cancer prevention trial. Selenum and Vitamin E Cancer Prevention Trial. J Urol 2001;166:1311-1315.

Kuban DA, Thames HD, Levy LB, et al. Long-term multi-institutional analysis of stage T1-T2 prostate cancer treated with radiotherapy in the PSA era. Int J Radiat Oncol Biol Phys 2003;57:915-928.

Kuban A, Potters L, Lawton C, et al. Prostate cancer. In: Gunderson LL, Tepper JE, editors. Clinical radiation oncology. 1st ed. Philadelphia: Churchill Livingstone; 2007. pp. 1165-1236.

Langen KM, Pouliot J, Anezinos C, et al. Evaluation of ultrasound-based prostate localization for image-guided radiotherapy. Int J Radiat Oncol Biol Phys 2003;57:635-644.

Laverdiere J, Nabid A, De Bedoya LD, et al. The efficacy and sequencing of a short course of androgen suppression on freedom from biochemical failure when administered with radiation therapy for T2-T3 prostate cancer. J Urol 2004;171:1137-1140.

Lawton CA, Winter K, Byhardt R, et al. Androgen suppression plus radiation versus radiation alone for patients with D1 (pN+) adenocarcinoma of the prostate (results based on a national prospective randomized trial, RTOG 85-31). Radiation Therapy Oncology Group. Int J Radiat Oncol Biol Phys 1997;38:931-939.

Lawton CA, Winter K, Grignon D, et al. Androgen suppression plus radiation versus radiation alone for patients with stage d1/pathologic node-positive adenocarcinoma of the prostate: updated results based on national prospective randomized trial radiation therapy oncology group 85-31. J Clin Oncol 2005;23:800-807.

Lawton CA, Winter K, Murray K, et al. Updated results of the phase III Radiation Therapy Oncology Group (RTOG) trial 85-31 evaluating the potential benefit of androgen suppression following standard radiation therapy for unfavorable prognosis carcinoma of the prostate. Int J Radiat Oncol Biol Phys 2001;49:937-946.

Martinez AA, Pataki I, Edmundson G, et al. Phase II prospective study of the use of conformal high-dose-rate brachytherapy as monotherapy for the treatment of favorable stage prostate cancer: a feasibility report. Int J Radiat Oncol Biol Phys 2001;49:61-69.

National Comprehensive Cancer Network. Clinical Practice Guidelines in Oncology: Prostate Cancer. Available at: http://www.nccn.org/professionals/physician_gls/PDF/prostate.pdf Accessed on January 19, 2005.

Partin AW, Mangold LA, Lamm DM, et al. Contemporary update of prostate cancer staging nomograms (Partin Tables) for the new millennium. Urology 2001;58:843-848.

Petrylak DP, Tangen CM, Hussain MH, et al. Docetaxel and estramustine compared with mitoxantrone and prednisone for advanced refractory prostate cancer. N Engl J Med 2004;351: 1513-1520.

Pickett B, Kurhanewicz J, Coakley F, et al. Efficacy of external beam radiotherapy compared to permanent prostate implant in treating low risk prostate cancer based on endorectal magnetic resonance spectroscopy imaging and PSA. Int J Radiat Oncol Biol Phys 2004;60(1 Suppl 1):S185-S186.

Pickett B, Kurhanewicz J, Coakley F, et al. Use of MRI and spectroscopy in evaluation of external beam radiotherapy for prostate cancer. Int J Radiat Oncol Biol Phys 2004;60:1047-1055.

Pickett B, Ten Haken RK, Kurhanewicz J, et al. Time to metabolic atrophy after permanent prostate seed implantation based on magnetic resonance spectroscopic imaging. Int J Radiat Oncol Biol Phys 2004;59:665-673.

Pollack A. The prostate. In: Cox JD, Ang KK, editors. Radiation oncology: rationale, technique, results. 8th ed. St. Louis: Mosby; 2003. pp. 629-680.

Quinn DI, Henshall SM, Haynes AM, et al. Prognostic significance of pathologic features in localized prostate cancer treated with radical prostatectomy: implications for staging systems and predictive models. J Clin Oncol 2001;19:3692-3705.

Roach III M, Wallner K. Cancer of the Prostate. In: Leibel SA, Phillips TL, editors. Textbook of radiation oncology. 2nd ed. Philadelphia: Saunders; 2004. pp. 959-1030.

Roach M 3rd, DeSilvio M, Lawton C, et al. Phase III trial comparing whole-pelvic versus prostate-only radiotherapy and neoadjuvant versus adjuvant combined androgen suppression: Radiation Therapy Oncology Group 9413. J Clin Oncol 2003;21:1904-1911.

Roach M 3rd. Hormonal therapy and radiotherapy for localized prostate cancer: who, where and how long? J Urol 2003;170:S35-S40; discussion S40-S31.

Roach M 3rd. Regarding the influence of adjuvant suppression therapy for prostate cancer on the frequency and timing of fatal myocardial infarction: how real is the risk? J Clin Oncol 2007;25 (33):5325-5326; author reply 5326.

Roach M, 3rd, Lu J, Pilepich MV, et al. Predicting long-term survival, and the need for hormonal therapy: a meta-analysis of RTOG prostate cancer trials. Int J Radiat Oncol Biol Phys 2000;47:617-627.

Roach M, Lu J, Pilepich MV, et al. Four prognostic groups predict long-term survival from prostate cancer following radiotherapy alone on Radiation Therapy Oncology Group clinical trials. Int J Radiat Oncol Biol Phys 2000;47:609-615.

Schroder FH, Hugosson J, Roobol MJ, et al. Screening and Prostate-Cancer Mortality in a Randomized European Study. N Engl J Med. 2009;360(13):1320-1328.

Shariat SF, Karakiewicz PI, Margulis V, Kattan MW. Inventory of prostate cancer predictive tools. Curr Opin Urol 2008;18(3):279-296.

Stephenson AJ, Shariat SF, Zelefsky MJ, et al. Salvage radiotherapy for recurrent prostate cancer after radical prostatectomy. JAMA 2004;291:1325-1332.

Stock RG, Stone NN, Cesaretti JA. Prostate-specific antigen bounce after prostate seed implantation for localized prostate cancer: descriptions and implications. Int J Radiat Oncol Biol Phys 2003;56:448-453.

Storey MR, Pollack A, Zagars G, et al. Complications from radiotherapy dose escalation in prostate cancer: preliminary results of a randomized trial. Int J Radiat Oncol Biol Phys 2000;48:635-642.

Sylvester JE, Blasko JC, Grimm PD, et al. Ten-year biochemical relapse-free survival after external beam radiation and brachytherapy for localized prostate cancer: the Seattle experience. Int J Radiat Oncol Biol Phys 2003;57:944-952.

Thames H, Kuban D, Levy L, et al. Comparison of alternative biochemical failure definitions based on clinical outcome in 4839 prostate cancer patients treated by external beam radiotherapy between 1986 and 1995. Int J Radiat Oncol Biol Phys 2003;57:929-943.

Thompson IM, Goodman PJ, Tangen CM, et al. The influence of finasteride on the development of prostate cancer. N Engl J Med 2003;349:215-224.

Valicenti RK, Gomella LG, Perez CA. Radiation therapy after radical prostatectomy: a review of the issues and options. Semin Radiat Oncol 2003;13:130-140.

Zelefsky MJ, Valicenti RK, Hunt M et al. Low-risk prostate cancer. In: Perez CA, Brady LW, Halperin EC, et al., editors. Principles and practice of radiation oncology. 5th ed. Philadelphia: Lippincott Williams & Wilkins; 2008. pp. 1439-1482.

Chapter 27
Cancer of the Penis

Alice Wang-Chesebro, William Foster, and Alexander R. Gottschalk

PEARLS

- Penile cancer is rare in Western countries (<1% of cancers in men), but accounts for 10–20% of male malignancies in Africa, Asia, and South America.
- LN drainage: skin of penis – bilateral superficial inguinal nodes; glans penis – bilateral inguinal or iliac nodes; penis corporal tissue – bilateral deep inguinal and iliac; 20% chance of LN+ at surgery if clinically node negative.
- Risk factors: uncircumcised status, phimosis, poor local hygiene, HPV-16, 18.
- Pathology: 95% squamous cell; others very rare – melanoma, lymphoma, basal cell, Kaposi's sarcoma.

WORKUP

- H&P with careful palpation and exam; if deep, consider cystourethroscopy with biopsy; bimanual exam under anesthesia.
- Labs: CBC, chemistries, BUN, Cr, LFTs including alkaline phosphatase.
- Imaging: ultrasound (penis) or MRI for extent of local extension; pelvic/abdominal CT for nodes; CXR for all, bone scan if advanced/suspicious.
- Biopsy of the lesion.
- Needle biopsy for suspicious nodes.

STAGING: CANCER OF THE PENIS

Editors' note: All TNM stage and stage groups referred to elsewhere in this chapter reflect the 2002 AJCC staging nomenclature unless otherwise noted as the new system below was published after this chapter was written.

(AJCC 6TH ED., 2002)

Primary tumor (T)

TX: Primary tumor cannot be assessed
T0: No evidence of primary tumor
Tis: Carcinoma in situ
Ta: Noninvasive verrucous carcinoma
T1: Tumor invades subepithelial connective tissue
T2: Tumor invades corpus spongiosum or cavernosum
T3: Tumor invades urethra or prostate
T4: Tumor invades other adjacent structures

Regional lymph nodes (N)

NX: No regional lymph node metastasis cannot be assessed
N0: No regional lymph node metastasis
N1: Metastasis in single, superficial, inguinal node
N2: Metastasis in multiple or bilateral superficial inguinal lymph nodes
N3: Metastasis in deep inguinal or pelvic lymph node(s), unilateral or bilateral

Distant metastasis (M)

MX: Distant metastasis cannot be assessed
M0: No distant metastasis
M1: Distant metastasis

Stage grouping		**~3-Year OS by Stage**	
0:	TisN0M0, TaN0M0	I:	70–100%
I :	T1N0M0	II:	65–100%
II:	T2N0M0, T1-2N1M0	III:	60–90%
III:	T3N0-1M0	IV	50–70%
	T1-3N2M0		

(AJCC 7TH ED., 2010)

Primary tumor (T)

TX: Primary tumor cannot be assessed
T0: No evidence of primary tumor
Tis: Carcinoma in situ
Ta: Noninvasive verrucous carcinoma*
T1a: Tumor invades subepithelial connective tissue without lymph vascular invasion and is not poorly differentiated (i.e., grades 3–4)
T1b: Tumor invades subepithelial connective tissue with lymph vascular invasion or is poorly differentiated
T2: Tumor invades corpus spongiosum or cavernosum
T3: Tumor invades urethra
T4: Tumor invades other adjacent structures

**Note*: Broad pushing penetration (invasion) is permitted; destructive invasion is against this diagnosis.

Regional lymph nodes (N)

*Clinical stage definition**

cNX: Regional lymph nodes cannot be assessed
cN0: No palpable or visibly enlarged inguinal lymph nodes
cN1: Palpable mobile unilateral inguinal lymph node

cN2: Palpable mobile multiple or bilateral inguinal lymph nodes
cN3: Palpable fixed inguinal nodal mass or pelvic lymphadenopathy unilateral or bilateral

**Note*: Clinical stage definition based on palpation, imaging.

*Pathologic stage definition**

pNX: Regional lymph nodes cannot be assessed
pN0: No regional lymph node metastasis

continued

IV:	T4 Any N M0
	Any T N3 M0
	Any T Any N M1

Used with the permission from the American Joint Committee on Cancer (AJCC), Chicago, IL. The original source for this material is the AJCC Cancer Staging Manual, Sixth Edition (2002), published by Springer Science+Business Media.

pN1:	Metastasis in a single inguinal lymph node
pN2:	Metastasis in multiple or bilateral inguinal lymph nodes
pN3:	Extranodal extension of lymph node metastasis or pelvic lymph node(s) unilateral or bilateral

**Note*: Pathologic stage definition based on biopsy or surgical excision.

Distant metastasis (M)

M0: No distant metastasis

M1: Distant metastasis*

**Note*: Lymph node metastasis outside of the true pelvis in addition to visceral or bone sites.

Additional Descriptor. The m suffix indicates the presence of multiple primary tumors and is recorded in parentheses – e.g., pTa (m) N0M0

Anatomic stage/prognostic groups

0:	Tis N0 M0
	Ta N0 M0
I:	T1a N0 M0
II:	T1b N0 M0
	T2 N0 M0
	T3 N0 M0
IIIa:	T1-3 N1 M0
IIIb:	T1-3 N2 M0
IV:	T4 Any N M0
	Any T N3 M0
	Any T Any N M1

Used with the permission from the American Joint Committee on Cancer (AJCC), Chicago, IL. The original source for this material is the AJCC Cancer Staging Manual, Seventh Edition (2010), published by Springer Science+Business Media.

continued

TREATMENT RECOMMENDATIONS

2002 Stage	Recommended treatment
CIS	Circumcision, local excision, Moh's surgery, topical 5-FU, Imiquimod
Early limited lesions (For RT alone, lesions should be T1-2, <4 cm size)	Options: penectomy noted to have high psychosocial morbidity; therefore, organ preservation is gaining popularity ■ *Penis preservation*: circumcise first, then EBRT or brachytherapy alone, or chemo-RT *EBRT*: 40–50 Gy to whole penile shaft ± lymph nodes (see surgical management below), then boost to primary lesion + 2 cm margin (total 60–65 Gy) ■ *Brachytherapy alone*: contraindicated if >1 cm invasion into corpus cavernosa or >4 cm size. Two methods: radioactive mold – 60 Gy to tumor, 50 Gy to urethra, or interstitial (IS) with Ir-192 to 65 Gy (treatment of choice in Europe) ■ *Chemo-RT*: gaining popularity based on data from anal and cervical cancers ■ Consider prophylactic inguinal node RT ■ *Surgery* – from circumcision to local excision to radical penectomy. Recommend >1.5–2 cm margin. For clinically node negative, EUA guidelines recommend prophylactic inguinal node dissection for tumors T2 and over and/or G3. For T1G2, consider dissection depending on other factors (LVI status). If no node dissection, requires very close monitoring. Pelvic dissection if 2+ inguinal nodes, + ECE or + nodes on imaging. Post-op RT for LN+ based on vulvar cancer data
More advanced lesions	Options: ■ *EBRT*: 60 Gy in 2 Gy fractions. Chemo-RT preferred to RT alone based on data from other cancers; include pelvic and bilateral inguinal nodes; consider LND for bulky nodes ■ *Surgery*: save for salvage; partial to radical penectomy; consider prophylactic inguinal node dissection with tumors extending onto shaft of penis/poorly differentiated; if node positive, need inguinal and pelvic LND; post-op RT for LN+ based on vulvar cancer data ■ *Investigational*: neoadjuvant chemo to render unresectable disease resectable; chemo (various regimens) for +LN or metastatic disease

STUDIES

- There are no randomized trials for primary penile cancers.
- Selected results for early penile cancer treated with EBRT.
  - Grabstald and Kelley (1980) report of 10 patients with stage I–II treated with EBRT; at 6–10-year follow-up, LC 90%, DFS 90%, and OS 90%.
  - McLean et al. (1993): 26 patients with stages I–II treated with "radical" EBRT, range 35–50 Gy, most 50 Gy in 20 fx with cobalt-60; median follow-up 9.7 years; 5-year OS 62% (for N0–79%, for N+12%), 5-year CSS 69%, 5-year DFS 50%.
- Selected results for early penile cancer treated with brachytherapy.
  - Crook et al. (2005): 49 patients with T1 (51%), T2 (33%), and T3 (8%) penile SCC treated with Ir-192 to 55–65 Gy; median follow-up 33 months; 5-year OS 78%, 5-year CSS 90%, 5-year FFS 64%, 5-year LF 15%, 5-year penile preservation rate 86.5%, 5-year soft tissue necrosis rate 16%, and urethral stenosis rate 12%.
  - Updated results Crook et al. (2008): 67 patients treated with Ir-192 to 55–65 Gy; median follow-up 48 months; 10-year OS 59%, 5 and 10-year CSS 83.6%, 5-FFLF 87.3%, and 10-FFLF 72.3%. Penile preservation rate at 5 years is 88%, at 10 years 67.3%; necrosis rate 12%, meatal stenosis 9%.
  - Mazeron et al. (1984): 50 patients with T1–T3 treated with Ir-192 to median dose 65 (60–70 Gy); LC-78%, penis conservation 74%.
- Selected series with all stages of penile cancer.
  - Krieg et al. (1981): 17 patients with stage I–IV treated with surgery ± LND and 12 patients with stages I–III treated with EBRT alone (dose 50–65 Gy, no prophylactic node RT); LC 88% with surgery, 75% with RT alone, and 92% with surgical salvage; 88% (8/9) of patients not treated prophylactically to groin did not develop pelvic/inguinal node recurrence; 2 patients developed stricture, 1 developed penile necrosis (66 Gy).
  - Sarin et al. (1997): 101 patients with stages I–IV, median age 64 years, treated with primary EBRT (59), brachytherapy (13), penectomy (29); median follow-up 5.2 years; 5/10-year OS 56.5/39%, 5/10-year CSS 66/57%; 5/10-year LC 60/55%; no difference between surgery and RT in LC after salvage; note: 2 attempted suicides after penectomy, 1 successful.

VII

RADIATION TECHNIQUES

SIMULATION AND FIELD DESIGN

- EBRT
  - Simulate patient supine; apply foley catheter and suspend penis; surround penis by tissue bolus for MV RT. If treating inguinal nodes, pt is treated in the frog-leg position. If treating pelvic nodes, may secure penis cranially into pelvic field
  - Volumes
    - GTV: palpable/visible disease (physical exam, CT, MRI)
    - CTV:
      - (a) GTV + whole shaft of penis
      - (b) ±superficial and deep inguinal nodes
      - (c) ±pelvic nodes (internal + external iliacs, obturator nodes)
    - PTV: depends on technique, 1 cm appropriate
  - Dose: 45–50 Gy in 1.8–2 Gy fx to CTV, then conedown boost to GTV of 10–20 Gy for total 65–70 Gy
  - If treating inguinal nodes, techniques may be used to protect the femoral heads
- Plesiobrachytherapy/molds
  - Penis is placed into a cylinder loaded with Ir-192 sources; pt wears mold for calculated amount of time; target dose 60 Gy, urethra dose 50 Gy; requires very compliant patient
- Interstitial brachytherapy:
  - Implant requires general or spinal anesthesia, takes 30–45 min
  - Catheterize to assist urethra identification to avoid transfixing with needles/catheters; patients remain catheterized for duration of treatment
  - May use rigid steel needles held in predrilled parallel acrylic templates or parallel flexible nylon catheters, placed 1–1.5 cm apart
  - HDR with afterloaded Ir-192
  - Patients wear supporting Styrofoam collar around penis, may need mild analgesia with per OS meds, DVT prophylaxis if stay in bed

DOSE LIMITATIONS

- Doses >60 Gy increase risk of urethral stenosis and fibrosis
- Sterilization occurs with 2–3 Gy
- For pelvic fields, limit bladder ≤75 Gy and rectum ≤70 Gy

COMPLICATIONS

- Dermatitis, dysuria, urethral stricture (10–40%), urethral fistula, impotence (10–20%), late skin telangiectasia (nearly universal), penile fibrosis, penile necrosis (3–15%, higher with IS), small bowel obstruction (rare).

FOLLOW-UP

- Need close follow-up, especially if no prophylactic nodal treatment in cN0 patients.
- H&P every 1–2 months for 1 year, every 3 months for second year, every 6 months for third to fifth years, then annually.

REFERENCES

Crook J, Jezioranski J, et al. Penile brachytherapy: results for 49 patients. IJROBP 2005;62:460-467.

Crook J, Clement M, Grimard L. Radiation therapy in the management of the primary penile tumor: an update. World J Urol 2008; DOI 10.1007/s00345-008-0309-5.

Grabstald H, Kelley C. Radiation therapy of penile cancer six to ten year follow-up. Urology 1980;15:575-576.

Krieg R, Hoffman R. Current management of unusual genitourinary cancers part 1: penile cancer. Oncology 1999;13:1347-1352.

Mazeron JJ, Langlois D, et al. Interstitial radiation therapy for carcinoma of the penis using iridium 192 wires: The Henri Mondor experience (1970-79). IJROBP 1984;10:1891-1895.

McLean M, et al. The results of primary radiation therapy in the management of squamous cell carcinoma of the penis. IJROBP 1993;25:623-628.

Sarin R, Norman AR, et al. Treatment results and prognostic factors in 101 men treated for squamous carcinoma of the penis. Int J Radiat Oncol Biol Phys 1997;38:713-722.

VII

FURTHER READING

Krieg R, Luk K. Carcinoma of the penis: review of cases treated by surgery and radiation therapy 1960-70. Urology 1981;18:149-154.

Mansur DB, Chao KSC. Penis and Male Urethra. In: Perez CA, Brady LW, Halperin EC, editors. Principles and Practice of Radiation Oncology. 5th ed. Philadelphia: Lippincott Williams & Wilkins; 2008. pp. 1519-1531.

Solsona E, Algaba F, et al. European Urology Association (EUA) Guidelines on Penile Cancer. Update March 2004.

Yamada Y. Cancer of the Male Urethra and Penis. In: Leibel SA, Phillips TL, editors. Textbook of Radiation Oncology. 2nd edn. Philadelphia: Saunders; 2004. pp. 1047-1053.

Chapter 28
Testicular Cancer

Brian Missett and Alexander R. Gottschalk

PEARLS

- Spermatogenesis: spermatogonia → spermatocytes → spermatids → spermatozoa. Takes ~2 months in adult men.
- LN drainage.
  - L testicle: testicular vein → L renal vein → paraaortic LN.
  - R testicle: testicular vein → IVC below level of renal vein → paracaval and aortocaval nodes.
  - Prior inguinal surgery may disrupt drainage and redirect through iliac nodes.
- *Pathology*: >95% are germ cell tumors (GCTs) = seminomas and nonseminomatous germ cell tumors (NSGCTs).
- Sixty percent of tumors are mixed and 40% are pure (seminoma most common pure).
- Seminoma is the most common single histology, but together NSGCTs are more common.
- Seminoma subtypes: classic (>90% of cases, stains + for PLAP) and spermatocytic (older age, cured by orchiectomy, rarely metastasizes, stains negative for PLAP). Anaplastic no longer considered a subtype.
- NSGCTs subtypes: embryonal carcinoma (most common NSGCT), yolk sac tumor (elevated AFP, Schiller Duval bodies), choriocarcinoma (elevated β-hCG, rarest pure GCT), teratoma, and mixed GCTs.
- Other tumors: Sertoli cell tumors (produce estrogen, present with gynecomastia); Leydig cell tumors (produce androgens and estrogen, present with early puberty, gynecomastia); lymphoma; embryonal rhabdomyosarcoma.
- Risk factors: undescended testicle, first-born, pre/perinatal estrogen exposure, polyvinyl chloride exposure, advanced maternal age, Down's syndrome, Klinefelter's syndrome (47XXY), CIS, HIV/AIDS.

VII

WORKUP

- H&P, bilateral testicular ultrasound, β-hCG, AFP, LDH, CBC, chemistries, fertility assessment ± sperm banking, CXR, CT abdomen and pelvis, CT chest if ≥ stage II
- Repeat tumor markers if elevated preoperatively
  - β-hCG half-life is 24–36 h; AFP half-life is 3.5–6 days
  - β-hCG is rarely elevated in seminoma. If AFP elevated, not pure seminoma
- Bone scan and/or MRI brain if clinically indicated

STAGING (AJCC 7TH ED., 2010): TESTICULAR CANCER

- The definition of TNM and the stage grouping for this chapter have not changed from the AJCC 6th Ed., 2002.

Primary tumor (T)*

The extent of primary tumor is usually classified after radical orchiectomy, and for this reason, a pathologic stage is assigned

pTX: Primary tumor cannot be assessed
pT0: No evidence of primary tumor (e.g., histologic scar in testis)
pTis: Intratubular germ cell neoplasia (carcinoma in situ)
pT1: Tumor limited to the testis and epididymis without vascular/lymphatic invasion; tumor may invade into the tunica albuginea, but not the tunica vaginalis
pT2: Tumor limited to the testis and epididymis with vascular/lymphatic invasion, or tumor extending through the tunica albuginea with involvement of the tunica vaginalis
pT3: Tumor invades the spermatic cord with or without vascular/lymphatic invasion
pT4: Tumor invades the scrotum with or without vascular/lymphatic invasion

**Note*: Except for pTis and pT4, extent of primary tumor is classified by radical orchiectomy. TX may be used for other categories in the absence of radical orchiectomy.

Regional lymph nodes (N)

Clinical

NX: Regional lymph nodes cannot be assessed
N0: No regional lymph node metastasis
N1: Metastasis with a lymph node mass 2 cm or less in greatest dimension; or multiple lymph nodes, not more than 2 cm in greatest dimension
N2: Metastasis with a lymph node mass more than 2 cm, but not more than 5 cm in greatest dimension; or multiple lymph nodes, any one mass greater than 2 cm, but not more than 5 cm in greatest dimension
N3: Metastasis with a lymph node mass more than 5 cm in greatest dimension

Pathologic (pN)

pNX: Regional lymph nodes cannot be assessed
pN0: No regional lymph node metastasis
pN1: Metastasis with a lymph node mass 2 cm or less in greatest dimension and less than or equal to five nodes positive, not more than 2 cm in greatest dimension
pN2: Metastasis with a lymph node mass more than 2 cm, but not more than 5 cm in greatest dimension; or more than five nodes positive, not more than 5 cm; or evidence of extranodal extension of tumor
pN3: Metastasis with a lymph node mass more than 5 cm in greatest dimension

Distant metastasis (M)

M0: No distant metastasis
M1: Distant metastasis
  M1a: Nonregional nodal or pulmonary metastasis
  M1b: Distant metastasis other than nonregional lymph nodes and lung

continued

Anatomic stage/prognostic groups

Group	T	N	M	S (serum tumor markers)
0:	pTis	N0	M0	S0
I:	pT1–4	N0	M0	SX
IA:	pT1	N0	M0	S0
IB:	pT2	N0	M0	S0
	pT3	N0	M0	S0
	pT4	N0	M0	S0
IS:	Any pT/Tx	N0	M0	S1–3 (measured post orchiectomy)
II:	Any pT/Tx	N1–3	M0	SX
IIA:	Any pT/Tx	N1	M0	S0
	Any pT/Tx	N1	M0	S1
IIB:	Any pT/Tx	N2	M0	S0
	Any pT/Tx	N2	M0	S1
IIC:	Any pT/Tx	N3	M0	S0
	Any pT/Tx	N3	M0	S1
III:	Any pT/Tx	Any N	M1	SX
IIIA:	Any pT/Tx	Any N	M1a	S0
	Any pT/Tx	Any N	M1a	S1
IIIB:	Any pT/Tx	N1–3	M0	S2
	Any pT/Tx	Any N	M1a	S2
IIIC:	Any pT/Tx	N1–3	M0	S3
	Any pT/Tx	Any N	M1a	S3
	Any pT/Tx	Any N	M1b	Any S

Used with the permission from the American Joint Committee on Cancer (AJCC), Chicago, IL. The original source for this material is the AJCC Cancer Staging Manual, Seventh Edition (2010), published by Springer Science+Business Media.

Royal Marsden staging

System

I:	Limited to testis
IIA:	Nodes <2 cm
IIB:	Nodes 2–5 cm
IIC:	Nodes 5–10 cm
IID:	Nodes >10 cm
III =	Nodes above and below diaphragm
IV =	Extralymphatic mets

~10-Year survival (seminoma)

I:	RFS 96–98%, CSS 99–100%
IIA:	RFS 92%, CSS 96–100%
IIB:	RFS 86%, CSS 96–100%
IIC:	RFS 70%, OS 90% (RT alone)
IID:	RFS 50% (RT alone), 90% (chemo)
IIIA/B:	OS 90%
IIIC:	OS 80%

VII

TREATMENT RECOMMENDATIONS FOR SEMINOMA

Stage	Recommended treatment
All patients	■ Radical inguinal orchiectomy with high ligation of spermatic cord
I Seminoma	■ Post resection: surveillance (relapse rate 16%) or RT (20 Gy to paraaortic ± pelvic LN), or carboplatinum × 1–2 cycles
IIA/IIB Seminoma	■ RT 20 Gy to pelvic and paraaortic LN with boost to gross disease (30 Gy for IIA, 36 Gy for IIB). Consider etoposide, cisplatin (EP) chemo × 4c for select IIB patients

continued

IIC/D and III Seminoma	■ Chemo (etoposide, cisplatinum, ± bleomycin): EP × 4c or BEP × 3c
NSGCT	■ IA: open nerve-sparing retroperitoneal LN dissection (nsRPLND) or surveillance in compliant patients ■ IB: open nsRPLND or BEP chemo × 2c or surveillance if T2 and compliant pt ■ IS: EP chemo × 4c or BEP chemo × 3c ■ IIA: if markers negative, open nsRPLND or EP chemo × 4c or BEP chemo × 3c. If persistent tumor marker elevation, chemo ■ IIB: if markers negative, open nsRPLND or EP chemo × 4c or BEP chemo × 3c. If persistent tumor marker elevation or multifocal LN mets with aberrant drainage, chemo ■ IIC/IIIA: primary chemo. RT for brain metastases

STUDIES

SURVEILLANCE

- Warde et al. (2002): 638 patients with stage I seminoma followed with surveillance with 7-year follow-up. Increased relapse with tumors >4 cm, LVSI, and rete testis involvement. Relapses: 0 risk factors = 12%, 1 risk factor = 16%, 2 risk factors = 30%. Prior study showed age <34 years also increased risk of failure

RT FIELD AND DOSE FOR STAGE I

- MRC (Fossa et al. 1999): 478 patients with stage I seminoma randomized to dogleg vs. paraaortic RT. No difference in 3-year RFS/OS with dogleg (97/96%) vs. paraaortic (99/100%). Three-year pelvic RFS was 100% with dogleg vs. 98% with paraaortic. Paraaortic had decreased nausea and vomiting, lower azospermia (11 vs. 35%), and more rapid recovery of sperm count. Two percent pelvic relapse in PA-only arm.
- MRC (Jones et al. 2005): 625 patients with stage I seminoma randomized to 20 vs. 30 Gy RT in 2 Gy fx. RT was paraaortic (with dogleg for patients with prior inguinal surgery). Five-year RFS was not different (97% 30 Gy, 96.4% 20 Gy). 20 Gy arm had decreased lethargy and inability to carry out normal work 1 month after treatment.

CHEMO FOR STAGE I

- MRC/EORTC (Oliver et al. 2005): 1,447 patients with stage I seminoma randomized to carboplatin × 1c vs. RT. RT was 20–30 Gy (87% PA, 13% dogleg). Median follow-up 4 years. 3-year RFS = RT 95.9%, carboplatin 94.8%. Relapse sites: carboplatin = 74% PA, 0% pelvic vs. RT = 9% PA, 28% pelvic. Carboplatin patients took less time off from work compared to RT. Update (Oliver et al. 2008): no difference in 5-year RFS (95% chemo, 96% RT), fewer new GCTs with chemo (2 patients vs. 15 with RT).

SECOND CANCER RISK

- Travis et al. (2005): review of >40,000 men with testicular cancer in 14 population registries in Europe and North America. For patients diagnosed by age 35 years, cumulative risk of second solid cancer 40 years later (i.e., to age 75 years) was 36% for seminoma and 31% for nonseminoma compared with 23% for the general population. Increased relative risk of solid cancers was noted for RT (RR = 2.0), chemotherapy alone (RR = 1.8), and both (RR = 2.9).

VII

RESIDUAL MASS

- Puc et al. (1996): 104 patients with stage IIC, III, or extragonadal primary who underwent surgery and had CR or PR of tumor markers. If a radiographic mass was <3 cm, only 3% of patients had pathologic evidence of failures. For masses >3 cm, 27% of patients had evidence of failure.
- De Santis et al. (2004): 51 patients with seminoma treated with chemo with residual masses. Compared pathologic predictive value of PET and CT. PET PPV 100% and NPV 96% for viable tumor. CT (≤3 vs. >3 cm) PPV 37% and NPV 97%.

RADIATION TECHNIQUES

SIMULATION AND FIELD DESIGN

- Prior to simulation, fertility assessment ± sperm bank
- Simulate supine
- Need IVP or CT to block out kidneys and rule out horseshoe kidney
- Place clamshell on uninvolved testicle. Position penis out of field
- Borders: PA = T10/T11 superiorly to L5/S1 inferiorly. Dogleg,

inferior border is top of obturator foramen. Lateral = tips of transverse processes of lumbar vertebra or 2 cm margin on all nodes (about 10–12 cm wide). For left-sided tumors, widen field to include left renal hilar nodes

- If prior inguinal surgery, treat contralateral inguinal and iliac regions (Figs. 28.1 and 28.2)

DOSE PRESCRIPTIONS

- 20 Gy at 2.0 Gy/fx. Alternatively, 25.5 Gy at 1.5 Gy/fx
- Boost IIA nodes to 30 Gy and IIB nodes to 36 Gy

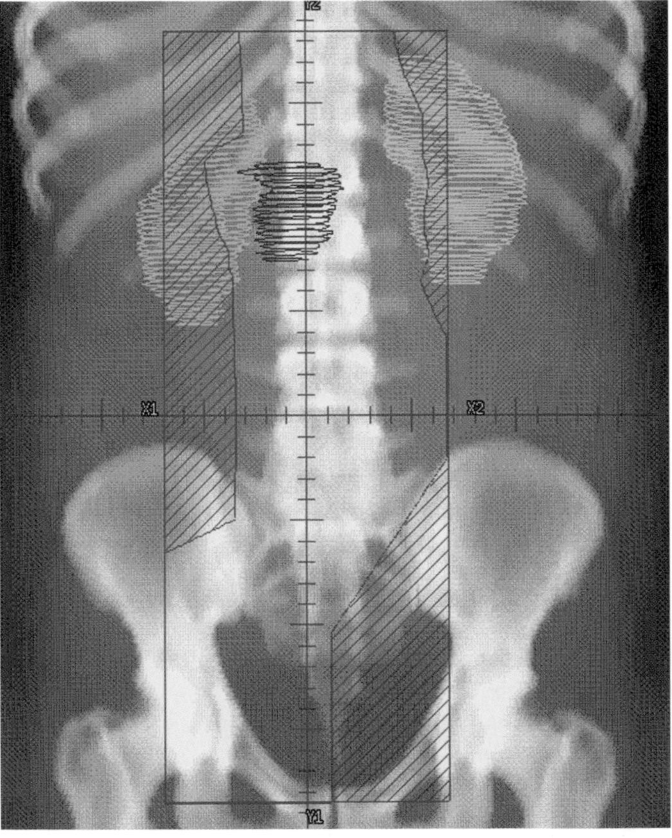

Fig. 28.1 DRR of a dogleg field used to treat a stage IIB seminoma

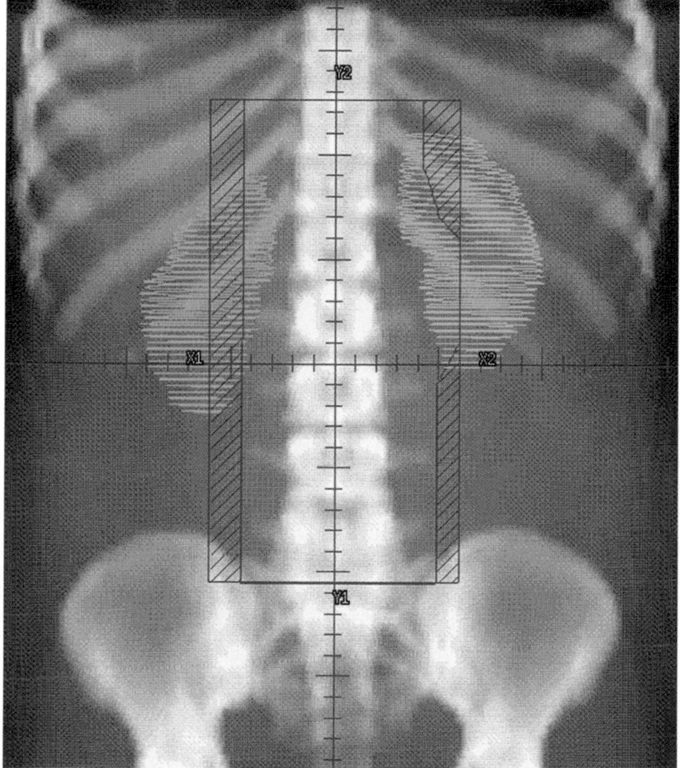

Fig. 28.2 DRR of a paraaortic field used to treat a stage I seminoma

DOSE LIMITATIONS

- 50 cGy causes transient azospermia with recovery at 1 year, but only 50% of patients reach their baseline
- 80–100 cGy causes total azospermia with recovery 1–2 years later for some patients
- 200 cGy causes sterilization
- Clamshell reduces testicle dose by 2–3× (dogleg without shield ~4 cGy/fx, with shield ~1.5 cGy/fx; paraaortic without shield ~2 cGy/fx, with shield ~0.7 cGy/fx)
- Kidneys: limit at least 70% <20 Gy

COMPLICATIONS

- Acute nausea, vomiting, diarrhea
- Late small bowel obstruction, chronic diarrhea, peptic ulcer disease (<2% with <35 Gy)
- With testicular shielding, most patients will have oligospermia by 4 months that lasts ~1 year
- Infertility: 50% of patients have subfertile counts on presentation or after surgery. After RT, 30% able to have children
- BEP causes immediate azospermia, but >50% recover sperm count
- Chemo side effects = alopecia, nausea, myelosuppression, pulmonary fibrosis, ototoxicity
- Second cancers: 5–10% increased risk vs. general population after RT

FOLLOW-UP

- See NCCN Guidelines (www.nccn.org)
- After RT for stage I seminoma
  - H&P, labs (AFP, β-HCG, LDH), and CXR every 3–4 months for year 1, every 6 months for year 2, then annually. Pelvic CT annually for 3 years for patients treated with PA-only RT (not needed if PA and pelvic RT)
- Stage I surveillance
  - H&P, labs every 3–4 months for years 1–3, every 6 months for years 4–7, then annually. CT abdomen and pelvis at each visit. CXR at alternate visits up to 10 years
- PET/CT can predict viable tumor in postchemotherapy residual disease.

REFERENCES

De Santis M, Becherer A, Bokemeyer C, et al. 2-18fluoro-deoxy-D-glucose positron emission tomography is a reliable predictor for viable tumor in postchemotherapy seminoma: an update of the prospective multicentric SEMPET trial. J Clin Oncol 2004;22:1034-1039.

Fossa SD, Horwich A, Russell JM, et al. Optimal planning target volume for stage I testicular seminoma: A Medical Research Council randomized trial. Medical Research Council Testicular Tumor Working Group. J Clin Oncol 1999;17:1146.

Jones WG, Fossa SD, Mead GM, et al. Randomized trial of 30 versus 20 Gy in the adjuvant treatment of stage I Testicular Seminoma: a report on Medical Research Council Trial TE18, European Organisation for the Research and Treatment of Cancer Trial 30942 (ISRCTN18525328). J Clin Oncol 2005;23:1200-1208.

Morton G, Thomas G. Testis. In: Halperin EC, Perez CA, Brady LW, et al., editors. Principles and practice of radiation oncology. 5th ed. Philadelphia: Lippincott Williams & Wilkins; 2008. pp. 1503-1518.

National Comprehensive Cancer Network. Clinical Practice Guidelines in Oncology: Testicular Cancer. Available at: http://www.nccn.org/professionals/physician_gls/PDF/testicular.pdf. Accessed on June 1, 2009.

Oliver RTD, Mason MD, Mead GM, et al. Radiotherapy versus single-dose carboplatin in adjuvant treatment of stage I seminoma: a randomized trial. Lancet 2005;266:293-300.

Oliver RT, Mead GM, Fogarty PJ, et al. Radiotherapy vs carboplatin for stage I seminoma: updated analysis of the MRC/EORTC randomized trial. J Clin Oncol 2008;26:abstr 1.

Puc HS, Heelan R, Mazumdar M, et al. Management of residual mass in advanced seminoma: results and recommendations from the Memorial Sloan-Kettering Cancer Center. J Clin Oncol 1996;14:454-460.

Travis LB, Fossa SD, Schonfeld SJ, et al. Second cancers among 40,576 testicular cancer patients: focus on long-term survivors. J Natl Cancer Inst 2005;97:1354-1365.

Warde P, Specht L, Horwich A, et al. Prognostic factors for relapse in stage I seminoma managed by surveillance: a pooled analysis. J Clin Oncol 2002;20:4448-4452.

FURTHER READING

Becherer A, De Santis M, Karanikas G, et al. FDG PET is superior to CT in the prediction of viable tumour in post-chemotherapy seminoma residuals. Eur J Radiol 2005;54(2): 284-248.

Garwood D. Cancer of the Testis. In: Leibel SA, Phillips TL, editors. Textbook of radiation oncology. 2nd ed. Philadelphia: Saunders; 2004. pp. 1031-1046.

Hussey D, Meistrich M. The Testicle. In: Cox JD, Ang KK, editors. Radiation oncology: rationale, technique, results. 8th ed. St. Louis: Mosby; 2003. pp. 605-628.

PART VIII
Gynecologic Sites

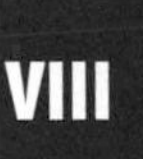

Chapter 29
Cervical Cancer

R. Scott Bermudez, Kim Huang, and I-Chow Hsu

PEARLS

- Leading cause of cancer mortality in women in developing countries and third most common gynecological cancer in the US.
- Screening with Pap smear decreases mortality by 70%, accounting for the steady decline in incidence in developed nations.
- ACS recommends screening for all women who are sexually active or >20 years old. Following three normal annual exams after age 30, screening may be performed less frequently, at least once every 3 years.
- Fifty percent of newly diagnosed cancers occur in women who have never been screened.
- Risk factors: early first intercourse, multiple partners, history of other STD's, high parity, smoking, immunosuppression, and prenatal DES exposure (clear cell CA).
- Ninety to ninety-five percent of cases are associated with HPV infection.
- HPV types 16 and 18 confer the highest risk of SCC and adenocarcinoma, respectively. HPV 6 and 11 are associated with benign warts.
- In 2006, the FDA approved the quadrivalent HPV recombinant vaccine for prevention of cancers caused by HPV types 6, 11, 16, and 18 for women aged 9–26 years.
- Eighty to ninety percent of invasive tumors are SCC, 10–20% are adenocarcinoma, and 1–2% are clear cell.
- SCC originates in the squamocolumnar junction with invasive disease frequently associated with adjacent CIS.
- Preinvasive disease: atypical squamous cells of uncertain significance (ASCUS), low-grade squamous intraepithelial lesion (LGSIL), and high-grade squamous intraepithelial lesion (HGSIL).
- ASCUS: 2/3 resolve spontaneously. Repeat Pap in 6 months and, if abnormal, perform colposcopy.

- LGSIL = Mild dysplasia/CIN 1. Half resolve spontaneously. Repeat Pap in 6 months and, if abnormal, perform colposcopy.
- HGSIL = Severe dysplasia / CIN 2/3/CIS. One-third resolve spontaneously. All undergo colposcopy with biopsy.
- The mean age of women diagnosed with cervical intraepithelial neoplasia (CIN) is 15–20 years younger than those diagnosed with invasive disease.
- Prognostic factors include LN metastases, tumor size, stage, uterine extension, and Hgb level <10.
- Risk of pelvic LN involvement for stage I, II, and III disease is approximately 15%, 30%, and 45%, respectively.
- Most common site for metastases are pelvic lymph nodes followed by lungs and paraaortic nodes.

WORKUP

- H&P including gynecologic history, abnormal vaginal bleeding or discharge, and pelvic pain. Examine abdomen, nodes (SCV, groins). Perform pelvic EUA, including bimanual palpation, jointly with a Gynecologic Oncologist.
- Pap smear if not bleeding.
- Colposcopy with 15× magnification, cold conization if no gross lesion noted and cannot visualize entire lesion with colposcope. Alternatively, four quadrant punch biopsies or D&C for pathology.
- Cystoscopy, sigmoidoscopy, and/or barium enema for IIB, III, or IVA disease, or for symptoms.
- Laboratories: CBC, LFTs, chemistries, BUN/Cr, urinalysis.
- Imaging: CT/MRI of abdomen and pelvis and CXR. Consider lymphangiogram and IVP (if no CT).
- PET scans are sensitive (~85–90%) and specific (~95–100%).
- If stage IIIB, place renal stent prior to starting chemo.
- Note: FIGO clinical staging does not allow CT, MRI, bone scan, PET, lymphangiography, or laparotomy.

STAGING: CERVICAL CANCER

Editors' note: All TNM stage and stage groups referred to elsewhere in this chapter reflect the 1988 FIGO/2002 AJCC staging nomenclature unless otherwise noted as the new system below was published after this chapter was written.

(AJCC 6TH ED., 2002/FIGO 1988)

FIGO/AJCC Clinical Staging

TX:	Primary tumor cannot be assessed
T0:	No evidence of primary tumor
0/Tis:	Carcinoma in situ*
I/T1:	Cervical carcinoma confined to uterus (extension to corpus should be disregarded)
IA/T1a**:	Invasive carcinoma diagnosed only by microscopy. Stromal invasion with a maximum depth of 5.0 mm measured from the base of the epithelium and a horizontal spread of 7.0 mm or less. Vascular space involvement, venous or lymphatic, does not affect classification
IA1/T1a1:	Measured stromal invasion 3 mm or less in depth and 7 mm or less in horizontal spread
IA2/T1a2:	Measured stromal invasion more than 3 mm and not more than 5.0 mm with a horizontal spread 7 mm or less
IB/T1b:	Clinically visible lesion confined to the cervix or microscopic lesion greater than IA2 / T1a
IB1/T1b1:	Clinically visible lesion 4.0 cm or less in greatest dimension
IB2/T1b2:	Clinically visible lesion more than 4.0 cm in greatest dimension
II/T2:	Cervical carcinoma invades beyond uterus, but not to pelvic wall or lower third of vagina
IIA/T2a:	Tumor without parametrial invasion
IIB/T2b:	Tumor with parametrial invasion
IIIA/T3a:	Tumor involves lower third of vagina, no extension to pelvic wall
IIIB/T3b:	Tumor extends to pelvic wall and/or causes hydronephrosis or nonfunctioning kidney

(AJCC 7TH ED., 2010/FIGO 2008)

Primary tumor (T)

TNM Categories	*FIGO Stages*	
TX		Primary tumor cannot be assessed
T0		No evidence of primary tumor
Tis*		Carcinoma in situ (preinvasive carcinoma)
T1	I	Cervical carcinoma confined to uterus (extension to corpus should be disregarded)
T1a**	IA	Invasive carcinoma diagnosed only by microscopy. Stromal invasion with a maximum depth of 5.0 mm measured from the base of the epithelium and a horizontal spread of 7.0 mm or less. Vascular space involvement, venous or lymphatic, does not affect classification
T1a1	IA1	Measured stromal invasion 3.0 mm or less in depth and 7.0 mm or less in horizontal spread
T1a2	IA2	Measured stromal invasion more than 3.0 mm and not more than 5.0 mm with a horizontal spread 7.0 mm or less
T1b	IB	Clinically visible lesion confined to the cervix or microscopic lesion greater than T1a/IA2
T1b1	IB1	Clinically visible lesion 4.0 cm or less in greatest dimension
T1b2	IB2	Clinically visible lesion more than 4.0 cm in greatest dimension

continued

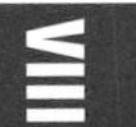

IVA/T4:	Tumor invades mucosa of bladder, rectum, and/or extends beyond true pelvis (bullous edema is not sufficient to classify a tumor as T4)
NX:	Regional lymph nodes cannot be assessed
N0:	No regional lymph node metastasis
N1:	Regional pelvic lymph node metastasis
MX:	Distant metastasis cannot be assessed
M0:	No distant metastasis
IVB/M1:	Distant metastasis (including paraaotic and inguinal nodal metastases)

*Bethesda or WHO system is used to further classify
**All macroscopically visible lesions – even with superficial invasion – are T1b/IB

AJCC stage		**~LC**		**~Survival**	
0:	TisN0M0	IA:	95–100%	IA:	95–100%
I:	T1N0M0	IB1:	90–95%	IB1:	85–90%
IA:	T1aN0M0	IB2:	60–80%	IB2:	60–70%
IA1:	T1a1N0M0	IIA:	80–85%	IIA:	75%
IA2:	T1a2N0M0	IIB:	60–80%	IIB:	60–65%
IB:	T1bN0M0	IIIA:	60%	IIIA:	25–50%
IB1:	T1b1N0M0	IIIB:	50–60%	IIIB:	25–50%
IB2:	T1b2N0M0	IVA:	30%	IVA:	15–30%
II:	T2N0M0			IVB:	<10%
IIA:	T2aN0M0				
IIB:	T2bN0M0				
III:	T3N0M0				
IIIA:	T3aN0M0				
IIIB:	T3b any NM0, T1-T3aN1M0				
IVA:	T4 any NM0				
IVB:	Any T any N M1				

T2	II	Cervical carcinoma invades beyond uterus, but not to pelvic wall or to lower third of vagina
T2a	IIA	Tumor without parametrial invasion
T2a1	IIA1	Clinically visible lesion 4.0 cm or less in greatest dimension
T2a2	IIA2	Clinically visible lesion more than 4.0 cm in greatest dimension
T2b	IIB	Tumor with parametrial invasion
T3	III	Tumor extends to pelvic wall and/or involves lower third of vagina, and/or causes hydronephrosis or nonfunctioning kidney
T3a	IIIA	Tumor involves lower third of vagina, no extension to pelvic wall
T3b	IIIB	Tumor extends to pelvic wall and/or causes hydronephrosis or nonfunctioning kidney
T4	IVA	Tumor invades mucosa of bladder or rectum, and/or extends beyond true pelvis (bullous edema is not sufficient to classify a tumor as T4)

*Note: FIGO no longer includes Stage 0 (Tis).
**Note: All macroscopically visible lesions – even with superficial invasion – are T1b/IB.

Regional lymph nodes (N)

TNM Categories	*FIGO Stages*	
NX		Regional lymph nodes cannot be assessed
N0		No regional lymph node metastasis
N1	IIIB	Regional lymph node metastasis

continued

Distant metastasis (M)

TNM Categories	*FIGO stages*	
M0		No distant metastasis
M1	IVB	Distant metastasis (including peritoneal spread, involvement of supraclavicular, mediastinal, or paraaortic lymph nodes, lung, liver, or bone)

Anatomic stage/prognostic groups (FIGO 2008)

0*:	Tis N0 M0
I:	T1 N0 M0
IA:	T1a N0 M0
IA1:	T1a1 N0 M0
IA2:	T1a2 N0 M0
IB:	T1b N0 M0
IB1:	T1b1 N0 M0
IB2:	T1b2 N0 M0
II:	T2 N0 M0
IIA:	T2a N0 M0
IIA1:	T2a1 N0 M0
IIA2:	T2a2 N0 M0
IIB:	T2b N0 M0
III:	T3 N0 M0
IIIA:	T3a N0 M0
IIIB:	T3b Any N M0
	T1-3 N1 M0
IVA:	T4 Any N M0
IVB:	Any T Any N M1

**Note*: FIGO no longer includes Stage 0 (Tis)

Used with the permission from the American Joint Committee on Cancer (AJCC), Chicago, IL. The original source for this material is the AJCC Cancer Staging Manual, Seventh Edition (2010), published by Springer Science–Business Media.

SUMMARY OF STAGING CHANGES

- Stage IIA is subdivided into stage IIA1 and IIA2 based on size (≤4 vs. >4 cm).
- Microinvasive and invasive adenocarcinoma should be staged as squamous cell carcinoma of the cervix.
- The use of diagnostic imaging techniques to assess the size of the primary tumor is encouraged, but not mandatory.
- For those institutions with access to MRI/CT scanning, radiological tumor volume and parametrial invasion should be recorded and sent to the FIGO Annual Report Editorial Office for data entry and inclusion in the Annual Report. Other investigations (i.e., examination under anesthesia, cystoscopy, sigmoidoscopy, and intravenous pyelography) are optional and no longer mandatory.

~LOCAL CONTROL AND SURVIVAL BY STAGE

~LC		~Survival	
IA:	95–100%	IA:	95–100%
IB1:	90–95%	IB1:	85–90%
IB2:	60–80%	IB2:	60–70%
IIA:	80–85%	IIA:	75%
IIB:	60–80%	IIB:	60–65%
IIIA:	60%	IIIA:	25–50%
IIIB:	50–60%	IIIB:	25–50%
IVA:	30%	IVA:	15–30%
		IVB:	<10%

TREATMENT RECOMMENDATIONS

SURGICAL TECHNIQUES

- Class I: total abdominal hysterectomy (extrafascial). Removal of cervix, small rim of vaginal cuff, and outside of the pubocervical fascia.
- Class II: modified radical hysterectomy (extended). Unroofing of ureters to resect parametrial and paracervical tissue medial to ureters (cardinal and uterosacral ligaments) and vaginal cuff (1–2 cm).
- Class III: radical abdominal hysterectomy (Wertheim-Meigs). Mobilization of ureters, bladder, and rectum to remove parametrial tissue to pelvic sidewall and vaginal cuff (upper 1/3–1/2), and lymphadenectomy.
- Class IV: extended radical hysterectomy. Removal of superior vesicular artery, part of ureter and bladder, and more vaginal cuff.

INDICATIONS FOR POST-OP RT/CHEMO-RT.

- Post-op pelvic RT: LVSI, >1/3 stromal invasion, or >4 cm tumor.
- Post-op chemo-RT: +margin, +LN, or parametrial or greater extension.

2002 Stage	Recommended treatment
Preinvasive	■ Conization or loop electrosurgical excisional procedure (LEEP) or laser or cryotherapy ablation or simple hysterectomy
IA	■ Total abdominal hysterectomy or trachelectomy or large cone biopsy with negative margins and close follow-up (if fertility preservation desired). Radical hysterectomy preferred for IA2 lesions OR ■ Brachytherapy alone (LDR 65–75 Gy or HDR 7 Gy × 5–6 fx). If high-risk pathologic features, treat as IB
IB1	■ Radical hysterectomy with pelvic LN dissection OR ■ Definitive RT: EBRT to WP (45 Gy) and brachytherapy (HDR 6 Gy × 5 fx, 7 Gy × 4 fx or LDR 15–20 Gy × 2 fx)
IB2–IIA	■ Concurrent chemo-RT with cisplatin. WP RT (45 Gy). Brachytherapy = HDR 6 Gy × 5 fx, 7 Gy × 4 fx or LDR 15–20 Gy × 2 fx
IIB	■ Concurrent chemo-RT with cisplatin. WP RT (45–50.4 Gy). Brachytherapy = HDR 6 Gy × 5 fx, 7 Gy × 4 fx or LDR 15–20 Gy × 2 fx
IIIA	■ Concurrent chemo-RT with cisplatin. RT to WP, vagina, and inguinal LN (45 Gy-50.4 Gy). Brachytherapy = HDR 6 Gy × 5 fx, 7 Gy × 4 fx or LDR 17–20 Gy × 2 fx
IIIB–IVA	■ Concurrent chemo-RT with cisplatin. WP RT (50–54 Gy). Brachytherapy = HDR 6 Gy × 5, 7 Gy × 4 fx or LDR 20 Gy × 2. If LN+, add paraaortic LN IMRT (45–60 Gy)
IVB	■ Combination chemotherapy

STUDIES

SURGERY VS. RADIATION

- Landoni et al. (1997): 343 patients with IB–IIA randomized to RT vs. surgery ± RT. Surgery was radical hysterectomy + pelvic LND with optional adjuvant RT to 50.4 Gy for stage > IIA, <3 mm uninvolved cervix, +margin or LN+. Fourty-five Gy given to + PAN. Sixty-three percent of patients in surgery arm received adjuvant RT, including 83% with tumors >4 cm. RT alone arm was 47 Gy EBRT + LDR 76 Gy point A dose. No significant differences in 5-year OS (83%), DFS (74%), or recurrence (25%). Morbidity worse with surgery ± RT arm vs. RT alone arm (28 vs. 12%).

EXTENDED-FIELD RT (EFRT)

- *RTOG 79-20* (Rotman et al., 1995, 2006): 337 patients with IIB without clinical or radiographically involved PAN randomized to WP 45 Gy or EFRT 45 Gy. EFRT improved 10-year OS (55 vs. 44%), but no difference on LRC (65%) or DM (25–30%). Toxicity increased with EFRT (8 vs. 4%).

CHEMO-RT

- *RTOG 90-01* (Morris et al., 1999; Eifel et al., 2004): 386 patients with surgically staged IIB–IVA, IB–IIA ≥ 5 cm, or LN + randomized to EFRT + brachytherapy (total 85 Gy point A dose) or to WPRT + brachytherapy (total 85 Gy point A dose) + cisplatin/5FU. Chemo-RT improved 8-year OS (67 vs. 41%), DFS (61 vs. 46%), and decreased LRF (18 vs. 35%) and DM (20 vs. 35%). Chemo-RT had a nonsignificant increase in PAN failures (8 vs. 4).
- *GOG 120* (Rose et al., 1999, 2007): 526 patients with IIB–IVA (surgically staged -PAN) randomized to WP + LDR brachytherapy (total 81 Gy point A dose) + 3 different chemo regimens: weekly cisplatin vs. cisplatin/5FU/hydroxyurea vs. hydroxyurea alone. Cisplatin arms decreased stage IIB and III 10-year LR (21–22 vs. 34%) and improved PFS (43–46 vs. 26%), OS (53 vs. 34%). No difference in grade 3–4 late toxicities among three regimens.
- *NCIC* (Pearcey et al., 2002): 353 patients with IA, IIA >5 cm, or IIB randomized to WP45 Gy + LDR 35 Gy ×1 or HDR 8 Gy ×3 vs. same RT + weekly cisplatin 40 mg/m² x6c. No difference in 5-year OS (62 vs. 58%).
- *GOG 123* (Stehman et al., 2007; Keys et al., 1999): 369 patients with IB2 randomized to WP + LDR RT (total 75 Gy to point A) followed by adjuvant simple hysterectomy vs. same RT + concurrent weekly cisplatin (40 mg/m²) × 6c followed by same surgery. Chemo-RT improved 5-year PFS (71 vs. 60%) and OS (78 vs. 64%), without increasing serious late adverse effects.

- *GOG 165* (Lanciano et al., 2005): 316 patients with IIB, IIIB, and IVA randomized to WP 45 Gy + parametrial boost + IC brachytherapy with standard weekly cisplatin (40 mg/m^2) vs. same RT with six cycles protracted venous infusion (PVI) 5-FU. Study closed prematurely when planned interim analysis demonstrated a 35% higher distant failure rate with RT + PVI 5-FU.

ADJUVANT HYSTERECTOMY AFTER RT

- *GOG 71* (Keys, 1997, 2003): 282 patients with >4 cm tumors randomized to EBRT + brachytherapy (80 Gy point A dose) vs. same RT (except 75 Gy point A dose) followed by adjuvant hysterectomy. No difference in OS (61 vs. 64%), but trend for higher LR without surgery (26 vs. 14%, $p = 0.08$).

POST-OP RT

- *GOG 92 / RTOG 87-06* (Rotman et al., 2006; Sedlis et al., 1999): 277 patients with bulky IB treated with radical hysterectomy with negative margins and LNs, but with ≥2 risk factors (LVSI, >1/3 stromal invasion, or ≥4 cm tumors) randomized to observation vs. post-op WP RT (46–50.4 Gy). Post-op RT reduced local and distant recurrences (31→18%), and improved PFS (65→78%).

POST-OP CHEMO-RT

- *GOG 109/SWOG 8797* (Peters et al., 2000): 243 patients s/p radical hysterectomy with IA2, IB, IIA, and + LN or + margin or + parametria randomized to WP RT (49.3 Gy with 45 Gy to PAN if common iliac LN+) vs. WP RT + cisplatin/5FU every 3 weeks × 4c. Post-op chemo-RT improved 4-year PFS (80 vs. 63%) and OS (81 vs. 71%). Re-analysis demonstrated that chemo-RT decreased LR by 50% and DM by 30%. Approximately 20% OS benefit from chemo for tumors >2 cm and patients with ≥2 + LN.

VIII

RADIATION TECHNIQUES

EBRT SIMULATION AND FIELD DESIGN

- Place two radiopaque gold seed markers in cervix and at distal margin of any vaginal disease. Use vaginal and anal markers as needed.
- There is no standard pelvic EBRT field. Blocking should be based on 3D imaging when treating with four field or AP/PA technique.
- Simulate patient supine with CT planning. Borders: superior = L4/5; inferior = 3 cm below most inferior vaginal involvement as marked by gold seeds (often at inferior obturator

foramen); lateral = 2 cm lateral to pelvic brim; posterior = include entire sacrum; anterior = 1 cm anterior to pubic symphysis.

- Treat inguinal nodes if stage IIIA (lower 1/3 vagina). Inferior border is vaginal introitus or flash.
- If common iliac nodes involved, raise superior border to allow for at least a 4 cm margin (~L3/4 level).
- EFRT for paraaortic nodes: superior border = T12/L1, lateral = encompass tips of transverse processes. Block kidneys as determined by CT planning. Use IMRT to minimize dose to kidneys and small bowel.
- When used, midline block is to avoid excess dose adjacent to the implant and to deliver higher dose to potential tumor bearing regions outside the implant. Midline block reduces dose to bladder and rectum, but may underdose sacrum. Since T&O has 100% dose through point A, which is ~2 cm from midline, a 4 cm midline block would be at the 100% IDL. Superior border of midline block = midsacroiliac joint. If concerned about toxicity, use a wider midline block (6 cm, ~50% IDL), or if concerned about tumor dose, use a narrower block. Midline blocks narrower than 5 cm may include the ureters which are ~2–2.5 cm from midline.
- At some institutions, it is preferred to deliver higher EBRT doses with a midline block for advanced lesions. After 45 Gy to the WP, the superior border may be lowered to the midsacroiliac joint and EBRT continued to 50 Gy. At 50 Gy, the superior border is further lowered to the bottom of the sacroiliac joint and treated to 54 Gy. If parametrial tumor persists after 50–54 Gy, it may boost parametria to 60 Gy.
- If bulky Unresectable LN+, use 3DCRT or IMRT boost to 60 Gy to involved nodes.

BRACHYTHERAPY

- If possible, proceed when tumor <4 cm (so point A dose covers) without prolonging overall treatment time.
- Unless greater shrinkage is needed, first intracavitary insertion is after 10–20 Gy EBRT. Second application is 1–2 weeks later. Smitt sleeve may be left in cervical canal between insertions.
- If small lesion and narrow vagina, treat first with IC RT before EBRT causes vaginal narrowing.
- If large lesion and narrow vagina, use EBRT first to shrink the tumor.
- If superficial vaginal involvement, use a combination of a T&O applicator alternating with a tandem and vaginal cylinder appli-

cator (with packing to spare rectum or bladder). Alternatively, use two tandem and vaginal cylinder insertions.

- For deep or thicker vaginal involvement, use IS brachytherapy.
- Use gauze packing imbedded with radiopaque wire to push bladder and rectum away. Always Use Triple-Sulfate soaked gauze for LDR and K-Y Jelly for HDR.
- LDR is generally Cs-137 at 0.4–0.8 Gy/h. 0.4–0.6 Gy/h may have less complications then 0.8– Gy/h.
- HDR is generally an Ir-192 high activity (~10 Ci) source with dose rate ~12 Gy/h.
- ICRU system: report applicator type, source type, loading, and orthogonal radiographs. Use reference air-kerma strength, volume treated to 60 Gy.
- Prescribe to point A = 2 cm superior to external cervical OS (or vaginal fornices) and 2 cm lateral to central canal / tandem. Point A dose is very sensitive to ovoid position relative to the tandem.
- Point B = 3 cm lateral to point A, represents parametrial (obturator nodes). Receives ~1/3–1/4 of dose to point A.
- Bladder point = posterior surface of foley balloon on lateral X-ray and center of balloon on AP film. Foley balloon filled with 7 cm^3 radiopaque fluid and pulled down against urethra.
- Rectal point = 5 mm behind posterior vaginal wall between ovoids at inferior point of last intrauterine tandem source, or midvaginal source.
- Vaginal point = lateral edge of ovoid on AP film and midovoid on lateral film.
- Tandem placement: use a looping suture through the cervix for countertraction. Hegar uterine dilators are used to dilate the os to 6 mm. Tandem length is usually 6–8 cm (4 cm for postmenopausal women). For tandems >8 cm, avoid loading/active source at end to protect small bowel. Tandem should be located centrally between the ovoids on the AP view and bisect the ovoids on the lateral view.
- Typical tandem loading with Cs-137 = 30–40 mgRaEq with three 10–15 mgRaEq sources (e.g., 15-15-10 cephalad to caudad).
- Ovoids: cervix should be marked with 2 gold seeds (usually at 12 and 6 o'clock). Use largest ovoids possible separated by 0.5–1 cm. Standard ovoid loadings = 10–15 mgRaEq for 2 cm (small) ovoids, 15–20 mgRaEq for 2.5 cm (medium) ovoids, or 5–10 mgRaEq for miniovoids.
- Pack anteriorly and posteriorly to spare the bladder and rectum.
- Take plain films in the OR so that system may be repositioned and/or repacked if suboptimal.
- Implant evaluation:

VIII

- Anterior film: tandem bisects ovoids and tandem not rotated; phlange close to cervical marker seeds; ovoids high in fornices <1 cm from marker seeds with 0.5–1 cm spacing between them.
- Lateral film: tandem bisects ovoids and is midway between sacrum and bladder, at least 3 cm from sacral promontory; sufficient anterior and posterior packing; foley balloon firmly pulled down.

- With optimally placed system, LDR dose rate at point A is ~45–55 cGy/h.
- Attempt to keep overall treatment time <7 weeks; prolongation of treatment time increases failure rate by 0.6%/d in IB–IIA and by 0.9%/d in IIB.
- Image-guided brachytherapy requires modification of dwell time based on 3D images. Treatment delivery is accomplished by HDR and PDR remote afterloaders. Recommendations regarding 3D MRI/CT image-guided brachytherapy treatment planning have been published by the GEC-ESTRO Working Group (Pötter et al., 2006; Haie-Meder et al., 2005).

DOSE PRESCRIPTIONS

- EBRT: 1.8 Gy/fx. Whole pelvis = 45 Gy. Side wall boost = 50–54 Gy. Persistent or bulky parametrial tumor = 60 Gy. Paraaortic LN (if treated) = 45 Gy. Bulky LN = 60 Gy
- Brachytherapy
  - LDR = 15–20 Gy × 2 fx
  - HDR = 6 Gy × 5 fx or 7 Gy × 4 fx
- Desired cumulative doses
  - Point A: IA = 65–75 Gy, IB1–IIB 75–85 Gy, III–IVA 85–90 Gy
  - Sidewall dose: IB–IIA = 45–50 Gy, IIB = 45–54 Gy, III–IVA = 54–60 Gy

DOSE LIMITATIONS

- HDR: limit bladder and rectal points to <70% of point A dose with HDR.
- LDR: limit rectal point <70 Gy and bladder point <75 Gy.
- Limit upper vaginal mucosa <120 Gy, midvaginal mucosa <80–90 Gy, and lower vaginal mucosa <60–70 Gy. Vaginal doses >50–60 Gy cause significant fibrosis and stenosis.
- Ovarian failure with 5–10 Gy and sterilization with 2–3 Gy.
- Limit uterus <100 Gy, ureters <75 Gy, and femoral heads <50 Gy.

COMPLICATIONS

- Acute: pruritis, dry/moist desquamation, nausea, colitis, cystitis, and vaginitis.
- HDR and LDR morbidity are equivalent: uterine perforation (<3%), vaginal laceration (<1%), DVT (<1%).
- Late: vaginal stenosis, ureteral stricture (1–3%), vesicovaginal or rectovaginal fistula (<2%), intestinal obstruction or perforation (<5%), femoral neck fracture (<5%).
- Recommend vaginal dilation as needed to maintain vaginal vault size and sexual function.
- Standard post-op complications. Surgical mortality 1%.

FOLLOW-UP

- H&P every month for 3 months, then every 3 months for 9 months, then every 4 months for 1 year, then every 6 months for 2 years, then annually.
- Follow-up Pap smears controversial due to post-RT change.
- CXR annually × 5 years.

REFERENCES

Eifel PJ, Winter K, Morris M, et al. Pelvic irradiation with concurrent chemotherapy versus pelvic and para-aortic irradiation for high-risk cervical cancer: an update of radiation therapy oncology group trial (RTOG) 90-01. J Clin Oncol 2004;22:872-880.

Haie-Meder C, Pötter R, Van Limbergen E, et al. Recommendations from Gynaecological (GYN) GEC-ESTRO Working Group (I): concepts and terms in 3D image based 3D treatment planning in cervix cancer brachytherapy with emphasis on MRI assessment of GTV and CTV. Radiother Oncol 2005;74(3):235-245.

Keys HM, Bundy BN, Stehman FB, et al. Adjuvant hysterectomy after radiation therapy reduces detection of local recurrences in "bulky" stage IB cervical without improving survival: results of a prospective randomized GOG trial. Cancer J Sci Am 1997;3:117(abstr).

Keys HM, Bundy BN, Stehman FB, et al. Cisplatin, radiation, and adjuvant hysterectomy compared with radiation and adjuvant hysterectomy for bulky stage IB cervical carcinoma. N Engl J Med 1999;340:1154-1161.

Keys HM, Bundy BN, Stehman FB, et al. Radiation therapy with and without extrafascial hysterectomy for bulky stage IB cervical carcinoma: a randomized trial of the Gynecologic Oncology Group. Gynecol Oncol 2003;89:343-353.

Lanciano R, Calkins A, Bundy BN, et al. Randomized comparison of weekly cisplatin or protracted venous infusion of fluorouracil in combination with pelvic radiation in advanced cervix cancer: a Gynecologic Oncology Group study. J Clin Oncol 2005;23:8289-8295.

Landoni F, Maneo A, Colombo A, et al. Randomised study of radical surgery versus radiotherapy for stage Ib-IIa cervical cancer. Lancet 1997;350:535-540.

Morris M, Eifel PJ, Lu J, et al. Pelvic radiation with concurrent chemotherapy compared with pelvic and para-aortic radiation for high-risk cervical cancer. N Engl J Med 1999;340:1137-1143.

Pearcey R, Brundage M, Drouin P, et al. Phase III trial comparing radical radiotherapy with and without cisplatin chemotherapy in patients with advanced squamous cell cancer of the cervix. J Clin Oncol 2002;20:966-972.

Peters WA III, Liu PY, Barrett RJ II, et al. Concurrent chemotherapy and pelvic radiation therapy compared with pelvic radiation therapy alone as adjuvant therapy after radical surgery in high-risk early-stage cancer of the cervix. J Clin Oncol 2000;18:1606-1613.

Pötter R, Haie-Meder C, Van Limbergen E, et al. Recommendations from gynaecological (GYN) GEC ESTRO working group (II): concepts and terms in 3D image-based treatment planning in cervix cancer brachytherapy-3D dose volume parameters and aspects of 3D image-based anatomy, radiation physics, radiobiology. Radiother Oncol 2006;78(1):67-77.

Rose PG, Ali S, Watkins E, et al. Long-term follow-up of a randomized trial comparing concurrent single agent cisplatin, cisplatin-based combination chemotherapy, or hydroxyurea during pelvic irradiation for locally advanced cervical cancer: a Gynecologic Oncology Group study. J Clin Oncol 2007;25:2804-2810.

Rose PG, Bundy BN, Watkins EB, et al. Concurrent cisplatin-based radiotherapy and chemotherapy for locally advanced cervical cancer. N Engl J Med 1999;340:1144-1153.

Rotman M, Sedlis A, Piedmonte MR, et al. A phase III randomized trial of postoperative pelvic irradiation in stage IB cervical carcinoma with poor prognostic features: follow-up of a gynecologic oncology group study. Int J Radiat Oncol Biol Phys 2006;65:169-176.

Rotman M, Pajak TF, Choi K, et al. Prophylactic extended-field irradiation of para-aortic lymph nodes in stages IIB and bulky IB and IIA cervical carcinomas. Ten-year treatment results of RTOG 79-20. JAMA 1995;274:387-393.

Sedlis A, Bundy BN, Rotman MZ, et al. A randomized trial of pelvic radiation therapy versus no further therapy in selected patients with stage IB carcinoma of the cervix after radical hysterectomy and pelvic lymphadenectomy: A Gynecologic Oncology Group Study. Gynecol Oncol 1999;73:177-183.

Stehman FB, Ali S, Keys HM, et al. Radiation therapy with or without weekly cisplatin for bulky stage 1B cervical carcinoma: follow-up of a Gynecologic Oncology Group trial. Am J Obstet Gynecol 2007;197(5):503.e1-6.

FURTHER READING

Greene FL, American Joint Committee on Cancer., American Cancer Society. AJCC cancer staging manual. 6th ed. New York: Springer; 2002.

Koh W, Moore DH. Cervical Cancer. In: Gunderson LL, Tepper JE, et al., editors. Clinical radiation oncology. 2nd ed. Philadelphia: Churchill Livingstone; 2007. pp. 1323-1357.

National Comprehensive Cancer Network. Clinical Practice Guidelines in Oncology: Cervical Cancers. Available at: http://www.nccn.org/professionals/physician_gls/PDF/cervical.pdf. Accessed on May 28 2009.

Perez CA, Kavanagh BD. Uterine Cervix. In: Halperin CE, Perez CA, Brady LW, et al., editors. Principles and practice of radiation oncology. 5th ed. Philadelphia: Lippincott Williams & Wilkins; 2008. pp. 1532-1609.

Swift PS, Hsu IC. Cancer of the Uterine Cervix. In: Leibel SA, Phillips TL, editors. Textbook of radiation oncology. 2nd ed. Philadelphia: Saunders; 2004. pp. 1055-1100.

Chapter 30
Endometrial Cancer

R. Scott Bermudez, Kim Huang, and I-Chow Hsu

PEARLS

- Most common gynecological cancer in the U.S; fourth most common malignancy in women after breast, lung, and colorectal.
- Risk factors: unopposed estrogen, postmenopausal (median age at diagnosis is 61 years), nulliparity, early menarche, late menopause, obesity, tamoxifen (7.5×), oral contraceptives use.
- Grade is determined by percentage of dedifferentiated solid growth pattern: Grade 1: ≤5%, Grade 2: 5–50%, Grade 3: >50%.
- Seventy-five percent of tumors are endometrioid endometrial adenocarcinomas, which are estrogen-dependent tumors that commonly present with postmenopausal bleeding and are frequently preceded by endometrial hyperplasia.
- Rate of progression to invasive cancer from simple hyperplasia is rare (<2%) with progression to carcinoma in patients with simple and complex hyperplasia with atypia being more common (30–40%).
- Twenty percent of endometrial carcinomas are nonendometrioid including papillary serous (UPSC), clear cell, and mucinous.
- Papillary serous and clear cell carcinomas are often diagnosed with more advanced disease and have a poorer prognosis.
- Up to 5% of uterine cancers are sarcomas, including carcinosarcoma (most common), leiomyosarcoma, and endometrial stromal sarcomas.
- Prognostic factors = stage (#1), cell type, grade, LVSI, depth of invasion, cervical extension, and patient age.
- Primary lymphatic drainage is to pelvic LN (internal and external iliac, obturator, common iliac, presacral, parametrial); direct spread may occur to paraaortic LN.
- ~1/3 of patients with + pelvic LN have + paraaortic LN.

WORKUP

- H&P with attention to uterine size, cervical and vaginal involvement, ascites, nodes.

VIII

- Labs: CBC, blood chemistries, LFTs, CA-125 (elevated in 60%), UA.
- Endometrial biopsy is diagnostic gold standard with >90% sensitivity and 85% specificity, thereby largely obviating need for D&C.
- D&C if endometrial biopsy is nondiagnostic.
- Pap smear has limited sensitivity (as low as 40%).
- Imaging: CXR, CT, or MRI of abdomen and pelvis or transvaginal ultrasound to evaluate symptomatic disease.
- Cystoscopy and/or sigmoidoscopy as clinically indicated.

STAGING (AJCC 6TH ED., 2002/FIGO 1988 PATHOLOGIC STAGING): ENDOMETRIAL CANCER

TX:	Primary tumor cannot be assessed
T0:	No evidence of primary tumor
Tis/0:	Carcinoma in situ
T1/I:	Tumor confined to corpus uteri
T1a/IA:	Tumor limited to endometrium
T1b/IB:	Tumor invades less than one-half of the myometrium
T1c/IC:	Tumor invades one-half or more of the myometrium
T2/II:	Tumor invades cervix, but does not extend beyond uterus
T2a/IIA:	Tumor limited to glandular epithelium of endocervix. There is no evidence of connective tissue stromal invasion
T2b/IIB:	Invasion of the stromal connective tissue of the cervix
T3/III:	Local and/or regional spread as defined below
T3a/IIIA:	Tumor involves serosa and/or adnexa (direct extension or metastasis) and/or cancer cells in ascites or peritoneal washings
T3b/IIIB:	Vaginal involvement (direct extension or metastasis)
T4/IVA:	Tumor invades bladder mucosa and/or bowel mucosa (bullous edema not sufficient to classify tumor as T4)
NX:	Regional lymph nodes cannot be assessed
N0:	No regional lymph node metastasis
N1/IIIC:	Regional lymph node metastasis to pelvic and/or paraaortic nodes
MX:	Distant metastasis cannot be assessed
M0:	No distant metastasis
M1/IVB:	Distant metastasis (includes metastasis to abdominal lymph nodes other than paraaortic, and/or inguinal lymph nodes; excludes metastasis to vagina, pelvic serosa, or adnexa)

A small number of patients may be treated with primary radiation. Such patients should be staged with the clinical staging system adopted by FIGO in 1971 (Int J Gynaecol Obstet 1971;9:172)

STAGING (AJCC 7TH ED., 2010/FIGO 2008)

Editors' note: All TNM stage and stage groups referred to elsewhere in this chapter reflect the 1988 FIGO/2002 AJCC staging nomenclature unless otherwise noted as the new system below was published after this chapter was written.

SUMMARY OF CHANGES

- The FIGO 1988 Stage IA and IB have been combined, so that Stage IA now involves the endometrium and/or less than one-half myometrial invasion, and IB is now equal to or greater than the outer one-half of the myometrium (previously IC).
- Stage II no longer has a subset A and B. Involvement of the endocervical glandular portion of the cervix (previously IIA) is now considered stage I. Previous stage IIB is now simply stage II.
- Stage IIIC pelvic and paraaortic node involvement have been separated, rather than combined in a single substage. As a result, stage IIIC is now categorized as IIIC1 (indicating positive pelvic nodes) and IIIC2 (indicating positive paraaortic nodes with or without positive pelvic nodes).
- A separate staging schema for uterine sarcoma has been added.

UTERINE CARCINOMAS

Primary tumor (T) (surgical-pathologic findings)

TNM categories	*FIGO stages*	
TX		Primary tumor cannot be assessed
T0		No evidence of primary tumor
Tis*		Carcinoma in situ (preinvasive carcinoma)
T1	I	Tumor confined to corpus uteri
T1a	IA	Tumor limited to endometrium or invades less than one-half of the myometrium
T1b	IB	Tumor invades one-half or more of the myometrium
T2	II	Tumor invades stromal connective tissue of the cervix, but does not extend beyond uterus**
T3a	IIIA	Tumor involves serosa and/or adnexa (direct extension or metastasis)
T3b	IIIB	Vaginal involvement (direct extension or metastasis) or parametrial involvement
T4	IVA	Tumor invades bladder mucosa and/or bowel mucosa (bullous edema is not sufficient to classify a tumor as T4)

**Note*: FIGO no longer includes Stage 0 (Tis).
**Endocervical glandular involvement only should be considered Stage I and not Stage II.

Regional lymph nodes (*N*)

TNM categories	*FIGO stages*	
NX		Regional lymph nodes cannot be assessed
N0		No regional lymph node metastasis
N1	IIIC1	Regional lymph node metastasis to pelvic lymph nodes
N2	IIIC2	Regional lymph node metastasis to paraaortic lymph nodes, with or without positive pelvic lymph nodes

continued

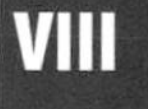

Distant metastasis (M)

TNM Categories	*FIGO Stages*	
M0		No distant metastasis
M1	IVB	Distant metastasis (includes metastasis to inguinal lymph nodes intraperitoneal disease, or lung, liver, or bone. Excludes metastasis to paraaortic lymph nodes, vagina, pelvic serosa, or adnexa)

Anatomic stage/prognostic groups

*Carcinomas**

0**: Tis N0 M0
I: T1 N0 M0
IA: T1a N0 M0
IB: T1b N0 M0
II: T2 N0 M0
III: T3 N0 M0
IIIA: T3a N0 M0
IIIB: T3b N0 M0
IIIC1: T1-T3 N1 M0
IIIC2: T1-T3 N2 M0
IVA: T4 Any N M0
IVB: Any T Any N M1

*Carcinosarcomas should be staged as carcinoma.
**Note: FIGO no longer includes Stage 0 (Tis).

LEIOMYOSARCOMA, ENDOMETRIAL STROMAL SARCOMA

Primary tumor (T)

TNM Categories	*FIGO Stages*	
TX		Primary tumor cannot be assessed
T0		No evidence of primary tumor
T1	I	Tumor limited to the uterus
T1a	IA	Tumor 5 cm or less in greatest dimension
T1b	IB	Tumor more than 5 cm
T2	II	Tumor extends beyond the uterus, within the pelvis
T2a	IIA	Tumor involves adnexa
T2b	IIB	Tumor involves other pelvic tissues
T3	III*	Tumor infiltrates abdominal tissues
T3a	IIIA	One site
T3b	IIIB	More than one site
T4	IVA	Tumor invades bladder or rectum

Note: Simultaneous tumors of the uterine corpus and ovary/pelvis in association with ovarian/pelvic endometriosis should be classified as independent primary tumors.
*Lesions must infiltrate abdominal tissues and not just protrude into the abdominal cavity.

Regional lymph nodes (N)

TNM Categories	*FIGO Stages*	
NX		Regional lymph nodes cannot be assessed
N0		No regional lymph node metastasis
N1	IIIC	Regional lymph node metastasis

continued

Distant metastasis (M)

TNM Categories	*FIGO stages*	
M0		No distant metastasis
M1	IVB	Distant metastasis (excluding adnexa, pelvic, and abdominal tissues)

Used with permission from the American Joint Committee on Cancer (AJCC), Chicago, IL. The original source for this material is the AJCC Cancer Staging Manual, Seventh Edition (2010), published by Springer Science+Business Media.

ADENOSARCOMA

Primary tumor (T)

TNM Categories	*FIGO stages*	
TX		Primary tumor cannot be assessed
T0		No evidence of primary tumor
T1	I	Tumor limited to the uterus
T1a	IA	Tumor limited to the endometrium/endocervix
T1b	IB	Tumor invades to less than half of the myometrium
T1c	IC	Tumor invades more than half of the myometrium
T2	II	Tumor extends beyond the uterus, within the pelvis
T2a	IIA	Tumor involves adnexa
T2b	IIB	Tumor involves other pelvic tissues
T3	III*	Tumor involves abdominal tissues
T3a	IIIA	One site
T3b	IIIB	More than one site
T4	IVA	Tumor invades bladder or rectum

Note: Simultaneous tumors of the uterine corpus and ovary/pelvis in association with ovarian/pelvic endometriosis should be classified as independent primary tumors.
*In this stage lesions must infiltrate abdominal tissues and not just protrude into the abdominal cavity

Regional lymph nodes (N)

TNM Categories	*FIGO stages*	
NX		Regional lymph nodes cannot be assessed
N0		No regional lymph node metastasis
N1	IIIC	Regional lymph node metastasis

Distant metastasis (M)

TNM Categories	*FIGO stages*	
M0		No distant metastasis
M1	IVB	Distant metastasis (excluding adnexa, pelvic and abdominal tissues)

Used with permission from the American Joint Committee on Cancer (AJCC), Chicago, IL. The original source for this material is the AJCC Cancer Staging Manual, Seventh Edition (2010), published by Springer Science+Business Media.

UTERINE SARCOMA

Anatomic stage/prognostic groups

I: T1 N0 M0
IA*: T1a N0 M0
IB*: T1b N0 M0
IC**: T1c N0 M0
II: T2 N0 M0
IIIA: T3a N0 M0
IIIB: T3b N0 M0
IIIC: T1, T2, T3 N1 M0
IVA: T4 Any N M0
IVB: Any T Any N M1

**Note*: Stages IA and IB differ from those applied for leiomyosarcoma and endometrial stromal sarcoma.
***Note*: Stage IC does not apply for leiomyosarcoma and endometrial stromal sarcoma.

TREATMENT RECOMMENDATIONS

2002 Stage	Recommended treatment
All patients	■ All medically operable patients should have surgery. Perform TAH/BSO or radical hysterectomy if cervical stromal involvement and obtain peritoneal cytology. Generally, exploratory laparotomy with inspection and palpation ± biopsy of the omentum, liver, peritoneal surfaces, and adnexae is performed. Consider selective pelvic and paraaortic LN dissection for myometrial invasion or if grade 2–3, and include nodes from paraaortic, common iliac, external iliac, internal iliac, and obturator chains. Adjuvant treatment as below:
IA, IB	■ Observation, or if grade 2–3 and adverse features present (age >60 years, LVSI, large tumor size, lower uterine involvement), pelvic RT and/or vaginal cuff brachytherapy (VC)
IC	■ Observation, or if other adverse features present (grade 2–3, advanced age >50–70 years, LVSI, large tumor size, lower uterine segment involvement) pelvic RT and/or vaginal cuff brachytherapy (VC). Consider chemotherapy for grade 3
IIA, IIB	■ Consider pelvic RT ±VC. Consider chemotherapy for grade 3
IIIA	■ Positive cytology only: Observation for grade 1–2, chemotherapy for grade 3. Consider pelvic RT and/or VC. All other IIIA: Chemotherapy and/or tumor-directed RT

continued

Stage III-IV	■ Surgery → chemotherapy and/or tumor-directed RT
Medically inoperable	■ Tumor-directed EBRT to uterus, cervix, upper vagina, pelvic LN, and other involved areas (~45–50.4 Gy), followed by intracavitary brachytherapy boost (e.g., 6 Gy × 3 HDR to uterine serosal surface). Consider dose-escalation to gross disease using image-guided brachytherapy or IMRT with CT or MRI planning
Recurrence	■ If no prior RT → EBRT and IC or IS brachytherapy boost to total dose 60–70 Gy. Consider IS salvage brachytherapy for select previously irradiated patients
Papillary serous/clear cell	■ Surgery. For stage IA, consider chemotherapy and/or tumor-directed RT. For stage IB, IC, II, and debulked stage III-IV, give chemotherapy ± tumor-directed RT.
Sarcomas, carcinosarcoma [malignant mixed mesodermal (Mullerian) tumor]	■ Surgery. Post-op RT for high-grade sarcomas, leiomyosarcomas, and carcinosarcomas to improve LC. Pelvic RT ± VC for stages I–II and tumor-directed RT for stages III–IV. Consider chemotherapy for high-grade undifferentiated sarcoma and leiomyosarcoma

VIII

STUDIES

LYMPHADENECTOMY

- *MRC ASTEC* (2009): 1,408 women thought preoperatively to have corpus confined disease randomized to surgery (TAH/BSO/washings/PALN palpation) ± lymphadenectomy. With adjustment for baseline characteristics and pathology, lymphadenectomy provided no significant OS or RFS.

ADJUVANT RADIOTHERAPY

- *GOG 99* (Keys et al. 2004): Three hundred and ninety-two patients with IB (60%), IC (30%), and occult II (10%) treated with TAH/BSO, pelvic and PALN sampling, and peritoneal cytology with 6-year F/U. Patients randomized to observation vs. post-op WP RT (50.4 Gy). Two-third of patients had low–intermediate risk disease and one-third of patients were high-intermediate risk (G2-3, outer 1/3 involvement, and LVSI or age >50 years + 2 factors, or age >70 years + 1 factor). WP RT improved LRR (12→3%), mostly among high-intermediate risk patients

(26→6%) compared to low–intermediate risk patients (6→2%). No difference in OS (86→92%), but not powered to detect OS change. Majority of pelvic recurrences were in the vaginal cuff.

- *PORTEC-1* (Creutzberg et al. 2000; Scholten et al. 2005): Seven hundred and fourteen patients with IB G2–3 or IC G1–2 treated with TAH/BSO randomized to observation vs. WP RT (46 Gy). No LN dissection (only sampling of suspicious LN). Ninety percent of patients had G1–2 and 40% were IB. WP RT decreased LRR (14→4%), with 75% of failures occuring in the vaginal vault. No difference in OS (81 vs. 85%) or DM (8 vs. 7%). Update with 10-year f/u and central pathology review for 80% of patients confirmed WP RT continued to reduce LRR (14→5%) without an OS benefit (66 vs. 73%), even after excluding IB grade 1 patients. Patients with 2 or more risk factors (age ≥60 years, grade 3, and ≥50% myometrial invasion) had greatest LRR benefit with RT (23→5%).
- *ASTEC EN.5* (2009): Nine hundred and nine patients with IA/B grade 3, IC any grade, or I-II papillary serous or clear cell histology randomized after surgery to observation or WP RT (40–46 Gy). However, vaginal cuff brachytherapy was used in 51% of patients randomized to the observation arm. There was no difference in 5-year OS (84%) or DSS (89–90%). WP RT reduced isolated pelvic or vaginal recurrences (6.1→3.2%), and increased acute toxicity (27→57%) and late severe toxicity (3→7%).
- Aalders et al. (1980): Five hundred patients with IB-IC any grade treated with TAH/BSO without LN sampling. Sixty-five percent of patients had IB G1-2 Randomized to VC vs. VC → WP RT. VC = LDR 60 Gy to surface. WP RT = 2/40 Gy with central shielding at 20 Gy. Addition of WP RT decreased pelvic and vaginal recurrences (7→2%), but did not change OS (90%) because more DM in WP RT arm. On subset analysis, most improvement in LRR with IC G3 (20→5%). Poor prognostic factors = IC, G3, LVSI, age >60 years.
- *PORTEC 2* (Nout 2008 – abstract only): Four hundred and twenty-seven patients with high-intermediate risk (age >60 years and IC grade 1–2 or IB grade 3; any age and IIA grade 1–2 or grade 3 with <50% invasion) randomized to WP RT (46 Gy) or VC brachytherapy (21 Gy HDR in 3 fx or 30 Gy LDR). Although WP RT reduced pelvic relapse (3.6→0.7%), there was no significant difference in 3-year VC relapse (0.9% VC vs. 2% WP), OS (90–91%), or RFS (89–90%). Patient-reported quality of life was better with VC brachytherapy.
- *Metaanalyses* (Johnson 2007; Kong et al., 2007) suggest that pelvic EBRT may improve DFS for high-risk patients, such as those with IC grade 3 disease.

- *SEER* (Lee et al. 2006). Review of 21,249 patients with stage I disease treated with (19.2%) or without (80.8%) adjuvant RT. Adjuvant RT improved OS and RFS for IC grade 1 and IC grade 3–4 patients, similar to results among patients who had a surgical LN examination.

ROLE OF CHEMOTHERAPY

- *GOG 122* (Randall et al. 2006): Three hundred and ninety-six patients with III/IV disease treated with surgery with maximal residual disease ≤2 cm randomized to WART (30 Gy + 15 Gy pelvic boost + 15 Gy paraaortic boost if pelvic LN+ or no sampling of pelvic and paraaortic LN) vs. chemo (doxorubicin + cisplatin every 3 weeks × 7c → cisplatin × 1c). 21% of patients had UPSC in each arm. Chemo improved 5-year OS (42→55%) and DFS (38→50%), but increased grade 3–4 hematologic, gastrointestinal, and cardiac toxicity.
- *Ontario Canada group* (Lupe et al. 2007): Thirty-three patients with III/IV disease treated with carboplatin/paclitaxel every 3 weeks × 4c, then pelvic RT 45 Gy, then 2 more cycles chemo. PA RT and/or VC HDR were optional. 2-year DFS and OS 55%, with only 3% pelvic relapse.
- *RTOG 9708* (Greven et al. 2006): Phase II trial of 46 patients with grade 2–3 disease with either >50% myometrial invasion and cervical stromal invasion or pelvic-confined extrauterine disease treated with WP RT (45 Gy) and cisplatin on days 1 and 28. Four-year pelvic, regional, and distant recurrence rates were 2%, 2%, and 19%, respectively. Four-year OS and DFS were 85% and 81%, respectively. There were no recurrences for stages IC, IIA, or IIB.
- *Italian* (Maggi et al. 2006): Three hundred and forty-five patients with IC G3, II G3 with >50% myometrial invasion, and IIIA-IIIC randomized to pelvic RT 45–50 Gy vs. CAP chemo (cyclophosphamide/doxorubicin/cisplatin) monthly x 5c. Note 64% of the patient had stage III disease. No difference in 7-year OS 62% or PFS 56–60%. RT delayed LF (11→7%) and chemo delayed DM (21→16%)
- *Japanese* (Susumu et al. 2008): 385 patients with stage IC-III with >50% myometrial invasion treated with surgery and pelvic LN dissection randomized to pelvic RT (45–50 Gy) vs. CAP chemo (cyclophosphamide, doxorubicin, cisplatin) every 4 weeks for 3c. Only 3% received brachytherapy. No difference in 5-year PFS (82–84%) or OS (85–87%). On subset analysis, no difference for ICG1-2 <70 years (low–intermediate risk), but chemo improved PFS (66→84%) and OS (74→90%) for

higher-risk group (ICG3 or IC >70 years or stage II or IIIA (+cytology)). Seven percent pelvic failures in each arm, but fewer vaginal recurrences in RT arm. No differences in extrapelvic recurrences (~15%).

- *NSGO-EC-9501/EORTC 55991* (Hogberg 2007 – abstract only): Three hundred and seventy-two patients with surgical stage I, II, IIIA (+cytology only), or IIIC (+pelvic LN only) randomized to pelvic RT (≥44 Gy) ± VC brachytherapy vs. chemotherapy before or after RT. Chemotherapy included options of doxorubicin/cisplatin, carboplatin/paclitaxel, or carboplatin/paclitaxel/epirubicin. Most patients had 2 or more risk factors of grade 3, deep myometrial invasion, or DNA nondiploidy. Patients with serous, clear cell, or anaplastic histology were eligible regardless of risk factors. Addition of chemotherapy to RT improved 5-year PFS by 7% (75→82%).

SARCOMA

- *EORTC 55874* (Reed et al. 2008): Two hundred and twenty-four women with stage I/II of all uterine sarcoma subtypes after TAH/BSO/washings with optional nodal sampling randomized to observation vs. post-op WP RT (50.4 Gy). RT reduced LRR (22% vs. 40%), but had no effect on OS, PFS, or DM. In subset analysis, WP RT increased LC for carcinosarcomas, but not leiomyosracomas.
- *GOG 150* (Wolfson et al. 2007): Two hundred and thirty-two patients with stage I-IV uterine carcinosarcoma ≤ 1 cm residual and/or no extraabdominal spread randomized to WART (whole abdomen 30 Gy/pelvis 49.8-50 Gy at 1 Gy bid or 1.5 Gy QD) vs. chemotherapy (cisplatin/ifosfamide/mesna × 3c). No significant difference in recurrence rate or survival between the two arms.

RADIATION TECHNIQUES

SIMULATION AND FIELD DESIGN

- Simulate patient supine with CT planning; administer presimulation enema.
- WP borders: superior = L5-S1; inferior = below obturator canal and including upper 1/2–2/3 of vagina; lateral = 2 cm lateral to pelvic brim; posterior = split sacrum to S3; anterior = pubic symphysis. Consider using IMRT (Fig. 30.1)
- EFRT borders: Extend superior border to top of L1 with CT planning to avoid kidneys. Recommend IMRT.

- If IMRT is used, careful attention to target delineation is necessary, and consider using internal target volume (ITV) or volume of vagina that is in both the empty and full bladder CT. Refer to RTOG CTV consensus guidelines (Small et al. 2008).

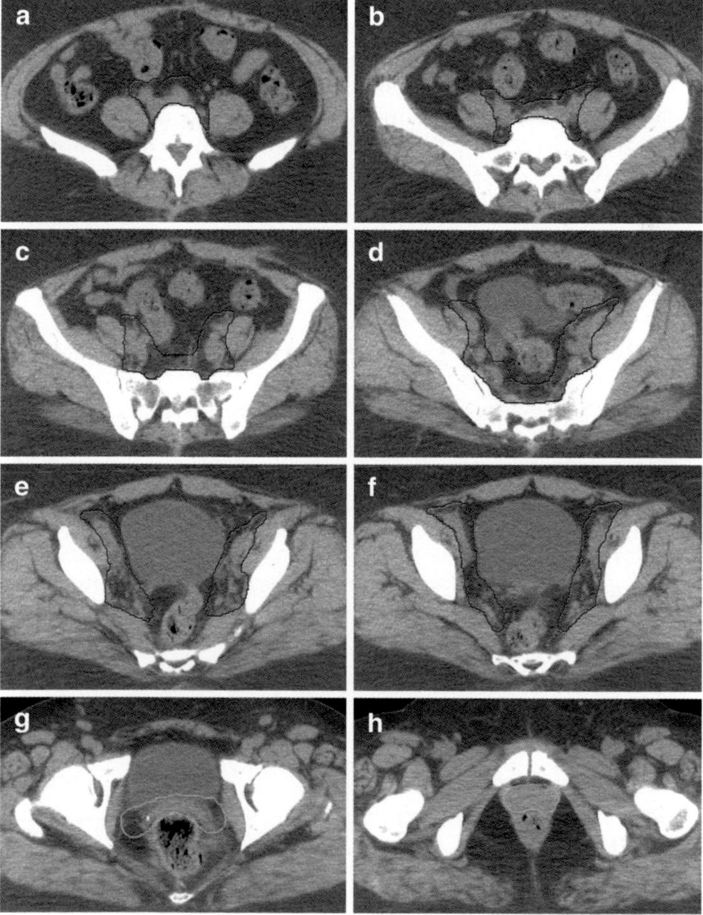

Fig. 30.1 Example pelvic nodal IMRT clinical tumor volumes on representative axial CT slices: (**a**) upper common iliacs, (**b**) midcommon iliacs and presacral area, (**c**) lower common iliacs and presacral area, (**d**) upper internal and external iliacs and presacral area, (**e** and **f**) internal and external iliacs, (**g**) vagina and parametrium, (**h**) vagina

- Vaginal brachytherapy: Place two marker seeds in vaginal cuff at both ends of hysterectomy scars. Use largest vaginal cylinder possible (2.5–3.5 cm). Target upper two-third of vaginal cuff. Consider CT planning. We recommend prescribing dose to vaginal surface because it represents the Dmax of normal tissue. However, some institutions prescribe to 0.5 cm, and dose and fractionation should be modified based on institutional their experience.
- Brachytherapy for intact uterus: Use Martinez-Y applicator or combination of tandem and cylinder with interstitial catheters. Consider using US guidance and 3D image-guided brachytherapy. Use tandem with ring or ovoids for pre-op stage II.
- WART = Use CT or fluoroscopy to determine 1 cm above diaphragmatic dome. Consider using IMRT (Fig. 30.1).

DOSE PRESCRIPTIONS

- Post-op
  - WP: 1.8 Gy/fx to 45–50.4 Gy.
  - VC boost: 6 Gy × 3 at vaginal surface (HDR) or 20 Gy at vaginal surface (LDR).
  - VC alone: 6 Gy × 5–6 or 10–10.5 Gy × 3 at vaginal surface (HDR) or 50–60 Gy at vaginal surface (LDR).
- Pre-op: WP 1.8 Gy/fx to 45 Gy and T&R or T&O 6 Gy × 3 (HDR).
- Vaginal extension: WP 45 Gy plus interstitial implants 6–7 Gy × 3 (HDR).
- Paraaortic LN+: EFRT to 45–50 Gy, enlarged unresectable nodes should be boosted to 60 Gy. IMRT recommended. Consider IORT at surgery.
- WART: 1.5 Gy/fx to 30 Gy to whole abdomen → boost paraaortic LN and WP to 45 Gy. Consider IMRT to improve target coverage and marrow sparing.
- Inoperable: WP 45–50 Gy and 6–7 Gy × 3 (HDR).

DOSE LIMITATIONS

- Upper vaginal mucosa 150 Gy, midvaginal mucosa 80–90 Gy, lower vaginal mucosa 60–70 Gy.
- Ovarian failure with 5–10 Gy. Sterilization with 2–3 Gy.
- Small bowel <45–50.4 Gy, Rectal point dose <70 Gy, bladder point <75 Gy based on 2D planning.
- For WART, use blocks to restrict kidneys <15 Gy, liver block to shield R lobe of liver after 25 Gy.

COMPLICATIONS

- TAH/BSO complications – mortality (<1%), infection, wound dehiscence, fistula, bleeding
- Frequency and urgency of urine and/or stool
- Vaginal stenosis – use dilators
- Thrombocytopenia with WART

FOLLOW-UP

- Physical exam every 3 months × 2 years, then every 6 months × 3 years, then annually. Vaginal cytology every 6 months for 2 years, then annually. CA-125 optional. Annual chest X-ray. CT/MRI as clinically indicated.

REFERENCES

Aalders JG, Abeler V, Kolstad P, et al. Postoperative external irradiation and prognostic parameters in stage I endometrial carcinoma: clinical and histopathologic study of 540 patients. Gynecol Oncol. 1980;56:419.

Alektiar KM, Nori D. Cancer of the endometrium. In: Leibel SA, Phillips TL, editors. Textbook of radiation oncology. 2nd ed. Philadelphia: Saunders; 2004. pp. 1101-1131.

ASTEC/EN.5 study group, Blake P, Swart AM, Orton J, et al. Adjuvant external beam radiotherapy in the treatment of endometrial cancer (MRC ASTEC and NCIC CTG EN.5 randomised trials): pooled trial results, systematic review, and meta-analysis. Lancet 2009;373:137-146.

ASTEC study group, Kitchener H, Swart AM, et al. Efficacy of systematic pelvic lymphadenectomy in endometrial cancer (MRC ASTEC trial): a randomized study. Lancet 2009; 373: 125-136.

Creutzberg CL. Endometrial Cancer. In: Gunderson LL, Tepper JE, et al., editors. Clinical radiation oncology. 2nd ed. Philadelphia: Churchill Livingstone; 2007. pp. 1359-1384.

Creutzberg CL, van Putten WL, Koper PC, et al. Surgery and postoperative radiotherapy versus surgery alone for patients with stage-1 endometrial carcinoma: multicentre randomised trial. PORTEC Study Group. Post operative radiation therapy in endometrial carcinoma. Lancet 2000;355:1404-1411.

Cardenes HR, Look K, Michael H, et al. Endometrium. In: Halperin CE, Perez CA, Brady LW, et al., editors. Principles and practice of radiation oncology. 5th ed. Philadelphia: Lippincott Williams & Wilkins; 2008. pp. 1610-1628.

FIGO Committee on Gynecologic Oncology. FIGO staging for uterine sarcomas. Int J Gynaecol Obstet. 2009;104:179.

Greene FL, American Joint Committee on Cancer. American Cancer Society. AJCC cancer staging manual. 6th ed. New York: Springer; 2002.

Greven K, Winter K, Underhill K, et al. Final analysis of RTOG 9708: adjuvant postoperative irradiation combined with cisplatin/paclitaxel chemotherapy following surgery for patients with high risk endometrial cancer. Gynecol Oncol. 2006;103:155-159.

Hogberg T, Rosenberg P, Kristensen G, et al. A randomized phase-III study on adjuvant treatment with radiation (RT) ± chemotherapy (CT) in early-stage high-risk endometrial cancer (NSGO-EC-9501/EORTC 55991). J Clin Oncol. 2007;25(18S):5503.

Int J Gynaecol Obstet, 105(2), Pecorelli S, Revised FIGO staging for carcinoma of the vulva, cervix, and endometrium, pgs 103-4, Copyright 2009, with permission from Elsevier.

Int J Gynaecol Obstet, 104, FIGO Committee on Gynecologic Oncology, FIGO staging for uterine sarcomas, pg 179, Copyright 2009, with permission from Elsevier.

Johnson N, Cornes P. Survival and recurrent disease after Postoperative radiotherapy for early endometrial cancer: Systematic review and meta-analysis. BJOG. 2007;114(11):1313-1320.

Keys HM, Roberts JA, Brunetto VL, et al. A phase III trial of surgery with or without adjunctive external pelvic radiation therapy in intermediate risk endometrial adenocarcinoma: a Gynecologic Oncology Group study. Gynecol Oncol. 2004;92:744-751.

Kong A, Simera I, Collingwood M, et al. Adjuvant radiotherapy for stage I endometrial cancer: systematic review and meta-analysis. Ann Oncol. 2007;18(10):1595-604.

Lee CM, Szabo A, Shrieve DC, et al. Frequency and effect of adjuvant radiation therapy among women with stage I endometrial adenocarcinoma. JAMA 2006;295:389-397

Lupe K, Kwon J, D'Souza D, et al. Adjuvant paclitaxel and carboplatin chemotherapy with involved field radiation in advanced endometrial cancer: a sequential approach. Int J Radiat Oncol Biol Phys. 2007;67(1):110-116.

Maggi R, Lissoni A, Spina F, et al. Adjuvant chemotherapy vs radiotherapy in high-risk endometrial carcinoma: results of a randomised trial. Br J Cancer. 2006;95(3):266-271.

National Comprehensive Cancer Network. Clinical Practice Guidelines in Oncology: Endometrial cancers. Available at: http://www.nccn.org/professionals/physician_gls/PDF/uterine.pdf. Accessed on May 19, 2009.

Nout RA, Putter H, Jurgenliemk-Schulz IM, et al. Vaginal brachytherapy versus external beam pelvic radiotherapy for high-intermediate risk endometrial cancer: results of the randomized PORTEC-2 trial [abstract]. J Clin Oncol. 2008;26:LBA5503.

Pecorelli S. Revised FIGO staging for carcinoma of the vulva, cervix, and endometrium. Int J Gynaecol Obstet. 2009;105(2):103-104.

Randall ME, Filiaci VL, Muss H, et al. Randomized phase III trial of whole-abdominal irradiation versus doxorubicin and cisplatin chemotherapy in advanced endometrial carcinoma: a Gynecologic Oncology Group study. J Clin Oncol. 2006;24:36-44.

Reed NS, Mangioni C, Malstrom H, et al. Phase III randomized study to evaluate the role of adjuvant pelvic radiotherapy in the treatment of uterine sarcomas stages I and II: an European organization for research and treatment of cancer gynaecological cancer group study (protocol 55874). Eur J Cancer. 2008;44:808-818.

Scholten AN, van Putten WLJ, Beerman H, et al. Postoperative radiotherapy for stage 1 endometrial carcinoma: long-term outcome of the randomized PORTEC trial with central pathology review. Int J Radiat Oncol Biol Phys. 2005;63:834-838.

Small W, Mell LK, Anderson P, et al. Consensus guidelines for delineation of clinical target volume for intensity-modulated pelvic radiotherapy in postoperative treatment of endometrial and cervical cancer. Int J Radiat Oncol Biol Phys. 2008;71(2):428-434.

Susumu N, Sagae S, Udagawa Y, et al. Randomized phase III trial of pelvic radiotherapy versus cisplatin-based combined chemotherapy in patients with intermediate- and high-risk endometrial cancer: a Japanese Gynecologic Oncology Group study. Gynecol Oncol. 2008;108(1): 226-233.

Wolfson A, Brady M, Rocereto T, et al. Gynecologic oncology group. Randomized phase III trial of whole abdominal irradiation (WAI) vs. cisplatin-ifosfamide and mesna (CIM) as post-surgical therapy in stage I-IV carcinosarcoma (CS) of the uterus. Gynecol Oncol. 2007;107(2):177-185.

Chapter 31
Ovarian Cancer

R. Scott Bermudez, James Rembert, and I-Chow Hsu

PEARLS

- Fourth leading cause of cancer death in women; leading cause of gynecologic cancer death.
- Average lifetime risk is 1 in 70 with median age at diagnosis of 63 years.
- Highly curable if diagnosed at an early stage, but 75% present with stage III or IV disease.
- Early diagnosis is frequently difficult because of vague abdominal symptoms at presentation and a lack of a good screening test.
- Risk factors: nulliparity, first parity >35 years, infertility, early menarche, late menopause, ovulation inducing drugs, hormone replacement therapy, obesity.
- Strongest risk factor is a family history of ovarian cancer , yet only 5–10% of tumors result from a known genetic disposition.
- Lifetime risk: general population 1.8%, one first-degree relative: 5%, two first-degree relatives: 25–50%.
- Consider genetic testing and/or prophylactic salpingo-oophorectomy for a strong family history.
- Familial syndromes tend to occur earlier and have a more indolent course than sporadic variants:
  - BRCA1 (lifetime risk 45%). BRCA2 (lifetime risk 25%), HNPCC.
- Pathology: epithelial 65%, germ cell 25%, sex cord-stromal 5%, metastases 5%.
  - Epithelial histologic types: serous 50%, endometrioid 20%, undifferentiated 15%, mucinous 10%, clear cell <5%.
- Patterns of spread: exfoliation into peritoneal cavity, hematogenous and lymphatic (mainly pelvic/paraaortic, but inguinals also at risk via round ligament).
- 90% recurrences occur within 5 years; only 15% relapse extraabdominally.
- Most patients die from local disease (small bowel obstruction, ascites, abdominal organ infiltration, etc.).

VIII

- Most important negative prognostic factors: stage, grade, residual volume of disease.
  - Other negative factors: age>65, pre-op ascites, CA125 elevated after 3c chemo or nadir >20 U/mL after first-line therapy.

WORKUP

- H&P with complete gynecologic exam and Pap smear.
  - Common signs/symptoms: abdominal discomfort/pain, increasing girth, change in bowel habits, early satiety, dyspepsia, nausea, ascites, adnexal mass, pleural effusion, Sister Mary Joseph's nodule, Blumer's shelf, Leser–Trelat sign (sudden appearance of seborrheic keratoses), hypercalcemia with clear cell, and subacute cerebellar degeneration.
- Labs: CBC, LFT, BUN/Cr, serum tumor markers as follows:
  - CA125: elevated in 80% of epithelial ovarian tumors; may serve as an early marker for disease recurrence.
    - False positives possible, especially in premenopausal women.
  - CA 19–9: low sensitivity but may be positive in GI or Müllerian tumors.
  - CEA: elevated in 58% with stage III disease.
  - AFP and βHCG: measure if <30 years old to help rule out germ cell tumors.
- Imaging:
  - Transvaginal US (more useful than transabdominal US for adnexal masses)
    - Ovarian enlargement during reproductive years usually benign.
    - Simple cyst <3 cm can be followed by serial US.
    - Complex ovarian cyst or postmenopausal women with simple cyst and CA-125 >65 U/mL suggestive of cancer → surgery indicated.
  - CT/MRI abdomen/pelvis: especially helpful preoperatively if advanced disease.
- Cystoscopy, sigmoidoscopy, barium enema, upper GI series, or endoscopy as clinically indicated.
- Endometrial biopsy preoperatively in women with abnormal vaginal bleeding.
- Pre-op percutaneous assessment of ascites or mass not recommended as it may lead to tumor seeding along tract or peritoneum and delay surgical staging/management.
- Surgical exploration: EUA, excise intact suspicious mass, frozen sections → if malignant, proceed to complete surgical staging.

- Surgical staging: vertical incision, collect ascites/washings, TAH/BSO*, complete abdominal exploration, omentectomy, random peritoneal biopsies (including diaphragm), aortic/pelvic lymph node sampling, optimal debulking, ±appendectomy.

*If proven stage IA, may preserve fertility with unilateral salpingo-oophrectomy (USO).

STAGING (AJCC 7TH ED., 2010/FIGO 2008): OVARIAN CANCER

- The definition of TNM and the stage grouping for this chapter have not changed from the AJCC 6th Ed., 2002.

Primary tumor (T)

TNM Categories	*FIGO* Stages	
TX		Primary tumor cannot be assessed
T0		No evidence of primary tumor
T1	I	Tumor limited to ovaries (one or both)
T1a	IA	Tumor limited to one ovary; capsule No malignant cells in ascites or peritoneal washings
T1b	IB	Tumor limited to both ovaries; capsules intact, no tumor on ovarian surface. No malignant cells in ascites or peritoneal washings
T1c	IC	Tumor limited to one or both ovaries with any of the following: capsule ruptured, tumor on ovarian surface, malignant cells in ascites or peritoneal washings
T2	II	Tumor involves one or both ovaries with pelvic extension
T2a	IIA	Extension and/or implants on uterus and/or tube(s). No malignant cells in ascites or peritoneal washings
T2b	IIB	Extension to and/or implants on other pelvic tissues. No malignant cells in ascites or peritoneal washings
T2c	IIC	Pelvic extension and/or implants (T2a or T2b) with malignant cells in ascites or peritoneal washings
T3	III	Tumor involves one or both ovaries with microscopically confirmed peritoneal metastasis outside the pelvis
T3a	IIIA	Microscopic peritoneal metastasis beyond pelvis (no macroscopic tumor)
T3b	IIIB	Macroscopic peritoneal metastasis beyond pelvis 2 cm or less in greatest dimension
T3c	IIIC	Peritoneal metastasis beyond pelvis more than 2 cm in greatest dimension and/or regional lymph node metastasis

Note: Liver capsule metastasis T3/Stage III; liver parenchymal metastasis M1/Stage IV. Pleural effusion must have positive cytology for M1/Stage IV.

Regional lymph nodes (N)

TNM Categories	*FIGO Stages*	
NX		Regional lymph nodes cannot be assessed
N0		No regional lymph node metastasis
N1	IIIC	Regional lymph node metastasis

Distant metastasis (M)

TNM Categories	*FIGO Stages*	
M0		No distant metastasis
M1	IV	Distant metastasis (excludes peritoneal metastasis)

continued

VIII

Anatomic stage/prognostic groups

I: T1 N0 M0
IA: T1a N0 M0
IB: T1b N0 M0
IC: T1c N0 M0
II: T2 N0 M0
IIA: T2a N0 M0
IIB: T2b N0 M0
IIC: T2c N0 M0
III: T3 N0 M0
IIIA: T3a N0 M0
IIIB: T3b N0 M0
IIIC: T3c N0 M0
Any T N1 M0
IV: Any T any N M1

TREATMENT RECOMMENDATIONS

Stage	Recommended treatment
IA/B Gr 1	■ Surgery→observation
IA/B Gr 2	■ Surgery→observation or ■ Surgery→taxane/carboplatin × 3–6c
IA/B Gr 3, IC, II	■ Surgery→taxane/carboplatin × 3–6c or ■ Surgery→WART (if not a chemo candidate and <2 cm residual) (Dembo 1985)
III	■ Surgery→taxane/carboplatin × 6–8c. Alternatively, surgery → intraperitoneal chemo (IP) in <1 cm optimally debulked patients. Completion surgery as indicated by tumor response and potential resectability in select patients or ■ Surgery→WART (if not a chemo candidate and <2 cm residual) (Dembo 1985)
IV	■ Manage abdominal disease as for stage III and Palliative management of metastatic disease
Abdominal or pelvic recurrence	■ >6 months from primary therapy – can retreat with same agents ■ <6 months from primary therapy – consider additional agents and/or ■ EBRT for palliation of symptomatic tumor deposits

STUDIES

ADJUVANT CHEMO: EARLY STAGE

- ICON and EORTC-ACTION investigators (2003): 925 patients, ICON included mainly stage I–II, ACTION included IA/BG2–3,

IC, IIA randomized to observation vs. 4–6c immediate adjuvant platinum-based chemo (57% single agent carboplatin, 27% combo cisplatin). Immediate chemo improved 5-year OS 8% (82 vs. 74%) and 5-year RFS 11% (76 vs. 65%).

- *GOG 157* Bell et al. (2006): 457 patients, included IA/BG2–3, IC, II randomized to 3c (considered standard arm) vs. 6c adjuvant paclitaxel/carboplatin. No significant difference in 5-year recurrence between 3c and 6c chemo (25.4 vs. 20.1%), but 6c associated with greater toxicity.

ADJUVANT CHEMO: ADVANCED STAGE

- *GOG 111* (McGuire et al. 1996): 410 patients, stage III/IV with <1 cm residual randomized to cisplatin with either cyclophosphamide or paclitaxel. Paclitaxel improved response rate (73 vs. 60%), PFS (18 vs. 13 months), and median survival (38 vs. 24 months). Results confirmed in large European/Canadian Intergroup trial (Piccart et al. 2000)
- *GOG 158* (Ozols et al. 2003): 792 patients, advanced stage with <1 cm residual randomized to paclitaxel with either cisplatin or carboplatin. Carboplatin regimen was less toxic, easier to administer, and equally effective.
- *GOG 172* (Bundy et al. 2001): 462 patients, stage III <1 cm residual randomized to 2c IV carboplatin followed by 6c intraperitoneal (IP) cisplatin and IV paclitaxel vs. 6c IV paclitaxel/cisplatin. PFS improved and LR and OS trend favored IP over IV, but higher toxicity with IP.

VIII

ADJUVANT WHOLE ABDOMINAL RADIATION THERAPY (WART)

- Dembo (1985): 190 patients with IB, II, asymptomatic III randomized to pelvic RT vs. pelvic RT + chlorambucil vs. WART. In patients with complete resection, WART improved 5 and 10-year OS vs. pelvic RT ± chlorambucil (5 years 78 vs. 51%, 10 year 64 vs. 40%); 30% decrease in abdominal recurrences with WART.

CHEMO VS. WART FOR PRIMARY ADJUVANT THERAPY

No randomized trial comparing best modern chemo and WART techniques has been performed.

RADIATION TECHNIQUES

SIMULATION AND FIELD DESIGN

- Supine, alpha cradle or knee sponge, planning CT scan.
- Include entire peritoneal cavity; pelvic RT alone is never adequate as primary adjuvant therapy (Dembo 1985).

- Open field currently accepted over moving strip technique.
- Treat AP/PA. Borders: superior = above diaphragm; inferior = below obturator foramen; lateral = outside peritoneal reflection.
- Shield kidneys at 15 Gy and liver at 25 Gy (UCSF does not use liver blocks).
- Consider IMRT to reduce dose to bone marrow and kidneys.

DOSE PRESCRIPTIONS

- 30 Gy at 1.2–1.5 Gy/fx whole field; kidney blocks at 15 Gy, liver blocks at 25 Gy.
- Paraaortic boost to 45 Gy.
- Pelvis boost to 45–55 Gy.

DOSE LIMITATIONS (TD 5/5)

- Kidney <20 Gy
- Liver <25 Gy
- Lung: limit volume receiving ≥20 Gy (V20) <20%
- Spinal cord <45 Gy
- Bone marrow <30 Gy
- Stomach <45 Gy
- Small bowel <45–50 Gy
- Rectum <60 Gy
- Bladder <60 Gy

WART COMPLICATIONS

- Fyles et al. (1992): 598 patients received WART 1971–1985.
  - Acute: diarrhea (~70%), nausea/vomiting (60%), leukopenia (11%), thrombocytopenia (11%); 23% required treatment breaks, primarily for hematologic toxicity.
  - Late: transient LFT elevation (44%), chronic diarrhea (14%), basal pneumonitis (4%), serious bowel obstruction (4.2%).

FOLLOW-UP

- H&P every 2–4 months for 2 years, then every 6 months for 3 years, then annually.
- CBC annually, CA-125 at each visit if initially elevated, other labs and imaging as indicated.
- US as indicated in patients who underwent USO.

REFERENCES

Bell J, Brady MF, Young RC, et al. Randomized phase III trial of three versus six cycle of adjuvant carboplatin and paclitaxel in early stage epithelial ovarian carcinoma: A Gynecologic Oncology Group study. Gyn Oncol 2006;102:432-439.

Bundy B, Alberts DS, et al. Phase III Trial of Standard-Dose Intravenous Cisplatin plus Paclitaxel versus moderately high-dose Carboplatin followed by intravenous Paclitaxel and Intraperitoneal Cisplatin in Small-Volume Stage III Ovarian Carcinoma: An Intergroup Study of the Gynecologic Oncology Group, Southwestern Oncology Group, and Eastern Cooperative Group. J Clin Oncol 2001;19:1001-1007.

Dembo AJ. Abdominopelvic radiotherapy in ovarian cancer. A 10-year experience. Cancer 1985;55(9 Suppl):2285-2290.

Fyles AW, Dembo AJ, Bush RS, et al. Analysis of complications in patients treated with abdomino-pelvic radiation therapy for ovarian carcinoma. Int J Radiat Oncol Biol Phys 1992;22(5):847-851.

ICON and EORTC-ACTION investigators: International Collaboration on Ovarian Neoplasm Trial 1 and Adjuvant Chemotherapy in Ovarian Neoplasm Trial: Two parallel randomized phase III trials of adjuvant chemotherapy in patients with early stage ovarian cancer. J Natl Cancer Inst 2003;95:105-112.

McGuire WP, Hosking WJ, Brady MF, et al. Taxol and cisplatin improves outcome in patients with advanced ovarian cancer as compared to cytoxan/cisplatin. N Engl J Med 1996;334(1):1-6.

Ozols RF, Bundy BN, Greer E, et al. Phase III trials of carboplatin and paclitaxel compared with cisplatin and paclitaxel in patients with optimally resected stage III ovarian cancer: A Gynecology Oncology Group Study. J Clin Oncol 2003;21:3194-3200.

Piccart M, Bertelsen K, James K, et al. Randomized intergroup trial of cisplatin-paclitaxel versus cisplatin-cyclophosphamide in women with advanced epithelial ovarian cancer: Three-year results. J Natl Cancer Inst 2000;92:699-708.

FURTHER READING

Alektiar K, Fuks Z. Cancer of the Ovary. In: Leibel SA, Phillips TL, editors.Textbook of radiation oncology. 2nd ed. Philadelphia: Saunders; 2004.pp. 1131-1156.

Cardenas H, Schilder J. Ovarian Cancer. In: Gunderson L, Tepper J, editors. Clinical Radiation Oncology. Philadelphia: Churchill Livingstone; 2007. pp. 1423-1451.

Gehrig PA, Varia M, Apsarnthanarax S, et al. Ovary. In: Halperin EC, Perez CA, Brady LW, et al., editors. Principles and practice of radiation oncology. 5th ed. Philadelphia: Lippincott Williams & Wilkins; 2008. pp. 1629-1649.

Greene FL. American Joint Committee on Cancer. American Cancer Society. AJCC Cancer Staging Manual. 6th ed. New York: Springer; 2002.

National Comprehensive Cancer Network. Clinical Practice Guidelines in Oncology: Ovarian Cancer. Available at: http://www.nccn.org/professionals/physician_gls/PDF/ovarian.pdf. Accessed on May 1, 2009.

Chapter 32
Vaginal Cancer

Thomas T. Bui, Eric K. Hansen, and Joycelyn L. Speight

PEARLS

- Rare (only 1–2% of all gynecologic malignancies).
- Twenty percent of vaginal tumors are detected incidentally as a result of Pap smear cytologic screening for cervical cancer.
- Eighty to ninety percent of cases are squamous cell carcinomas; most common location is the upper posterior 1/3 of the vagina.
- Lymph node drainage from the upper 2/3 of the vagina is to the pelvic nodes and from the lower 1/3 of the vagina is to the inguinal/femoral nodes.
- VAIN (vaginal intraepithelial neoplasia) associated with human papilloma virus (HPV); frequently multifocal, and progresses to invasive disease.
- Melanoma comprises 5% and most frequently occur in the lower 1/3 of the vagina. Adenocarcinoma comprises 5–15% and frequently presents in the Bartholin's or Skene's glands. Verrucous carcinomas tend to recur locally, but rarely metastasize. Rare histologies include papillary serous adenocarcinoma, small cell carcinoma, botryoid variant of embryonal rhabdomyosarcoma, lymphoma, and clear cell adenocarcinoma (which is associated with in utero exposure to diethylstilbestrol (DES)).
- Pelvic disease control worse in primary non-DES–associated adenocarcinoma of the vagina compared to squamous cell carcinoma (31 vs. 81%; $p < 0.01$) (Frank et al. 2007).
- Risk factors: carcinoma in situ, HPV, chronic vaginal irritation, previous abnormal Pap smears, early hysterectomy, multiple lifetime sex partners, early age at first intercourse, current smoker, in utero exposure to DES, partner with penile cancer.
- Most significant prognostic factor is FIGO stage; other adverse prognostic factors: age >60 years, middle or lower 1/3 location, poorly differentiated, size, and anemia (Chyle et al. 1996; Perez et al. 1999; Tran et al. 2006).

- External beam radiotherapy in combination with brachytherapy has been shown to improve survival compared to external beam treatment alone.
- The role for chemotherapy (usually cisplatin-based) is based on small phase I and II studies and extrapolated from cervical cancer literature (Morris et al. 2004; Samant et al. 2007; National Cancer Institute, 2009).
- Combined analysis of three randomized clinical trials of the FDA-approved human papillomavirus quadrivalent (Types 6, 11, 16, 18) vaccine shows 50% efficacy (95% CI) for HPV18-related VAIN2/3 in the intention-to-treat population (Joura et al. 2007).

WORKUP

- H&P with bimanual and rectal exam, speculum examination and Pap smear. On speculum exam, rotate the speculum while withdrawing to visualize the posterior wall. Examination under anesthesia, preferably with the Gynecologic Oncologist, and with biopsy if not previously performed or definitive diagnosis not yet established.
- Colposcopy with Schiller's test and multiple directed biopsies including the cervix and vulva to rule out primary cervical and/or vulvar cancer.
- Fine needle aspiration or excision of clinically or radiographically suspicious inguinal nodes.
- Cystoscopy and sigmoidoscopy for stage ≥ II or symptoms.
- Labs: CBC, electrolytes, BUN, Cr, LFTs including alkaline phosphatase.
- Imaging: CXR, CT ± PET, and/or MRI depending on extent (but not to be used for FIGO clinical staging).
- Risk of nodal involvement generally increases with stage: I = 5%, II = 25%, III = 75%, IV = 85%. Consider biopsy of enlarged LN to confirm involvement as may be inflammatory. Conversely, normal size LN may be pathologically involved.

STAGING (AJCC 7TH ED., 2010/FIGO 2008): VAGINAL CANCER

- The definition of TNM and the Stage Grouping for this chapter have not changed from the AJCC 6th Ed., 2002.

Primary tumor (T)

TNM Categories	*FIGO* Stages*	
TX		Primary tumor cannot be assessed
T0		No evidence of primary tumor
Tis*		Carcinoma in situ (preinvasive carcinoma)
T1	I	Tumor confined to vagina
T2	II	Tumor invades paravaginal tissues, but not to pelvic wall
T3	III	Tumor extends to pelvic wall**
T4	IVA	Tumor invades mucosa of the bladder or rectum and/or extends beyond the true pelvis (bullous edema is not sufficient evidence to classify a tumor as T4)

**Note*: FIGO no longer includes Stage 0 (Tis).
***Note*: Pelvic wall is defined as muscle, fascia, neurovascular structures, or skeletal portions of the bony pelvis. On rectal examination, there is no cancer-free space between the tumor and pelvic wall.

Regional lymph nodes (N)

TNM Categories	*FIGO Stages*	
NX		Regional lymph nodes cannot be assessed
N0		No regional lymph node metastasis
N1	III	Pelvic or inguinal lymph node metastasis

Distant metastasis (M)

TNM Categories	*FIGO Stages*	
M0		No distant metastasis
M1	IVB	Distant metastasis

Anatomic stage/prognostic groups

0*:	Ti N0 M0
I:	T1 N0 M0
II:	T2 N0 M0
III:	T1–T3 N1 M0
	T3 N0 M0
IVA:	T4 Any N M0
IVB:	Any T Any N M1

**Note*: FIGO no longer includes Stage 0 (Tis).

VIII

TREATMENT RECOMMENDATIONS

Stage	**Recommended treatment**	**~Outcomes**
CIS	■ CO_2 laser or topical 5-FU or wide local excision. Close follow-up required because of multifocality and frequent progression. For recurrent cases, intracavitary (IC) brachytherapy 60–70 Gy to the entire vaginal mucosa	LC: >90% DSS: >90%

continued

I (<0.5 cm thick, <2 cm, and low-grade)	■ *Surgery* (wide local excision or total vaginectomy with vaginal reconstruction). Preserves ovarian function. Post-op RT for close/+ margins ■ *Alternative: IC ± IS RT*. Treat entire vaginal mucosa to surface dose 65 Gy (60–70 Gy). Tumor with 2 cm radial margin boosted to 90 Gy mucosal dose (corresponding to ~67 Gy at 0.5 cm depth)	LC: 90% DSS: 80–85% Pelvic control: 80% DM: 10–20%
I (>0.5 cm thick, >2 cm, or high-grade)	■ *Surgery*: radical vaginectomy and pelvic lymphadenectomy (for upper 2/3) or inguinal lymphadenectomy (for lower 1/3). Post-op RT for close/+ margins ■ *Alternative: RT*. EBRT to whole pelvis ± inguinal LN to 45 Gy. IS ± IC boost to tumor with 2 cm radial margin to 75–80 Gy (corresponding to ~100–105 Gy tumor mucosal dose)	
II	■ EBRT to whole pelvis ± inguinal LN to 45 Gy (± midline block after 20 Gy, for non-IMRT plans). IS ± IC boost to tumor with 2 cm radial margin to 75–80 Gy (corresponding to ~100–105 tumor mucosal dose)	LC: 65–90% Pelvic: 65–85% DM: 20% DSS: 75–80%
III, IVA	■ EBRT to whole pelvis to 45–50 Gy (for non-IMRT plans, consider midline block after 40 Gy). If lower 1/3 involvement, treat inguinal nodes to 45–50 Gy ■ IS ± IC boost tumor with 2 cm radial margin to 75–85 Gy (corresponding to 100–110 Gy tumor mucosal dose)	*III* LC: 50–75% Pelvic: 65–70% DM: 25% DSS: 30–60%
	■ For lesions involving >50% of vagina, rectovaginal (RV) septum, and/or bladder, use brachytherapy with caution due to the risk of fistula formation *Alternative*: EBRT boost to 65–70 Gy	*IVA* LC: 20–40% Pelvic: 40% DM: >30% DSS: <10–20%

continued

- For parametrial and paravaginal extension, EBRT or IS boost to 65–70 Gy
- For +LN, boost to 60 Gy with EBRT
- Consider concomitant cisplatin-based chemo (based on cervix and vulvar literature) for tumors >4 cm and III–IVA
- If fistula or high risk of fistula, options include total vaginectomy, exenteration, and repair of fistula, if possible. LND generally performed. Avoid primary RT, especially brachytherapy

Clear cell adeno-carcinoma

- Surgery may preserve ovarian function, but it is morbid because it includes radical hysterectomy, vaginectomy, pelvic lymphadenectomy, and paraaortic lymph node sampling. If elected, definitive radiation techniques are the same as those described for stages II, III, IV

Metastasis

- Palliative RT ± chemo

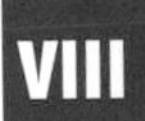

Recurrence

- Pelvic exenteration if no extension to side wall (removes vulva, vagina, uterus, anorectum, bladder, urethra, and pelvic and groin lymph node dissections). Interstitial brachytherapy with or without supplementary external beam radiotherapy can effectively salvage vaginal recurrence (Nag et al. 2002). Isolated vaginal recurrences can be salvaged with radiation therapy (Huh et al. 2007). HDR interstitial brachytherapy may be effective means of dose escalation, and HDR brachytherapy is efficacious for primary or recurrent vaginal cancer (Beriwal et al. 2008).

STUDIES

- Most trials are retrospective and have small patient numbers. Data concerning chemotherapy are limited, and their use is based on the cervix and vulvar literature.
- There are no prospective trials comparing HDR to LDR brachytherapy.
- In general, RT is preferred over surgery, except for early or posterior stage I lesions, distal lesions, or in the presence of a fistula.
- *Univ of Alberta experience* (Lian et al. 2008): Retrospective review of 68 patients. Vaginal morbidity low if BT alone (0%), and highest in the EBRT and BT group (82.1%). Five-year DSS by stage: I 90%, II 87%, III 32%, IV 26%.
- *Gustave-Roussy Instit experience* (D Crevoisier et al. 2007): Retrospective review of 91 patients. Five-year DSS by stage: I 83%, II 76%, III 52%. Pelvic control by stage: I 79%, II 62%, III 62%.
- *MDACC experience* (Frank et al. 2005): Retrospective review of 193 patients. Tumors >4 cm did worse. Most relapse was LR (68–83%). Major complications increased with stage (4–21%). Five-year DSS by stage: I 85%, II 78%, III–IVA 58%. Vaginal control by stage: I–II 91%, III–IVA 83%. Pelvic control by stage: I 86%, II 84%, III–IVA 71%.

RADIATION TECHNIQUES

SIMULATION AND FIELD DESIGN

EBRT

- Simulate the patient supine with tumor and introitus markers. Bolus on inguinal nodes may be needed (correlate with CT scan). If treating the inguinal nodes, treat patient in the frog-leg position.
- AP/PA field borders are as follows: *superior* = L5/S1 interspace (node negative patients); *inferior* = cover entire vagina and 3 cm below lowest extent of disease as marked with a radiopaque marker; *lateral* = 2 cm lateral to the pelvic brim.
- If distal 1/3 vaginal involvement, lateral borders widened to include the inguinofemoral nodes (*lateral* = greater trochanter; *inferior* = inguinal crease or 2.5 cm below ischium; *superolateral* = anterior superior iliac spine).
- If treating inguinal nodes, techniques may be used to protect the femoral heads as described for vulvar and anal cancer.
- A midline block is optional to decrease the dose to the bladder and rectum. If a midline block is not used, the brachytherapy dose must be reduced.

- If 4-field technique is used, care must be taken to avoid underdosing the presacral, perirectal, and anterior external iliac LN. On the lateral fields: *anterior border* = pubic symphysis and *posterior border* = S2/S3 or behind sacrum depending on stage.
- IMRT techniques require great care in treatment planning and careful attention to primary tumor and LN mapping (Frumovitz et al. 2008).
- Reevaluate patient after ~30 Gy to determine boost technique, but never wait until completely finished with EBRT to reevaluate for boost treatment.
- For extensive lesions and those involving rectovaginal septum or bladder, EBRT boost to total 64–70 Gy is used instead of brachytherapy.
- Concurrent chemotherapy may be considered for high-risk patients (tumors >4 cm or stage III–IVA) with good performance status.

Brachytherapy

- Brachytherapy monotherapy may be used for early stage, well-defined lesions involving <50% vagina and not involving rectovaginal septum.
- IC brachytherapy uses largest possible vaginal cylinder to improve the ratio of mucosa to tumor dose.
- Dome cylinders are used for homogenous irradiation of the vaginal cuff.
- Upper 1/3 lesions may be treated with an intrauterine tandem and vaginal colpostats, followed by treatment of the middle and lower 1/3 of the vagina with a vaginal cylinder with a blank source at the top of the cylinder if full dose has already been reached at the apex.
- Never carry a source at the level of the ovoids in the tandem or vaginal cylinder to prevent damage to the rectum and bladder.
- IS brachytherapy is preferred for lesions >0.5 cm to improve coverage. Favor CT planning.
- HDR dose is ~60% of LDR dose.
- Typical HDR boost dose after 45 Gy EBRT = 6 Gy × 3 (~30 Gy LDR equivalent).

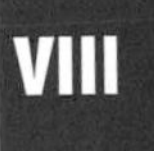

DOSE LIMITATIONS

- Upper vaginal mucosa tolerance is 120 Gy, mid-vaginal mucosal tolerance is 80–90 Gy, and lower vaginal mucosa tolerance is 60–70 Gy. Vaginal doses >50–60 Gy increase risk of significant vaginal fibrosis and stenosis.

- Ovarian failure occurs with 5–10 Gy. Sterilization occurs with 2–3 Gy.
- Limit bladder ≤65 Gy and rectum ≤60 Gy.

COMPLICATIONS

- Complications are dose related and include vaginal dryness and atrophy, pubic hair loss, vaginal stenosis and fibrosis (~50%), cystitis (~50%), proctitis (~40%), rectovaginal or vesicovaginal fistula (<5%), vaginal necrosis (<5–15%), lymphedema (increased risk in post-op setting), urethral stricture (rare), and small bowel obstruction (rare in the absence of prior abdominal surgery).
- Post-radiotherapy, vaginal dilators, and topical estrogen should be used to minimize stenosis.
- Radiation-induced menopause may occur. Therefore, consider surgical ovarian transposition prior to pelvic radiation.
- Smoking cessation should be encouraged to reduce risk of late radiation toxicity.
- Hyperbaric oxygen therapy may be used for the treatment of radiation-induced severe late side-effects.

FOLLOW-UP

- H&P (with pelvic exam and pap smear) every 3 months for 1 year, every 4 months for second year, every 6 months for third and fourth years, then annually. CXR annually for 5 years.

REFERENCES

Beriwal S, Heron DE, Mogus R, et al. High-dose rate brachytherapy (HDRB) for primary or recurrent cancer in the vagina. Radiat Oncol 2008 Feb 13;3:7.

Chyle V, Zagars GK, Wheeler JA, et al. Definitive radiotherapy for carcinoma of the vagina: outcome and prognostic factors. Int J Radiat Oncol Biol Phys 1996;35:891-905.

D Crevoisier R, Sanfilippo N, et al. Exclusive radiotherapy for primary squamous cell carcinoma of the vagina. Radiother Oncol 2007;85(3):362-370.

Frank SJ, Deaver MT, Jhingran A, et al. Primary adenocarcinoma of the vagina not associated with diethylstilbestrol (DES) exposure. Gynecol Oncol 2007;105(2):470-474.

Frank SJ, Jhingran A, Levenback C, et al. Definitive radiation therapy for squamous cell carcinoma of the vagina. Int J Radiat Oncol Biol Phys 2005;62:138-147.

Frumovitz M, Gayed IW, Jhingran A, et al. Lymphatic mapping and sentinel lymph node detection in women with vaginal cancer. Gynecol Oncol 2008;108(3):478-481.

Huh WK, Straughn JM Jr, Mariani A, et al. Salvage of isolated vaginal recurrences in women with surgical stage I endometrial cancer: a multiinstitutional experience. Int J Gynecol Cancer 2007;17(4):886-889.

Joura EA, Leodolter S, Hernandez-Avila M, et al. Efficacy of a quadrivalent prophylactic human papillomavirus (types 6, 11, 16, and 18) L1 virus-like-particle vaccine against high-grade vulval and vaginal lesions: a combined analysis of three randomised clinical trials. Lancet 2007;369(9574):1693-1702.

Lian J, Dundas G, Carlone M, Ghosh S, Pearcey R. Twenty-year review of radiotherapy for vaginal cancer: an institutional experience. Gynecol Oncol 2008;111(2):298-306.

Morris M, Blessing JA, Monk BJ, et al. Phase II study of cisplatin and vinorelbine in squamous cell carcinoma of the cervix: a Gynecologic Oncology Group Study. J Clin Oncol 2004;22(16):3340-3344.

Nag S, Yacoub S, Copeland LJ, Fowler JM. Interstitial brachytherapy for salvage treatment of vaginal recurrences in previously unirradiated endometrial cancer patients. Int J Radiat Oncol Biol Phys 2002;54:1153–1159.

National Cancer Institute. Vaginal Cancer (PDQ): Treatment. Available at: http://cancer.gov/cancertopics/pdq/treatment/vaginal/healthprofessional/. Accessed on March 3, 2010.

Samant R, Lau B, Choan E, et al. Primary vaginal cancer treated with concurrent chemoradiation using cis-platinum. Int J Radiat Oncol Biol Phys 2007;69:746-750.

Tran PT, Su Z, Lee P, et al. Prognostic factors for outcomes and complications for primary squamous cell carcinoma of the vagina treated with radiation. Int J Radiat Oncol Biol Phys 2006;S66:1052.

FURTHER HEADING

Cardenes HR, Perez CA. Vagina. In: Perez CA, Brady LW, Halperin EC, et al., editors. Principles and practice of radiation oncology. 5th ed. Philadelphia: Lippincott Williams & Wilkins; 2008. pp. 1657-1681.

Edge SB, American Joint Committee on Cancer. American Cancer Society. AJCC cancer staging manual. 7th ed. New York: Springer Science+Business Media; 2010.

Eifel PJ. The Vulva and Vagina. In: Cox JD, Ang KK, editors. Radiation oncology: rationale, technique, results. 8th ed. St. Louis: Mosby; 2003. pp. 743-756.

Eifel PJ, Koh WJ (2008). Vaginal and Vulvar Cancer (#304). Presented at American Society of Therapeutic Radiology and Oncology Annual Meeting, Boston, MA.

Perez CA, Grigsby PW, Garipagaoglu M, et al. Factors affecting long-term outcome of irradiation in carcinoma of the vagina. Int J Radiat Oncol Biol Phys 1999;44:37-45.

Russell AH. Vulvar and Vaginal Carcinoma. In: Gunderson LL, Tepper JE, editors. Clinical radiation oncology. 2nd ed. Philadelphia: Churchill Livingstone; 2007. pp. 1319-1410.

Stock RG, Green S. Cancer of the Vagina. In: Leibel SA, Phillips TL, editors. Textbook of radiation oncology. 2nd ed. Philadelphia: Saunders; 2004. pp. 1157-1176.

Chapter 33
Vulvar Cancer

Stephen Shiao, Brian Missett, and Joycelyn L. Speight

PEARLS

- Anatomy = mons pubis, clitoris, labia majora, labia minora, vaginal vestibule, Bartholin's glands (at posterior labia majora), prepuce over clitoris, posterior forchette, perineal body.
- Most common presenting symptoms = pruritis, pain, and/or a palpable mass.
- Approximately 70% arise in the labia and ~15% arise in the clitoris or perineal body.
- LN spread is to inguino-femoral nodes (superficial and deep). Most superior deep femoral node = Cloquet's node.
- Clitoris can theoretically drain directly to pelvic LN, but rare without inguino-femoral LN involvement.
- Risk factors = HPV 16, 18, 33 (condyloma acuminatum), vulvar intraepithelial neoplasia (2–5% progress to CA), Bowen's disease, Paget's disease, erythroplasia, chronic irritant vaginitis (e.g., with pessary), leukoplakia, employment in laundry and cleaning industry, smoking.
- Risk of nodal involvement correlates with stage and depth of tumor invasion:
  - IA <1 mm deep <5%, 1–3 mm deep 8–10%, 3–5 mm deep 20%
  - More than 5 mm deep or >2 cm size 40%
  - III 30–80%
  - IV 80–100%
- Approximately 20–25% of cN0 patients are pN+.
- If inguinal LN+, ~30% risk of pelvic LN+.

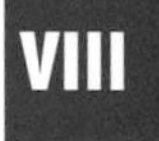

WORKUP

- H&P with examination under anesthesia (EUA).
- Colposcopy and biopsy of primary and FNA or excisional biopsy of clinically positive inguinal nodes.

- Pap smear of cervix and vagina.
- Cystoscopy, sigmoidoscopy may be indicated for advanced stages and/or bladder/bowel symptoms.
- CBC, UA.
- Pelvic CT or MRI. PET/CT may be better for the evaluation of nodal involvement.
- CXR.

STAGING: VULVAR CANCER

Editors' note: All TNM stage and stage groups referred to elsewhere in this chapter reflect the 1988 FIGO/2002 AJCC staging nomenclature unless otherwise noted as the new system below was published after this chapter was written.

(AJCC 6TH ED., 2002/FIGO 1988)

FIGO/AJCC primary tumor (T)

0/Tis:	Carcinoma in situ (preinvasive carcinoma)
IA/T1a:	Tumor confined to the vulva or vulva and perineum, 2 cm or less in greatest dimension, and with stromal invasion no greater than 1 mm
IB/T1b:	Tumor confined to the vulva or vulva and perineum, 2 cm or less in greatest dimension, and with stromal invasion greater than 1 mm
II/T2:	Tumor confined to the vulva or vulva and perineum, more than 2 cm in greatest dimension
III/T3:	Tumor of any size with contiguous spread to the lower urethra and/or vagina or anus
IVA/T4:	Tumor invades any of the following: upper urethra, bladder mucosa, rectal mucosa, or is fixed to the pubic bone

FIGO/AJCC regional lymph nodes (N)

III/N1:	Unilateral regional lymph node metastasis (inguinal/femoral LN)
IVA/N2:	Bilateral regional lymph node metastasis (inguinal/femoral LN)

FIGO/AJCC metastases (M)

IVB/M1:	Distant metastasis (including pelvic LN)

~5 yr OS by 2002 Stage (GOG 36, Landrum Gynecol Oncol 2007)

I:	>95%
II:	85%
III:	75%
IV:	25-30%

(AJCC 7TH ED., 2010/FIGO 2008)

Primary tumor (T)

TNM Categories	*FIGO Stages*	
TX		Primary tumor cannot be assessed
T0		No evidence of primary tumor
Tis*		Carcinoma in situ (preinvasive carcinoma)
T1a	IA	Lesions 2 cm or less in size, confined to the vulva or perineum and with stromal invasion 1.0 mm or less**
T1b	IB	Lesions more than 2 cm in size *or* any size with stromal invasion more than 1.0 mm, confined to the vulva or perineum
T2***	II	Tumor of any size with extension to adjacent perineal structures (lower/distal 1/3 urethra, lower/distal 1/3 vagina, anal involvement)
T3****	IVA	Tumor of any size with extension to any of the following: upper/proximal 2/3 of urethra, upper/proximal 2/3 vagina, bladder mucosa, rectal mucosa, or fixed to pelvic bone

**Note*: FIGO no longer includes Stage 0 (Tis).
***Note*: The depth of invasion is defined as the measurement of the tumor from the epithelial–stromal junction of the adjacent most superficial dermal papilla to the deepest point of invasion.
***FIGO uses the classification T2/T3. This is defined as T2 in TNM.
****FIGO uses the classification T4. This is defined as T3 in TNM.

Regional lymph nodes (N)

TNM Categories	*FIGO Stages*	
NX		Regional lymph nodes cannot be assessed
N0		No regional lymph node metastasis

continued

Used with the permission from the American Joint Committee on Cancer (AJCC), Chicago, IL. The original source for this material is the AJCC Cancer Staging Manual, Sixth Edition (2002), published by Springer Science+Business Media.

N1		One or two regional lymph nodes with the following features
N1a	IIIA	one lymph node metastasis each 5 mm or less
N1b	IIIA	One lymph node metastasis 5 mm or greater
N2	IIIB	Regional lymph node metastasis with the following features
N2a	IIIB	Three or more lymph node metastases each less than 5 mm
N2b	IIIB	Two or more lymph node metastases 5 mm or greater
N2c	IIIC	Lymph node metastasis with extracapsular spread
N3	IVA	Fixed or ulcerated regional lymph node metastasis

Distant metastasis (M)

TNM Categories	*FIGO Stages*	
M0		No distant metastasis
M1	IVB	Distant metastasis (including pelvic lymph node metastasis)

Anatomic stage/prognostic groups

0*: Tis N0 M0
I: T1 N0 M0
IA: T1a N0 M0
IB: T1b N0 M0
II: T2 N0 M0
IIIA: T1, T2 N1a, N1b M0
IIIB: T1, T2 N2a, N2b M0
IIIC: T1, T2 N2c M0
IVA: T1, T2 N3 M0
T3 Any N M0
IVB: Any T Any N M1

**Note*: FIGO no longer includes Stage 0 (Tis).

Used with the permission from the American Joint Committee on Cancer (AJCC), Chicago, IL. The original source for this material is the AJCC Cancer Staging Manual, Seventh Edition (2010), published by Springer Science+Business Media.

FIGO staging: Pecorelli 2009, Copyright 2009, with permission from Elsevier.

TREATMENT RECOMMENDATIONS

2002 Stage	Recommended treatment
CIS	■ Local excision or CO_2 laser
IA	■ Wide local excision (WLE). Post-op RT (50 Gy) to vulva for + margin, margin <8 mm, LVSI, or depth >5 mm. [Sample lymph nodes for lesion with >1 mm depth of invasion]
IB/II	■ WLE with ipsilateral (superficial) LN dissection or sentinel lymph node biopsy for lateralized lesions. Bilateral (superficial) LN dissection for central lesions, lesions >5 mm deep, LVSI, or poorly differentiated lesions. If LN+, add deep inguinal dissection. Post-op RT to vulva for + margin, margin <8 mm, LVSI, or lesions >5 mm deep. Post-op RT to inguinal and pelvic nodes for >1 LN+, or nodal ECE ■ Alternatively, consider pre-op chemo-RT (50 Gy for cN- or 54 Gy for cN+) for lesions close to urethra, clitoris, or rectum because margin may be difficult to obtain. Either elective chemo-RT to groins or planned LN dissection (before or after chemo-RT). If bilateral LN dissection performed initially, pathologic LN findings dictate whether or not RT needed to groins. However, chemo-RT to primary lesion could be delayed. If primary lesion has CR to chemo-RT, consider biopsy, and if negative observation. If <CR or biopsy demonstrates persistent disease, resect with functional preservation if possible, or boost primary to 65–70 Gy or consider radical vulvectomy
III/IVA	■ If cN0, perform bilateral LN dissection first followed by chemo-RT to vulva or vulva and inguinal/pelvic nodes (for ECE, >1 LN+) ■ If cN+ fixed or ulcerated, pre-op chemo-RT (45–50 Gy with cisplatin, 5-FU, and/or mitomycin C) provides about 50% CR. Follow with bilateral LN dissection. Surgical salvage for persistent or recurrent disease. If nodal ECE boost to 60 Gy; if gross residual take to 65–70 Gy (Eifel 2003, Russell 2004, Montana and Kang 2008)

STUDIES

INDICATIONS FOR POST-OP VULVAR RT

- Heaps et al. (1990): review of surgical-pathologic factors predictive of LR for 135 patients with vulvar CA. Increased LR with + margin, margin <8 mm pathologically or <1 cm clinically, LVSI, and depth >5 mm.

INDICATIONS FOR PELVIC/INGUINAL RT

- GOG 36 (Homesley et al. 1986): 114 patients treated with radical vulvectomy and bilateral inguinal lymphadenectomy. If inguinal LN+, randomized to pelvic LN dissection vs. post-op RT with 45–50 Gy to pelvic and inguinal LN (but not to vulva). RT decreased groin recurrence (5 vs. 24%) and improved 2-year OS (68 vs. 54%). Subset analysis showed benefit only in cN+, patients with >1 pN+ or +LN with ECE. No difference in pelvic recurrence.

NODAL EVALUATION AND MANAGEMENT

- Kirby et al. (2005): retrospective review of 65 patients with Stage I/II vulvar cancer treated with vulvectomy and superficial inguinal lymphadenectomy (SupIL). Patients with pathologically negative SupIL had 4.6% recurrence rate in the inguinal region and 16.9% recurrence on the vulva. Five-year DFS and OS were 66 and 97%, respectively.
- Van der Zee et al. (2008): observational study looking at 623 groins in 403 patients. Two hundred and fifty-nine patients with unifocal vulvar disease and negative sentinel node (SN). Three-year groin recurrent rate was 2.3% and OS 97%. Short-term and long-term morbidity significantly decreased with sentinel node removal vs. sentinel node removal + inguino-femoral lymphadenectomy. Basis for current ongoing trial, GOG 173, to validate use of SN biopsy in stage I/II vulvar cancer.
- *GOG 88* (Stehman et al. 1992): 121 patients with IB–III cN0 treated with radical vulvectomy randomized to bilateral inguinal RT (50 Gy to D3, without pelvic RT) vs. bilateral radical LN dissection. If pLN+, then received RT (50 Gy) to bilateral groin and pelvis. Interim analysis of only 58 patients demonstrated improved 2-year OS (90 vs. 70%) with surgery and decreased inguinal recurrences.
  - Criticisms: RT addressed only inguinal nodes, whereas surgery included pelvic LN dissection if inguinal LN+; arms biased since no CT used for staging; poor technique of RT (prescribed

to D3, all inguinal recurrences received < prescribed dose); 50 Gy should sterilize microscopic disease as evidenced by University of Wisconsin retrospective review with good technique (Petereit, *Int J Radiat Oncol Biol Phys* 1993).

CHEMO-RT

- *GOG 101* (Moore et al. 1998): phase II trial of 41 patients with T3 unresectable or T4, any LN status treated with pre-op chemo-RT with 1.7 Gy b.i.d. d1–4, 1.7 Gy qd d5–12 to 23.8 Gy with cisplatin on d1 and 5-FU on d1–4 → 2week break → repeat to total dose 47.6 Gy. For cN0, RT was to vulvar area only and for cN+ included inguinal and pelvic LN. Surgery 4–8 weeks after chemo-RT. Pre-op chemo-RT had 47% CR and 55% 4-year OS (expect 20–50%). Fifty-four percent of patients had gross residual disease, but only 3% were unresectable.
- GOG 101 Montana et al. (2000): 46 patients with advanced disease in the inguino-femoral nodes (stage IVA) N2/N3 received a split course of radiation (47.6 Gy) to the primary and LN with concurrent cisplatin/5-FU followed by surgery. Ninety-five percent were deemed resectable after chemo-RT. Local control of primary and lymph nodes was 76 and 97%, respectively.
- Landrum et al. (2008): 63 patients with stage III/IV disease treated with primary surgery or chemo-RT. Primary chemo-RT patients were younger (61 vs. 72 years), had fewer nodal metastasis (54 vs. 83%), and larger tumors (6 vs. 3.5 cm). No difference in OS, PFS, or recurrence rates.
- Beriwal et al. (2008): 18 patients with stage II–IVA disease treated twice-daily IMRT and with 5-FU/cisplatin chemotherapy during the first and last weeks of treatment. No patients had RT-related acute or late toxicity >grade 3. Seventy-eight percent patients had surgery 6–8 weeks after chemo-IMRT, with 64% pCR rate. Two-year CSS 75%, OS 70%.

VIII

MIDLINE BLOCK

- Dusenberry et al. (1994): 27 patients with stage III/IV disease with +LN treated with post-op RT with a midline block status post resection. Forty-eight percent central recurrence rate with the use of the midline block. Authors recommended discontinuing routine use of the midline block.

RADIATION TECHNIQUES

SIMULATION AND FIELD DESIGN

- Simulate supine, frog-leg position with custom immobilization.
- Wire LN, vulva, anus, scars.
- Borders: superior = L5/S1 or mid SI if clinically no involved pelvic LN (L4/5 if pelvic LN+); inferior = flash vulva and 3 cm inferior to bottom of ischium; lateral = 2 cm beyond pelvic brim and greater trochanter (anterior superior iliac spine) to include inguinal LN.
- Energy = 6 MV AP, 18 MV PA. Bolus groins and vulva prn.
- CT plan depth of groin nodes.
- May need to boost groins with en face electrons.
- Consider IMRT in experienced centers to reduce dose to normal structures.

DOSE PRESCRIPTIONS

- 1.8 Gy/fx
- 45–50.4 Gy to vulva and pelvic LN
- 45–50.4 Gy for cN0 inguinal nodes, and boost to 60 Gy for LN+ or ECE
- For residual disease, boost to 65–70 Gy (may require brachytherapy)

DOSE LIMITATIONS

- Small bowel <45–55 Gy
- Femoral heads <45 Gy
- Bladder <60 Gy
- Rectum <60 Gy
- Lower vagina <75–80 Gy

COMPLICATIONS

- Acute: epilation of pubic hair, hyperpigmentation, skin reaction. Moist desquamation by third–fifth weeks. Treat with Domeboro's solution, loose garments, Sitz baths. Also treat candida superinfections, if any. Diarrhea, cystitis.
- Late = atrophy of skin and telangiectasia, shortening and narrowing of vagina, vaginal dryness. Femoral neck fracture <5%, associated with osteoporosis and smoking.

Chapter 34
Urethral Cancer

Siavash Jabbari, Eric K. Hansen, and Alexander R. Gottschalk

PEARLS

- Female urethra is ~4 cm long.
- Muscular layer is continuous with that of the bladder.
- Two sphincters: internal at bladder neck and voluntary sphincter at plane of urogenital diaphragm.
- Proximal 1/3 epithelium = transitional cells.
- Distal 2/3 epithelium = nonkeratinizing squamous cells.
- Periurethral Skene's glands secrete mucous near meatus (and extend along distal urethra).
- Carcinoma of urethra is rare (<0.1% of cancers).
  - 70% = squamous cell CA
  - 10–15% = TCC
  - 10–15% = adenoCA
  - Rare = melanoma, lymphomas, mets, adenoid cystic
- Average age is 60 (50–80) years.
- May be associated with HPV 16.
- Female urethra cancer more common than male urethral cancer (4:1).
- Male urethral CA.
  - Urethral location: bulbomembranous 60%, penile 30%, prostatic 10%
  - Histology: 75% squamous cell CA
- LN spread is to inguinal and pelvic LN (including presacral and obturator).
  - T1 lesions = uncommon.
  - T2–T3 lesions = 35–50% of cases.
  - For urethra, clinically involved LN are almost always pathologically involved (vs. penile carcinoma only ~50% are pathologically involved).
- At presentation, ~10% of patients have DM.
- Most important prognostic factors = tumor size, local invasion, and location (distal more favorable).

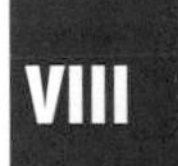

WORKUP

- H&P: Symptoms include bleeding, pain, dysuria, urinary frequency. Less commonly, mass, inguinal LN, perineal pain, dyspareunia.
- Detailed pelvic EUA.
- Urethroscopy and cystoscopy.
- CT/MRI of pelvis. CXR.
- Biopsy.

STAGING (AJCC 7TH ED., 2010): URETHRAL CANCER

Primary tumor (T): male and female

TX: Primary tumor cannot be assessed
T0: No evidence of primary tumor
Ta: Noninvasive papillary, polypoid, or verrucous carcinoma
Tis: Carcinoma in situ
T1: Tumor invades subepithelial connective tissue
T2: Tumor invades any of the following: corpus spongiosum, prostate, periurethral muscle
T3: Tumor invades any of the following: corpus cavernosum, beyond prostatic capsule, anterior vagina, bladder neck
T4: Tumor invades other adjacent organs

Urothelial (Transitional Cell) Carcinoma of the Prostate

Tis pu: Carcinoma in situ, involvement of the prostatic urethra
Tis pd: Carcinoma in situ, involvement of the prostatic ducts
T1: Tumor invades urethral subepithelial connective tissue
T2: Tumor invades any of the following: prostatic stroma, corpus spongiosum, periurethral muscle
T3: Tumor invades any of the following: corpus cavernosum, beyond prostatic capsule, bladder neck (extraprostatic extension)
T4: Tumor invades other adjacent organs (invasion of the bladder)

Regional lymph nodes (N)

NX: Regional lymph nodes cannot be assessed
N0: No regional lymph node metastasis
N1: Metastasis in a single lymph node 2 cm or less in greatest dimension
N2: Metastasis in a single node more than 2 cm in greatest dimension, or in multiple nodes

Distant metastasis (M)

M0: No distant metastasis
M1: Distant metastasis

Anatomic stage/prognostic groups

0a: Ta N0 M0
0is: Tis N0 M0
Tis pu N0 M0
Tis pd N0 M0
I: T1 N0 M0
II: T2 N0 M0
III: T1 N1 M0
T2 N1 M0
T3 N0 M0
T3 N1 M0
IV: T4 N0 M0
T4 N1 M0
Any T N2 M0
Any T Any N M1

continued

~LOCAL CONTROL AND SURVIVAL BY STAGE

~LC	~5-year OS
I–II: 70–90%	I–II: 70–90%
III: 20–60%	III: 20–40%
IV: 10–20%	IV: 10–20%

TREATMENT RECOMMENDATIONS

2002 Stage	Recommended treatment
CIS	■ Surgical options: Laser coagulation, open excision, or partial or total urethrectomy
I-II	■ Distal lesions ■ Surgical resection of primary ± regional LN dissection ■ IS brachytherapy alone ■ EBRT (including prophylactic regional LN) + IS brachy boost (± concurrent chemotherapy for squamous cell histology) ■ Proximal lesions or those of entire urethra ■ Pre-op RT → surgery with urinary diversion
III, IV	■ Distal lesions ■ Surgical resection of primary + inguinal LND ■ EBRT (including prophylactic regional LN) + IS brachy boost (± concurrent chemotherapy for squamous cell histology) ■ Proximal lesions or those of entire urethra ■ Pre-op RT -> surgery (radical cystourethrectomy or cystoprostatectomy, or female anterior exenteration with the removal of gynecologic organs too) with pelvic LND and urinary diversion. May require exenteration if extensive
Mets	■ Investigational chemo protocols
Recurrence	■ After RT, surgical excision or exenteration ■ After surgery, RT + further surgery

VIII

STUDIES

- Because of its rarity, most trials are retrospective and have small patient numbers.
- Data concerning chemotherapy are limited. Some use cisplatin or 5-fu/mitomycin-based concurrent chemo with EBRT for squamous cell histology, with extrapolation from cervix and anal cancer literature.

RADIATION TECHNIQUES

SIMULATION AND FIELD DESIGN

- Interstitial implant most often used for distal or meatal lesions with 4–8 IS catheters arranged around urethral orifice.
- CT or radiographs used to verify needle placement.
- Larger, more invasive, or proximal tumors should be treated with a combination of EBRT and IS brachy.
- Use CT planning for EBRT.
- Bolus may be required to ensure adequate dose for superficial tumors and/or inguinal LN.
- EBRT borders = whole pelvis and inguinal LN.
  - Superior = L5/S1
  - Inferior = flash perineum
  - Lateral = cover inguinal LN
- EBRT dose.
  - WP = 50 Gy
  - Involved LN = boost to 60–66 Gy
- Brachy dose.
  - With implant alone for early lesions = 60–70 Gy (LDR equivalent)
  - As boost after 50 Gy WP = 10–30 Gy boost to 60–80 Gy (LDR equivalent)

DOSE LIMITATIONS

- Perineal skin reaction is limiting factor for EBRT, and thus, limit to ~50–66 Gy.
- Upper vaginal mucosa tolerance is 120 Gy, midvaginal mucosal tolerance is 80–90 Gy, and lower vaginal mucosa tolerance is 60–70 Gy.
- Vaginal doses >50–60 Gy cause significant vaginal fibrosis and stenosis.
- Ovarian failure occurs with 5–10 Gy. Sterilization occurs with 2–3 Gy.
- Limit bladder ≤65 Gy, and rectum ≤60 Gy.

COMPLICATIONS

- Complications are dose related and include skin reaction, urethral stricture (that could necessitate dilatation or urinary diversion), urinary incontinence, cystitis, vaginal dryness and atrophy, vaginal stenosis and fibrosis, vaginal necrosis, vesicovaginal fistula, proctitis, pubic hair loss, small bowel obstruction (rare).
- Vaginal dilators should be used to minimize stenosis.

FOLLOW-UP

- H&P with careful pelvic exam every 3 months for 1 year, every 4 months for second year, every 6 months for third and fourth years, then annually. CXR annually for 5 years.

FURTHER READING

Amin MB, Young RH. Primary carcinomas of the urethra. Semin Diagn Pathol. 1997;14(2):147-160.

Cohen MS, Triaca V, Billmeyer B, et al. Coordinated chemoradiation therapy with genital preservation for the treatment of primary invasive carcinoma of the male urethra. J Urol. 2008;179(2):536-541; discussion 541.

Dalbagni G, Zhang ZF, Lacombe L, Herr HW. Male urethral carcinoma: analysis of treatment outcome. Urology. 1999;53(6):1126-1132.

Davis JW, Schellhammer PF, Schlossberg SM. Conservative surgical therapy for penile and urethral carcinoma. Urology. 1999;53(2):386-392.

Eng TY. Female Urethra. In: Perez CA, Brady LW, Halperin EC, editors. Principles and Practice of Radiation Oncology. 5th ed. Philadelphia: Lippincott Williams & Wilkins; 2008. pp. 1682-1691.

Foens CS, Hussey DH, Staples JJ, Doornbos JF, Wen BC, Vigliotti AP. A comparison of the roles of surgery and radiation therapy in the management of carcinoma of the female urethra. Int J Radiat Oncol Biol Phys. 1991;21(4):961-968.

Forman JD, Lichter AS. The role of radiation therapy in the management of carcinoma of the male and female urethra. Urol Clin North Am. 1992;19(2):383-389.

Jemal A, Siegel R, Ward E, et al. Cancer statistics, 2008. CA Cancer J Clin. 2008;58(2):71-96.

Kuettel MR, Parda DS, Harter KW, Rodgers JE, Lynch JH. Treatment of female urethral carcinoma in medically inoperable patients using external beam irradiation and high dose rate intracavitary brachytherapy. J Urol. 1997;157(5):1669-1671.

Manur DB, Chao KS. Penis and Male Urethra. In: Perez CA, Brady LW, Halperin EC, editors. Principles and Practice of Radiation Oncology. 5th ed. Philadelphia: Lippincott Williams & Wilkins; 2008. pp. 1519-1531.

Micaily B, Dzeda MF, Miyamoto CT, Brady LW. Brachytherapy for cancer of the female urethra. Semin Surg Oncol. 1997;13(3):208-214.

Mostofi FK, Davis CJ, Jr., Sesterhenn IA. Carcinoma of the male and female urethra. Urol Clin North Am. 1992;19(2):347-358.

VanderMolen LA, Sheehy PF, Dillman RO. Successful treatment of transitional cell carcinoma of the urethra with chemotherapy. Cancer Invest. 2002;20(2):206-207.

PART IX
Lymphomas and Myeloma

IX

Chapter 35
Hodgkin's Lymphoma

Hans T. Chung, Stephen L. Shiao, and Naomi R. Schechter

EPIDEMIOLOGY

- Incidence/mortality in the US for 2008 is 8,220/1,350.
- Males slightly greater than females (1.1:1).
- Bimodal peak: ages 25–30 and >55.
- First-degree relatives of patients have fivefold increase in risk for Hodgkin's disease.
- Associated with Epstein–Barr virus, which is associated with mixed cellularity subtype. EBV DNA has been detected in Reed-Sternberg cells.
- Associated with HIV infection.

HISTOLOGY

- Hallmark is Reed-Sternberg cells (binucleate CD15+, CD30+), derived from monoclonal populations of B-cells.
- Eighty percent present with cervical lymphadenopathy.
- Fifty percent present with mediastinal disease (most likely NSHL).
- Thirty-three percent present with B symptoms overall, but only 15–20% of stage I–II have B symptoms.
- WHO classification.
  - Nodular lymphocyte predominance (NLPHL; CD15−, CD30−, CD20+, CD45+)
  - Classic (CHL; CD15+, CD30+, CD20±)
    - Nodular sclerosis (NSHL) = 70% (more common in adolescents and young adults)
    - Mixed cellularity (MCHL) = 20% (more common in young children)
    - Lymphocyte rich (LRCHL) = 10%
    - Lymphocyte depletion (LDHL) ≤ 5%
- NLPHL: occasional late relapse, but best OS. Often stage I–II, B symptoms <10%, more common patients >40 years.

IX

- NS: mediastinum often involved. One-third have B symptoms.
- MC: presents more commonly with advanced disease, often subclinical subdiaphragmatic disease in patients with clinically staged I–II above diaphragm.
- LD: rare, mostly advanced with B symptoms in older patients, worst prognosis, associated with HIV.

WORKUP

- H&P, including B symptoms, performance status, alcohol-induced pain, pruritis. Most common presentation is painless lymphadenopathy. Careful complete lymph node exam.
- Labs: CBC with differential, LFTs, BUN/Cr, ESR, chemistries, alkaline phosphatase, LDH, albumin. Pregnancy test. HIV test (if risk factors).
- MUGA test and LVEF before ABVD chemo.
- Pathology: Excisional LN biopsy. Bone marrow biopsy only for patients with B symptoms, stage III–IV, bulky disease, recurrent disease.
- Imaging: CXR; CT chest, abdomen and pelvis; PET–CT scan (sensitivity 75–91%) is considered standard (included in NCCN guidelines) and is performed pretreatment and after two cycles to assess response (predictive of outcome; Sieniawski et al. 2007).
- Consider oophoropexy for women to preserve ovarian function.
- Pretreatment dental evaluation if going to treat neck.

STAGING (AJCC 7TH ED., 2010): HODGKIN'S LYMPHOMA

- The definition of TNM and the stage grouping for this chapter have not changed from the AJCC 6th Ed., 2002.

Anatomic stage/prognostic groups	
I:	Involvement of a single lymphatic site (i.e., nodal region, Waldeyer's ring, thymus, or spleen) (I); or localized involvement of a single extralymphatic organ or site in the absence of any lymph node involvement (IE) (rare in Hodgkin's lymphoma)
II:	Involvement of two or more lymph node regions on the same side of the diaphragm (II); or localized involvement of a single extralymphatic organ or site in association with regional lymph node involvement with or without involvement of other lymph node regions on the same side of the diaphragm (IIE). The number of regions involved may be indicated by a subscript, as in, for example, II 3

continued

III: Involvement of lymph node regions on both sides of the diaphragm (III), which also may be accompanied by extralymphatic extension in association with adjacent lymph node involvement (IIIE) or by involvement of the spleen (IIIS) or both (IIIE,S). Splenic involvement is designated by the letter S

IV: Diffuse or disseminated involvement of one or more extralymphatic organs, with or without associated lymph node involvement; or isolated extralymphatic organ involvement in the absence of adjacent regional lymph node involvement, but in conjunction with disease in distant site(s). Stage IV includes any involvement of the liver or bone marrow, lungs (other than by direct extension from another site), or cerebrospinal fluid

Used with the permission from the American Joint Committee on Cancer (AJCC), Chicago, IL. The original source for this material is the AJCC Cancer Staging Manual, Seventh Edition (2010), published by Springer Science+Business Media.

Lymph node groups: Waldeyer's ring; occipital/cervical/preauricular/supraclavicular; infraclavicular; axillary; epitrochlear; mediastinal; right and left hilar (separate); paraaortic; splenic; mesenteric; iliac; inguinal/femoral; popliteal.

PROGNOSIS

- B symptoms, bulky mediastinal disease
- Early stage treated with chemo-RT, 5-year FFF 95% and OS >95%
- Advanced stage (Hasenclever et al. 1998):
  - Poor prognostic factors: male gender, age >45 years, stage IV, Hgb <10.5, WBC >15 k, lymphocyte $<0.6 \times 10^9$/L, albumin <40 g/L.
  - If ≤3 factors, 5-year FFP 70%, whereas >3 factors is 50%.

TREATMENT

CHEMO AGENTS

- MOPP = mechlorethamine, Oncovin (vincristine), procarbazine, prednisone
- ABVD = Adriamycin (doxorubicin), bleomycin, vinblastine, dacarbazine. (Decreased sterility and second malignancies vs. MOPP)
- BEACOPP (Diehl et al. 2003) = bleomycin, etoposide, Adriamycin (doxorubicin), cyclophosphamide, Oncovin (vincristine), prednisone, procarbazine
- Stanford V (Horning et al. 2004) mechlorethamine = mechlorethamine, vincristine, prednisone, doxorubicin, bleomycin, vinblastine, etoposide. Administered weekly for 8–12 weeks. (Decreased bleomycin and doxorubicin toxicity vs. ABVD.)

TREATMENT RECOMMENDATIONS

Stage	Recommended treatment
Favorable IA/IIA (no bulky disease, ≤3 sites, ESR<50), NLPD HL	■ ABVD ×4 then IFRT [30 Gy (subclinical) –36 Gy (clinical)] ■ Alternative chemo = 8 week Stanford V + IFRT (30 Gy) ■ STLI 40–44 Gy ■ For LP IA, may give IFRT or regional RT alone (30–36 Gy) Stage I–IIA: IFRT 30 Gy with boost to 36 for residual disease. Then, restage with PET/CT. If <CR, observe or give chemo (ABVD±R; CHOP±R) ■ Other stages: treat similar to classic HL ■ Preliminary phase II data support Rituximab since CD20+ ■ ~10-year EFS/OS: 85–90%
Unfavorable IA/IIA (bulky disease, >3 sites, or ESR>50), IB/IIB	■ ABVD ×4–6 then IFRT [30–36 Gy (subclinical) –36 Gy (clinical)] ■ Alternative: 12 weeks Stanford V + IFRT 36 Gy (to any node >5 cm If refuses chemo, STNI (mantle → PA + splenic) or mantle alone may be considered. 36–44 Gy ■ ~10-year FFP 85%, OS 90%
III–IV	■ ABVD ×4 then restage with PET/CT. If CR, ABVD ×2 + IFRT 20–36 Gy to bulky sites (optional). If PR, ABVD ×2–4c,-6 then IFRT 30–36 Gy to bulky sites (optional) ■ Alternative: 12 week Stanford V + IFRT 36 Gy (to any node >5 cm and residual PET + sites). Or, dose-escalated BEACOPP with IFRT 30 Gy to initial sites > 5 cm and 40 Gy to residual PET + areas ~ 10-year FFP Stage III 75% Stage IV 65%, OS Stage III80%, Stage IV 75% ■ ~10-year FFP 85%, OS 90%
Primary refractory disease	■ High-dose chemo + stem cell transplant (30–60% salvage)
Relapse	■ Chemo or chemo-RT salvages ~50–80% of patients initially treated with RT alone. After chemo, may give 15–25 Gy to previously irradiated sites or 30–40 Gy to not previously irradiated sites

- For patients who relapse after chemo, only 40–60% salvage
- Most chemo-alone failures occur in sites of initial disease
- If relapse after initial stage III/IV, then autologous bone marrow transplant or autologous peripheral stem cell transplant

STUDIES

EARLY FAVORABLE

Staging laparotomy

- *EORTC H6F* (Carde et al. 1993): 262 patients with clinical stage I–II and favorable factors [1–2 sites, no bulky disease, ESR <50 (or <30 if B symptoms)] randomized to: (1) no laparotomy with STLI; (2) negative laparotomy and NS or LP with mantle 40 Gy or STLI alone if MC or LD; (3) positive laparotomy then chemo-RT. No difference in 6-year DFS (83 vs. 78%) or OS (89 vs. 93%) with or without laparotomy. Therefore, laparotomy is unnecessary with chemo-RT or STLI.

ROLE OF CHEMOTHERAPY AND REDUCED RT FIELD SIZE

- *EORTC H7VF* (Noordijk et al. 1997): 40 patients with very favorable group (women <40 years with IA nonbulky NS or LP with ESR <50) treated with mantle RT alone. Although OS was 96%, RFS was 73%, suggesting that mantle alone is insufficient. Most relapses were in the abdomen.
- *EORTC H7F* (Noordijk et al. 1997, 2005): 333 patients with favorable group randomized to EBVP chemo ×6 and IFRT vs. STNI + splenic RT. Chemo-RT improved 10-year EFS (88 vs. 78%), but not OS (92 vs. 92%).
- *GHSG HD7* (Sieber et al. 2002; Engert et al. 2007): 627 patients with favorable clinical stage IA–IIB (no bulky disease, extranodal disease, elevated ESR, >2 LN regions) randomized to EFRT (30 Gy) + boost 10 Gy vs. ABVD×2 and EFRT + boost 10 Gy. Chemo-RT increased 7-year DFS (88 vs. 67%), but no difference in OS (94 vs. 92%). Difference in DFS mainly due to failures in RT alone arm, but treatment of relapses significantly more successful in RT alone vs. chemo-RT.

IX

- *SWOG 9133/CALGB 9391* (Press et al. 2001): 348 patients with favorable clinical stage I–IIA (no bulky disease, infradiaphragmatic disease, B symptoms) randomized to three cycles of doxorubicin and vinblastine and STLI (36–40 Gy) or STLI alone (36–40 Gy). Chemo-RT increased overall response and 3-year FFS (94 vs. 81%), but not OS.
- *Stanford G4* (ASH 2004 Horing et al. 2004): 87 patients with non-bulky favorable I/IIA received 8 weeks of Stanford V followed by IFRT (30 Gy). Median follow-up 5.7 year. Eight-year FFP and OS were 96 and 98%.
- *GHSG HD10* (ESH 2004 Diehl et al. 2005a); Diehl et al. 2005b): 1,131 patients with favorable I–II with no risk factors randomized to ABVD ×2c vs. ×4c, followed by IFRT 20 vs. 30 Gy. At medium follow-up 2 years, no difference between any of the arms (freedom from failure 97%, OS 98.5%).
- *EORTC-GELA H8F* (Ferme et al. 2007): 542 patients with favorable stage I–II randomized to STLI (36+4 Gy IF boost) vs. MOPP-ABV×3 + IFRT (36 Gy for CR, 40 Gy for PR). Median follow-up 92 months. Five-year EFS (98 vs. 74%) and 10-year OS (97 vs. 92%) better with MOPP-ABV + IFRT.
- *Stanford G4* (ASH 2004, Horing et al. 2004): 87 patients with non-bulky favorable I/IIA received 8 weeks of Stanford V followed by IFRT (30 Gy). Median follow-up 5.7 year. Eight-year FFP and OS were 96 and 98%.

Radiation dose and chemo cycles

- *GHSG HD10* (ESH 2004, Diehl et al. 2005b): 1,131 patients with favorable I–II with no risk factors randomized to ABVD ×2c vs. ×4c, followed by IFRT 20 vs. 30 Gy. At medium follow-up 2 years, no difference between any of the arms (freedom from failure 97%, OS 98.5%).
- *EORTC H9F* (Diehl et al. 2005b, Thomas et al. 2007): 783 patients with favorable IA–IIB randomized to no IFRT, IFRT (20 Gy), or IFRT (36 Gy), after attaining CR with EBVP ×6c (79% of patients had CR and were randomized). Median follow-up 33 months. Four-year EFS decreased without IFRT (70%) vs. 84 (20 Gy) and 87% (36 Gy), no RT arm stopped because of unacceptable failure rate (>20%). No difference in OS (98% all three arms).
- *Stanford G5* Currently still accruing patients with favorable I–IIA to risk-adapted Stanford V-C and low-dose IFRT.
- *EORTC 20051/GELA H10:* Currently accruing patients with favorable I–II to ABVD×3+INRT vs. ABVD×2 → FDG-PET, if

PET positive, then escalated BEACOPP×2+INRT; if PET negative then ABVD×2.

- *GHSG HD13:* Currently accruing patients with favorable I–II to ABVD×2, ABV×2, AVD×2, or AV×2, then IFRT (30 Gy). Interim analysis showed significant increase in events in the ABV and AV arms which were then subsequently closed.

EARLY UNFAVORABLE

Role of chemotherapy and reduced RT field size

- *Specht metaanalysis* (Specht et al. 1998). RT alone vs. chemo-RT. Chemo-RT decreases 10-year recurrence by 50% (IA 20–10%, IB 30–15%). No difference in OS (RT 77%, chemo-RT 79%), or CSS (85–88%).
- *EORTC-GELA H8U* (ASH 2000, Ferme et al. 2000, Ferme et al. 2007): 996 patients with unfavorable clinical stage I–II disease randomized to: (1) MOPP/ABV×6 + IFRT; (2) MOPP/ABV×4 + IFRT; (3) MOPP/ABV×4 + STLI. IFRT = 36–40 Gy. No difference in five-year EFS (84, 88, 87%) or OS (88, 85, 84%), therefore four cycles equivalent to six cycles and IFRT equivalent to STLI.
- Milan (Laskar et al. 2004). Randomized 136 patients with clinical stage IA bulky, IB, IIA, or IIA bulky to ABVD×4 then STLI vs. IFRT. Dose 36 Gy for CR, 40 Gy for PR, and 30.6 Gy for STNI prophylactic. No difference in 12-year FFP (93 vs. 94%) or OS (96 vs. 94%). Three patients had second CA with STNI vs. 0 with IFRT.
- *GHSG HD8* (Eng ert et al. 2003): 1,064 patients with clinical stage I–II and at least one unfavorable factor (bulky mediastinal disease, massive splenomegaly, >2 nodal sites, extranodal disease, high ESR) to four cycles of COPP/ABVD and EFRT or IFRT (30 Gy + 10 Gy boost). There was no difference in EFS or OS.
- *NCCTG HD-6/ECOG JHD06* (Gobbi et al. 2005): 399 patients with nonbulky CS I–IIA HD were randomized to STLI ± ABVD×2 or ABVD×4–6. Patients in the STLI arm were stratified into favorable and unfavorable risk (MC or LD histology, ≥4 sites, ESR ≥50 or age ≥40). Unfavorable patients received STLI + ABVD×2. For all patients, STLI improved 5-year FFP (93 vs. 87%), but not EFS and OS. Subgroup analysis of unfavorable risk patients showed improved FFP (95 vs. 88%), but not OS. No difference seen in favorable risk patients. Second cancers (10 vs. 4) and CAD (12 vs. 4) were increased in STLI arm.

Chemotherapy regimens and duration

- *EORTC H6U* (Carde et al. 1993): 316 patients clinical stage I–II and unfavorable factors treated with split course chemo with mantle RT (35 Gy ± boost 5–10 Gy) and no laparotomy were randomized to MOPP×6 vs. ABVD×6. ABVD improved 10-year DFS (88 vs. 77%), but not OS (87 vs. 87%). ABVD had higher pulmonary toxicity, but less sterility and hematologic complications.
- *EORTC H7U* (Noordijk et al. 2006): 389 patients with clinical stage I–II and any unfavorable factor, randomized to MOPP/ABV×6 vs. EBVP×6, followed by IFRT (36–40 Gy). MOPP/ABV improved both 10-year RFS (88 vs. 68%) and OS (87 vs. 79%).
- *EORTC-GELA H8U* (ASH 2000); (Ferme et al. 2000); Ferme et al. 2007: 996 patients with unfavorable clinical stage I–II disease randomized to: (1) MOPP/ABV×6 + IFRT; (2) MOPP/ABV×4 + IFRT; (3) MOPP/ABV×4 + STLI. IFRT = 36–40 Gy. No difference in 5-year EFS (84, 88, 87%) or OS (88, 85, 84%), therefore four cycles equivalent to six cycles and IFRT equivalent to STLI.
- Milan (Laskar et al. 2004). Randomized 136 patients with clinical stage IA bulky, IB, IIA, or IIA bulky to ABVD×4, then STLI vs. IFRT. Dose 36 Gy for CR, 40 Gy for PR, and 30.6 Gy for STNI prophylactic. No difference in 12-year FFP (93 vs. 94%) or OS (96 vs. 94%). Three patients had second CA with STNI vs. 0 with IFRT79%).
- *EORTC-GELA H9U* (ASCO 2005, Noordijk et al. 2005): 808 patients with unfavorable stage I–II randomized to ABVD×6 vs. ABVD×4 vs. BEACOPP×4 + 30 Gy IF-RT in all arms. No difference in 4-year EFS (94, 89, and 91%) or OS (96, 95, and 93%). Toxicity worse with BEACOPP compared to ABVD.
- *GHSG HD8* (Engert et al. 2003): 1,064 patients with clinical stage I–II and at least one unfavorable factor (bulky mediastinal disease, massive splenomegaly, >2 nodal sites, extranodal disease, high ESR) to four cycles of COPP/ABVD and EFRT or IFRT (30 + 10 Gy boost). There was no difference in EFS or OS.
- *GHSG HD11* (Diehl et al. 2005b): 1,570 patients with clinical stage I–II randomized to ABVD×4 + IF-RT (30 Gy) vs. ABVD×4 + IF-RT (20 Gy) vs. BEACOPP×4 IF-RT (30 Gy) vs. BEACOPP×4 + IF-RT (20 Gy). Median follow-up 3 years. No difference in overall freedom from treatment failure (FFTF) or OS between ABVD (87, 97%) vs. BEACOPP (88, 96%) or 20 Gy (87, 97%) vs. 30 Gy (90, 97%), though there was more toxicity with BEACOPP and more relapses in the 20 Gy arm requiring salvage.

- *NCCTG HD-6/ECOG JHD06* (Gobbi et al. 2005): 399 patients with nonbulky CS I–IIA HD were randomized to STLI ± ABVD×2 or ABVD×4–6. Patients in the STLI arm were stratified into favorable and unfavorable risk (MC or LD histology, ≥4 sites, ESR ≥50 or age ≥40). Unfavorable patients received STLI + ABVD×2. For all patients, STLI improved 5-year FFP (93 vs. 87%), but not EFS and OS. Subgroup analysis of unfavorable risk patients showed improved FFP (95 vs. 88%), but not OS. No difference seen in favorable risk patients. Second cancers (10 vs. 4) and CAD (12 vs. 4) were increased in STLI arm.
- *GHSG HD14*. Currently accruing patients with unfavorable I–II to dose-escalated BEACOPPx2+ABVDx2+IFRT (30 Gy) vs. ABVD×4+IFRT (30 Gy). Rationale is that despite excellent initial CR rates, 10–15% will recur within 5 year.
- *EORTC 20051/GELA H10*. Currently accruing patients with unfavorable I–II to ABVD×4+INRT vs. ABVD×2 → FDG-PET, if PET positive, then escalated BEACOPP +and INRT; if PET negative, then ABVD×4.
- *GHSG HD17*. Currently accruing patients with unfavorable I–II to EACOPP14 with ABVD, and INRT (involved-node RT) with IFRT.

CHEMOTHERAPY ± RT FOR EARLY-STAGE

- *EORTC H9F* (ASCO abstr 2005, Noordijk et al. 2005, Thomas et al. 2007). See above.
- *NCIC/ECOG* (Meyer et al. 2005; Macdonald et al. 2007): 399 patients with I–IIA low-risk (LP, NS, age <40 years, <3 sites, ESR <50) randomized to STNI vs. ABVD ×4–6c alone. Higher risk patients were randomized to ABVD ×2c + STNI vs. ABVD ×4–6c. Chemo-alone had poorer 5-year PFS (93→87%), but no change in OS.
- *MSKCC* (Straus et al. 2004): 152 patients nonbulky CS IA–IIB, IIIA treated with ABVD ×6c randomized to modified EFRT 36 Gy vs. no RT. RT improved 5-year FFP (81→86%), but not OS (90→97%).
- *CCG* (Nachman et al. 2002): 829 patients <21 years risk-adapted treatment. Favorable CS I–II COPP/ABV ×4c. Unfavorable CS I–II and III COPP/ABV ×6c. IV: Intensive chemo. If CR randomized to 21 Gy IFRT vs. none. If PR, all got 21 Gy IFRT. IFRT improved 3-year EFS (85→93%), but not OS.
- *GATLA* (Pavlovsky et al. 1988): 277 patients CS I–II treated with CVPP ×6c randomized to 30 Gy IFRT vs. none. IFRT improved DFS (62→71%) for unfavorable patients (34→75%), but not favorable patients (70→77%). No OS difference. Used inferior chemo regimen. 45% patients <16 years.

IX

- CR after ABVD×6, then randomized to no RT or consolidation RT. IFRT was given in 84%. Forty-seven percent were <15 years and 68% had MC histology. RT improved 8-year EFS (76 vs. 88%) and OS (89 vs. 100%).
- Picardi et al. 2007): 260 patients with bulky >5 cm got VEBEP chemo. One hundred and sixty patients became PET- after chemo, but had residual CT mass >1.3 cm randomized to observation vs. IFRT 32 Gy. Median follow-up 40 months. IFRT reduced failures 14→4% and all chemo-alone failures were in initial site and contiguous nodal regions.

ADVANCED

- *CALGB 8251* (canellos et al. 1992, 2002): 361 patients with stage III–IV randomized to MOPP × 6–8c, ABVD × 6–8c, or MOPP-ABVD × 12 months. No RT. Both ABVD and MOPP-ABVD improved 5-year FFS, but not OS. ABVD less toxic than MOPP-ABVD.

ROLE OF IFRT

- *SWOG 7808* (Fabian et al. 1994). CS III–IV MOP-BAP × 6 months. If CR, randomized to observation vs. 20 Gy IFRT. Improved FFP for NSHD (60–82%), bulky >6 cm (57–75%) and patients who actually completed assigned treatment (67–85%). No difference in OS.
- *GHSG HD3* (Diehl et al. 1995). CS IIIB/IV COPP/ABVD × 6 months. If CR, randomized to 2 months COPP/ABVD or 20 Gy IFRT. No diff RFS (77%) or OS (90%).
- *EORTC 20884/GPMC H34* (Aleman et al. 2003, Eichet et al. 2007). CS III/IV MOPP-ABV × 6–8c. If CR, randomized to observation vs. consolidative IFRT (24 Gy). IFRT did not improve RFS or OS and had higher rate of myelodysplastic syndrome and leukemia. For those in PR (33%, all received RT), 8-year EFS 76% and OS 84% not significantly different from those with CR ± RT (75 and 82%), therefore role for RT in patients with PR.
- *GHSG HD9* (Engert et al. 2009): 1,196 patients with CS IIB/IIIA and risk factors or stage IIIB/IV randomized to COPP/ABVD×4+IFRT vs. std BEACOPP×8+IFRT or increased-dose BEACOPP×8+IFRT. Median follow-up 111 months. Ten-year FFTF 64, 70, 82% with 10-year OS 75, 80, and 86%. Significant improvement in FFTF and OS with increased-dose BEACOPP, but higher risk of secondary AML.
- *GHSG HD12* (Eich et al. 2007; ASH 2008; Diehl et al. 2008; Diehl et al. 2009): 1,571 patients with CS IIB/IIIA and risk factors or stage IIIB/IV randomized to escalated BEACOPP×8 vs. escalated

BEACOPP×4 +and std BEACOPP×4 with IFRT to residual vs. no RT to residual for both arms. Second randomization of IFRT (30 Gy) vs. no IFRT to initial bulky or residual enlarged nodes. At 5 years, no statistical difference between any of the four arms. RT improved 4-year FFTF (88→95%), but no difference in survival. Because RT was given to 10% of patients in "non-RT" arms, equivalency of a non-RT strategy cannot be proved.

- *India* (Laskar et al. 2004): 179 (71%) of 251 patients with stage I–IV achieved *GHSG HD3* (Diehl et al. 1995). CS IIIB/IV COPP/ABVD × 6 months. If CR after ABVD×6, then randomized to no RT2 months COPP/ABVD or consolidation RT. IFRT (20 Gy) was given in 84%. Forty-seven percent were <15 years and 68% had MC histology. RT improved 8-year EFS (76 vs. 88%) and OS (89 vs. 100%). No diff RFS (77%) or OS (90%).
- *GELA H89* (Ferme et al. 2000): 418 patients CS IIIB/IV who achieved CR/PR after six cycles of MOPP/ABV or ABVPP were randomized to STLI or two more cycles of chemo. Five-year DFS (79 vs. 74%) and OS (88 vs. 85%) were not different.

Chemotherapy regimens and duration

- *CALGB 8251* (Canellos et al. 1992, 2002): 361 patients with stage III–IV randomized to MOPP × 6–8c, ABVD × 6–8c, or MOPP-ABVD × 12 months. No RT. Both ABVD and MOPP-ABVD improved 5-year FFS, but not OS. ABVD less toxic than MOPP-ABVD.
- *GHSG HD9* (Diehl et al. 2007): 1,196 patients with CS IIB/IIIA and risk factors or stage IIIB/IV randomized to COPP/ABVD×4+IFRT vs. standard-dose BEACOPP×8+IFRT or dose-escalated BEACOPP×8+IFRT. Median follow-up 113 months. Ten-year FFTF 64, 70, 82% with 10-year OS 75, 80, and 86%. Significant improvement in FFTF and OS with increased-dose BEACOPP, but higher risk of secondary AML.
- *Stanford G3* (ASH 2004, Horing et al. 2004): 108 patients with stage III–IV were prospectively treated with 12 weeks of Stanford V and IFRT 36 Gy to any sites ≥5 cm. Median follow-up was 6.8 year. Eight-year FFP and OS were 85.9 and 95.2%.
- *IIL HD9601 Italy* (Gobbi et al. 2005): 334 patients with IIB–IV randomized to ABVD ×6 vs. MOPPEBVCAD ×6 vs. 12 week modified Stanford V. RT (36–42 Gy) to residual mass or previously bulky disease (>6 cm), and to no more than two sites (different than original Stanford V). Median follow-up was 61 months. Modified Stanford V had lower CR (89v94v76%), 5-year FFS (78v81v54%), and FFP (85v94v73%), but no difference in OS (90v89v82%). In ascending order of severity, hematologic toxicity was least in ABVD, Stanford V than MOPPEBVCAD.

IX

- *ECOG 2496/CALGB 59905*. Now closed. Patients with bulky stage I–IIA/B or III–IV disease randomized to either Stanford V with IFRT to bulky disease, or ABVD with IFRT for bulky mediastinal disease.
- *GHSG HD18*. Currently accruing patients. Patients with bulky IIB–IV disease receive escalated BEACOPP×3 with PET after second cycle, if PET+ then patients randomized to escBEACOPP×5 + RT to residual (30 Gy) or escBEACOPP×5 + Rituximab + RT to residual (30 Gy). If PET–, then patients randomized to escBEACOPP×5 or escBEACOPP×1.

PRIMARY REFRACTORY OR RELAPSED HD

- *GHSG relapse patterns in early-stage HD* (Sieniawski et al. 2007) Early-Stage Favorable – 1,129 patients with early-stage favorable Hodgkin's lymphoma from GHSG HD7/HD10/HD13 trials who were treated with ABVD×2+EFRT/IFRT. Forty-two patients with treatment failure treated with either salvage chemo (24), chemo+SCT (14), or RT alone (4). Median follow-up 36 months. FFTF2 and OS were 52 and 67%, respectively. High treatment-related mortality rate. Overall prognosis dependent duration of first remission, clinical stage, and anemia at relapse with two of three factors having significantly worse prognosis.
- *Vancouver experience* (Lavoie et al. 2005): 100 patients with primary refractory or relapsed HD underwent high-dose chemo and autologous stem cell transplantation. After median follow-up of 11.4 year, 15-year OS was 54%. OS higher in relapsed HD (67%) vs. primary refractory HD (39%). Treatment-related mortality, including death from second malignancy, was 17% at 15 year. Fifteen-year cumulative second malignancy was 9%.

ROLE OF PET

- *Italy* (Rigacci et al. 2007). Prospective, multicenter study of 186 patients to evaluate the addition of PET scan in the staging of HD by CT. PET imaging led to 14% upstaging and 1% downstaging as compared to CT staging alone. Among the patients with CT-staged localized disease, 8% were upstaged to advanced disease with PET.
- *PET for staging/prognosis* (Gallmini et al. 2007): 260 patients with stage IIA–IVB treated with ABVD + RT to bulky disease or residual mass. PET done at baseline and then after two cycles and compared to IPS to for prognostic value. Median follow-up 2 years. Two-year PFS for PET+ = 12.8% and for PET– = 95.0%; in multi-

variate analysis only PET significantly associated with treatment outcome. Basis for EORTC H10 and GHSG HD15 trial design.

- *Prognostic value of PET after chemo* (Advani et al. 2007). Retrospective analysis of 81 patients with stage I–IV had PET at baseline and again after the completion of Stanford V chemotherapy before planned RT. Four-year FFP 96 vs. 33% for PET− vs. PET+ patients irregardless of RT. PET highly predictive of FFP after chemotherapy whether or not patients receive RT.
- *GHSG HD15* (Kobe et al. 2007). Negative prognostic value of PET after chemo was investigated. Patients with a negative PET scan were not irradiated, whereas patients with a positive PET scan were irradiated. Ninety-five percent of patients with negative PET scan have not relapsed after 12 months.
- International Harmonization Project (Juweid et al. 2008) was convened to develop guidelines for performing and interpreting PET scans for treatment assessment. Sensitivity and specificity postchemo for detection of residual disease are 84 and 90%, respectively. Recommendations included: (1) PET scans after the completion of therapy should be performed ≥3 weeks, and preferably 6–8 weeks, after chemo, and 8–12 weeks after RT or chemo-RT, to distinguish between viable tumor necrosis or fibrosis; (2) pretreatment PET scans are not obligatory as HD is FDG-avid, but may be used to facilitate interpretation of posttreatment PET; (3) abnormal PET can be defined as focal or diffuse FDG uptake above background in a location incompatible with normal anatomy/physiology (please refer to reference for exceptions); (4) PET scans performed during treatment should be performed as close as possible (i.e., within 4 days) before the subsequent cycle.

FUTURE DIRECTIONS

Radiotherapy dose: 20 Gy is being investigated in stage I–II, favorable (GHSG HD10, EORTC H9F, Stanford G5), and stage I–II, unfavorable (GHSG HD11).

Radiotherapy volume: INRT (involved-node RT) is being investigated in GHSG HD17 (Gallmini et al. 2007, 2008).

RADIATION TECHNIQUES

SIMULATION AND FIELD DESIGN (3DCRT)

- Simulate supine with custom immobilization. Wire nodes. Consider PET–CT simulation
- Consider custom compensator for neck, mediastinal, or SCV fields

- Extended RT fields
  - Mantle: bilateral cervical, SCV, infraclavicular, mediastinal, hilar, and axilla
  - Mini-mantle: mantle without mediastinum, hila
  - Modified mantle: mantle without axilla
  - Inverted Y: paraaortic, bilateral pelvic and inguino-femoral, ± splenic
  - Total lymphoid irradiation (TLI): both mantle and inverted Y-fields
  - Subtotal lymphoid irradiation (STLI): TLI with exclusion of pelvis
- Mantle
  - Simulate with arms-up (to pull axillary LN from chest to allow for more lung blocking) or arms akimbo (to shield humeral heads and minimize tissue in SCV folds). Head extended. Use CT planning
  - Borders: lateral = beyond humeral heads; inferior = bottom of diaphragm (T11/12); superior = inferior mandible
  - Blocks: larynx on AP field. Humeral heads on AP and PA fields. PA cord block (if dose >40 Gy). Lung block at top of fourth rib to cover infraclavicular LN. If pericardial or mediastinal extension, include entire heart to 15 Gy, then block apex of heart. After 30 Gy, block heart beyond 5 cm inferior to carina (unless residual disease)
  - Margins: Prechemo cranio-caudad + 2–5 cm; postchemo lateral + 1.5 cm (Fig. 35.1)
- If plan to treat subdiaphragmatic disease, start 7–10 days after mantle
- Definition for IFRT (ASTRO 2002):
  - IFRT encompasses a region, not an individual LN
  - Major involved-field regions are: neck (unilateral), mediastinum (including bilateral hilum), axilla (including supraclavicular and infraclavicular LN), spleen, PA, inguinal (femoral and iliac nodes)
  - Initially involved prechemo sites and volume are treated, except for the transverse diameter of mediastinal and PA LN for which the reduced post-CHT volume is treated
- Neck: Include ipsilateral cervical and SCV regions. Consider IMRT (refer to RTOG H&N contouring atlas for nodal locations)
- Mediastinum: include bilateral hilar regions. If SCV involved, include bilateral SCV and cervical regions. Consider respiratory gating
- Axilla: include ipsilateral SCV and infraclavicular regions (Fig. 35.2)

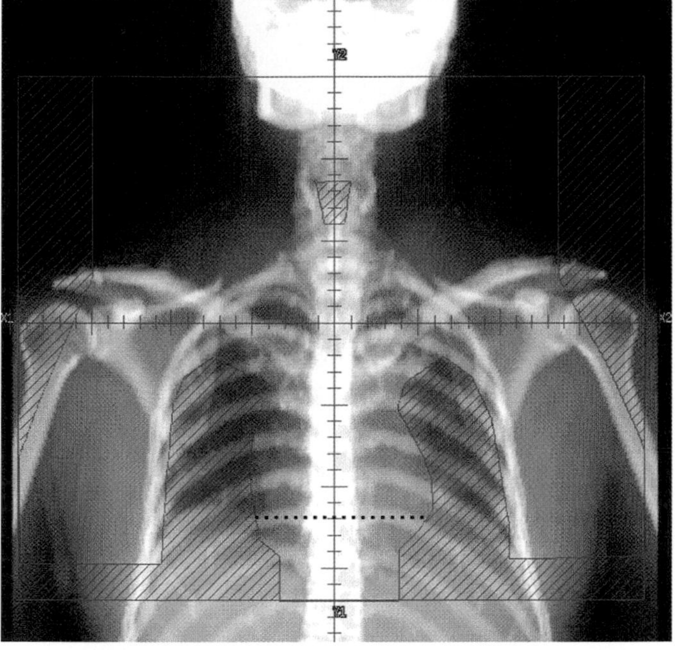

Fig. 35.1 DRR of an AP mantle field with cardiac block after 30 Gy (black dotted line)

- Inguinal: Include external iliac and femoral regions
- Margins: generally 2 cm superior and inferior to prechemo volume and 2 cm lateral to postchemo volume for mediastinal and para-aortic fields
- Shield testes for men and consider oophoropexy for women (Fig. 35.3)
- Match fields with half-beam or gap techniques

IX

DOSE PRESCRIPTIONS

- See treatment algorithm

DOSE LIMITATIONS

- Femoral head: <25 Gy to prevent slipped capital femoral epiphysis; avascular necrosis with steroids or >30–40 Gy
- Mandible dental abnormalities with 20–40 Gy
- Thyroid: <20% to <26 Gy

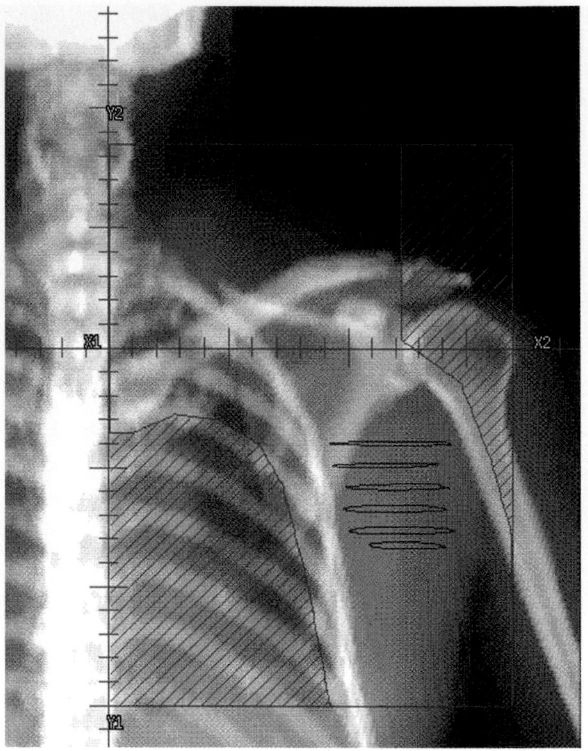

Fig. 35.2 DRR of IFRT for a stage I axillary Hodgkin's lymphoma

- Lung blocks
- Entire cardiac silhouette <15 Gy, block at apex, after 30–35 Gy add subcarinal block (5 cm below the carina)
- Renal and liver blocks if necessary

COMPLICATIONS

- Acute: fatigue, dermatitis, esophagitis, nausea, diarrhea
- Subacute: radiation pneumonitis, Lhermitte's syndrome
- Late: coronary artery disease, hypothyroidism, gastric ulcer, pulmonary toxicity, decreased immunity, second malignancies (leukemia RR 22.3×, usually AML peaking at 5–9 years; solid tumors RR 2.8×, usually thyroid, lung, breast, GI occurring >5 years after treatment), infertility

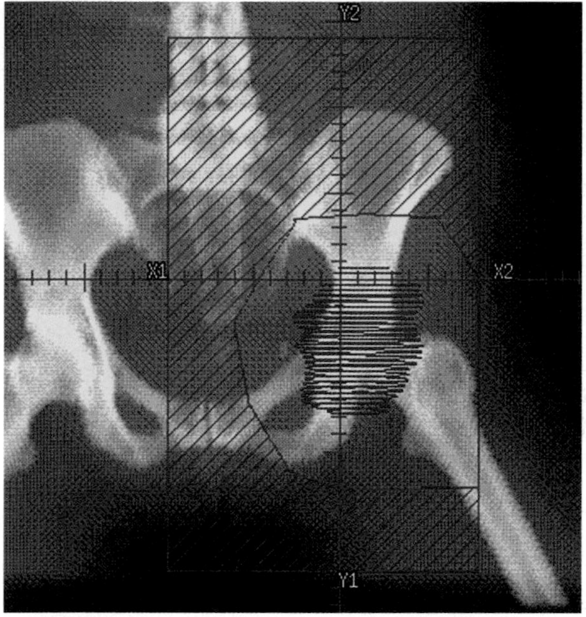

Fig. 35.3 DRR of IFRT for a stage I inguinal-femoral Hodgkin's lymphoma

FOLLOW-UP

- Every 3 months for 2 year, then every 6 months for 3–4 years, then annually with H&P, labs, CXR ± CT/PET/gallium. Follow thyroid function (annual TSH and T4) if in irradiated field. Annual mammogram for women <30 years starting 5–8 years after RT

IX

REFERENCES

Advani R, Maeda L, Lavori P, et al. Impact of positive positron emission tomography on prediction of freedom from progression after Stanford V chemotherapy in Hodgkin's Disease. J Clin Oncol 2007;25(25):3902–3907.

Aleman BM, Raemaekers JM, Tomasic R, et al. Involved field radiotherapy for patients in partial remission after chemotherapy for advanced Hodgkin's lymphoma. Int J Radiat Oncol Biol Phys 2007;67(1):19–30.

Aleman BMP, Raemaekers JMM, Tirelli U, et al. Involved-field radiotherapy for advanced Hodgkin's lymphoma. N Engl J Med 2003;348:2396–2406.

Canellos GP, Anderson JR, Propert KJ, et al. Chemotherapy of advanced Hodgkin's disease with MOPP, ABVD, or MOPP alternating with ABVD. N Eng J Med 1992;327:1478–1484.

Canellos GP, Niedzwiecki D. Long-term follow-up of Hodgkin's disease trial. N Engl J Med 2002;346:1417–1418.

Carde P, Hagenbeek A, Hayat M, et al. Clinical staging versus laparotomy and combined modality with MOPP versus ABVD in early-stage Hodgkin's disease: the H6 twin randomized trials from the European Organization for Research and Treatment of Cancer Lymphoma Cooperative Group. J Clin Oncol 1993;11:2258–2272.

Diehl V, Brillant C, Engert A, et al. HD10: Investigating reduction of combined modality treatment intensity in early stage Hodgkin's lymphoma. Interim analysis of a randomized trial of the German Hodgkin Study Group (GHSG). J Clin Oncol (Meeting abstracts) 2005a; 23:6506.

Diehl V, Brillant C, Engert A, et al. Recent interim analysis of the HD11 trial of the GHSG: intensification of chemotherapy and reduction of radiation dose in early unfavorable stage Hodgkin's lymphoma. Blood 2005b;106:(abstract no. 816)

Diehl V, Franklin J, Pfistner B, et al. Ten-year results of a German Hodgkin Study Group randomized trial of standard and increased dose BEACOPP chemotherapy for advanced Hodgkin lymphoma (HD9). J Clin Oncol (Meeting abstracts) 2007;25:LBA8015.

Diehl V, Franklin J, Pfreundschuh M, et al. Standard and increased-dose BEACOPP chemotherapy compared with COPP-ABVD for advanced Hodgkin's disease. NEJM 2003;348:2386–2395.

Diehl V, Franklin J, Tesch H, et al. Dose escalation of BEACOPP chemotherapy for advanced Hodgkin's disease in the HD9 trial of the German Hodgkin's Lymphoma Study Group (GHSG). Proc ASCO 2007 (abstract no. 7).

Diehl V, Haverkamp H, Mueller R, et al. Eight cycles of BEACOPP escalated compared with 4 cycles of BEACOPP baseline with or without readiotherapy in patients in advanced stage Hodgkin lymphoma (HL): final analysis of the HD12 trial of the Germa Hodgkin Study Group (GHSG). J Clin Oncol 2009;27:15s (Suppl; abstr 8544).

Diehl V, Loeffler M, Pfreundschuh M, et al. Further chemotherapy versus low-dose involved-field radiotherapy as consolidation of complete remission after six cycles of alternating chemotherapy in patients with advance Hodgkin's disease. German Hodgkins' Study Group (GHSG). Ann Oncol. 1995;6(9):901–910.

Eich H, Gossmann A, Engert A, et al. A contribution to solve the problem of the need for consolidative radiotherapy after intensive chemotherapy in advanced stages of Hodgkin's lymphoma – analysis of a quality control program initiated by the Radiotherapy Reference Center of the German Hodgkin Study Group (GHSG). Int J Radiat Oncol Biol Phys 2007;69:1187–1192.

Engert A, Diehl V, Franklin J, et al. Escalated-dose BEACOPP in the treatment of patients with advanced-stage Hodgkin's lymphoma: 10 years of follow-up of the GHSG HD9 study. J Clin Oncol 2009;27(27):4548–4554.

Engert A, Schiller P, Josting A, et al. Involved-field radiotherapy is equally effective and less toxic compared with extended-field radiotherapy after four cycles of chemotherapy in patients with early-stage unfavorable Hodgkin's lymphoma: results of the HD8 trial of the German Hodgkin's Lymphoma Study Group. J Clin Oncol 2003;21:3601–3608.

Engert, A, Franklin, J, Eich H, et al. Two cycles of doxorubicin, bleomycin, vinblastine and dacarbazine plus extended-field radiotherapy is superior to radiotherapy alone in early favorable Hodgkin's lymphoma: final results of the GHSG HD7 Trial. J Clin Oncol 2007;25(23): 3495–3502.

Fabian CJ, Mansfield CM, Dahlberg S, et al. Low-dose involved field radiation after chemotherapy in advanced Hodgkin disease. A Southwest Oncology Group randomized study. Ann Intern Med 1994;120(11):903–912.

Ferme C, Eghbali H, Meerwaldt JH, et al. Chemotherapy plus involved-field radiation in early-stage Hodgkin's disease. N Engl J Med 2007;357(19):1916–1927.

Ferme C, Sebban C, Hennequin C, et al. Comparison of chemotherapy to radiotherapy as consolidation of complete or good partial response after six cycles of chemotherapy for patients with advanced Hodgkin's disease: results of the Groupe d'etudes des Lymphomes de l'Adulte H89 trial. Blood 2000;95:2246–2252.

Gallmini A, Hutchings M, Rigacci L, et al. Early Interim 2-[^{18}F]Fluoro-2-deoxy-D-glucose positron emission tomography is prognostically superior to international prognostic score in advanced-stage Hodgkin's lymphoma: a report from a joint Italian-Danish study. J Clin Oncol 2007;25:3746–3752.

Girinsky T, Specht L, Ghalibafian M, et al. The conundrum of Hodgkin lymphoma nodes: To be or not to be included in the involved node radiation fields. The EORTC-GELA lymphoma group guidelines. Radiother Oncol 2008;88:202–210.

Gobbi PG, Levis A, Chisesi T, et al. ABVD versus modified Stanford V versus MOPPEBVCAD with optional and limited radiotherapy in intermediate- and advanced stage Hodgkin's lymphoma. Final results of a multicenter randomized trial by the Intergruppo Italiano Linfomi. J Clin Oncol 2005;23:9198–9207.

Hasenclever D, Diehl V, Armitage JO, et al. A prognostic score for advanced Hodgkin's disease. N Engl J Med 1998;339:1506–1514.

Horning SJ, Hoppe RT, Advani R, et al. Efficacy and late effects of Stanford V chemotherapy and radiotherapy in untreated Hodgkin's disease: mature data in early and advanced stage patients. Blood 2004;104(abstr 308).

Juweid ME, Stroobants S, Hoekstra OS, et al. Use of positron emission tomography for response assessment of lymphoma: consensus of the imaging subcommittee on Internation Harmonization Project in Lymphoma. J Clin Oncol 2007;25(5):571–578.

Kobe C, Dietlein M, Franklin J *et al.* FDG-PET for assessment of residual tissue after completion of chemotherapy in Hodgkin lymphoma – report on the second interim analysis of the PET investigation in the trial HD15 of the GHSG. Haematologica 2007;92(Suppl 5):CO21.

Laskar S, Gupta T, Vimal S, et al. Consolidation radiation after complete remission in Hodgkin's disease following six cycles of doxorubicin, bleomycin, vinblastine, and dacarbazine chemotherapy: is there a need? J Clin Oncol 2004;22:62–68.

Lavoie JC, Connors JM, and Phillips GL, et al. High-dose chemotherapy and autologous stem cell transplantation for primary refractory or relapsed Hodgkin lymphoma: long-term outcome in the first 100 patients treated in Vancouver. Blood 2005;106(4):1473–1478.

Macdonald DA, Ding K, Gospodarowicz MK, et al. Patterns of disease progression and outcomes in a randomized trial testing ABVD alone for patients with limited-stage Hodgkin lymphoma. Ann Oncol 2007;18(10):1680–1684.

Meyer RM, Gospodarowicz MK, Connors JM, et al. Randomized comparison of ABVD chemotherapy with a strategy that includes radiation therapy in patients with limited-stage Hodgkin's lymphoma: National Cancer Institute of Canada Clinical Trials Group and the Eastern Cooperative Oncology Group. J Clin Oncol 2005;23:4634–4642.

Noordijk E, Carde P, Hagenbeek A. Combination of radiotherapy and chemotherapy is advisable in all patients with clinical stage I-II Hodgkin's disease. Six-year results of the EORTC-GPMC controlled clinical trials "H7-VF", "H7-F" and "H7-U". Presented at ASTRO; 1997.

Noordijk EM, Thomas J, Ferme C, et al. First results of the EORTC-GELA H9 randomized trials: the H9-F trial (comparing 3 radiation dose levels) and H9-U trial (comparing 3 chemotherapy schemes) in patients with favorable or unfavorable early stage Hodgkin's lymphoma (HL). J Clin Oncol (Meeting abstracts) 2005;23:6505.

Noordijk, EM, Carde P, Dupouy N, et al. Combined-modality therapy for clinical stage I or II Hodgkin's lymphoma: long-term results of the European Oranization for Research and Treatment of Cancer (EORTC) H7 randomized controlled trials. J Clin Oncol 2006;24:3128–3135.

Pavlovsky S, Maschio M, Santarelli MT, et al. Randomized trial of chemotherapy versus chemotherapy plus radiotherapy for stage I–II Hodgkin's disease. J Natl Cancer Inst 1988;80(18): 1466–1473.

Picardi M, De Renzo A, Pane F, et al. Randomized comparison of consolidation radiation versus observation in bulky Hodgkin's lymphoma with post-chemotherapy negative positron emission tomography scans. Leuk Lymphoma 2007;48(9):1721–1727.

Press OW, LeBlanc M, Lichter AS, et al. Phase III randomized intergroup trial of subtotal lymphoid irradiation versus doxorubicin, vinblastine, and subtotal lymphoid irradiation for stage IA to IIA Hodgkin's disease. J Clin Oncol 2001;19:4238–4244.

Rigacci L, Vitolo U, Nassi L, et al. Positron emission tomography in the staging of patients with Hodgkin's lymphoma. Ann Hematol 2007;86:897–903.

Sieber M, Franklin J, Tesch H. Two Cycles ABVD plus extended field radiotherapy is superior to radiotherapy alone in early stage Hodgkin's disease: results of the German Hodgkin's Lymphoma Study Group (GHSG) Trial HD7. Leuk Lymphoma 2002;43(Suppl 2):52.

Sieniawski, M, Franklin J, Nogova, L et al. Outcome of patientS experiencing progression or relapse after primary treatment with two cycles of chemotherapy and radiotherapy for early-stage favorable Hodgkin's Lymphoma. J Clin Oncol 2007;25(15):2000–2005.

Specht L, Gray RG, Clarke MJ, et al. Influence of more extensive radiotherapy and adjuvant chemotherapy on long-term outcome of early-stage Hodgkin's disease: a meta-analysis of 23 randomized trials involving 3,888 patients. International Hodgkin's Disease Collaborative Group. J Clin Oncol 1998;16:830–843.

Straus DJ, Portlock CS, Qin J, et al. Results of a prospective randomized clinical trial of doxorubicin, bleomycin, vinblastine, and dacarbazine (ABVD) followed by radiation therapy (RT) versus ABVD alone for stages I, II, and IIIA nonbulky Hodgkin disease. Blood 2004;104: 3483–3489.

Thomas J, Ferme C, Noordijk EM, et al. EORTC lymphoma group; groupe d'études des lymphomes adultes (GELA). Results of the EORTC-GELA H9 randomized trials: The H9-F trial (comparing 3 radiation dose levels) and H9-U trial (comparing 3 chemotherapy schemes) in patients with favorable or unfavorable early stage Hodgkin's lymphoma (HL). Haematologica 2007;92(s5):27.

FURTHER READING

Bonadonna G, Bonfante V, Viviani S, et al. ABVD plus subtotal nodal versus involved-field radiotherapy in early-stage Hodgkin's disease: long-term results. J Clin Oncol 2004;22: 2835–2841.

Carde P, Noordijk EM, Hagenbeek A, et al. Superiority of EBVP chemotherapy in combination with involved field irradiation (EBVP/IF) over subtotal nodal irradiation (STNI) in favorable clinical stage (CS) I-II Hodgkin's disease: the EORTC-GPMC H7F randomized trial (Meeting abstract). J Clin Oncol 1997;16:16.

Chisesi T, Federico M, Levis A, et al. ABVD versus stanford V versus MEC in unfavourable Hodgkin's lymphoma: results of a randomised trial. Ann Oncol 2002;13(Suppl 1):102–106.

Cosset J. MOPP/ABV hybrid and irradiation in unfavourable supradiaphragmatic clinical stages I-II Hodgkin's lymphoma: preliminary results of the EORTC-GELA H8-U randomized trial (no. 20931) in 995 patients. Leuk Lymphoma 2001;42:12.

Girinsky T, van der Maazen, Specht L, et al. Involved-node radiotherapy (INRT) in patients with early Hodgkin lumphoma: concepts and guidelines. Radiother Oncol 2006;79:270–277.

Sieber M, Tesch H, Pfistner B, et al. Treatment of advanced Hodgkin's disease with COPP/ABV/IMEP versus COPP/ABVD and consolidating radiotherapy: final results of the German Hodgkin's Lymphoma Study Group HD6 trial. Ann Oncol 2004;15:276–282.

The NCCN Hodgkin Disease/Lymphoma Guidelines (Version 2.2008) in The Complete Library of NCCN Clinical Practice Guidelines in Oncology™ [CD-ROM] (March 2009). Fort Washington, Pennsylvania: © 2008 National Comprehensive Cancer Network, Inc; 2009.

Chapter 36
Non-Hodgkin's Lymphoma

Hans T. Chung, Stephen L. Shiao, and Naomi R. Schechter

PEARLS
EPIDEMIOLOGY

- Rising in incidence (2008 US incidence 66,120 and mortality 19,160); median age 60–65 years.
- Causative conditions:
  - Immunodeficiency – congenital (SCID, ataxia telangiectasia), acquired (HIV, organ transplant), autoimmune (Sjogren's, Hashimoto's disease, rheumatoid arthritis, systemic lupus erythematosus).
  - Environmental – chemicals (pesticides and solvents).
  - Viral – EBV (Burkitt's lymphoma and NK/T cell), HTLV-1 (human lymphotrophic virus, type I; adult T-cell leukemia in southern Japan and Caribbean, spread by breastfeeding, sex and blood products), HHV-8 (Kaposi's sarcoma), HCV (extra-nodal B-cell NHL).
  - Bacterial – *Helicobacter pylori* (MALT).
  - Radiation – weak association.
  - Chemo – alkylating agents.

HISTOLOGY

- *WHO classification*: B-cell neoplasms vs. T-cell and natural killer (NK) cell neoplasms.
- B cell (80%) = DLBCL (31%), follicular (22%), MALT (5%), B-cell CLL (6%), and mantle cell (6%).
- T cell (13%) = T/NK cell, peripheral T-cell lymphoma (6%), mycosis fungoides (<1%), anaplastic large cell (2%).
- *Low grade*: follicular (grade 1–2), CLL, MALT, mycosis fungoides.
- *Intermediate grade*: follicular (grade 3), mantle cell, DLBCL, T/NK cell, peripheral T-cell lymphoma, anaplastic large cell.
- *High grade*: Burkitt's lymphoma, lymphoblastic.
- DLBCL: 30–40% present with stage I–II disease. Extranodal disease is common.

- Follicular presentation = stage I–II (21%), III (19%), IV (60%). Histologic grade: 1 = follicular small cleaved, 2 = follicular mixed, 3 = follicular large.
- MALT (or extranodal marginal zone B-cell lymphoma) commonly involves stomach, ocular adnexae, skin, thyroid, parotid gland, lung, and breast. Most present as stage I–II (65–70%).
- Mantle cell: commonly presents with disseminated disease with spleen, bone marrow, and gastrointestinal involvement.
  - Associated with t(11;14)(q13;q32) translocation with overexpression of cyclin D1.
  - M:F 4:1, median age 60 years.
  - Associated with poor prognosis; median survival time 3 years.
- Immunophenotyping: see Appendix D.
- Cytogenetics: see Appendix D.

WORKUP

- H&P. Performance status. B symptoms. Thorough node examination. ENT examination if suprahyoid cervical LN involvement. Ophthalmologic examination for CNS lymphoma.
- Excisional LN biopsy with H&E, immunophenotyping, genotyping, and molecular profiling with microarrays.
- Labs: CBC, LFTs, creatinine, ESR, alkaline phosphatase, uric acid, LDH, HBsAg, HCV Ab, and HIV.
- Imaging: CXR, CT (chest/abdomen/pelvis ± neck). FDG-PET/CT scan (if unavailable, gallium scan; Tsukamoto 2007). Consider MRI.
- Bone marrow biopsy.
- CSF cytology if indicated (CNS or epidural lymphoma).
- Discuss fertility issues and sperm banking if pertinent.

STAGING

- *AJCC Ann Arbor staging system* used (see Chap. 35).
- *Limited stage*: stage I–II (≤3 adjacent LN regions), no B symptoms, and nonbulky (<10 cm).
- *Advanced stage*: stage II with more than three contiguous LN regions, stage III–IV, B symptoms, or bulky (≥10 cm).
- Sites that are extranodal, but not extralymphatic (therefore, not classified as E): Waldeyer's ring, thymus, and spleen.

International Prognostic Index (Fisher et al. 1993).

- For intermediate- and high-grade NHL.
- Adverse factors: age ≥60 years, stage III/IV, elevated LDH, reduced performance status (e.g., ECOG ≥2), and more than one site of extranodal involvement.
- Five-year OS by number adverse factors: 0–1 (73%), 2 (51%), 3 (43%), 4–5 (26%).

Follicular Lymphoma International Prognostic Index (FLIPI) (Solal-Céligny et al. 2004).

- Adverse factors: age (>60 years), stage III/IV, hemoglobin level (<120 g/L), number of nodal areas (>4), and elevated LDH.
- Five-year OS by number of adverse factors: 0–1 (91%), 2 (78%), ≥3 (53%).

Mantle Cell Lymphoma International Prognostic Index (MIPI) (Hoster et al. 2008).

- For advanced stage mantle cell lymphoma.
- Adverse factors: age (<50 = 0, 50–59=1, 60–69=2, ≥70=1), performance status (ECOG ≥2 = 2), lactate dehydrogenase (<0.67*upper limit of normal (ULN) = 0, 0.67–0.99*ULN=1, 1–1.49*ULN=2, ≥1.5*ULN = 3), and leukocyte count (<6.7 = 0, 6.7–9.9=1, 10–14.9=2, ≥15 = 3).
- Five-year OS by risk: low risk = 0–3 (70%), intermediate risk = 4–5 (45%), high risk = 6–11 (10%).

International response criteria for NHL (Cheson 2007): standardized response criteria for clinical trials with new guidelines for incorporating PET, immunohistochemistry, and flow cytometry. Standardized definitions of end points are provided as well.

IX

TREATMENT RECOMMENDATIONS

LOW-GRADE B-CELL NHL

Stage	Recommended treatment
Limited (10% of cases)	■ IFRT (25–36 Gy at 1.5–1.8 Gy/fx, depending on volume) ■ Median survival 10–15 years. 10-year DFS 40–50%. LC 90–100% ■ Transformation to DLBCL occurs in 10–15%
Advanced (90%)	■ Asymptomatic: observation

continued

	■ Symptomatic: decision to treat based on international criteria (GELF or FLIPI), which consider symptoms, threatened end-organ dysfunction, cytopenias, bulky disease at presentation, steady progression of disease, or patient preference. Treatment options include rituximab (R) ± chemotherapy (CHOP, CVP, or – fludarabineR-), radioimmunotherapy (RIT), or palliative local RT (4 Gy × 1 or 2 Gy × 2; Haas et al. 2003) Median survival 8–9 years (among <60 years, 10–12 years)
Relapse	■ High-dose chemo plus stem cell transplant, or radioimmunotherapy
Transformed Disease	■ Treat as per intermediate-grade disease ■ Rituxan is investigational in maintenance therapy ■ Transplant is also investigational

RADIOIMMUNOTHERAPY

- Indications
  - Relapsed or refractory low-grade, follicular, or transformed B-cell NHL, CD20+
  - Sixty to eighty percent response rate with 20–40% CR
- Contraindications
  - Known hypersensitivity to murine proteins
  - ≥25% marrow involvement by lymphoma
  - Platelets <100,000
  - Pregnancy, nursing mothers

Name	Decay	Half-life, dose	Dosimetry	Toxicity
Y-90 Ibritumomab (Zevalin)	Pure beta (2.3 MeV, 1.1 cm tissue range)	2.7 days 65–75 cGy	Pretreatment biodistribution scan, then treat day 7. Biodistribution improved with pretreatment nonlabeled tositumomab or rituximab	85% Grade 3–4 cytopenia nadir 8 weeks. MDS/AML 2%
I-131 Tositumomab (Bexaar)	Beta (0.6 MeV, 2.3 mm tissue range) and gamma (~0.33 MeV)	8 days 0.3–0.4 mCi/kg up to 32 mCi		70% grade 3–4 cytopenia nadir 6 weeks. MDS/AML 2% Hypothyroid 5%

continued

INTERMEDIATE-GRADE B-CELL NHL

Stage	Recommended treatment
Limited (30% of cases)	■ Favorable (nonbulky < 10 cm; stage I; < 60 years, PS 0–1, normal LDH) ■ R-CHOP (rituximab, cyclophosphamide, doxorubicin, vincristine, prednisone) × 3c, then IFRT (30–36 Gy) ■ Alternative: R-CHOP × 6–8c if RT contraindictated ■ Unfavorable (bulky; stage II; >60 years; PS ≥2; elevated LDH) ■ R-CHOP × 6–8c ± IFRT (30–36 Gy) ■ Alternative: R-CHOP × 3c + IFRT (30–36 Gy) ■ Bulky: R-CHOP × 6–8c + IFRT (30–40 Gy)
Advanced (70%)	■ R-CHOP × 6–8 ± radioimmunotherapy ■ Consider IFRT to initially bulky sites in select cases ■ Upfront transplant is investigational ■ Mantle cell lymphoma – R-CHOP or hyperCVAD ± R
Relapse	■ High-dose chemo plus stem cell transplant
Palliative	■ Solitary recurrence – RT ■ Diffuse disease – chemo (rituximab, etoposide, etc.)

*In testicular lymphoma, after completion of chemotherapy, RT (30–36 Gy) should be given to the contralateral testis.

HIGH-GRADE NHL

Stage	Recommended treatment
All cases	Combination chemo or clinical trial

Gastric MALT

Stage	Recommended treatment
Stage I–II	■ For *H. pylori* positive patients, 3–4 drug current antibiotic regimen with proton pump inhibitor for 2 weeks. CR 97–99%, but median time to CR is 6–8 months. t(11:18) is a predictor for lack of response to antibiotic therapy and these patients should be considered for RT. If disease persists despite antibiotic therapy or if H pylori negative, IFRT to entire stomach and perigastric nodes (30 Gy in 20 fractions). Local control >95%. If RT contraindicated, rituximab may be considered
Stage III–IV	■ Induction chemoimmunotherapy or IFRT indicated for symptoms, GI bleeding, threatened end-organ dysfunction, bulky disease, steady progression, or patient preference

IX

STUDIES

LIMITED STAGE LOW-GRADE LYMPHOMA

- Stanford (1996): 177 patients with stage I–II follicular lymphoma (FL) treated with RT alone. Twenty-five percent had staging laparotomy. Ten-year RFS and OS were 44 and 64%, respectively. Median survival was 13.8 years.
- *Royal Marsden Hospital* (Spier et al. 2004, 1994): 208 patients with clinical stage I/IE low-grade lymphoma treated with RT alone. Ten-year DFS/CSS was 47%/71%.
- *Princess Margaret Hospital* (*ASCO* 2004): 460 patients with clinical stage I–II FL treated with IFRT alone. Median follow-up 12.5 years. Ten-year DFS, CSS, and OS were 41, 79, and 62%. Late relapses after 10 years were infrequent.

ADVANCED STAGE LOW-GRADE LYMPHOMA

- *BNLI* (Ardeshna et al. 2003): 309 patients with stage III–IV. A low-grade lymphoma was randomized to immediate chlorambucil or observation. There was no difference in OS. MS was 5.9 years (chlorambucil) vs. 6.7 years (observation).
- *GLSG* (Hiddemann et al. 2005): 428 patients with symptomatic stage III–IV FL grades I–II randomized to either CHOP vs. R-CHOP. Median follow-up 18 months. R-CHOP significantly improved Time to treatment failure (TTF) and 2-year OS (95 vs. 90%).
- *EORTC 20921* (2006): 381 patients with treatment-naïve, advanced stage, low-grade lymphoma were randomized to CVP (cyclophosphamide, vincristine, and prednisone) or fludarabine. Fludarabine increased overall response rate from 58 to 75%, but had no effect on OS or TTP.
- *CVP±R* (Marcus et al. 2008): 321 patients with symptomatic stage III–IV FL grades I–II randomized to CVP vs. R-CVP. Median follow-up 53 months. TTF and OS (83 vs. 77%) were significantly improved with R-CVP vs. CVP.
- *Morschhauser Ibritumomab Trial* (Morschhauser et al. 2008): phase III trial of 414 patients with advanced FL treated with first-line chemotherapy with a complete or partial response were randomized to receive Y-90-Ibritumomab or no further treatment. Median observation of 3.5 years. Y-90-Ibritumomab significantly prolonged PFS in all patients (36.5 vs. 13.3 months); no difference between CR or PR after first-line chemo. Seventy-seven percent of patients with PR converted to CR. Main toxicity was grade III–IV hematologic toxicity.

LIMITED STAGE INTERMEDIATE-GRADE LYMPHOMA

- *SWOG 8736* (Spier et al. 2004): 401 patients with intermediate-grade, stage I/IE/II/IIE, or bulky stage I lymphoma were randomized to CHOP × 3 + IFRT (40–50 Gy) or CHOP × 8 alone. Five-year results (Miller et al. 1998) showed improved OS and FFS with CHOP-IFRT. Seven and 10-year results no longer show any difference in OS or FFS.
- *ECOG E1484* (2004): 352 patients with intermediate-grade, bulky or extranodal stage I, nonbulky stage II/IIE disease received CHOP × 8, then randomized to observation or IFRT (30–40 Gy). IFRT improved 6-year DFS (73 vs. 56%), but no OS difference.
- *GELA LNH93-1* (2005): 647 patients ≤ 60 years, stage I–II, IPI = 0 intermediate-grade NHL were randomized to ACVBP × 3 followed by consolidation chemo (no RT) or CHOP × 3 + IFRT (40 Gy). ACVBP significantly improved 5-year EFS and OS, regardless of bulky disease or not.
- *GELA LNH93-4* (Bonnet et al. 2007): 576 patients >60 years, stage I–II, IPI = 0 randomized to CHOPx4 + IFRT (40 Gy) vs. CHOP × 4. Median follow-up 7 years. Five-year EFS (64 vs. 61%) and OS (68 vs. 72%) showed no difference between the groups.
- *SEER* (2007): 6,743 patients with I–II DLBCL treated with RT (39%) or without RT (61%). RT improved 5 and 10-year OS (62→70%; 48→56%), regardless of age <60 or >60. Also, RT reduced 10 and 15-year risk of cardiac death (10→8%; 15→12%) for patients ≥60 years likely due to reduced athracycline chemo exposure, but not for patients <60 years.

ADVANCED STAGE INTERMEDIATE-GRADE LYMPHOMA

IX

- *SWOG 8516* (Fisher et al. 1993): 899 patients with bulky stage II, stage III–IV disease randomized to CHOP vs. three newer and more intensive chemo regimens (m-BACOD, ProMACE-CytaBOM, MACOP-B). No difference in OS, CR, or DFS.
- *GELA LNH98-5* (Coiffier et al. 2002, 2007): 399 patients >60 years with stage II–IV disease randomized to CHOP × 8 or CHOP × 8 plus rituximab. Median follow-up 7 years. R-CHOP improved CR (76 vs. 63%), 7-year EFS (42 vs. 25%) and OS (53 vs. 35%).
- *MINT* (2006): 824 patients ≤ 60 years with IPI 0–1, stage II–IV or bulky stage I DLBCL randomized to CHOP-like × 6 or CHOP-like + rituximab × 6. CHOP-like + R improved 3-year EFS (79 vs. 59%) and 3-year OS (93 vs. 84%).
- *Intergroup/ECOG 4494* (2006): 632 patients >60 years with stage I–IV DLBCL randomized to CHOP vs. R-CHOP and responders randomized to maintenance R vs. obs. R-CHOP

increased 3-years FFS (46→53%) and maintenance R increased 2-year FFS (61–76%), but not after prior R-CHOP. Therefore, R may be given as induction or maintenance tx.

- *RICOVER-60* (Pfreundschuh et al. 2008): 1,222 patients 61–80 years with stage I–IV DLBCL (50% stage III/IV) randomized to six vs. eight cycles of CHOP-14 (given at 2 week intervals) ± rituximab. Patients with initial bulky disease (diameter ≥7.5 cm) or extranodal involvement received 36 Gy RT. Six-cycle R-CHOP improved 3-year EFS (47→66%) and OS (68→78%) vs. CHOP alone, and there was no benefit of increasing to eight cycles of R-CHOP even for patients with only a PR after four cycles of chemo.
- *SWOG Tositumomab Trial S9911* (2006): phase II trial of 91 patients with advanced FL treated with CHOP × 6, then tositumomab/I-13. Median follow-up 5.1 years. Est 5-year OS and PFS are 87 and 67%, respectively, ~20% improvement of historical results with CHOP × 6. Basis for Phase III Intergroup Trial S0016 comparing CHOP + I-131 tositumomab and CHOP + Rituxan.

RELAPSED INTERMEDIATE-GRADE LYMPHOMA

- Milpied et al. (2004): 197 patients <60 years randomized to CHOP vs. high-dose chemo and stem cell transplant. High-dose improved 5-year EFS (37→55%) and also OS for patients with two adverse IPI risk factors (44→74%).
- *PARMA* (*ASCO* 1998): 109 of 215 patients with relapsed intermediate- or high-grade and responsive to induction DHAP × 2 were randomized to high-dose chemo (BEAC) + autologous bone marrow transplant or DHAP × 4. IFRT was indicated in both arms for bulky disease (>5 cm). Median follow-up was 100 months. Eight-year EFS and OS were significantly improved in the BMT arm. Relapses were decreased with the addition of IFRT in the BMT arm (36 vs. 55%).

GASTRIC MALT

- LY03 (Hancock et al. 2009) – chlorambucil vs. observation after anti-*H. pylori* treatment. No benefit to the addition of chlorambucil.
- GIT NHL 02/96 (2005) – shows that radical surgery not needed.

RADIATION TECHNIQUES

SIMULATION AND FIELD DESIGN

- IFRT fields are used. See descriptions in Chap. 35

DOSE PRESCRIPTIONS

- See treatment algorithm

DOSE LIMITATIONS

- Same as in Chap. 35

COMPLICATIONS

- Same as in Chap. 35

FOLLOW-UP

- Same as in Chap. 35

REFERENCES

Ardeshna KM, Smith P, Norton A, et al. Long-term effect of a watch and wait policy versus immediate systemic treatment for asymptomatic advanced-stage non-Hodgkin lymphoma: a randomised controlled trial. Lancet 2003;362:516-522.

Armitage JO. Defining the stages of aggressive non-Hodgkin's lymphoma – a work in progress. N Engl J Med 2005;352:1250-1252.

Ballonoff A, McCammon R, Schwer A, et al. Increased overall survival in patients with stages i and ii diffuse large b-cell lymphoma treated with radiation therapy: a surveillance, epidemiology, and end results (SEER) analysis. Int J Radiat Oncol Biol Phys 2007;69S:S15-S16.

Bonnet C, Fillet G, Mounier N, et al. CHOP alone compared with CHOP plus radiotherapy for localized aggressive lymphoma in elderly patients: a study by the Groupe d'Etude des Lymphomes de l'Adulte. J Clin Oncol 2007;25(7):787-792.

Brice P, Bastion Y, Lepage E, et al. Comparison in low-tumor-burden follicular lymphomas between an initial no-treatment policy, prednimustine, or interferon alfa: a randomized study from the Groupe d'Etude des Lymphomes Folliculaires. Groupe d'Etude des Lymphomes de l'Adulte. J Clin Oncol 1997;15:1110–1117.

Cheson BD, Pfistner B, Juweid ME, et al. Revised response criteria for malignant lymphoma. J Clin Oncol. 2007;25(5):579-586.

Coiffier B, Feugier P, Mounier N, et al. Long-term results of the GELA study comparing R-CHOP and CHOP chemotherapy in older patients with diffuse large B-cell lymphoma show good survival in poor-risk patients. J Clin Oncol 2007;25(suppl 18S):443s. Abstract 8009.

Coiffier B, Lepage E, Briere J, et al. CHOP Chemotherapy plus rituximab compared with CHOP alone in elderly patients with diffuse large-b-cell lymphoma. N Engl J Med 2002;346:235-242.

Feugier P et al. Long-term results of the r-chop study in the treatment of elderly patients with diffuse large B-cell lymphoma: a study by the Groupe d'Etude des Lymphomes de l'Adulte. J Clin Oncol 2005;23:4117-4126.

Fisher RI, Gaynor ER, Dahlberg S, et al. Comparison of a standard regimen (CHOP) with three intensive chemotherapy regimens for advanced non-Hodgkin's lymphoma. N Engl J Med 1993;328:1002-1006.

Guglielmi C, Gomez F, Philip T, Hagenbeek A, Martelli M, Sebban C, et al. Time to relapse has prognostic value in patients with aggressive lymphoma enrolled onto the Parma trial. J Clin Oncol 1998;16:3264-3269.

Haas R, Poortmans P, de Jong D, et al. High response rates and lasting remissions after low-dose involved field radiotherapy in indolent lymphomas. J Clin Oncol 2003;21(13):2474-2480.

Habermann T, Weller E, Morrison V, et al. Rituximab-CHOP versus CHOP alone or with maintenance rituximab in older patients with diffuse large B-cell lymphoma. J Clin Oncol 2006;24:3121-3127.

Hagenbeek A, Eghbali H, Monfardini S, et al. Phase III intergroup study of fludarabine phosphate compared with cyclophosphamide, vincristine, and prednisone chemotherapy in newly diagnosed patients with stage iii and IV low-grade malignant non-Hodgkin's lymphoma. J Clin Oncol 2006;24:1590-1596.

Hancock BW, Qian W, Linch D et al. Chlorambucil versus observation after anti-Helicobacter therapy in gastric MALT lymphomas: results of the international randomised LY03 trial. Br J Hematol 2009;144(3):367-375.

Hiddemann W, Kneba M, Dreyling M, et al. Frontline therapy with rituximab assed to the combination of cyclophosphamide, doxorubicin, vincristine and prednisone (CHOP) significantly improves the outcome for patient with advanced-stage follicular lymphoma compared with therapy with CHOP alone: results of a prospective randomized study of the German low-grade lymphoma study group. Blood 2005;106:3725-3732.

Horning SJ, Weller E, Kim K, et al. Chemotherapy with or without radiotherapy in limited-stage diffuse aggressive non-Hodgkin's lymphoma: Eastern Cooperative Oncology Group Study 1484. J Clin Oncol 2004;22:3032-3038.

Hoster E, Dreyling M, Klapper W et al. A new prognostic index (MIPI) for patients with advanced-stage mantle cell lymphoma. Blood 2008;111:558-565.

Koch P, Probst A, Berdel WE et al. Treatment results in localized primary gastric lymphoma: data of patients registered within the German Multicenter Study (GIT NHL 02/96). J Clin Oncol 2005;23(28):7050-7059.

Mac Manus MP, Hoppe RT. Is radiotherapy curative for stage I and II low-grade follicular lymphoma? Results of a long-term follow-up study of patients treated at Stanford University. J Clin Oncol 1996;14:1282-1290.

Marcus R, Imrie K, Solal-Celigny P, et al. Phase III study of R-CVP compared cyclophosphamide, vincristine and prednisone alone in patients with previously untreated advanced follicular lymphoma. J Clin Oncol 2008;26(28):4579-4586.

Miller TP, Dahlberg S, Cassady JR, et al. chemotherapy alone compared with chemotherapy plus radiotherapy for localized intermediate- and high-grade non-Hodgkin's lymphoma. N Engl J Med 1998;339:21-26.

Milpied N, Deconinck E, Gaillard F, et al. Initial treatment of aggressive lymphoma with high-dose chemotherapy and autologous stem-cell support. N Engl J Med 2004;350:1287-1295.

Pfreundschuh M, Trümper L, Österborg A, et al. CHOP-like chemotherapy plus rituximab versus CHOP-like chemotherapy alone in young patients with good-prognosis diffuse large-B-cell lymphoma: a randomised controlled trial by the MabThera International Trial (MInT) Group. Lancet Oncol 2006;7:379-391.

Morschhauser F, Radford J, Van Hoof A, et al. Phase II trial of consolidation therapy with yttrium-90-ibritumomab tiuxetan compared with no additional therapy after first remission in advanced follicular lymphoma. J Clin Oncol 2008;26(32):5156-5164.

Park SI, Press OW. Radioimmunotherapy for treatment of B-cell lymphomas and other hematologic malignancies. Curr Opin Hematol 2007;14(6):632-638.

Petersen PM, Gospodarowicz MK, Tsang RW, et al. Long-term outcome in stage I and II follicular lymphoma following treatment with involved field radiation therapy alone. J Clin Oncol 2004;22:6521.

Pfreundschuh M, Schubert J, Ziepert M, et al. Six versus eight cycles of bi-weekly CHOP-14 with or without rituximab in elderly patients with aggressive CD20+ B-cell lymphomas: a randomised controlled trial (RICOVER-60). Lancet Oncol 2008;9(2):105-116.

Pfreundschuh M, Trümper L, Ma D, et al. Randomized intergroup trial of first line treatment for patients <=60 years with diffuse large B-cell non-Hodgkin's lymphoma (DLBCL) with a CHOP-like regimen with or without the anti-CD20 antibody rituximab – early stopping after the first interim analysis. J Clin Oncol 2004;22:6500.

Philip T, Guglielmi C, Hagenbeek A, et al. Autologous bone marrow transplantation as compared with salvage chemotherapy in relapses of chemotherapy-sensitive non-Hodgkin's lymphoma. N Engl J Med 1995;333:1540-1545.

Press OW, Unger JM, Braziel RM, et al. Phase II trail of CHOP chemotherapy followed by tositumomab/iodine I-131 tositumomab for previously untreated follicular non-Hodgkin's lymphoma: fiver-year follow-up of Southwest Oncology Group Protocol S9911. J Clin Oncol 2006;24(25):4143-4149.

Reyes F, Lepage E, Ganem G, et al. ACVBP versus CHOP plus radiotherapy for localized aggressive lymphoma. N Engl J Med 2005;352:1197-1205.

Solal-Céligny P, Roy P, Colombat P, et al. Follicular lymphoma international prognostic index. Blood 2004;104(5):1258-1265.

Spier CM, LeBlanc M, Chase E, et al. Histologic subtypes do not confer unique outcomes in early-stage lymphoma: long-term follow-up of SWOG 8736. Blood 2004;104:abst 3263.

Tsukamoto N, Kojima M, Hasegawa M et al. The usefulness of (18)F-fluorodeoxyglucose positron emission tomography ((18)F-FDG-PET) and a comparison of (18)F-FDG-pet with (67)gallium scintigraphy in the evaluation of lymphoma: relation to histologic subtypes based on the World Health Organization classification. Cancer 2007;110(3):652-659.

Vaughan Hudson B, Vaughan Hudson G, MacLennan KA, et al. Clinical stage 1 non-Hodgkin's lymphoma: long-term follow-up of patients treated by the British National Lymphoma Investigation with radiotherapy alone as initial therapy. Br J Cancer 1994;69:1088-1093.

Chapter 37
Cutaneous Lymphomas

Amy Gillis, Thomas T. Bui, and Mack Roach III

PEARLS

- Primary cutaneous lymphomas (PCL) are subdivided according to cell lineage. These include cutaneous B-cell lymphomas (CBCL) – 30% and cutaneous T-cell lymphomas (CTCL) – 70%.
- Overall, 1–1.5 new cases per 100,000/year. Annual age-adjusted incidence of CBCL was 4 per million; CTCL was 6 per million persons (Hoppe et al. 2004; Yahalom et al. 2004).
- Skin is the most common extranodal site of non-Hodgkin's lymphoma (NHL), representing 2% of new cases of NHL.
- Affects older adults (55–60 years), 2:1 male predominance, blacks > whites.
- Hypothesized links with environmental factors or viral etiology not substantiated (de Jong et al. 2008)
- Presentation: skin lesions, but long natural history. Median time from skin lesion to diagnosis ~5 years.
- Sézary cells: malignant T-cells. Sézary syndrome: erythroderma, lymphadenopathy, and Sézary cells in peripheral blood.
- Treatment should be tailored to specific subtype of PCL.
- Unlike other NHL's, which use the Ann Arbor staging system, Mycosis fungoides/Sézary syndrome (MF/SS) uses a TNM staging system that correlates to prognosis (Kim et al. 2007; Horwitz et al. 2008).
- EORTC and WHO have classification schemes as well (Willemze et al. 2005; Golling et al. 2008).

WORKUP

- Complete history and physical examination. Include examination of entire skin LN examination.
- Incisional or excisional skin biopsies (several often needed to diagnose; dermatopathology review essential). Include immunophenotyping as appropriate.
- LN biopsy, if clinically indicated.

- Laboratory studies: CBC with manual differential, Sézary cell count, Sézary flow cytometry, CMP, LDH, ALT, AST, PCR for T-cell receptor gene rearrangement.
- Imaging studies: Chest X-ray (if limited disease only), CT neck/chest/abdomen/pelvis, or integrated whole body PET/CT.
- May also need peripheral blood smear for Sézary cells or bone marrow biopsy as appropriate, depending on histology.

WHO-EORTC CLASSIFICATION WITH SURVIVAL (WILLEMZE ET AL. 2005)[a]

WHO-EORTC	Frequency (%)	5-year DS survival (%)
Cutaneous T-cell lymphomas		
Indolent		
Mycosis fungoides	44	88
Primary cutaneous anaplastic large cell	8	95
Lymphatoid papulosis	12	100
Aggressive		
Sézary Syndrome	3	24
Primary cutaneous T-cell, peripheral or aggressive CD8+	~2	16–18
Cutaneous B-cell lymphomas		
Indolent		
Follicle center lymphoma	11	95
Marginal Zone B-cell lymphoma	7	99
Intermediate		
Large B-cell lymphoma of the leg	4	55
Other diffuse large B-cell	<1	50

[a]Adapted from Willemze et al. 2005. Copyright American Society of Hematology, used with permission. See reference for complete classification.

STAGING

TNM staging systems exist for Mycosis Fungiodes/Sézary Syndrome. See the AJCC Cancer Staging Manual, 7th Edition (2010) published by Springer, New York, www.springer.com. There is no change from the 2002 Edition. A modified and updated TNM staging system has been published (Olsen et al. 2007).

TNM staging systems also exist for cutaneous lymphomas other than MF/Sézary Syndrome, as developed by the EORTC and International Society for Cutaneous Lymphomas. (Kim et al. 2007).

TREATMENT RECOMMENDATIONS AND STUDIES BY CELL TYPE

B-cell cutaneous lymphomas

Typical treatment for cutaneous marginal zone and follicular center lymphomas

- Locoregional disease: treat with locoregional RT or excision; in selected cases, observation or topical medications
- Generalized disease within skin: observation or rituximab; for palliation use locoregional RT or chemotherapy

Primary cutaneous marginal zone lymphoma: B-cell

- Typically presents with deep-seated nodular or papular lesions on the upper extremities or trunk
- Lacks extracutaneous involvement at the time of diagnosis
- Indolent disease course for localized disease as reviewed in 18 studies showing typical CR
- When RT used primarily, excellent prognosis with a 5-year OS and DSS of 90% and 95%, respectively
- Dutch Cutaneous Lymphoma Working Group registry analysis (Senff et al. 2007): MZL managed with RT as primary treatment had cutaneous relapses only at nonirradiated sites

Primary cutaneous follicular center lymphoma: B-cell

- Affects the scalp, neck, and trunk indolently
- Typically express CD20, CD79a, and bcl-6
- Radiation used as first-line treatment
- When RT used primarily, excellent prognosis with a 5-year OS and DSS were 90% and 97%, respectively

Primary cutaneous diffuse large B-cell

- Leg presentation ("leg type") portends poorer prognosis
- Expression of bcl-2, Mum-1, and OCT2 was significantly associated with a poor OS and DSS
- Treat with R-CHOP ± IFRT; consider using dose-dense R-CHOP
- RT alone should not be considered first choice. M.D. Anderson experience (Sarris et al. 2001): RT alone has poorer prognosis: OS 25% RT alone vs. 77% with RT + doxorubicin-based chemo

IX

T-cell cutaneous lymphomas

Lymphatoid papulosis: T-cell

- Fourteen percent of PCL, 100% 5-year survival
- Distributed mainly at trunk and proximal portions of limbs
- Diffuse papular, papulonecrotic, or nodular skin lesions
- Often generalized, common to have spontaneous remissions, and lesions can wax and wane
- Transition to other lymphoma rare
- Often no treatment needed
- Palliation can be achieved with PUVA, methotrexate, interferon, topical/intralesional steroids, and topical bexarotene

continued

ALCL (anaplastic large-cell lymphoma): T-cell

- Rarely fatal
- Possible link between silicone breast prostheses and ALCL requires further study; absolute risk is exceedingly low due to the rare occurrence of ALCL of the breast
- Systemic ALCL associated with translocation [t(2;5)(p23;q35)], which occurs in 40–60% of patients
- Localized diseases are typically treated with RT (40 Gy) or local excision;10-year survival >90%
- Treat relapse with additional RT or low-dose methotrexate

CTCL: mycosis fungoides (MF) and Sézary syndrome (SS): T-cell

- Median duration from lesion onset to diagnosis: 8–10 years
- Median survival from diagnosis: 5–10 years
- With lymph node involvement: median survival <2 years
- Visceral organ involvement: median survival <1 year
- Occurs more frequently in men than women
- Usually located at trunk and proximal thigh
- Diagnosis of SS based on the triad of erythroderma, lymphadenopathy, and the presence of Sézary cells (atypical cells with convoluted nuclei) in the peripheral blood exceeding 10–15%
- At autopsy: 80% have extracutaneous involvement

TREATMENT RECOMMENDATIONS: MYCOSIS FUNGIODES

Disease extent	Recommended treatment
Limited patch/ plaque	■ Local/Topical treatment: Steroids, retinoids, imiquimod, topical chemotherapeutics, and/or phototherapy [narrow-band UVB given 3 ×/week for an initial clearing regimen for patch or thin-plaque disease; Psoralen plus UVA (PUVA) given 2–3 ×/week for thicker plaques] ■ Local electron beam therapy (EBT) 24–36 Gy
Multiple patches <1 cm in diameter ± abnormal LN	■ Local/Topical treatment: as above ■ Total skin electron beam therapy (TSEBT) to 30–36 Gy
One or more tumors ≥1 cm ± abnormal LN	Few tumors ■ Local EBT ■ Systemic treatment: retiniods, IFNs, HDAC inhibitors, extracorporeal photopheresis, MTX ± local EBT Generalized tumors ■ TSEBT ■ Systemic treatment as above, or other chemotherapies ± local EBT

continued

Confluence of patches >80% BSA ± abnormal LN	■ Systemic treatment as above ± local EBT ■ Total skin electron beam therapy (TSEBT) to 30–36 Gy ■ Systemic treatment ± local treatment ± local EBT
Abnormal LN with poor path features; Sézary syndrome or visceral dz	■ Combined modality treatment may include systemic treatment, local treatment, and RT

RADIATION TECHNIQUES

TREATMENT AND DOSE

- Low doses effective, 24–36 Gy.
- Palliative: 100–200 kV X-rays or 6–9 MeV electrons, often 15 Gy (3 Gy × 5 fx or 5 Gy × 3 fx).
- Individualize treatment to the site of disease. Local or locoregional field typically treated to 30–36 Gy (1.5–2 Gy/fx).

TOTAL SKIN ELECTRON BEAM (TSEB)

- Six patient positions: Anterior, posterior, 2 posterior obliques, and 2 anterior obliques.
- Six-dual field technique = 6 patients positions, each with superior and inferior fields.
- Patient standing, 3.5 m from electron source.
- Lucite plate near patient surface to scatter electrons.
- Machine angled at 18°, up/down for homogeneity at patient surface; dose inhomogeneity in air at treatment distance should be <10% within vertical and lateral dimensions.
- Eighty percent isodose line should be ≥4 mm deep to the skin surface to ensure epidermis and dermis fall within high-dose region.
- Twenty percent isodose line should be <20 mm from the skin surface to minimize dose to underlying structures.
- Total dose to bone marrow from photon contamination should be less than 0.7 Gy.
- 30–36 Gy in 1.5–2 Gy/fx with 1-week break midtreatment, if significant skin erythema occurs.
- Thicker or tumorous lesions may require boost; supplemental patch fields used to ensure surface dose ≥50% of prescribed TSEB dose.
- Treat three patient positions each day, 2-day treatment cycle, 4 days/week for 9 weeks.

COMPLICATIONS

- Local RT, Acute side effects: erythema, dry desquamation, pruritis locally. If regional, RT may also include edema of affected limb.
- Intermediate: fatigue, alopecia (temporary if scalp dose limited to 25 Gy), hyperpigmentation.
- TSEB: Temporary loss of toe/finger nails, localized anhydrosis, rarely mild epistaxis, and parotiditis.
- TSEB, Chronic side effects: persistent nail dystrophy, xerosis, telangiectasias, permanent partial alopecia, fingertip anesthesia, and possible infertility in male patients.
- Secondary cutaneous malignancies possible: SCC, BCC, and malignant melanoma.

FOLLOW-UP

- Regular clinic visits with complete history and physical.
- With RT, expect continued regression 6–8 weeks posttreatment.

REFERENCES

Olsen E, Vonderheid E, Pimpinelli N, et al. Revisions to the staging and classification of mycosis fungoides and Sézary syndrome: a proposal of the International Society for cutaneous lymphomas (ISCL) and the cutaneous lymphoma task force of the European Organization of Research and Treatment of Cancer (EORTC). Blood. 2007;110:1713-1722.

Sarris AH, Braunschweig I, et al. Primary cutaneous non-Hodgkin's lymphoma of Ann Arbor stage I: preferential cutaneous relapses but high cure rate with doxorubicin-based therapy. J Clin Oncol. 2001;19(2):398-405.

Senff NJ, Hoefnagel JJ, Neelis KJ, et al. for the Dutch Cutaneous Lymphoma Group. Results of radiotherapy in 153 primary cutaneous B-cell lymphomas classified according to the WHO-EORTC classification. Arch Dermatol. 2007;143(12):1520-1526.

Willemze R, Jaffe ES, et al. WHO-EORTC classification for cutaneous lymphomas. Blood. 2005;105(10): 3768-3785.

FURTHER READINGS

Carter J, Zug K. Phototherapy for cutaneous T-cell lymphoma: Online survey and literature review. J Am Acad Dermatol. 2009;60:39-50.

de Jong D, Vasmel W, de Boer JP, et al. Anaplastic large-cell lymphoma in women with breast implants. JAMA. 2008;300(17):2030-2035.

Golling P, Cozzio A, Dummer R, et al. Primary cutaneous B-cell lymphomas – clinicopathological, prognostic and therapeutic characterisation of 54 cases according to the WHO-EORTC classification and the ISCL/EORTC TNM classification system for primary cutaneous lymphomas other than mycosis fungoides and Sézary syndrome. Leuk Lymphoma. 2008;49(6):1094-1103.

Hoppe RT, Kim Y. Mycosis Fungiodes. In: Leibel SA, Phillips TL, editors. Textbook of radiation oncology. 2nd ed. Philadelphia: Saunders; 2004. pp. 1417-1431.

Horwitz S, Olsen E, Duvic M, et al. Review of the treatment of mycosis fungoides and Sézary syndrome: a stage-based approach. JNCCN. 2008;6:436-442.

Kim Y, Willemze R, Pimpinelli N, et al. TNM classification system for cutaneous lymphomas other than mycosis fungoides and sézary syndrome: a proposal of the International Society for Cutaneous Lymphomas (ISCL) and the Cutaneous Lymphoma Task Force of the European Organization of Research and Treatment of Cancer (EORTC). Blood. 2007;110:479-484.

National Comprehensive Cancer Network. Clinical Practice Guidelines in Oncology v1.2010: Multiple Myeloma. Available at http://www.nccn.org/professionals/physician_gls/PDF/nhl.pdf. Accessed on March 3, 2010.

Yahalom J. Non-Hodgkin's lymphoma. In: Leibel SA, Phillips TL, editors. Textbook of radiation oncology. 2nd ed. Philadelphia: Saunders; 2004. pp. 1393-1416.

Chapter 38
Multiple Myeloma and Plasmacytoma

Thomas T. Bui, Kavita Mishra, and Mack Roach III

PEARLS

- Plasma cell tumors are monoclonal tumors of immunoglobulin-secreting cells, derived from B-cell lymphocytes.
- Incidence is low overall, ~1–2% of U.S. cancers diagnosed yearly are plasma cell tumors. More than 90% of these are multiple myeloma (MM); ~2–10% are solitary plasmacytoma (SP).
- MM incidence higher in blacks than whites (~2:1). Median age at diagnosis 70 years.
- SP more common in men than women (4:1). Median age at diagnosis 50–55 years.
- Etiology is unknown, may involve occupational exposures, RT, solvents (Nau et al. 2008).
- 20% of patients are free of clinical symptoms at diagnosis.
- Osseous SP and MM may manifest as bone pain, neurologic symptoms, pathologic fracture, cord compression, anemia, hypercalcemia, renal insufficiency (Schechter et al. 2003).
- ~80% of extraosseous SP occur in upper aerodigestive tract. Common presenting signs include epistaxis, nasal discharge, nasal obstruction.
- 50–80% of patients with osseous SP progress to MM at a median ~2–3 years after treatment. Factors that predict for conversion are controversial, but may include lesion size ≥5 cm, age >40 year old, presence of M spike, spinal location, persistence of M-protein after RT.
- 10–40% of patients with extraosseous SP progress to MM at 10 years (Hodgson et al. 2008).
- Bone marrow in MM >10% plasma cells. Immunoperoxidase staining detects either kappa or lambda light chains, but not both, in the cytoplasm of bone marrow plasma cells.

WORKUP

- H&P.
- CBC and differential with examination of peripheral smear, chemistries, LFTs, albumin, calcium.
- SPEP with immunofixation and quantitation of immunoglobulins, 24-hr UPEP and immunofixation. Twenty-four-hour urine for Bence-Jones proteins (National Comprehensive Cancer Network, 2010).
- Serum viscosity if M-protein concentration >5 g/dL.
- Beta-2 microglobulin, LDH, and C-reactive protein reflect tumor burden.
- Unilateral bone marrow aspirate and biopsy.
- Bone marrow immunohistochemistry and/or bone marrow flow cytometry.
- Skeletal survey. Bone scan often noncontributory since purely lytic lesions with low isotope uptake.
- Cytogenetics.
- FISH [del 13, del 17, t(4;14), t(11;14), t(14;16)].
- CXR.
- Consider MRI for suspected vertebral compression.
- Consider CT (avoid contrast per NCCN Practice Guidelines) if painful weightbearing areas.
- Consider PET/CT scan for suspicion of plasmacytoma of bone.
- Solitary plasmacytoma: need confirmatory tissue biopsy of single lesion; normal BM biopsy (<10% plasma cells), negative skeletal survey, and no signs or symptoms of systemic disease (Smith et al. 2006).
- Smoldering myeloma (asymptomatic myeloma): serum M-protein ≥30 g/L *and/or* BM clonal plasma cells ≥10%; no end organ damage (including bone lesions), anemia, hypercalcemia, or symptoms (Kyle et al. 1980).

STAGING

Durie-Salmon myeloma staging system[1]

Stage	*Criteria*	*Measured myeloma cell mass (cells × $10^{12}/m^2$)*
I	All of the following: 1. Hemoglobin value >10 g/100 mL 2. Serum calcium value normal (≤12 mg/100 mL) 3. Bone X-ray, normal bone structure, or solitary bone plasmacytoma only 4. Low M-component production rates	<0.6 (Low)

continued

	■ IgG value <5 g/100 mL ■ IgA value <3 g/100 mL ■ Urine light chain M-component on electrophoresis <4 g/24 h	
II	Fitting neither stage I nor stage III	0.6–1.20 (intermediate)
III	One or more of the following: 1. Hemoglobin value <8.5 g/100 mL 2. Serum calcium value >12 mg/100 mL 3. Advanced lytic bone lesions 4. High M-component production rates ■ IgG value >7 g/100 mL ■ IgA value >5 g/100 mL ■ Urine light chain M-component on electrophoresis >12 g/24 h	>1.20 (high)

Subclassification

A: Relatively normal renal function (serum creatinine value <2.0 mg/100 mL).

B: Abnormal renal function (serum creatinine value ≥2.0 mg/100 mL).

New international staging system[2]

Stage	*Criteria*	*MS (months)*
I	Serum β2-microglobulin <3.5 mg/L Serum albumin ≥3.5 g/dL	62
II	Neither stage I nor stage III	44
III	Serum β2-microglobulin ≥5.5 mg/L	29

[1]From Durie BGM, Salmon SE: A clinical staging system for multiple myeloma. *Cancer* 36:842-854, 1975. Copyright 1975 American Cancer Society. This material is reproduced with permission of Wiley-Liss, Inc., a subsidiary of Wiley, Inc.

[2]From Greipp PR, San Miguel J, Durie BG, et al. International staging system for multiple myeloma. *J Clin Oncol* 2005; 23: 3412-20. Reprinted with permission from the American Society of Clinical Oncology.

IX

TREATMENT RECOMMENDATIONS

Stage	**Recommended treatment**
I or systemic smoldering	■ Observe
SP – osseous	■ Involved field RT (≥45 Gy). LC ~90%, MS ~10 year, ~70% progress to MM
SP – extraosseous	■ Involved field RT (≥45 Gy) alone, surgery alone, or surgery + RT. LC >90%, MS >10 years, ~30% progress to MM

continued

II or III	■ Chemo (e.g., melphalan + prednisone) + bisphosphonate. ■ Consider allogenic or autologous stem cell transplant. Consider RT for palliation of local bone pain, prevention of pathologic fractures, relief of spinal cord compression.

STUDIES

- Hu (2000): Review article of SP literature, including total 338 patients with SP. Patients with osseous SP have LC rate 88–100%, rate of progression to MM 50–80% at 10 years, 10-year OS 45–70%. Patients with extraosseous SP have LC 80–100%, rate of progression to MM 10–40% at 10 years, 10-year OS 40–90%.
- Alexiou et al. (1999): Review article of 400+ publications with total 869 patients with extraosseous SP treated with RT alone, surgery alone, or combined surgery + RT. In upper aerodigestive (UAD) tract tumors, combined treatment resulted in higher OS; however, in non-UAD located tumors, there was no survival difference between treatment arms. Low risk of lymph node involvement (7.6% in UAD, 2.6% in non-UAD areas).
- Catell et al. (1998): Twenty-seven patients with MM affecting long bones received radiation to symptomatic lesion, plus a margin of 1–2 cm with no attempt to treat entire shaft. Only four patients developed progressive disease in the same bone, but outside the previously irradiated field.
- *IFM 9502* (2002): 282 patients with MM undergoing conditioning regimens before autologous stem-cell transplantation randomized to high-dose melphalan vs TBI (8 Gy in 4 fx) + lower dose melphalan. TBI arm had greater hematologic toxicity, higher toxic death rate, and decreased 45-month OS (45.5% vs. 66%).
- *Myeloma Aredia Study Group* (1996): 377n patients with stage III myeloma and at least 1 lytic lesion randomized to antimyeloma treatment plus either placebo or pamidronate (monthly infusions × 9 cycles). Pamidronate arm had significantly less skeletal events (24% vs. 41%) and had decreased bone pain.

RADIATION TECHNIQUES

SIMULATION AND FIELD DESIGN

- SP: Involved field RT including involved bone +2–3 cm margin. Use CT/MRI to delineate tumor extent, especially paravertebral extension. FDG-PET may help assess response after RT (Kim et al. 2008). For extraosseous SP, may include primary draining LN.

- MM: Main indication is for palliation. For symptomatic bony lesions, include entire bone if possible. May limit long bone/pelvis fields to decrease dose to bone marrow. If treating vertebral column, include involved vertebrae +2 vertebrae above and 2 below.
- Use limited involved fields to limit the impact of irradiation on stem-cell harvest or impact on potential future treatments.

DOSE PRESCRIPTIONS

- SP: 45–50 Gy over 4–5 weeks, 1.8–2 Gy/fx.
- MM is very radioresponsive, so lower doses can be given compared with standard palliative RT doses for bony mets from solid tumors (Ozsahin et al. 2006).
- MM: low-dose RT (10–30 Gy) in 1.5–2 Gy fractions can be used as palliative treatment for uncontrolled pain, for impending pathologic fracture, or impending cord compression. May increase dose to 30–36 Gy for cord compression, bulky soft tissue component, and incomplete palliation.

DOSE LIMITATIONS

- Varies based on organs within involved field
- Spinal cord <45 Gy at 1.8 Gy/fx

COMPLICATIONS

- Normal tissue toxicity within RT field
- Myelosuppression
- MM: hypercalcemia, anemia, renal insufficiency, infection, skeletal lesions

IX

FOLLOW-UP

- Systemic myeloma: Quantitative immunoglobulins + M-protein every 3 months. Follow CBC, serum BUN, Cr, Ca. Bone survey annually or for symptoms. Bone marrow biopsy as indicated.
- Smoldering multiple myeloma: Quantitative immunoglobulins + M-protein every 3 months. CBC, serum BUN, Cr, Ca every 3–4 months.
- SP osseous: As above + measure paraprotein every 3–6 months.
- SP extraosseous: Paraprotein every 3 months × 1 year, then annually. CT/MRI every 6 months × 1 year, then as clinically indicated.

REFERENCES

Alexiou C, Kau RJ, Dietzfelbinger H, et al. Extramedullary plasmacytoma: tumor occurrence and therapeutic concepts. Cancer 1999;85:2305-2314.

Catell D, Kogen Z, Donahue B, et al. Multiple myeloma of an extremity: must the entire bone be treated? Int J Radiat Oncol Biol Phys. 1998;40(1):117-119.

Creach CM, Foote RL, Netten-Wittich MA, et al. Radiotherapy for extramedullary plasmacytoma of the head and neck. Int J Radiat Oncol Biol Phys. 2009;73(3):789-794.

Hodgson DC, Mikhael J, Tsang RW. Plamsa cell myeloma and plasmacytomas. In: Halperin EC, Perez CA, Brady LW, editors. Principles and practice of radiation oncology. 5th ed. Philadelphia: Lippincott Williams & Wilkins; 2008.

Hu K,Yahalom J. Radiotherapy in the Management of Plasma Cell Tumors. Oncology. 2000;14(1): 100-111.

Intergroupe Francophone du Myelome. Comparison of 200 mg/m(2) melphalan and 8 Gy total body irradiation plus 140 mg/m(2) melphalan as conditioning regimens for peripheral blood stem cell transplantation in patients with newly diagnosed multiple myeloma: final analysis of the Intergroupe Francophone du Myelome 9502 randomized trial. Blood 2002;99:731-735.

Kim P, Hicks RJ, Wirth A, et al. Impact of (18)F-Fluorodeoxyglucose positron emission tomography before and after definitive radiation therapy in patients with apparently solitary plasmacytoma. Int J Radiat Oncol Biol Phys. 2008;74:740–746.

Kyle RA, Greipp PR. Smoldering multiple myeloma. N Engl J Med. 1980;302:1347.

Myeloma Aredia Study Group. Efficacy of pamidronate in reducing skeletal events in patients with advanced multiple myeloma. N Engl J Med. 1996;334:488-493.

National Comprehensive Cancer Network. Clinical Practice Guidelines in Oncology v3.2010: Multiple Myeloma. Available at http://www.nccn.org/professionals/physician_gls/PDF/myeloma.pdf. Accessed on March 3, 2010.

Nau K, Lewis W. Multiple myeloma: diagnosis and treatment. Am Fam Physician. 2008;78(7): 853-859, 860.

Ozsahin M, Tsang RW, Poortmans P, et al. Outcomes and patterns of failure in solitary plasmacytoma: a multicenter Rare Cancer Network study of 258 patients. Int J Radiat Oncol Biol Phys. 2006;64(1):210-217.

Schechter NR, Lewis VO. The Bone. In: Cox JD, Ang KK, editors. Radiation oncology: rationale, technique, results. 8th ed. St. Louis: Mosby; 2003. pp. 857-883.

Smith A, Wisloff F, Samson D. Guidelines on the diagnosis and management of multiple myeloma 2005. Br J Haematol. 2006;132(4):410-451.

FURTHER READINGS

Hu K,Yahalom J. Radiotherapy in the Management of Plasma Cell Tumors. Oncology. 2000;14(1): 100-111.

PART X
Musculoskeletal Sites

X

Chapter 39
Bone Tumors

Tania Kaprealian, Brian Lee, and Jean L. Nakamura

PEARLS

- Diaphysis = shaft; epiphysis = growth plate and end of bone; metaphysis = conical portion between diaphysis and epiphysis.
- Prevalence: Osteosarcoma > chondrosarcoma > Ewing's > malignant fibrous histiocytoma (MFH).
- Sixty percent cases occur between 10 and 20 years of age (most active age of skeletal growth).
- Eighty percent cases in long bones until epiphyseal closure (then ~occur with appendicular skeleton).
- In patients >60 years, >50% cases arise from other conditions (i.e., Paget's disease, fibrous dysplasia) → poor chemo response.
- Osteosarcoma: Malignant osteoid is hallmark (not seen in chondrosarcoma). Most common bone tumor in children. Seventy-five percent present in metaphyses of long bones with local pain/swelling. Eighty-five percent are grades 3–4. Osteosarcoma arising as second malignancy s/p chemo or RT does not necessarily have worse prognosis, but controversial. Associated with Li-Fraumeni Syndrome (p53) and retinoblastoma.
- Periosteal (juxtacortical) osteosarcomas are usually low-grade, localized with rare DM. Most present in popliteal fossa. Eighty to ninety percent curable with surgery alone.
- Osteosarcoma: Most common in femur > tibia > humerus. DM most common in lung > bone/BM.
- Chondrosarcoma: ~25% of all primary bone cancers. Most common in the femur. Frequent local recurrence, DM less common than osteosarcoma. 1/3 are high-grade.
- MFH: Very aggressive locally with frequent DM. Often presents with fracture.
- Fibrosarcoma: High-grade, behaves like osteosarcoma. Commonly presents with fractures.
- Chordoma: Physaliferous cell ("bubbly cell") is hallmark. Most often in sacrococcygeal area, base of skull, and spine. Presentation is location specific.

X

- Giant cell tumors = giant multinucleated osteoclast cells. Only 8–15% are malignant. Cyst formation, hemorrhage, necrosis are important with regard to radiosensitivity. Frequent LR (45–60%).
- Lung metastases common in osteosarcoma, chondrosarcoma, MFH.

WORKUP

- H&P.
- CBC, chemistries, urinalysis, ESR, alkaline phosphatase.
- Plain films (primary region and CXR) – Codman's triangle, periosteal bone spicules, 1° tumor often seen as cloud-like density.
- CT/MRI (primary area and chest) to evaluate soft tissue extensions.
- Bone scan – Intramedullary skip metastases. Consider PET scan.
- Biopsy lesion after complete radiologic evaluation and avoid incision over area not to be irradiated or re-excised. Biopsy should be performed at institution where treatment will occur.

DIFFERENTIATING EWING'S FROM OSTEOSARCOMA

Ewing's	Osteosarcoma
Lytic, destructive lesion	Sclerotic lesion
Diaphysis	Metaphysis
Onion skin effect	Sunburst pattern (periosteal new bone formation)

STAGING: BONE TUMORS

Editors' note: All TNM stage and stage groups referred to elsewhere in this chapter reflect the 2002 AJCC staging nomenclature unless otherwise noted as the new system below was published after this chapter was written.

(AJCC 6TH ED., 2002)

Primary tumor (T)
TX: Primary tumor cannot be assessed
T0: No evidence of primary tumor
T1: Tumor ≤8 cm in greatest dimension
T2: Tumor >8 cm in greatest dimension
T3: Discontinuous tumors in the primary bone site

Regional lymph nodes (N)
NX*: Regional lymph nodes cannot be assessed
N0: No regional lymph node metastasis
N1: Regional lymph node metastasis

*Because of the rarity of lymph node involvement in sarcomas, the designation NX may not be appropriate and could be considered N0 if no clinical involvement is evident.

Distant metastasis (M)
MX: Distant metastasis cannot be assessed
M0: No distant metastasis
M1: Distant metastasis
M1a: Lung
M1b: Other distant sites

Stage grouping
IA: T1N0M0 G1–2, low grade
IB: T2N0M0 G1–2, low grade
IIA: T1N0M0 G3–4, high grade
IIB: T2N0M0 G3–4, high grade
III: T3N0M0 any G

(AJCC 7TH ED., 2010)

Primary tumor (T)
TX: Primary tumor cannot be assessed
T0: No evidence of primary tumor
T1: Tumor 8 cm or less in greatest dimension
T2: Tumor more than 8 cm in greatest dimension
T3: Discontinuous tumors in the primary bone site

Regional lymph nodes (N)
NX: Regional lymph nodes cannot be assessed
N0: No regional lymph node metastasis
N1: Regional lymph node metastasis

Note: Because of the rarity of lymph node involvement in bone sarcomas, the designation NX may not be appropriate and cases should be considered N0 unless clinical node involvement is clearly evident.

Distant metastasis (M)
M0: No distant metastasis
M1: Distant metastasis
M1a: Lung
M1b: Other distant sites

Anatomic stage/prognostic groups
IA: T1 N0 M0 G1,2 low grade, GX
IB: T2 N0 M0 G1,2 low grade, GX
T3: N0 M0 G1,2 low grade, GX
IIA: T1 N0 M0 G3, 4 high grade
IIB: T2 N0 M0 G3, 4 high grade
III: T3 N0 M0 G3, 4

continued

X

IVA: Any T N0 M1a any G IVB: Any T N1 any M any G Any T any N M1b any G **~5-year OS by histology** Osteosarcoma: 60–75% (20% if M1) Chondrosarcoma: 50–70% MFH: 15–67% Fibrosarcoma: 25–50% Malignant giant cell tumor: 30% Used with the permission from the American Joint Committee on Cancer (AJCC), Chicago, IL. The original source for this material is the AJCC Cancer Staging Manual, Sixth Edition (2002), published by Springer Science+Business Media.	IVA: Any T N0 M1a any G IVB: Any T N1 any M any G Any T any N M1b any G Used with the permission of the American Joint Committee on Cancer (AJCC), Chicago, Illinois. The original source for this material is the AJCC Cancer Staging Manual, Seventh Edition (2010) published by Springer Science+Business Media.

HISTOLOGIC GRADE (G)

- A two-grade, three-grade, or four-grade system may be used.
- If a grading system is not specified, generally the following system is used:
  - GX Grade cannot be assessed
  - G1 Well differentiated – low grade
  - G2 Moderately differentiated – low grade
  - G3 Poorly differentiated
  - G4 Undifferentiated
  - Note : Ewing's sarcoma is classified as G4

~5-YEAR OS BY HISTOLOGY

- Osteosarcoma: 60–75% (20% if M1)
- Chondrosarcoma: 50–70%
- MFH: 15–67%
- Fibrosarcoma: 25–50%
- Malignant giant cell tumor: 30%

TREATMENT RECOMMENDATIONS

- In general, limb sparing strategies are preferred, which may involve a combination of neoadjuvant chemo, RT, and surgery.
- Input of orthopedic oncologist is essential in determining whether limb sparing is possible. Final limb function may sometimes be better with prosthesis than with partially resected and/or irradiated limb. In children, RT has added implications on growth of limb and future function.
- Osteosarcoma: Pre-op chemo → surgery → adjuvant chemo × 4–6 months.
  - Consider clinical trial.
  - Inoperable or close/+ margin → RT to 60–75 Gy with shrinking fields.
  - Pelvic tumors → Consider intraarterial chemo (cisplatin/doxorubicin) + RT 60–70 Gy.
  - M1a: Surgical resection of lung metastases improves survival.
- Chondrosarcoma/MFH/Giant cell: Surgery = 1° treatment (WLE, amputation). RT for inoperable tumors or close/+ margin.
  - EBRT = 60–70 Gy. IORT = 15–30 Gy
  - Giant Cell: 45–55 Gy

X

- Chordoma: Surgery → RT. RT alone for inoperable cases (66–70 Gy). Consider SRS or proton or charged particle treatment if available.
- Giant cell: Surgery. LR historically 45–60%, but as low as 10–20% with meticulous curettage or complete resection. RT for inoperable tumors, +margin, recurrent tumors, or if surgery would create significant functional disability. Dose 40–55 Gy.
- Aneurysmal bone cyst: Surgery. RT 25–30 Gy for recurrent disease and surgically inaccessible (e.g., vertebral).

STUDIES

OSTEOSARCOMA

- Randomized trials have established that neoadjuvant and adjuvant chemo help to prevent relapse or recurrence in patients with localized resectable primary tumors (Link et al. 1986; Eilber et al. 1987).
- *Cooperative German/Austrian Osteosarcoma Study Group* (Ozaki et al. 2003): Subset analysis of 67 patients with nonmetastatic, high-grade pelvic osteosarcomas. RT improved survival for patients with intralesional excision and unresectable tumors.
- DeLaney et al. (2005): Review of 41 patients with osteosarcoma who were either unresectable or had close or + margins and were treated with RT. No definitive dose-response, although doses >55 Gy had higher LC ($p = 0.11$). RT more effective for patients with microscopic or minimal residual disease.
- Machak et al. (2003): 31 patients with nonmetastatic osteosarcoma who refused surgery were treated with induction chemotherapy followed by RT, median dose 60 Gy. OS, PFS, and metastases-free survival (MFS) at 5 years were a mean of 61%, 56%, and 62%, respectively. Patients who were responders had OS and MFS at 5 years of 90% and 91%, respectively vs. nonresponders 35% and 42%, respectively ($p = 0.005$ and $p = 0.005$, respectively). PFS among nonresponders was 31% at 3 years and 0% at 5 years.
- Wagner et al. (2009): 48 patients had solid bone tumors (52% chordoma, 31% chondrosarcoma, 8% osteosarcoma, 4% Ewing's sarcoma) and were treated with preoperative RT, 20 Gy followed by resection and then postoperative RT, median dose of 50.4 Gy. Five-year OS, DFS, and LC were 65%, 53.8%, and 72%, respectively. No differences according to histology. This approach appears to inhibit tumor seeding and allows for dose escalation without high-dose preoperative RT or large-field postoperative RT.

CHORDOMA

- Several studies have indicated that charged particle treatment and/or radiosurgery may improve LC.

RADIATION TECHNIQUES

SIMULATION AND FIELD DESIGN

- Spare 1.5–2 cm strip of skin in extremity XRT, if possible, to prevent edema.
- Include entire surgical bed + scar + 2 cm margin, if possible.
- Bolus scar for first 50 Gy.
- CT/MRI data for tx planning.
- Try to exclude skin over anterior tibia, if possible, due to poor vascularity.
- Physical therapy instituted as early as possible during treatment to improve functional outcome.

DOSE LIMITATIONS

- >20 Gy can prematurely close epiphysis
- >40 Gy will ablate bone marrow
- ≥50 Gy to bone cortex significantly increases risk of fracture

COMPLICATIONS

- Abnormal bone and soft tissue growth and development, permanent weakening of affected bone, scoliosis, decreased range of motion due to fibrosis or joint involvement, vascular changes resulting in greater sensitivity to infection, fracture, lymphedema, skin discoloration or telangiectasia, osteoradionecrosis.
- Increased risk of 2° cancers (leukemia, sarcomas).

FOLLOW-UP

- Intensive physical rehabilitation very important, especially for pediatric cases.
- Regular H&P with functional assessment, CBC, chest imaging, and local imaging every 3 months for 2 years, every 4 months for third year, every 6 months for years 4 and 5, then annually.

X

REFERENCES

DeLaney TF, Park L, Goldberg SI, et al. Radiotherapy for local control of osteosarcoma. Int J Radiat Oncol Biol Phys 2005;61:492-498.

Eilber F, Giuliano A, Eckardt J, et al. Adjuvant chemotherapy for osteosarcoma: a randomized prospective trial. J Clin Oncol 1987;5:21-26.

Link MP, Goorin AM, Miser AW, et al. The effect of adjuvant chemotherapy on relapse-free survival in patients with osteosarcoma of the extremity. N Engl J Med 1986;314:1600-1606.

Machak GN, Tkachev SI, Solovyev YN, et al. Neoadjuvant chemotherapy and local radiotherapy for high-grade osteosarcoma of the extremities. Mayo Clin Proc 2003;78:147-155.

Ozaki T, Flege S, Kevric M, et al. Osteosarcoma of the pelvis: experience of the Cooperative Osteosarcoma Study Group. J Clin Oncol 2003;21:334-341.

Wagner TD, Kobayashi W, Dean S, et al. Combination short-course preoperative irradiation, surgical resection, and reduced-field high-dose postoperative irradiation in the treatment of tumors involving the bone. Int J Radiat Oncol Biol Phys 2009;73:259-266.

Further Reading

Bramwell VH, Burgers M, Sneath R, et al. A comparison of two short intensive adjuvant chemotherapy regimens in operable osteosarcoma of limbs in children and young adults: the first study of the European Osteosarcoma Intergroup. J Clin Oncol 1992;10:1579-1591.

Burgers JM, van Glabbeke M, Busson A, et al. Osteosarcoma of the limbs. Report of the EORTC-SIOP 03 trial 20781 investigating the value of adjuvant treatment with chemotherapy and/or prophylactic lung irradiation. Cancer 1988;61:1024-1031.

McNaney D, Lindberg RD, Ayala AG, et al. Fifteen year radiotherapy experience with chondrosarcoma of bone. Int J Radiat Oncol Biol Phys 1982;8: 187-190.

Montemaggi P BW, Horowitz SM. Bone. In: Perez CA, Brady LW, Halperin ED, Schmidt-Ullrich RK, editors. Principles and practice of radiation oncology. 4th ed. Philadelphia: Lippincott Williams & Wilkins; 2004. pp 2168-2184.

Romero J, Cardenes H, la Torre A, et al. Chordoma: results of radiation therapy in eighteen patients. Radiother Oncol 1993;29:27-32.

Schecter NR LV. The Bone. In: Cox JD, Ang KK, editors. Radiation Oncology: Rationale, technique, results. 8th ed. St. Louis: Mosby; 2003. pp. 857-883. 2003.

Schoenthaler R, Castro JR, Petti PL, et al. Charged particle irradiation of sacral chordomas. Int J Radiat Oncol Biol Phys 1993;26:291-298.

Schupak K. Sarcomas of Bone. In: Leibel SA, Phillips TL, editors. Textbook of Radiation Oncology. 2nd ed. Philadelphia: Saunders; 2004. pp. 1363-1374.

Chapter 40

Soft-Tissue Sarcoma

Brian Lee, Stuart Y. Tsuji, and Alexander R. Gottschalk

PEARLS

- ~10,400 cases/year and ~3,700 deaths/year in the US
- Median age 40–60 years.
- Slight male predominance, more frequent among African-Americans.
- Genetics: NF-1, Retinoblastoma, Gardner's syndrome, Li-Fraumeni syndrome.
- Environmental exposures: ionizing radiation, herbicides, thorotrast, chlorophenols, vinyl chloride, arsenic.
- Lower extremity (45%) > trunk (30%) > upper extremity (15%) > H&N (8%).
- Extremity = liposarcoma, MFH, synovial, fibrosarcoma, myxoid liposarcoma (upper medial thigh).
- Retroperitoneal = liposarcoma (fewer DM) > leiomyosarcoma (increased DM).
- H&N = MFH, usually high-grade (except myxoid MFH = intermediate grade).
- Frequency: MFH (20–30%), liposarcoma (10–20%), leiomyosarcoma (10–15%), fibrosarcoma (5–10%), synovial cell sarcoma (5–10%), rhabdomyosarcoma (5–10%), malignant peripheral nerve sheath tumor/malignant schwannoma (5%).
- Synovial sarcoma = usually high-grade, near (but not within) joints in tendon sheaths, bursae, and joint capsules.
- Grade based on cellularity, differentiation, pleomorphism, necrosis, #mitoses.
- Cytogenetics: See Appendix D.

X

PRESENTATION

- Painless mass. Typically 4–6 months from symptoms to diagnosis.
- Stewart-Treves syndrome = chronic lymphedema of upper extremity → lymphangiosarcoma.

- Approximately 10% have metastases at diagnosis. Extremity → lung, retroperitoneal → liver.
- Increased risk of LN spread: SCARE = synovial (14%), clear cell (28%), angiosarcoma (11%), rhabdomyosarcoma (15%), epithelioid (20%).

WORKUP

- H&P, CBC, BUN/Cr, ESR, LDH, CT/MRI of primary. Plain X-ray of primary. All patients get CT chest. If myxoid liposarcoma, include CT abdomen because it frequently metastasizes to retroperitoneum. MRI brain for alveolar type. Consider PET scan (investigational).
- Always perform imaging prior to biopsy or surgery because one cannot fully assess by clinical exam. Perform biopsy at institution where surgery will be performed.
- Incisional biopsy or core needle biopsy preferred. Core biopsy predicts type and grade 90% of time. Incision for biopsy should be oriented, so that it can be excised during the definitive surgery. Excisional biopsy often contaminates surrounding tissue.

PROGNOSIS

- Adverse factors for local recurrence: + margins, >50 years age, deep location, fibrosarcoma type including desmoid, malignant peripheral nerve sheath tumors.
- Adverse factors for distant metastasis: high-grade (at 5 years, <10% for low-grade, 50% for high grade), increasing size, deep location, leiomyosarcoma or malignant peripheral nerve sheath tumor, high Ki-67.

STAGING : SOFT-TISSUE SARCOMA

Editors' note: All TNM stage and stage groups referred to elsewhere in this chapter reflect the 2002 AJCC staging nomenclature unless otherwise noted as the new system below was published after this chapter was written.

(AJCC 6TH ED., 2002)

Primary tumor (T)

TX: Primary tumor cannot be assessed
T1: Tumor ≤5 cm in greatest dimension
 T1a: Superficial tumor
 T1b: Deep tumor
T2: Tumor >5 cm in greatest dimension
 T2a: Superficial tumor
 T2b: Deep tumor

Note: Superficial tumor is located exclusively above the superficial fascia without invasion of the fascia; deep tumor is located either exclusively beneath the superficial fascia, superficial to the fascia with invasion of or through the fascia, or both superficial yet beneath the fascia. Retroperitoneal, mediastinal, and pelvic sarcomas are classified as deep tumors.

Regional lymph nodes (N)

NX: Regional lymph nodes cannot be assessed
N0: No regional lymph node metastasis
N1: Regional lymph node metastasis. *Considered Stg IV

Distant metastasis (M)

MX: Distant metastasis cannot be assessed
M0: No distant metastasis
M1: Distant metastasis

Histologic grade (G)

GX: Grade cannot be assessed
G1: Well differentiated
G2: Moderated differentiated
G3: Poorly differentiated
G4: Poorly differentiated or undifferentiated (four-tiered systems only)

X

(AJCC 7TH ED., 2010)

Primary tumor (T)

TX: Primary tumor cannot be assessed
T0: No evidence of primary tumor
T1: Tumor 5 cm or less in greatest dimension*
 T1a: Superficial tumor
 T1b: Deep tumor
T2: Tumor more than 5 cm in greatest dimension*
 T2a: Superficial tumor
 T2b: Deep tumor

**Note*: Superficial tumor is located exclusively above the superficial fascia without the invasion of the fascia; deep tumor is located either exclusively beneath the superficial fascia, superficial to the fascia with invasion of or through the fascia, or both superficial yet beneath the fascia.

Regional lymph nodes (N)

NX: Regional lymph nodes cannot be assessed
N0: No regional lymph node metastasis
N1*: Regional lymph node metastasis

**Note*: Presence of positive nodes (N1) in M0 tumors is considered Stage III.

Distant metastasis (M)

M0: No distant metastasis
M1: Distant metastasis

Anatomic stage/prognostic groups

IA: T1a N0 M0 G1, GX
 T1b N0 M0 G1, GX
IB: T2a N0 M0 G1, GX
 T2b N0 M0 G1, GX

continued

Stage grouping

I: T1a, 1b, 2a, 2b N0 M0 G1-2 G1 low
II: T1a, 1b, 2a N0 M0 G3-4 G2-3 high
III: T2b N0 M0 G3-4 G2-3 high
IV: Any T N1 M0 any G any G high or low
IV: Any T N0 M1 any G any G high or low

**Not* included in AJCC soft-tissue sarcoma staging: angiosarcoma, malignant mesenchymoma, desmoid. *Included*: GI stromal tumors, Ewing's sarcoma/primitive neuroectodermal tumor have been added.

Used with the permission from the American Joint Committee on Cancer (AJCC), Chicago, IL. The original source for this material is the AJCC Cancer Staging Manual, Sixth Edition (2002), published by Springer Science+Business Media.

IIA: T1a N0 M0 G2, G3
T1b N0 M0 G2, G3
IIB: T2a N0 M0 G2
T2b N0 M0 G2
III: T2a, T2b N0 M0 G3
Any T N1 M0 any G
IV: Any T any N M1 any G

Used with the permission from the American Joint Committee on Cancer (AJCC), Chicago, IL. The original source for this material is the AJCC Cancer Staging Manual, Seventh Edition (2010), published by Springer Science+Business Media.

Histologic Grade (G) (French FNCLCC system preferred)

- The FNCLCC grade is determined by three parameters: differentiation (histology specific), mitotic activity, and extent of necrosis
- GX Grade cannot be assessed
- G1 Grade 1
- G2 Grade 2
- G3 Grade 3

Note: Kaposi's sarcoma, fibromatosis (desmoid tumor), and sarcomas arising from the dura mater, brain, parenchymatous organs, or hollow viscera are not included.

TREATMENT RECOMMENDATIONS

Stage	Recommended treatment
I extremity	■ Surgery alone (unless close (<1 cm) or + margin → post-op RT). ~5-year LC 90–100%, OS 90%
II–III extremity	■ Surgery + post-op RT or pre-op RT → surgery. Consider neoadjuvant/adjuvant chemo for large deep high-grade tumors since ~50% develop metastases. ~5-year LC 90%, OS 80% for stage II, 60% for stage III. For recurrence, amputation salvages ~75%
IV	■ For controlled primary, with ≤4 lung lesions and/or extended disease free interval, consider surgical resection. ~5-year OS ~25%. Otherwise, best supportive care, chemo, and/or palliative surgery or RT. ~5-year OS 10%
Retroperitoneal	■ Surgery + IORT (12–15 Gy) → post-op EBRT 45–50 Gy. Alternatively, pre-op RT +/- chemo → resection +/- IORT boost. ~5-year LC 50%, DM 20–30%, OS 50%
GIST	■ If resectable, surgery→imatinib (consider observation vs. imatinib if completely resected). If marginally or unresectable, imatinib→consider surgery→imatinib
Desmoid tumors	■ Surgery. If + margin, post-op RT (50 Gy). If inoperable, RT (56–60 Gy). ~5-year LC 60–70%. Consider chemotherapy (methotrexate/vinblastine) in certain cases as ~1/3 can have stable disease or a response

SURGERY

- Prefer wide en bloc resection with ≥2 cm margin in all directions.
- A radical resection removes entire anatomic compartment including neurovascular structures (LC >90%).
- Wide excision removes cuff of normal tissue (LC 40–70%).

- Excisional biopsy = marginal excision "shellout" of pseudocapsule only (LC <20%).
- Intralesional biopsy = inside pseudocapsule. Surgical scars should be oriented longitudinally, so circumferential RT can be avoided.
- Clips should be placed for RT planning.

CHEMO

- Approximately 50% of patients with high-grade tumors will die of DM, despite LC of primary.
- Most active single chemo agent = anthracycline, ifosfamide (15–30% response).
- Contradictory results in trials comparing single vs. combination chemo. No clear OS benefit to combination chemo.
- Post-op chemo controversial. If used, based on metaanalysis (doxorubicin/ifosfamide) or Italian study (epirubicin/ifosfamide).
- Consider neoadjuvant chemo → surgery for high-grade or unresectable tumors.
- Consider checking c-kit level as may respond to imatinib.

STUDIES

POST-OP RT

- Pisters et al. (1996): 160 patients with extremity and superficial trunk sarcoma s/p WLE. Randomized to brachytherapy (Ir-192 42–45 Gy over 4–6d) or observation. RT to tumor + 2 cm margin. Brachytherapy increased LC for high-grade lesions (65–90%), but not for low-grade lesions (~70%). No difference in DSS (80%) and DM.
- *NCI* (Yang et al. 1998): 140 patients with extremity sarcoma treated with WLE. Low-grade randomized to observation vs. post-op EBRT. High-grade randomized to post-op chemo vs. post-op chemo-RT. RT = large field to 45 Gy → boost to 63 Gy. RT increased LC for low-grade (60% vs. 95%) and high-grade (75% vs. 100%). No difference in OS (70%) or DMFS (75%).
- *NCI* (Rosenberg et al. 1982): 43 patients with high-grade STS of extremity randomized to WLE + post-op RT vs. amputation alone. RT = 45–50 Gy to compartment with boost to 60–70 Gy. No difference in LC, OS, or DFS. Sixty-five patients also randomized to WLE + post-op RT ± chemo. Chemo decreased LR and increased DFS (60% vs. 90%) and OS (75% vs. 95%).

PRE-OP OR POST-OP RT

- *NCIC* (O'Sullivan et al. 2002; Davis et al. 2005): 190 patients with extremity STS randomized pre-op RT (50 Gy) vs. post-op RT (66 Gy). If +margins, pre-op got 16 Gy boost. No difference in LC (93%), DM (25%), and PFS (65%). Initially, better OS with pre-op due to deaths other than sarcoma in post-op arm, but on 6-year follow-up, no difference in OS. More wound-healing problems with pre-op (35% vs. 15%), but increased late fibrosis with post-op RT (48% vs. 31%, $p = 0.07$).
- Pollack et al. (1998): Compared patients treated with post-op RT (60–66 Gy) or pre-op RT (50 Gy) before excision or reexcision. No difference in LC between pre vs. post-op (81%). For patients presenting with gross disease, best LC with pre-op RT (88% vs. 67%). For patients presenting after excision elsewhere, best treated with immediate reexcision and post-op RT (LC 91% vs. 72%). More wound-healing problems with pre-op (25% vs. 5%).

IORT

- *NCI* (Sindelar et al. 1993): 35 patients with resectable retroperitoneal STS randomized to surgery + IORT 20 Gy → post-op 35–40 Gy vs. surgery → post-op 50–55 Gy. No difference in 5-year OS (35%), but nonsignificant increase in LC (20% vs. 60%). IORT increased neuropathy if >15 Gy, but lower GI complications.
- Alektiar et al. (2000): 32 patients with primary or recurrent retroperitoneal STS treated with surgery + IORT 12–15 Gy → post-op EBRT 45–50 Gy. Results: 5-year OS 55%, DMFS 80%, LC 62%, 10% neuropathy.
- Oertel et al. (2006): 153 patients with primary or recurrent extremity STS treated with limb-sparing surgery + IORT 10–20 Gy → post-op EBRT 36–50 Gy. Five-year OS 77%, DMFS 48%, and LC 78%. IORT dose >15 Gy improved LC, but EBRT <45 or ≥45 Gy not significant for LC. Seventeen percent acute wound-healing toxicity.

X

CHEMO

- Metaanalysis update (Pervaiz et al. 2008): 1,953 patients with resectable STS treated with WLE ± RT randomized to observation vs. adjuvant doxorubicin-based chemo. Chemo improved LC (absolute 4%), DMFS (9%), RFS (10%), and OS (6%). Specifically doxorubicin/ifosfamide improved LC (absolute 5%, not significant), DMFS (10%), RFS (12%), and OS (11%).
- No trial of pre-op vs. post-op chemo.

RETROPERITONEAL

- Mendenhall (Cancer 2005): Reviewed literature on retroperitoneal STS. GTR feasible in ~50–67%, but most patients have close/+ margins. Major site of failure is local. With surgery and RT, 5-year LC is ~50%, 5-year DM ~20–30%, 5-year OS ~50%. Pre-op RT may increase resectability, allow normal tissues to be displaced by tumor, and decrease hypoxia. IORT may improve LC, but not OS.

RADIATION TECHNIQUES

POST-OP EBRT

- Start 10–20 days after surgery for healing.
- 4–6 MV for extremities.
- Bolus scar and drain sites for first 50 Gy unless in tangential beam.
- Field = tumor bed, scar, drainage sites + 5–7 cm longitudinal and 2–3 cm perpendicular margin in initial field. After 50 Gy, reduce field to surgical bed (outlined by clips, scar) + 2 cm margin.
- Dose=usually 2 Gy/fx with negative margins or microscopic residual to 60 Gy, +margins to 66 Gy, gross disease to 75 Gy.
- Always spare 1.5–2 cm strip of skin. Try to exclude skin over ant tibia, if possible, due to poor vascularity.
- Never treat whole circumference of extremity to >50 Gy.
- Try to spare 1/2 of cross-section of weight-bearing bone, entire or >1/2 of joint cavities, and major tendons (patellar, Achilles).
- IMRT may improve sparing of normal tissues, but careful planning with adequate margin and close attention to treatment set up are required to avoid marginal misses.
- Upper inner thigh best treated with frog-leg position.
- Buttock/post thigh best treated in prone position.
- Nodes: Gross nodes should be resected. No elective nodal radiation.
- For distal extremities, patients often have severe reaction with pain, edema, erythema. Usually heals within 1 months.

PRE-OP EBRT

- Dose = 2 Gy/fx to 50 Gy.
- Field = tumor + 5–7 cm longitudinal margin and 2 cm lateral margin. No conedown.
- Surgery 3 weeks after RT.
- Boost with EBRT, IORT, or brachytherapy: close/+margins to 65–66 Gy, gross disease to 75 Gy.

POST-OP BRACHYTHERAPY

- As monotherapy for high-grade tumors with negative surgical margins: 45–50 Gy.
- For low or high-grade tumors with +margin: 20 Gy brachytherapy followed by 50 Gy EBRT.
- Postoperatively after pre-op EBRT: 12–20 Gy depending on margin status.
- Brachytherapy target: tumor bed + 2 cm longitudinal margin + 1–1.5 cm circumferential margin over 4–6 days.
- Catheters placed in OR 1 cm apart. Load catheters on or after the sixth post-op day to allow time for wound healing.
- Do not include scar or drainage site.

IORT

- Dose = 12–15 Gy

EBRT ALONE

- 50 Gy to large field, conedown to 60 Gy, then to 75 Gy.
- Consider decreasing RT dose by 10%, if doxorubicin given.
- Delay RT >3 day from doxorubicin.
- Use gonadal shield to preserve fertility.
- Physical therapy instituted as early as possible during treatment to improve functional outcome.

DOSE LIMITATIONS

- >20 Gy can prematurely close epiphysis.
- ≥40 Gy ablates bone marrow.
- ≥50 Gy to bone cortex can cause fracture and healing problems.
- Exclude joint space after 40–45 Gy to avoid fibrotic constriction.

COMPLICATIONS

- Wound complications 5–15% with post-op RT vs. 25–35% with pre-op RT.
- Abnormal bone and soft-tissue growth and development.
- Limb length discrepancy (2–6 cm managed with shoe lift, otherwise need surgery).
- Permanent weakening of affected bone with highest risk for fracture within 18 month of RT.
- Decreased range of motion secondary to fibrosis.

- Lymphedema.
- Dermatitis and recall reaction with doxorubicin and dactinomycin.
- Skin discoloration, telangiectasia.
- Five percent patients may develop second malignancy.

FOLLOW-UP

- Exam with functional status, MRI of primary, CT chest every 3 months × 2 year, every 4 months in third year, every 6 months in fourth and fifth years, then annually.
- Consider bone scan or PET, if clinically indicated.

REFERENCES

Alektiar KM, Hu K, Anderson L, et al. High-dose-rate intraoperative radiation therapy (HDR-IORT) for retroperitoneal sarcomas. Int J Radiat Oncol Biol Phys 2000;47:157-163.

Davis AM, O'Sullivan B, et al. Late radiation morbidity following randomization to preoperative versus postoperative radiotherapy in extremity soft tissue sarcoma. Radiother Oncol 2005; 75:48-53.

Mendenhall WM, Zlotecki RA, Hochwald SN, et al. Retroperitoneal Soft Tissue Sarcoma. Cancer 2005;104:669-675.

Oertel S, Treiber M, Zahlten-Hinguranage A, et al. Intraoperative electron boost radiation followed by moderate doses of external beam radiotherapy in limb-sparing treatment of patients with extremity soft-tissue sarcoma. Int J Radiat Oncol Biol Phys 2006;64:1416-1423.

O'Sullivan B, Chung P, Euler C, et al. In Gunderson LL, Tepper JE, editors. Clinical Radiation Oncology. 2nd ed. Philadelphia: Elsevier; 2007. pp. 1519-1549. 2007.

O'Sullivan B, Davis AM, Turcotte R, et al. Preoperative versus postoperative radiotherapy in soft-tissue sarcoma of the limbs: a randomised trial. Lancet 2002;359:2235-2241.

Pervaiz N, Colterjohn N, Farrokhyar F, et al. A Systematic Meta-Analysis of Randomized Controlled Trials of Adjuvant Chemotherapy for Localized Resectable Soft-Tissue Sarcoma. Cancer 2008;113:573-581.

Pisters PW, Harrison LB, Leung DH, et al. Long-term results of a prospective randomized trial of adjuvant brachytherapy in soft tissue sarcoma. J Clin Oncol 1996;14:859-868.

Pollack A, Zagars GK, Goswitz MS, et al. Preoperative vs. postoperative radiotherapy in the treatment of soft tissue sarcomas: a matter of presentation. Int J Radiat Oncol Biol Phys 1998;42:563-572.

Rosenberg SA, Tepper J, Glatstein E, et al. The treatment of soft-tissue sarcomas of the extremities: prospective randomized evaluations of (1) limb-sparing surgery plus radiation therapy compared with amputation and (2) the role of adjuvant chemotherapy. Ann Surg 1982;196:305-31.

Sindelar WF, Kinsella TJ, Chen PW, et al. Intraoperative radiotherapy in retroperitoneal sarcomas. Final results of a prospective, randomized, clinical trial. Arch Surg 1993;128:402-410.

Yang JC, Chang AE, Baker AR, et al. Randomized prospective study of the benefit of adjuvant radiation therapy in the treatment of soft tissue sarcomas of the extremity. J Clin Oncol 1998;16:197-203.

FURTHER READING

Alektiar KM, Brennan MF, Healey JH, et al. Impact of intensity-modulated radiation therapy on local control in primary soft-tissue sarcoma of the extremity. J Clin Oncol 2008;26:3440-3444.

Ballo MT ZG. The Soft Tissue. In: Cox JD, Ang KK, editors. Radiation Oncology: Rationale, technique, results. 8th ed. St. Louis: Mosby; 2003. pp.884-911.

Jemal A, Siegel R, Ward E, et al. Cancer Statistics 2008. CA Cancer J Clin 2008; 58:71-96.

Le Q PT, Leibel SA. Sarcomas of Soft Tissue. In Leibel SA, Phillips TL, editors. Textbook of Radiation Oncology. 2nd ed. Philadelphia: Saunders; 2004. pp. 1335-1362. 2004.

National Comprehensive Cancer Network. Clinical Practice Guidelines in Oncology: Soft Tissue Sarcoma. Available at: http://www.nccn.org/professionals/physician_gls/PDF/sarcoma.pdf. Accessed on March 23, 2009.

Ray ME, McGinn CJ. In Halperin EC, Perez CA, Brady LW, editors. Principles and practice of radiation oncology. 5th ed. Philadelphia: Lippincott Williams & Wilkins; 2008. pp.1808-1821. 2008.

Tierney JF, Mosseri V, Stewart LA, et al. Adjuvant chemotherapy for soft-tissue sarcoma: review and meta-analysis of the published results of randomised clinical trials. Br J Cancer 1995;72:469-475.

PART XI
Pediatric (Non-CNS)

XI

Chapter 41
Pediatric (Non-CNS) Tumors

Stuart Y. Tsuji, Linda W. Chan, and Daphne A. Haas-Kogan

Special acknowledgement and thanks to Eric K. Hansen, co-author of the first edition of this chapter.

GENERAL PEARLS

- This chapter will discuss Wilms' tumor, neuroblastoma, rhabdomyosarcoma, Ewing's sarcoma, pediatric Hodgkin's disease, and retinoblastoma.
- The number one cause of death in children is accidents (44%), followed by cancer (10%), congenital abnormalities (8%), homicide (5%), and heart disease (4%).
- Of childhood cancers, leukemias are the most common (~30%, the majority of which are ALL) followed by CNS neoplasms (~20%), lymphomas (~15%, Hodgkin's > NHL > Burkitt's lymphoma), neuroblastoma (~8%), Wilms' tumor (~6%), osteosarcoma (~3%), rhabdomyosarcoma (~3%), nonrhabdomyosarcoma soft-tissue sarcomas (~3%), Ewing's sarcoma (~2%), retinoblastoma (~2%), and others.
- Of pediatric CNS neoplasms, gliomas are most common (low-grade astrocytomas ~35–50%, brainstem gliomas ~15%, malignant astrocytomas ~10%, optic pathway gliomas ~5%), followed by medulloblastoma (~20%), ependymomas (~10%), craniopharyngioma (~5–10%), and germ cell tumors (<5%). These are discussed in (Chapter 2).
- Whenever possible, we recommend that children be enrolled in cooperative group protocols.

WILMS' TUMOR

PEARLS

- Approximately 450 cases per year in the US.

PRESENTATION

- Presents with abdominal mass, pain, hematuria, HTN, fever, and/or malaise.

- Seventy-five percent of cases present before age 5. Median age at diagnosis is 3–4, or 2.5 years for bilateral tumors (only 4–8% of cases).
- Calcifications are uncommon (10%) in contrast to neuroblastoma (90%).

HISTOLOGY

- Ninety percent of cases are favorable histology (FH) = no anaplastic or sarcomatous components, while 10% are unfavorable histology (anaplastic [focal vs. diffuse], clear cell sarcoma, or rhabdoid tumor).
- Difference between focal and diffuse anaplasia is strongly significant for stage II–IV 4-year OS (90–100% vs. 4–55%).
- Clear cell sarcoma and rhabdoid tumors may not be true subtypes of Wilms' tumor, but they were included in early NWTS trials.

GENETICS

- Congenital anomalies associated with Wilms' tumor (~10%) include WAGR syndrome (Wilms', aniridia, genitourinary malformations, retardation due to del 11p13 and WT1 gene), Denys–Drash syndrome (pseudohermaphroditism, renal mesangial sclerosis, renal failure due to WT1 gene mutation), and Beckwith–Wiedemann syndrome (hemihypertrophy, macroglossia, GU abnormalities, gigantism due to 11p15 abnormality near WT2 gene).
- FH patients with LOH of 1p and/or 16q have poorer RFS and OS according to NWTS-5.

WORKUP

- H&P, abdominal US, CT or MRI of primary, CXR and/or CT chest, CBC, UA, BUN/Cr, LFTs.
- For clear cell variant, add bone scan, MRI brain, and bone marrow aspiration and biopsy (propensity for bone, bone marrow, and brain mets).
- For rhabdoid variant, may add MRI of brain (because 10–15% of patients have PNET of cerebellum or pineal regions).
- Do not biopsy unless unresectable or bilateral.

STAGING

COG staging system	NWTS 3 and 4 10-year OS
I: Tumor limited to kidney, completely resected. Renal capsule intact. Tumor not ruptured or biopsied prior to resection. Vessels of renal sinus not involved. Margins negative	Favorable histology: I: 97% II: 93% III: 90% IV: 80% V: 78%

continued

II: Tumor extends beyond kidney, but is completely excised with negative margins. Penetration of renal capsule or extensive invasion of the soft tissue of the renal sinus or involvement of blood vessels within nephrectomy specimen outside renal parenchyma, including renal sinus	Anaplastic II–III: 49% IV: 18% Clear cell sarcoma 77% Rhabdoid tumor 28%
III: Abdominal or pelvic LN+; penetration of peritoneal surface or peritoneal implants; +margins (gross or microscopic); unresectable due to infiltration of vital structures; tumor was biopsied before removal; tumor spillage either before or during surgery; tumor removed in >1 piece	
(*Note: Biopsy or tumor spillage confined to the flank was formerly stage II in NWTS-5, while diffuse peritoneal spillage was stage III. All are now classified stage III.*)	
IV: Hematogenous mets (except for adrenal gland) or LN mets outside of abdomen or pelvis	
V: Bilateral renal tumors at diagnosis. Stage each side separately	

TREATMENT RECOMMENDATIONS

- In the US, the standard is surgery for all cases (when possible). Ninety to ninety-five percent are resectable at diagnosis. Nodes must be sampled; liver and contralateral kidney should be evaluated. Perform radical nephrectomy. Clips should be placed in residual disease. If unresectable, biopsy, and give neoadjuvant therapy → resection if possible.
- Chemotherapy agents include vincristine (V), actinomycin (A), doxorubicin (D), cyclophosphamide (C), etoposide (E), carboplatin (P), and irinotecan (I). Actinomycin not given during RT.

Tumor risk classification		**Treatment**
Very low-risk FH	I, <2 years, and tumor <550 g	Nephrectomy and observation, only if central pathology review and LN sampling performed
Low-risk FH	I, ≥2 years, tumor ≥550 g II no LOH (both 1p and 16q)	Nephrectomy → VA. No RT

continued

Standard-risk FH	I–II with LOH 1p and 16q (except very low risk group)	Nephrectomy → VAD. No RT
	III, no LOH	Nephrectomy → RT → VAD
	IV , no LOH, rapid responders of lung mets at week 6 from VAD	Nephrectomy → RT → VAD. No whole lung radiation
Higher-risk FH	III with LOH 1p and 16q	Nephrectomy → RT → VAD/C/E
	IV with LOH 1p and 16q IV, no LOH, slow responders (lung and nonpulm mets)	Nephrectomy → RT → VAD/C/E + whole lung RT, and RT to mets
High-risk UH	I–IV focal anaplasia I diffuse anaplasia	Nephrectomy → RT → VAD
	I–III clear cell	Nephrectomy → RT → alternating VDC/CE
Highest risk	II–IV diffuse anaplasia IV clear cell I–IV rhabdoid	Nephrectomy → RT → alternating VDC/CPE → RT to mets

Bilateral Wilms: stage each side. Initial nephron-sparing resection only if >2/3 of each kidney can be preserved. Otherwise, induction chemo → surgery. Flank radiation indicated for I–II FH, only if unresectable disease after chemo, residual tumor, or + margins. Other stages including UH, RT given per above.

COG RT SUMMARY

General RT points	Start RT by day 9 post-op (day of surgery = day 0) CT plan to contour normal structures, but typically treat with APPA fields with 4–6 MV photons Fraction size is 1.8 Gy (except for whole abdomen and whole lung = 1.5 Gy)
Stage I–II FH	None
Stage III FH, I–III focal anaplasia, I–II diffuse anaplasia, I–III clear cell	10.8 Gy to flank Whole abdomen RT indicated if diffuse tumor spillage, pre-op or intraperitoneal tumor rupture, peritoneal tumor seeding, and cytology + ascites. Gross residual disease after surgery should receive 10 Gy boost
Stage III diffuse anaplasia, I–III rhabdoid	19.8 Gy (infants 10.8 Gy) to flank Whole abdomen RT indicated if diffuse tumor spillage, pre-op or intraperitoneal tumor rupture, peritoneal tumor seeding, and cytology + ascites.

continued

	Gross residual disease after surgery should receive 10 Gy boost
Recurrent abdominal tumor	12.6–18 Gy (for <12 months) or 21.6 Gy, if previous RT dose ≤10.8 Gy. Boost dose up to 9 Gy to gross residual tumor after surgery
Lung mets	12 Gy whole lung RT in 8 fx
Brain mets	30.6 Gy whole-brain RT in 17 fx, or 21.6 Gy whole-brain RT + 10.8 Gy IMRT or stereotactic boost
Liver mets	19.8 Gy whole liver RT in 11 fx
Bone mets	25.2 Gy to lesion + 3 cm margin
Unresected lymph node mets	19.8 Gy

TRIALS

- *NWTS-1* (D'Angio et al. 1976) demonstrated that RT is not needed for group 1 patients <2 years if chemo given; there was no radiation dose response seen for 10–40 Gy; RT should be started within 9 days of surgery; VCR/AMD is better than either alone for groups 2 and 3; pre-op chemo was not helpful in group 4.
- *NWTS 2* (D'Angio et al. 1981) demonstrated that RT is unnecessary for all group I patients; only 6 months of VCR/AMD are necessary for group 1; adding ADR for groups 2 and 3 improved OS.
- *NWTS 3* (D'Angio et al. 1989, Thomas et al. 1991) demonstrated that RT was not necessary for stage II when chemo was given; 10 Gy (instead of 20 Gy) was adequate for stage III if ADR used; only 11 weeks of chemo were necessary for stage I; ADR is unnecessary for stage II, but is necessary for stage III; CY did not benefit stage IV.
- *NWTS 4* (Green et al. 1998) demonstrated that pulse-intensive chemo has less hematologic toxicity and is less expensive than standard chemo and that it should be used in stage I–IV patients with favorable histology.
- *NWTS 5* (Green et al. *JCO* 2001; Grundy et al. *JCO* 2005; Dome et al. 2006) investigated treatment of stage I FH patients <2 years old with tumor <550 g with nephrectomy alone. Seventy-five patients entered, 11 patients relapsed with 2 yr DFS of 87% although OS was 100%. Among all FH patients, loss of heterozygosity (LOH) at chromosomes 1p and 16q is associated with increased risk of relapse and death. Patients with LOH 16q and/or 1p need treatment intensification. Stage I UH patients initially treated with only VCR/AMD had worse OS and EFS vs.similarly

XI

treated stage I FH (83 vs. 98%, 70 vs. 92%). For Stage II-IV UH, addition of etoposide improved OS compared to NWTS 3–4.

RADIATION TECHNIQUES

- The treatment volume is determined by the pre-op CT/MRI and includes the kidney and the tumor + 1–2 cm margin.
- When crossing midline, treat all of the vertebral body to avoid scoliosis.
- For paraaortic nodes, treat bilateral paraaortic chains to 10.8 Gy.
- Whole abdomen RT borders are the dome of the diaphragm superiorly, the bottom of the obturator foramen inferiorly, and flash laterally. The femoral heads are blocked out.
- Whole lung RT borders: flash the supraclavicular fossa bilaterally, extend 1–4 cm beyond the ribs laterally, and extend below the posterior aspect of the diaphragm inferiorly (usually ~L1). Patients treated with whole lung RT should receive TMP/SMX for PCP prophylaxis.

NWTS-5 DOSE LIMITATIONS

- Opposite kidney: ≤14.4 Gy.
- Liver: 1/2 of uninvolved liver ≤19.8 Gy. With liver mets 75% of liver ≤30.6 Gy.
- Bilateral whole lungs: 9 Gy (age <1.5 years) or 12 Gy (age >1.5 years).

COMPLICATIONS

- Scoliosis, kyphosis, soft-tissue hypoplasia, small bowel obstruction, iliac wing hypoplasia, liver/kidney hypoplasia, renal failure, pneumonitis, congestive heart failure (related to doxorubicin), and second malignancy.

NEUROBLASTOMA

PEARLS

- Neuroblastoma is the most common extracranial solid tumor in children and the most common malignancy in infants <1-year old. The median age at diagnosis is 17 months.
- It arises from primitive neural crest cells of the spinal ganglion, dorsal spinal nerve roots, and adrenal medulla.
- It is one of the small round blue cell tumors (along with lymphoma, all –"blastomas," small cell carcinoma of the lung, PNETs/Ewing's sarcoma, and rhabdomyosarcoma).

- Homer-Wright pseudorosettes are found in 15–50% of cases.
- Shimada Classification divides neuroblastoma into favorable (FH) and unfavorable (UH) histology based on age, amount of Schwann cell stroma, nodular vs. diffuse pattern, degree of differentiation, and mitotic index.
- Cytogenetic abnormalities associated with poorer prognosis include LOH 1p, N-myc protooncogene amplification, diploid tumors (DNA index 1), and increased telomerase activity.
- Screening does not change the mortality rate of neuroblastoma, as confirmed in international trials. The high spontaneous regression rate led to overdiagnosis of clinically insignificant disease.
- Neuroblastoma most commonly arises in the adrenal gland, followed by the abdomen and thorax.
- Sixty percent of patients <1 year present with localized disease, while 70% of patients >1 year present with metastases.
- London et al. (2005) retrospectively analyzed 3,666 patients on POG and CCG studies from 1986 to 2001 and demonstrated that the prognostic contribution of age to outcome is continuous in nature. A 460-day cutoff was selected to maximize the outcome difference between younger and older patients.
- Classic signs include the blueberry muffin sign (nontender blue skin nodules), raccoon eyes (orbital mets with proptosis and bruising), and opsoclonus-myoclonus-truncal ataxia (a paraneoplastic syndrome of myoclonic jerking and random eye movements that is associated with early stage and may persist after cure).

WORKUP

- H & P
- Labs include urine catecholamines vanillylmandelic acid, and homovanillic acid), CBC, BUN/Cr, and LFTs
- Imaging includes CT/MRI of primary, MIBG scan, and CXR. If CXR is +, then order CT chest. The primary is calcified on X-ray in 80–90% of cases (vs. 5–10% in Wilms'). Obtain bone scan if primary tumor is not MIBG+.
- Biopsy the primary or involved nodes.
- All patients should have a bilateral bone marrow biopsy and aspirate.

Note: The International Neuroblastoma Risk Group (INRG) classification system is used to develop pretreatment risk stratification to help standardize patients enrolled on trial. The International Neuroblastoma Staging System (INSS) is based on surgicopathologic findings.

INRG IMAGE DEFINED RISK FACTORS (IDRF)

Ipsilateral tumor extension within two body compartments	■ Neck-chest, chest-abdomen, abdomen-pelvis
Neck	■ Encasing carotid and/or vertebral artery, and/or internal jugular vein. Extending to the base of skull. Compressing the trachea
Cervico–thoracic junction	■ Encasing brachial plexus roots. Encasing subclavian vessels and/or vertebral and/or carotid artery. Compressing the trachea
Thorax	■ Encasing the aorta and/or major branches. Compressing the trachea and/or principal bronchi. Lower mediastinal tumor, infiltrating the costo-vertebral junction between T9 and T12
Thoraco-abdominal	■ Encasing the aorta and/or vena cava
Abdomen/pelvis	■ Infiltrating porta hepatis and/or the hepatoduodenal ligament. Encasing branches of the SMA at the mesenteric root. Encasing the origin of the celiac axis, and/or the SMA. Invading one or both renal pedicles. Encasing aorta and/or vena cava. Encasing iliac vessels. Pelvic tumor crossing the sciatic notch
Intraspinal tumor extension whatever the location provided that	■ More than one-third of the spinal canal in the axial plane is invaded and/or the perimedullary leptomeningeal spaces are not visible and/or the spinal cord signal is abnormal
Infiltration of adjacent organs/structures	■ Pericardium, diaphraghm, kidney, liver, duodeno-pancreatic block, and mesentery
Conditions to be recorded, but *not* considered IDRFs	■ Multifocal primary tumors. Pleural effusion, with or without malignant cells. Ascites, with or without malignant cells

INTERNATIONAL NEUROBLASTOMA RISK GROUP STAGING SYSTEM

L1	Localized tumor not involving vital structures as defined by the list of IDRFs and confined to one body compartment
L2	Locoregional tumor with the presence of one or more image-defined risk factors
M	Distant metastatic disease (except stage MS)
MS	Metastatic disease in children <18 months with metastases confined to skin, liver, and and/or bone marrow

INRG PRETREATMENT RISK GROUPS

INRG stage	Age (months)	Histologic category	Grade of tumor differentiation	MYCN	11q aberration	Ploidy	Pretreatment risk group
L1/L2		GN maturing; GNB intermixed					Very Low
L1		Any, except GN maturing or GNB intermixed		NA			Very Low
				Amp			High
L2	<18	Any, except GN maturing or GNB intermixed		NA	No	No	Low
					Yes		Intermediate
	≥18	GNB nodular; neuroblastoma	Differentiating	NA	No		Low
					Yes		Intermediate
			Poorly differentiated or undifferentiated	NA			
				Amp			High
M	<18			NA		Hyperdiploid	Low
	<18			NA		Diploid	Intermediate
	<18			Amp			High
	≥18						
MS	<18			NA	No		Very low
					Yes		High
				Amp			

GN ganglioneuroma; *GNB* ganglioneuroblastoma; *Amp* amplified

XI

- Five-year EFS cutpoints for the INRG pretreatment risk groups:
  - Very low: >85%
  - Low: 75–85%
  - Intermediate: 50–75%
  - High: <50%

INSS STAGING

1: Localized tumor with GTR ± microscopic residual. Adherent LN may be + but nonadherent ipsilateral LN−

2A: Localized tumor with incomplete gross resection, and ipsilateral nonadherent nodes negative

2B: Localized tumor with ipsilateral nonadherent LN+, but contralateral nodes negative

3: Unresectable tumor, tumor extends across midline (defined as opposite side of vertebral body), contralateral LN+, or a midline tumor with bilateral extension

4: Metastases to distant lymph nodes, bone, bone marrow, liver, skin, or other organs

4S: Age <1 year with an otherwise 1–2B primary tumor with metastases limited to skin, liver, and/or <10% of bone marrow. (MIBG scan, if performed, should be negative in bone marrow)

COG risk groups (based on INSS stage)

Low risk (3 year OS >90%)

Any stage I
Stage 2 <1 year
Stage 2 >1 year without N-myc amplification
Stage 2 >1 year with N-myc amplification and FH
Stage 4S <1 year without N-myc amplification, with FH and hyperdiploid

Intermediate risk (3-year OS 70–90%)

Stage 3 <1 year without N-myc amplification
Stage 3 >1 year without N-myc amplification with FH
Stage 4 <18 months without N-myc amplification
Stage 4S <1 year without N-myc amplification, with UH or diploid

High risk (3-year OS 30%)

Stage 2 >1 year with N-myc amplification and UH
Stage 3 <1 year with N-myc amplification
Stage 3 >1 year with N-myc amplification, or UH
Stage 4 <18 months with N-myc amplification
Stage 4 ≥18 months
Stage 4S <1 year with N-myc amplification

TREATMENT RECOMMENDATIONS

Risk group	Recommended treatment
Low risk	■ Surgery → observation if GTR. If STR, unresectable, or recurrence after GTR → chemo for 6–12 weeks. Chemo regimens consist of carboplatin, VP-16, CY, and/or ADR. However, if patient has severe symptoms from spinal cord compression, respiratory compromise, or GI/GU obstruction, give immediate chemo → surgery ■ RT (1.5/21 Gy) is used for symptoms that do not respond to chemo or for massive hepatomegaly causing respiratory distress (1.5/4.5 Gy). RT also used for rare local recurrences after chemo and surgery ■ For clinically-stable stage 4S low-risk patients, observe after biopsy unless massive hepatomegaly causes respiratory distress (then treat with chemo ± RT). Biopsy only is necessary as resection does not affect outcome
Intermediate risk	■ Maximal safe resection with lymphadenectomy → chemo for 12–24 weeks depending on biology. Chemo regimens consist of carboplatin, VP-16, CY, and/or ADR. Unresectable tumors may require pre-op chemo to convert them to resectable status ■ If PR to chemo → second look surgery. If viable residual disease present → RT to primary + 2 cm margin (1.5/24 Gy). If stage 4S with respiratory distress → RT to liver (1.5/4.5 Gy). Radiation controversial in intermediate-risk disease
High risk	■ High-dose chemo (same drugs often with ifosfamide and cisplatin) → attempt maximal safe resection. After surgery → high-dose chemo and ABMT. All patients then get RT (1.8/21.6 Gy) to the postchemo presurgical extent of tumor +2 cm margin → *cis*-retinoic acid for 6 months. If available, IORT may be used at the time of operation, although this is not standard-of-care

STUDIES

LOW RISK

XI

- *POG 8104* (Nitschke et al. 1988) treated 101 patients with POG A (INSS 1) disease with gross total resection → observation, and 2-year DFS was 89%.
- *CCG 3881* (Perez et al. 2000) treated 374 patients with Evans I–II (INSS 1–2B) with surgery alone (unless spinal cord compression

when RT allowed). For stage I, 4-year EFS and OS were 93 and 99%, and for stage II, they were 81 and 98%, respectively. Recurrences were managed successfully with surgery or multimodality therapy. Identified stage II patients with N-myc amplification or ≥2 years with either UH or + lymph nodes as patients at higher risk of death with surgery alone.

INTERMEDIATE RISK

- *Castleberry, POG* (Castleberry et al. *JCO* 1991) randomized 62 patients >1 year with POG C (INSS 2B-3) to post-op chemo ±concurrent RT → second look surgery → chemo. RT was to the primary and regional nodes (1.5/24 Gy for <2 years or 1.5/30 Gy for >2 years). Chemo-RT improved DFS (31→58%) and CR rate (45 → 67%).
- *POG 8742 and 9244* (*Eur J Cancer* 1997) treated 49 patients >1 year with INSS 2B-3 with surgery → chemo × 5c → second look surgery → RT for viable residual tumor → chemo-RT was 1.5/24 Gy for age 1–2 year, 1.5/30 Gy for age >2 year. Two-year EFS was 85% after GTR vs. 70% after STR, and 92% for FH vs. 58% for UH.

HIGH RISK

- *CCG 3891* (Matthay et al. 1999, Matthay 2009; Haas-Kogan et al. *IJROBP* 2003) treated 539 high-risk patients with chemo × 5 months →surgery (+ 10 Gy RT for gross residual disease), and then randomized them to myeloablative chemo, 10 Gy TBI, and ABMT vs. intensive chemo without TBI. If patients were disease-free, they were randomized to observation vs. 6 months of *cis*-retinoic acid. ABMT + TBI improved 5-year EFS (19 → 30%), and *cis*-retinoic acid trended toward an improved 5-year EFS (31→42%). There was a trend toward improved OS for both.

RADIATION TECHNIQUES

SIMULATION AND FIELD DESIGN

- CT and/or MRI used for planning 3DCRT or IMRT plans.
- Treat the postchemo presurgical tumor extent with a 2 cm margin. If lymph node involvement suspected or proven, cover primary + immediately adjacent nodal drainage areas. Do not give elective nodal RT because of morbidity.
- Always cover the full width of vertebrae to avoid scoliosis.
- After induction chemo, give RT to metastases if persistent active disease.

DOSE PRESCRIPTIONS

- Intermediate risk = 1.5/24 Gy (controversial)
- High risk = 1.8/21.6 Gy
- 4S liver involvement = 1.5/4.5 Gy

DOSE LIMITATIONS

- Contralateral kidney: ≥80% of volume <12 Gy
- Liver: ≥50% of volume <9 Gy, ≥2/3 of volume <15 Gy, or ≥75% of volume <18 Gy
- Lung: >2/3 of volume <15 Gy

COMPLICATIONS

- Disturbances of growth, infertility, neuropsychological sequelae, endocrinopathies, cardiac effects, pulmonary effects, bladder dysfunction, second malignancy.

RHABDOMYOSARCOMA

PEARLS

- Rhabdomyosarcoma accounts for ~3% of childhood cancers.
- The most common primary sites are the head and neck [40% = parameningeal (25%), orbit (9%), nonparameningeal sites (6%)], genitourinary tract (30%), extremity (15%), and trunk (15%).
- Primary sites are categorized as favorable or unfavorable (see table below).
- Most cases are sporadic, but predisposing conditions include Li-Fraumeni syndrome (germline p53 mutation), neurofibromatosis type 1, and Beckwith–Wiedemann syndrome (more commonly associated with Wilms' tumor).
- The classic histologic subtypes include: embryonal (60–70%), alveolar (20–40%), botyroid (10%), undifferentiated (5%), and spindle cell (<5%).
- Embryonal tumors, typically arise in the orbit, head and neck, or the genitourinary tract.
- Botyroid tumors arise in the vagina, bladder, nasopharynx, and biliary tract.
- Spindle cell tumors are most frequently observed in the paratesticular site.
- Alveolar tumors most commonly arise in the extremity, trunk, or retroperitoneum of adolescents.

- Positive prognostic histologic subtypes include botyroid (95% OS) and spindle cell (88% OS). Embryonal is an intermediate prognostic subtype (OS 66%). Poor prognostic subtypes include alveolar (OS 54%) and undifferentiated (OS 40%).
- Embryonal is associated with LOH on 11p15.5.
- Seventy percent of alveolar cases are associated with t(2;13) and 20% with t(1;13). The involved genes include FKHR (on chromosome 13), PAX3 (on chromosome 2), and PAX7 (on chromosome 1).

WORKUP

- H&P: EUA may be needed. Cystoscopy should be performed for GU sites.
- Labs include CBC, LFTs, BUN/Cr, LDH.
- Imaging includes CT/MRI of primary, CT of chest and abdomen, bone scan.
- If parameningeal site → lumbar puncture with cytology → if + → neuraxis MRI.
- Bone marrow biopsy.

STAGING

IRS preoperative staging system (dictates chemo)

Stage 1: Favorable site, any T, N0-1, M0
Stage 2: Unfavorable site, T1a/T2a, N0M0
Stage 3: Unfavorable site, T1b/T2b, N0M0, or any T, N1M0
Stage 4: Any M1

Favorable sites: Orbit, nonparameningeal H&N (scalp, parotid, OPX, oral cavity, larynx), GU nonbladder-prostate (paratestes, vagina, vulva, uterus), biliary tract.
Unfavorable sites: Parameningeal (NPX, nasal cavity, paranasal sinuses, middle ear, mastoid, pterygopalatine fossa, infratemporal fossa), bladder, prostate, extremity, other (trunk, retroperitoneum)

T1: Tumor is confined to site/organ of origin (a ≤5 cm, b >5 cm)
T2: Tumor extends beyond site/organ of origin (a ≤5 cm, b >5 cm)
N1: Regional lymph node involvement
M1: Distant metastases at diagnosis

IRS surgical-pathologic grouping system (dictates RT)

I: Localized disease, completely resected (~13% of all patients)
  A: Confined to organ or muscle of origin
  B: Infiltration outside organ or muscle of origin
II: Gross total resection (~20% of all patients)
  A: Microscopic residual disease, but no regional LN involvement
  B: Resected regional LN
  C: Both microscopic residual disease and resected regional LN

continued

III: Incomplete resection with gross residual disease (~48% of all patients)
- A: Due to biopsy
- B: After major resection (>50%)

IV: Distant metastases at diagnosis (~18% of all patients)

IRS risk groups

Low risk: Localized embryonal or botyroid histology at favorable sites (stage 1, Groups I–III) or at unfavorable sites with completely resected or microscopic residual disease (stages 2–3, Groups I–II).

Intermediate risk: Embryonal or botyroid histology at unfavorable sites with gross residual disease (stages 2–3 Group III); patients 2–10 years with metastatic embryonal histology (stage 4); nonmetastatic alveolar or undifferentiated histology (stages 1–3).

High risk: Any stage 4/Group IV (except for patients 2–10 years with embryonal histology).

~3-Year OS by risk group	~5-Year OS by histology	~5-Year OS by site
Low >90–95%	Botyroid 95%	Orbit >90%
Intermediate: 55–70%	Spindle cell 88%	Parameningeal 75%
High 30–50%	Embryonal 66%	H&N nonparamen: 80%
	Alveolar 54%	Bladder/prostate 82%
	Undifferentiated 40%	Paratesticular 69–96%
		Gynecologic sites 90–98%
		Extremity 70%

IRS-V TREATMENT

Stage/group	IRS-V treatment
All patients require multimodality therapy consisting of surgery (if possible) followed by chemo ±RT. Treatment is based on stage, group, and primary site. Chemotherapy agents include VCR, AMD, CY, topotecan, and irinotecan. VA=VCR/AMD. VAC=VCR/AMD/CY. VTC=VCR/topotecan/CY. VCPT=VCR/irinotecan	
Low risk	
Stage 1–3 Group I	■ Surgery → chemo (VA or VAC). No RT
Stage 1 Group II	■ Surgery → chemo (VA)+RT at week 3 (36 Gy for N0 or 41.4 Gy for N1)
Stage 1 Group III	■ Surgery (biopsy only for orbit) → chemo (VA)+RT (50.4 Gy except for orbit which is 45 Gy). Most get RT at week 3, but primary sites at vulva, uterus, biliary tract, and certain nonparameningeal H&N get RT at week 12 to allow for possible second look surgery. Vaginal primaries get RT at week 12 (N1) or 28 (N0)

continued

XI

Stage 2 Group II	■ Surgery → chemo (VAC) + RT at week 3 (36 Gy)
Stage 3 Group II	■ Surgery → chemo (VAC) + RT at week 3 (36 Gy for N0 or 41.4 Gy for N1)
Intermediate risk Embryonal stages 2–3, Group III; embryonal stage 4, age 2–10 years; alveolar/ undiff stages 1–3	■ Surgery → chemo (VAC or VAC alternating with VTC). At week 12, perform second look surgery or definitive RT if unresectable. Definitive RT dose at week 12 is 50.4 Gy. If second look surgery performed, post-op RT is given at week 15. Post-op RT doses depend on site, and are 0–36 Gy for complete resection, 36 Gy for microscopic residual and N0, 41.4 Gy for microscopic residual and N1, and 50.4 Gy for gross residual
High risk	■ Chemo (VCPT → VAC or VAC alternating with VCPT depending on response). RT is given at week 15 to primary and metastatic sites, except for patients with intracranial extension, spinal cord compression, or patients requiring emergency RT (day 0). Definitive RT dose is 50.4 Gy except for the orbit which is 45 Gy. If second look surgery is performed, post-op RT doses are 36 Gy for complete resection, 36 Gy for microscopic residual and N0, 41.4 Gy for microscopic residual and N1, and 50.4 Gy for gross residual
Site-specific recommendations	
Orbit	■ Only a biopsy is required to establish diagnosis → chemo → RT. RT is to the tumor + 2 cm margin. Dose depends on stage and group as above (45 Gy for stage 1 Group III). Orbital exenteration is reserved for salvage
Head and neck (nonparameningeal sites)	■ Follow stage/group guidelines above. For Group III, perform second look surgery or definitive RT if unresectable at week 12. Post-op dose is 36 Gy for complete resection and microscopic residual N0, 41.4 Gy for microscopic residual and N1, and 50.4 Gy for gross residual
Parameningeal sites	■ If intracranial extension or cranial neuropathy present, RT is given first. Otherwise, RT is given at week 12 or week 15 if second look surgery. For focal intracranial extension, include a 2 cm margin. If extensive intracranial involvement, treat with whole cranial RT
Biliary tract	■ Follow stage/group guidelines above. For Group III, perform second look surgery or definitive RT if unresectable at week 12. Post-op dose is 36 Gy for complete resection and microscopic residual, and 50.4 Gy for gross residual

continued

Extremity	■ Wide local excision with en bloc removal of a cuff of normal tissue with nodal sampling → chemo → local treatment as described in stage/group guidelines above
Trunk, retroperitoneum, perineum, GI	■ Follow stage/group guidelines above
Bladder/prostate	■ Follow stage/group guidelines above. Because one goal is bladder preservation, an initial biopsy is often performed rather than surgery → chemo + RT → surgery for residual disease
Paratesticular	■ Inguinal orchiectomy with resection of entire spermatic cord and ipsilateral lymph node dissection including high and low infrarenal and bilateral iliac nodes (except Group I patients). If scrotal violation, give RT to hemiscrotum. Contralateral testicle can be transposed into thigh prior to RT and later reimplanted. RT dose depends on stage and group as above (50.4 Gy for stage 1 Group III)
Uterus, cervix	■ Follow stage/group guidelines above. For Group III, perform second look surgery or definitive RT if unresectable at week 12. Post-op RT doses are 0 for completely resected N0, 41.4 Gy for completely resected N1, 36 Gy for microscopic residual and N0, 41.4 Gy for microscopic residual and N1, and 50.4 Gy for gross residual
Vulva	■ Follow stage/group guidelines above. For Group III, perform second look surgery or definitive RT if unresectable at week 12. Post-op RT doses are 36 Gy for complete resection and microscopic residual N0, 41.4 Gy for microscopic residual and N1, and 50.4 Gy for gross residual
Vagina	■ Follow stage/group guidelines above, but local treatment is at week 12 (N1) or 28 (N0) → reassess with biopsy. If biopsy negative, no further local treatment. If + biopsy → resect or RT if unresectable. Definitive RT doses are 36 Gy for Group II N0, 41.4 Gy for Group II N1, and 50.4 Gy for Group III. Post-op RT doses are 0 for complete resection, 36 Gy for microscopic residual and N0, 41.4 Gy for microscopic residual and N1, and 50.4 Gy for gross residual

IRS VI TREATMENT (IRS VI TRIAL CURRENTLY OPEN)

Stage/group	IRS-VI treatment
All patients require multimodality therapy consisting of surgery (if possible) followed by chemo ± RT. Chemotherapy agents include VCR, AMD, CY, irinotecan, Doxo, Etoposide	
Overall IRS VI summary	*Chemo* ■ Low risk: VAC × 22–46 weeks (46 weeks for stage III or Group III nonorbit) ■ Intermediate-risk (all alveolar, Group III unfavorable embryonal): VAC vs. VAC/VI × 42 weeks ■ High risk (met): Alternating between: V/Irinotecan, VDC, IE, and VAC *Timing of RT* ■ Direct extension into brain or cord compression or loss of vision: day 0 ■ Intermediate-risk (Group III unfavorable sites and all alveolar): Week 4 ■ Low risk: week 13 ■ Base of skull invasion or CN palsy: week 15 ■ High risk (metastatic): week 20 ■ Vagina Group II–III: week 25 ■ AMD is given just before, but not during RT. No doxo during RT *RT volumes* ■ GTV = prechemo, presurgical tumor and mets at diagnosis ■ CTV = GTV + 1 cm. If planning 50.4 Gy, cone-down to GTV + 0.5 cm after 36–41.4 Gy ■ If LN+, include entire LN chain ■ For orbit, CTV does not extend beyond bony orbit ■ If pushing border, do not need to cover displaced normal tissues that return to normal position after chemo. Do include entire pretreatment extent of disease ■ PTV = CTV + 0.5 cm *RT dose* ■ Stage 1–3 Group I = No RT, except alveolar = 36 Gy ■ Stage 1–3 Group II = 36 Gy N0, 41.4 Gy N+ ■ Stage 1 Group III = 45 Gy (orbit only). Otherwise, 50.4 Gy ■ IV = 50.4 Gy unless resected initially, as above. If second look surgery-margin, 36 Gy ■ If >1 lung met = whole lung RT 1.5/15 Gy

continued

RT dose limitations

- Optic nerve/chiasm: 46.8 Gy
- Lacrimal gland: 41.4 Gy
- Small bowel, spinal cord: 45 Gy
- Lung: <50% >18 Gy
- Kidney: <14.4 Gy
- Liver: Whole <23.4 Gy
- Heart Whole <30.6

Low risk
Stage 1 Group I–III
Stage 2 Group I–II
Stage 3 Group I–II

- All patients get surgery first (except orbit and vagina biopsy only) → VAC chemo × 22–46 weeks; 46 weeks chemo is given for stage III or Group III nonorbit

Timing of RT

- RT at week 13 for most patients, except Group I disease or node-negative Group III uterine/cervix primaries that are completely resected at week 13 (who do not receive RT), and patients with node-negative vaginal primaries (who begin RT following surgery at week 24)
- Patients with Group III disease may undergo second look surgery at week 13, followed by response-adjusted RT dosing (see Appendix VI of ARST 0331 protocol)

Volumes

- GTV = prechemo, presurgical tumor at diagnosis
- CTV = GTV + 1 cm. If Group III and CR to chemo, give 36 Gy to 1 cm margin, then conedown to 0.5 cm margin to complete 50.4 Gy. If LN+, include entire LN chain. There are special modifications of GTV and CTV for certain sites (see protocol).
- PTV = CTV + 0.5 cm

Dose

- Stage 1–3 Group I = No RT
- Stage 1–3 Group II = 36 Gy N0, 41.4 Gy N+
- Stage 1 Group III = 45 Gy (orbit only). Otherwise, 50.4 Gy

Intermediate risk
Stage 2–3, Group III embryonal unfavorable site; Nonmetastatic, Group I–III alveolar

- Surgery → chemo × 42 weeks (randomized to VAC vs. VAC alternating with VI for total of 14 cycles)

Timing of RT

- Simulation before week 4, RT begins at week 4
- Symptomatic spinal cord compression RT may begin during week 1
- No second look surgery for unfavorable site Group III or alveolar

continued

Volumes

- Same as low risk

Dose

- Stage 1–3 Group I alveolar = 36 Gy
- Stage 2–3 Group II = 36 Gy N0, 41.4 Gy N+
- Group III = 45 Gy (orbit only). Otherwise, 50.4 Gy. For patients receiving total dose of 50.4 Gy, conedown is permitted after 36 Gy. Volume reduction not recommended for invasive tumors

High risk (metastatic patients, patients with parameningeal paraspinal, or intracranial extension)

Chemo for 51 weeks (Alternating between: V/Irinotecan, VDC, IE, and VAC)

Timing of RT

- RT begins at week 20 to the primary and metastatic sites
- Exceptions

Intracranial extension consisting of direct extension into the brain, or emergent RT for spinal cord compression or loss of vision begin week 1 day 0, with RT to other metastatic sites at week 20

Volumes

- Same as low-risk, include all sites of metastases
- Patients with >1 lung met or pleural effusion receive bilateral whole lung RT

Dose

- All patients 50.4 Gy to primary and met sites
- Orbit limited to 45 Gy
- Whole lung RT for >1 met = 1.5/15 Gy. Boost residual if possible to 50.4 Gy
- If initial surgery, resected margins negative, embryonal = 0 Gy, alveolar = 36 Gy. Microscopic residual LN– 36 Gy, microscopic residual LN + 41.4 Gy
- If second look surgery, same except all patients with neg margins get 36 Gy

TRIALS

- *IRS-I* (Maurer et al. 1988): 1972–1978, 686 patients. All patients got chemo for 2 years. RT was given initially for groups I and II, and at week 6 for groups III and IV. RT dose was 40–60 Gy (<3 years = 40 Gy; <6 years and <5 cm = 50 Gy; >6 years or >5 cm = 55 Gy; >6 years and >5 cm = 60 Gy). Group I patients randomized to RT vs. no RT and no difference in OS/DFS for embryonal/botyroid. However, there was a benefit of post-op RT for Group I alveolar/undifferentiated histologies. Orbit and GU sites had the best prognosis, and retroperitoneal and alveolar histology had the worst prognosis. DM was much more common than LF.

- *IRS-II* (Maurer et al. 1993): 1978–1984, 990 patients. RT was modified from IRS-I as follows: RT given at week 0 for Group II, and week 6 for Groups III and IV. RT was to the tumor + 5 cm margin. Patients with CN palsies, base of skull (BOS) involvement, or intracranial disease got whole-brain RT ±intrathecal chemo to prevent meningeal relapse (improved from IRS-I). RT doses were: Group I = 0; Group II = 40–45 Gy; Group III = 40–45 Gy if <6 years and <5 cm, 45–50 Gy if >6 years or >5 cm, or 50–55 Gy if both. LC for all patients receiving >40 Gy was 93%. LC for Groups I and II was 90 vs. 80% for Group III. Worse LC and OS for patients with unfavorable histology and tumors >5 cm. Local-regional relapse was more common than distant relapse except for stage IV patients.
- *IRS-III* (*JCO* 1995): 1984–1991, 1,062 patients. All patients got post-op RT except Group I favorable histology and Group III special pelvic sites in CR after chemo. RT was given at day 0 for CN palsy, BOS erosion, intracranial extension; week 2 for Group II favorable sites and Group III orbit and H&N; otherwise RT at week 6. RT was to tumor + 2 cm. RT doses were: Group I unfavorable site or Group II = 41.4 Gy. Group III = 41.4 Gy if <6 years and <5 cm, 50.4 Gy if ≥6 years and ≥5 cm; 45 Gy for older children or large tumors. Five-year OS was superior in IRS-III (71%) compared to IRS-II (63%) and IRS-I (55%). LC was 90% for Group I and II patients, but only ~80% for Group III.
- *IRS-IV* (*JCO* 2001, Breitfeld et al. 2001): 1991–1997, 1,000 patients. Pretreatment staging assigned chemo, and clinical grouping assigned RT. Most patients got surgery → chemo day 0 → RT at week 9. RT was given at day 0 for CN palsy, BOS erosion, or intracranial extension; at week 3 for orbit and paratesticular; at week 18.5 for stage 4. RT was to the presurgery, prechemo tumor + 2 cm. Whole-brain RT omitted for patients with parameningeal primaries except when CSF+. Group I stages I–II did not get RT. Group I stage III and all Group II got 41.4 Gy. All Group III got 50.4 Gy in qd fractions vs. 1.1 Gy b.i.d. to 59.4 Gy. Orbital tumors were usually Group III due to biopsy only, so got 50.4 Gy.

Group/stage	Treatment	3-year OS	Findings
I para-testicular	VA	90%	No difference from IRS III
I orbit	VA	100%	No difference from IRS III
II orbit	VA + RT	100%	No difference from IRS III
I, Stage 1–2	VAC vs. VAI vs. VIE; no RT	84–88%	No difference between chemo regimens
I, Stage 3; all II	VAC vs. VAI vs. VIE + RT	84–88%	No difference between chemo regimens
III	VAC vs. VAI vs. VIE, + RT (qd vs. b.i.d.)	72–83% (3-year FFS)	No difference between chemo regimens. b.i.d. RT did not improve LC (~87%) or OS vs. qd RT
IV	VM vs. IE → VAC, + RT	27 vs. 55%	IE improved FFS, OS vs. VM chemo

- *COG D9803 Intermediate-risk protocol (IRS-V)* (Arndt, JCO 2009): 617 patients with intermediate-risk disease randomized to 39 weeks of VAC vs. VAC alternating with VTC. Local therapy after week 12 (see IRS-V treatment description above). Patients with parameningeal disease with intracranial extension received VAC and immediate RT. Treatment strata: stage 2/3 group III embryonal (33%), group IV embryonal <10 years (7%), stage 1 group I alveolar or undifferentiated (17%), alveolar or undifferentiated (27%), parameningeal extension (16%). No significant difference in 4-year FFS (73% VAC vs. 68% VAC/VTC) across risk groups or in frequency of second malignancies. No difference in 4-year LF (16.5–18.5%), regional failure (4.5–4.8%), or DM (10.5–13%).

RADIATION TECHNIQUES

SIMULATION AND FIELD DESIGN

- Many patients may require pediatric anesthesia.
- Excellent immobilization is required and 3DCRT and/or IMRT is encouraged to limit doses to normal structures.
- In IRS-V RT, volumes are to the initial prechemo, presurgical tumor + 2 cm margin. Involved lymph nodes are included in the RT field, but prophylactic RT is not used. For Group III patients requiring 50.4 Gy, the volume is reduced to the prechemo, presurgical tumor + 0.5 cm margin at 36 Gy for N0 patients or at 41.4 Gy for N1 patients.

- The timing of RT is described in the IRS-V treatment summary table above.
- Doses are 1.8 Gy/fraction to 36, 41.4, or 50.4 Gy.
- Dose limitations are as follows: kidney <14.4 Gy, whole liver <23.4 Gy, bilateral lungs <15 Gy in 1.5 Gy fractions, optic nerve and chiasm <46.8 Gy, spinal cord <45 Gy, GI tract <45 Gy, whole abdomen 24 Gy in 1.5 Gy fractions, heart <30.6 Gy, lens <14.4 Gy, lacrimal gland and cornea <41.4 Gy.
- The ovaries should be shielded, or moved in girls with pelvic primaries.
- The normal testicle can also be transposed prior to RT and later reimplanted.

COMPLICATIONS

- Complications are site dependent.
- Chemo complications include nausea, vomiting, mucositis, alopecia, and hematopoietic suppression. Ifosfamide and etoposide can cause renal and electrolyte imbalance. CY can cause hemorrhagic cystitis. ADR can cause cardiomyopathy. Cisplatin can cause hearing impairment. Topoisomerase inhibitors can cause second malignancies, particularly AML.
- AMD and ADR can accentuate radiation "recall" reaction if given during or immediately after RT.

FOLLOW-UP

- H&P and CXR every 2 months for first year with repeat imaging studies that were + at diagnosis every 3 months, then H&P and CXR every 4 months for second and third years, H&P annually for 5–10 years, and annual visit or phone contact after 10 years.

EWING'S SARCOMA

PEARLS

- Approximately 200 cases per year in the U.S. Put this on its own bullet Ewing's sarcoma is the second most common bone cancer of children (osteosarcoma is #1). Boys are affected more than girls (1.5–2:1). The median age at presentation is 14 years (usually 8–25 years). Ewing's sarcoma is rare in African Americans and Asians.

- Ewing's sarcoma commonly presents in the lower extremity (femur 15–20%, more common than tibia or fibula 5–10%), pelvis (20–30%), upper extremity (humerus 5–10%), ribs (9–13%), and spine (6–8%).
- Seventy-five to eighty percent of patients present with localized disease; 20–25% have metastases to lung, bone, or bone marrow. Nearly all patients have micromets at diagnosis, so all need chemo.
- Ewing's family of tumors includes Ewing's sarcoma (bone – 87%), extraosseous Ewing's sarcoma (8%), peripheral PNET (5%), and Askin's tumor (PNET of chest wall).
- More than 90% of patients have t(11;22) [or t(21;22)] involving the EWS gene on chromosome 22. The c-myc protooncogene is frequently expressed in Ewing's (whereas n-myc is often amplified in neuroblastoma).

WORKUP

- H&P. Labs include CBC, LFTs, LDH, and ESR.
- X-rays of the primary frequently show a moth-eaten lesion in the diaphysis. Lytic lesions are more common than blastic, and "onion-skinning" may be present for subperiosteal lesions.
- CT and/or MRI of primary, bone scan, CT chest, ±PET scan.
- Biopsy the lesion and obtain a bone marrow biopsy.
- Negative prognostic factors include metastases, pelvic or truncal primaries, proximal (vs. distal) extremity primaries, large tumors (>8 cm or >100–200 ml), age >17 years, high LDH or ESR, poor response to induction chemo, and no surgery.

STAGING

- There is no uniform staging system for Ewing's sarcomas. The AJCC staging systems for bone or soft-tissue sarcomas may be used. Please refer to the chapters on bone tumors (Chapter 39) and soft-tissue sarcomas (Chapter 40) for more details on staging.
- For localized disease, 5-year OS is ~60–70%.
- For patients with lung/pleural mets only, cure rates are ~30%.
- For patients with bone/bone marrow mets, cure rates are ~15%.

- For patients with both lung and bone/bone marrow mets, cure rates are <15%.
- Local treatment alone without chemo cures only ~10%.
- Local failure rates after definitive RT for Ewing's sarcoma generally range from ~10–25%, and are correlated with prognostic factors (above) such as site (extremity lesions LF 5–10% vs. pelvic lesions LF 15–70%) and size (<8 cm LF 10% vs. >8 cm LF 20%).

TREATMENT RECOMMENDATIONS

- Induction chemo (VDC(A) alternating with IE) × 48 weeks → local treatment (surgery or RT) at week 12 with concurrent multiagent VDC chemo often given → adjuvant chemo. Response rate to initial chemo is up to 90%.
  - Chemo agents = vincristine (V), doxorubicin (D), cyclophosphamide (C), actinomycin-D (A), ifosfamide (I), and etoposide (E).
  - Current Euro-Ewing 99 trial (*European portion of study randomized all patients, COG portion studying patients with isolated pulmonary mets only*): VIDE chemo q3 week × 6c → local therapy at week 18 → VAI or VAC chemo × 8c or busulfan–melphalan.
- Limb-salvage surgery is preferred over amputation. Adequate margins for surgery are: >1 cm for bone, >0.5 cm for soft tissue, and >0.2 cm for fascia.
- Post-op RT is given for gross residual disease (55.8 Gy) or + microscopic margins (45 Gy, as per EICESS-92 trial).
- Consider post-op RT if poor histologic response to induction chemo in resected specimen.
- Definitive RT is used for skull, face, vertebra, or pelvic primaries and for unresectable disease. The RT dose is 45 Gy to the prechemo GTV + 2 cm margin → boost to 55.8 Gy to the initial bony GTV + the postchemo soft-tissue extent.
- For a rib primary with a + pleural effusion, RT is given to the hemithorax (1.5/15 Gy) → RT to primary to 55.8 Gy as described above.
- For lung mets, give whole lung RT (1.5/15 Gy), or consider resection if ≤4 mets. If residual mets after whole lung RT, may boost to 45 Gy.
- Adding IE to VDCA does not improve survival for patients with metastatic disease at diagnosis.

TRIALS

- *IESS-1* (Nesbit Jr et al., 1990): Nonrandomized comparison of 342 patients with localized disease treated with VAC + D vs. VAC vs. VAC + prophylactic bilateral whole lung RT. The 5-year RFS was best with VAC + D (60%) vs. VAC (24%) vs. VAC + RT (44%).
- *IESS-2* (Evans, et al. *JCO* 1991): Randomized 214 patients with localized nonpelvic primaries to high-dose, intermittent VAC + D vs. moderate dose continuous VAC + D. Local treatment was surgery ± post-op RT, or RT alone to the whole bone 45 Gy → boost to 55 Gy. High-dose VAC + D improved OS (63 → 77%) and RFS, and there was no difference in OS for local control modalities.
- *IESS-3/INT 0091* (Grier et al. 2003): Randomized patients with localized or metastatic disease to VDCA vs. VDCA alternating with IE. Local treatment was given at week 9–15 with RT, surgery, or both. Adding IE improved 5-year OS (61→72%) for localized disease, but not for metastatic disease (25%).
- *CESS 86* (Paulussen et al. *JCO* 2001): 177 patients with localized Ewing's treated with chemo → nonrandomized local control arms of surgery alone, surgery + 45 Gy, or 60 Gy RT alone (randomized qd vs. b.i.d.). RT used 5 cm proximal/distal margins and 2 cm lateral and deep margins. The 5-year OS was 69%. There were no differences in OS or RFS according to local therapy. Local control was 100% for surgery, 95% for surgery + RT, and 86% for RT alone, and there was no difference for qd vs. b.i.d. RT. Sixteen to twenty-six percent of patients developed mets.
- *POG 8346* (Donaldson et al. 1998): 178 patients treated with chemo → surgery or RT. For 44 patients, RT volume was randomized to whole bone (39.6 Gy) → boost to initial tumor + 4 cm margin to 55.8 Gy vs. involved-field to boost volume alone to 55.8 Gy. The rest were treated with involved-field RT. There was no difference in LC or EFS when RT done properly. Five-year EFS was highest for distal extremity and central site (63–65%) vs. proximal extremity (46%) and pelvic/sacral (24%).
- *CESS 81, CESS 86, EICESS 92* (Schuck et al. 2003; Paulussen et al. 2008): Reviewed 1,058 patients treated on trial for localized disease. After surgery, LF was 7.5% with or without post-op RT, 5.3% after pre-op RT. After definitive RT, LF was 26.3%. RT patients were negatively selected with unfavorable tumor sites. Compared to surgery alone, post-op RT improved LC after intralesional resections and in tumors with wide resection and poor histologic response. After marginal resections, post-op

RT had similar LC to surgery alone despite poorer histologic response.

- There are no randomized trials that have directly compared RT to surgery for LC of Ewing's.

RADIATION TECHNIQUES

- The radiation fields are tailored depending on the primary site.
- MRI is recommended for treatment planning in all cases when available.
- For definitive RT for bone tumors with no soft-tissue involvement, treat the prechemo GTV + 2 cm margin to 55.8 Gy.
- For definitive RT for bone tumors with a soft-tissue component, treat the prechemo GTV + 2 cm margin to 45 Gy → boost to 55.8 Gy to the initial bony GTV + the postchemo soft-tissue extent.
- For post-op RT, treat the pretreatment GTV + 2 cm margin to 45 Gy → boost to the post-op residual disease + 2 cm margin (45 Gy for microscopic disease, or 55.8 Gy for gross residual disease).
- For N+, resect → 50.4 Gy to nodal bed. If not resected, give 55.8 Gy.
- Avoid bladder RT with CY or ifosfamide.

DOSE LIMITATIONS

- Depends on primary site.
- More than 20 Gy can prematurely close epiphysis.
- For extremity lesions, spare a 1–2 cm strip of skin to prevent lymphedema. 20–30 Gy usually can be given to entire circumference of an extremity, if necessary.
- Spinal cord <45 Gy.

COMPLICATIONS

- Dermatitis; recall-reaction may occur with ADR and dactinomycin.
- Abnormal bone and soft-tissue growth and development. Most of leg growth occurs at the distal femur and proximal tibia. Limb length discrepancy of 2–6 cm can be managed with a shoe lift, otherwise surgery is needed.
- Permanent weakening of affected bone. The highest risk for fracture is within 18 months of RT. Thus, avoid contact and high-impact sports.

- Decreased range of motion secondary to soft-tissue and/or joint fibrosis.
- Skin discoloration.
- Lymphedema.
- Cystitis (especially with CY or ifosfamide).
- Approximately 5% patients may develop a late second malignancy.

FOLLOW-UP

- H&P + CXR every 3 months for 2 years. X-ray primary every 3 months (and/or MRI of primary every 6 months) for 2 years. After 2 years, may increase follow-up intervals. Obtain CBC annually.

PEDIATRIC HODGKIN'S LYMPHOMA

PEARLS

- Hodgkin's lymphoma constitutes ~6% of childhood cancers. It shares many aspects of biology and natural history with adult Hodgkin's (see the chapter on adult Hodgkin's lymphoma for more details).
- Due to morbidity from RT, lower-dose RT with chemo is used to treat children.
- Hodgkin's lymphoma is most common among children >10 years and rare among children <4 years. For children <10 years, it is more common among boys than girls (3–4:1) but less so for children >10 years (1.3:1).
- Nodular sclerosing histology is the most common subtype in all age groups, but is less common among children (44%) than among adolescents and adults (72–77%). Lymphocyte-predominant histology is relatively more common among children <10 years (13%), whereas lymphocyte-depleted subtype is rare. Mixed-cellularity histology is more common in children (33%) than in adolescents or adults (11–17%).
- Approximately 80% of children present with cervical lymphadenopathy, ~25–30% have B symptoms, ~20% have bulky mediastinal adenopathy.
- Approximately 80–85% of patients present with stage I–III disease, and 15–20% present with stage IV.

WORKUP

- History (including B symptoms, pruritis, respiratory symptoms) and physical exam. Labs include CBC, LFTs, BUN/Cr, ESR.
- Imaging includes CXR, CT of chest, abdomen, and pelvis, and PET scan. Bone scan is ordered for patients with bone pain or elevated alkaline phosphatase.
- Pathologic diagnosis is obtained by excisional biopsy (to study architectural changes). Bone marrow biopsy is obtained for patients with B symptoms or stage III–IV. Histologic assessment is required to diagnose spleen and/or liver involvement.
- Adverse prognostic factors include stage IIB, IIIB, IV; bulky disease; B symptoms; male gender; WBC >11,500/mm^3; hemoglobin ≤11 g/dL.

STAGING

- *Ann Arbor Staging System* used (See Chap. 33).
- Ten-year OS is ≥90% for stages I–III and 75–80% for stage IV.

TREATMENT RECOMMENDATIONS

Stage	Recommended treatment
Low risk: IA, IIA favorable (no bulky disease, no extranodal disease, ≤3 sites)	■ Chemo × 2–4c → IFRT 15–25 Gy ■ Current AHOD 0431 trial investigating whether patients with CR after chemo can bypass IFRT.
Intermediate risk: stage I or II (not low-risk); IIIA	■ Chemo × 4–6c → IFRT 15–25 Gy ■ Current AHOD 0031 trial (which also included IVA patients) randomized patients with rapid response and CR to chemotherapy to: IFRT vs. no further tx.
High risk: IIIB, IVA/B, selected IIB with adverse associated features (e.g., bulky disease)	■ Chemo × 6–8c → IFRT 15–25 Gy.
Relapse	■ For patients with low-risk disease at diagnosis with relapse confined to an area of initial involvement after chemo and no RT, salvage chemo and IFRT is used. For postpubertal patients, standard dose RT may be used. For all other patients, induction chemo and high-dose chemo with peripheral blood stem cell rescue is used.

continued

XI

- Recently closed COG study (AHOD 0121) offered hyperfractionated RT, 21 Gy/ 1.5 b.i.d. to involved sites not previously treated, +ASCT.

Chemotherapy

- Hybrid regimens that utilize lower cumulative doses of alkylators, doxorubicin, and bleomycin are used [e.g., COPP/ABV, OEPA (males), OPPA (females), etc.]. Drugs include: cyclophosphamide (C), procarbazine (P), vincristine (O) and/or vinblastine (V), prednisone (P) or dexamethasone, doxorubicin (A) or epirubicin, bleomycin (B), dacarbazine (D), etoposide (E), methotrexate (M), and cytosine arabinoside.

TRIALS

- *CCG 5942* (Nachman et al. 2002): 501 patients with a CR to risk-adapted combination chemo randomized to IFRT or observation. In an as-treated analysis, 3-year EFS was increased with IFRT (85 → 93%), but OS was the same (98–99%).
- *GPOH-HD 95* (Ruhl et al. 2001; Ruhl et al. ASTRO 2004): 1,018 patients were treated with risk-adapted chemo (2–6 cycles) and RT. No RT was given for a CR, 20 Gy for a PR of >75% tumor regression, 30 Gy for PR <75%, or 35 Gy for residual mass >50 mL. DFS was superior for patients given RT after PR (92%) than for patients not given RT after CR (69–77%), but OS was the same (97%). No advantage for RT in low-risk patients, but this result conflicts with CCG-5942.
- Donaldson et al. (2007): 110 low-risk patients were treated with VAMP × 4 + IFRT (15 Gy for CR, 25.5 Gy for PR). Ten-year OS 96%, EFS 89%. Toxicity: hypothyroidism in 42%. One patient developed cardiac dysfunction; two patients developed secondary malignancies.
- Hudson et al. (2004): 159 unfavorable patients (I/II bulky or B symptoms, III, IV) were treated with alternating VAMP/COPP, then response-based IFRT. Five-year OS 93%, EFS 76%. Trial stopped early due to poor EFS. Poor result due either to chemotherapy regimen, or omitting RT.
- *AHOD0431* (closed to accrual): Low-risk patients treated with AV-PC (doxo, vincristine, prednisone, cyclophosphamide) × 3. If CR on PET after 3 cycles, no RT. Otherwise, IFRT (21 Gy in 14 fx). Interim analysis showed 1-year EFS 81% for CR on PET after 3 cycles. However, increased risk of events in these patients, if PET after 1 cycle less than a CR (COG memo 2008).

RADIATION TECHNIQUES

SIMULATION AND FIELD DESIGN

- Use immobilization for reproducibility and 6MV photons for better dose distribution.
- Involved fields are protocol specific, but generally include the initially involved lymph node region(s).
- Supradiaphragmatic fields may be simulated with the arms-up over the head or akimbo. Arms-up pulls the axillary nodes away from the lungs, allowing greater lung shielding, but the nodes are closer to the humeral heads. Attempts should be made to exclude as much lung, humeral head, and breast tissue as possible.
- For children <5 years, some consider bilateral RT to avoid growth asymmetry. However, with low doses, unilateral fields are usually appropriate.
- Treatment of a bulky mediastinal mass generally involves the initial craniocaudad dimension + 2 cm margin and the postchemo lateral margin + 1.5 cm. The supraclavicular fossa is generally included, but the axilla is not (unless involved).

DOSE PRESCRIPTIONS

- In general, the dose is 15–25 Gy (protocol specific). Occasionally, a 5 Gy boost is used. Dose may be determined by response to initial chemo.

DOSE LIMITATIONS

- Shield femoral head. Doses >25 Gy increase the risk slipped capital femoral epiphysis, and doses >30–40 Gy increase the risk of avascular necrosis.
- Dental abnormalities may occur with doses of 20–40 Gy.
- Radiation doses <30 Gy and cardiac shielding limit cardiac sequelae.
- Thyroid abnormalities are more common with doses >26 Gy.
- Pneumonitis is uncommon with doses <20 Gy except when used in combination with bleomycin.
- Shield testes to limit oligospermia or infertility.
- Consider oophoropexy for girls to preserve ovarian function.

COMPLICATIONS

- Chemo complications include bleomycin (pulmonary fibrosis/pneumonitis); doxorubicin (cardiomyopathy); alkylators and etoposide (AML and myelodysplasia); procarbazine (male infertility); prednisone (avascular necrosis).

- Acute side effects of mantle RT include epilation, dermatitis, dysgeusia, xerostomia, odynophagia, esophagitis. Paraaortic RT may cause acute nausea or vomiting.
- Subacute and late effects of RT include musculoskeletal hypoplasia, sterility, hypothyroidism, radiation pneumonitis, increased risk for myocardial atherosclerotic heart disease, and increased risk of second malignancy.
- The rate of second malignancies is ~8–15% at 20 years. Breast cancer is the most common solid 2nd malignancy following treatment.

RETINOBLASTOMA

Stuart Y. Tsuji, Linda W. Chan, Alice Wang-Chesebro, Eric K. Hansen, and Daphne A. Haas-Kogan

PEARLS

- Retinoblastoma (RB) is the most common intraocular tumor of childhood. Ninety-five percent of cases occur in children <5 years.
- The RB1 tumor suppressor gene on chromosome 13 causes RB only when both alleles are "hit."
- Forty percent of patients have a germline mutation of RB1; 60% of cases are sporadic.
  - Although autosomal recessive, RB is inherited in an autosomal dominant pattern due to penetrance approaching 100%.
- Up to 25–40% of cases are familial in that the affected gene is inherited, but only 10% have a + family history of RB.
- Genetic counseling should be given to all patients with RB and siblings should be examined.
- Sixty-five to eighty percent of cases are unilateral (mostly sporadic) and 20–35% are bilateral (mostly due to germline mutations).
- In the developing world, patients present with proptosis, orbital mass, or mets. In the US, the most common presentation is leukocoria, strabismus, painful glaucoma, irritability, failure to eat, and low-grade fever.
- The five patterns of spread are: continguous spread through the choroid/sclera/orbit; extension along the optic nerve into the brain; invasion of subarachnoid space/leptomeninges via CSF; hematogenous spread to bone, liver, and spleen; and lymphatic spread from the conjunctiva.
- The risk of metastases increases with tumor thickness and size.

- Trilateral RB refers to bilateral RB and midline CNS neuroblastic tumors (frequently of the pineal or suprasellar region).
- With germline RB, 15–35% of nonirradiated patients and 50–70% of irradiated patients develop second tumors by 50 years after diagnosis, mainly sarcomas or melanomas.
- Homer-Wright rosettes may be observed.

WORKUP

- H&P includes external ocular examination, slit lamp bimicroscopy, and biocular indirect ophthalmoscopy (often under anesthesia for mapping).
- Labs: CBC, chemistries, BUN, Cr, LFTs.
- Imaging: Fluorescein angiography, bilateral US (A&B mode), and MRI.
- Bone scan and/or lumbar puncture for symptoms or suspected metastatic disease.
- Risk factors for metastatic disease include optic nerve invasion, uveal invasion, orbital invasion, and choroidal involvement.

STAGING

- The most commonly used system is the Reese-Ellsworth system, which predicts the chance of visual preservation well, but not survival. The Abramson-Grabowski system addresses both intraocular and extraocular Rb. The International Classification ("ABCDE") system for intraocular Rb is under modification and is used in recent clinical protocols. The AJCC TNM system is new as of 2002.
- Five-year DFS is >90% for patients with intraocular disease, but <10% for patients with extraocular disease.

REESE-ELLSWORTH STAGING SYSTEM

Group I:	Very favorable (refers to chance of salvaging the affected eye) A: Solitary tumor, less than 4 disc diameters (DD) in size, at or behind the equator B: Multiple tumors, none over 4 DD in size, all at or behind the equator
Group II:	Favorable A: Solitary tumor, 4–10 DD in size, at or behind the equator B: Multiple tumors, 4–10 DD in size, behind the equator
Group III:	Doubtful A: Any lesion anterior to the equator B: Solitary tumors larger than 10 DD behind the equator

continued

XI

Group IV: Unfavorable
- A: Multiple tumors, some larger than 10 DD
- B: Any lesion extending anteriorly to the ora serrata

Group V: Very unfavorable
- A: Massive tumors involving over half the retina
- B: Vitreous seeding

Adapted from Reese AB, et al. 1963.

INTERNATIONAL CLASSIFICATION SYSTEM FOR INTRAOCULAR RETINOBLASTOMA

Group A

Small intraretinal tumors away from foveola and disc

- All tumors are 3 mm or smaller in greatest dimension, confined to the retina *and*
- All tumors are located further than 3 mm from the foveola *and* 1.5 mm from the optic disc

Group B

All remaining discrete tumors confined to the retina

- All other tumors confined to the retina not in Group A
- Tumor-associated subretinal fluid less than 3 mm from the tumor with no subretinal seeding

Group C

Discrete local disease with minimal subretinal or vitreous seeding

- Tumor(s) are discrete
- Subretinal fluid, present or past, without seeding involving up to 1/4 retina
- Local fine vitreous seeding may be present close to discrete tumor
- Local subretinal seeding less than 3 mm (2 DD) from the tumor

Group D

Diffuse disease with significant vitreous or subretinal seeding

- Tumor(s) may be massive or diffuse
- Subretinal fluid present or past without seeding, involving up to total retinal detachment
- Diffuse or massive vitreous disease may include "greasy" seeds or avascular tumor masses
- Diffuse subretinal seeding may include subretinal plaques or tumor nodules

Group E

Presence of any one or more of these poor prognosis features

- Tumor touching the lens

continued

- Tumor anterior to anterior vitreous face involving ciliary body or anterior segment
- Diffuse infiltrating retinoblastoma
- Neovascular glaucoma
- Opaque media from hemorrhage
- Tumor necrosis with aseptic orbital cellulites
- Phthisis bulbi

From COG Protocol ARET0331 (with permission): Trial of systemic neoadjuvant chemotherapy for Group B Intraocular Retinoblastoma: A Phase III Limited Institution Study. Available at: https://members.childrensoncologygroup.org/Prot/ARET0331/ARET0331DOC.pdf.

STAGING : RETINOBLASTOMA

Editors' note: All TNM stage and stage groups referred to elsewhere in this chapter reflect the 2002 AJCC staging nomenclature unless otherwise noted as the new system below was published after this chapter was written.

(AJCC 6TH ED., 2002)

Primary tumor (T)

- TX: Primary tumor cannot be assessed
- T0: No evidence of primary tumor
- T1a: Any eye in which the largest tumor is less than or equal to 3 mm in height and no tumor is located closer than 1 DD (1.5 mm) to the optic nerve or fovea
- T1b: All other eyes in which the tumor(s) are confined to the retina regardless of location or size (up to half the volume of the eye). No vitreous seeding. No retinal detachment or subretinal fluid >5 mm from the base of the tumor
- T2: Tumor with contiguous spread to adjacent tissues or spaces (vitreous or subretinal space)
  - T2a: Minimal tumor spread to vitreous and/or subretinal space. Fine local or diffuse vitreous seeding and/or serous retinal detachment up to total detachment may be present but no clumps, lumps, snowballs, or avascular masses are allowed in the vitreous or subretinal space. Calcium flecks in the vitreous or subretinal space are allowed. The tumor may fill up to 2/3 of the volume of the eye
  - T2b: Massive tumor spread to the vitreous and/or subretinal space. Vitreous seeding and/or subretinal implantation may consist of lumps, clumps, snowballs, or avascular tumor masses. Retinal detachment may be total. Tumor may fill up to 2/3 the volume of the eye
  - T2c: Unsalvageable intraocular disease. Tumor fills more than 2/3 the eye or there is no possibility of visual rehabilitation or one or more of the following are present: Tumor-associated glaucoma, either neovascular or angle closure; anterior segment extension of tumor; ciliary body extension of tumor; hyphema (significant); massive vitreous hemorrhage; tumor

(AJCC 7TH ED., 2010)

Clinical classification (cTNM)

Primary tumor (T)

- TX: Primary tumor cannot be assessed
- T0: No evidence of primary tumor
- T1: Tumors no more than 2/3 the volume of the eye with no vitreous or subretinal seeding
  - T1a: No tumor in either eye is greater than 3 mm in largest dimension or located closer than 1.5 mm to the optic nerve or fovea
  - T1b: At least one tumor is greater than 3 mm in largest dimension or located closer than 1.5 mm to the optic nerve or fovea. No retinal detachment or subretinal fluid beyond 5 mm from the base of the tumor
  - T1c: At least one tumor is greater than 3 mm in largest dimension or located closer than 1.5 mm to the optic nerve or fovea, with retinal detachment or subretinal fluid beyond 5 mm from the base of the tumor
- T2: Tumors no more than 2/3 the volume of the eye with vitreous or subretinal seeding. Can have retinal detachment
  - T2a: Focal vitreous and/or subretinal seeding of fine aggregates of tumor cells is present, but no large clumps or "snowballs" of tumor cells
  - T2b: Massive vitreous and/or subretinal seeding is present, defined as diffuse clumps or "snowballs" of tumor cells
- T3: Severe intraocular disease
  - T3a: Tumor fills more than 2/3 of the eye
  - T3b: One or more complications present, which may include tumor-associated neovascular or angle closure glaucoma, tumor extension into the anterior segment, hyphema, vitreous hemorrhage, or orbital cellulitis

continued

in contact with lens; orbital cellulites-like clinical presentation (massive tumor necrosis)
T3: Invasion of the optic nerve and/or optic coats
T4: Extraocular tumor

Regional lymph nodes (N)
NX: No regional lymph node metastasis cannot be assessed
N0: No regional lymph node metastasis
N1: Regional lymph node involvement (preauricular, submandibular, or cervical)
N2: Distant lymph node involvement

Distant metastasis (M)
MX: Distant metastasis cannot be assessed
M0: No distant metastasis
M1: Metastasis to central nervous system and/or bone, bone marrow, or other sites

Used with the permission from the American Joint Committee on Cancer (AJCC), Chicago, IL. The original source for this material is the AJCC Cancer Staging Manual, Sixth Edition (2002), published by Springer Science+Business Media.

T4: Extraocular disease detected by imaging studies
 T4a: Invasion of optic nerve
 T4b: Invasion into the orbit
 T4c: Intracranial extension not past chiasm
 T4d: Intracranial extension past chiasm

Regional lymph nodes (N)
NX: Regional lymph nodes cannot be assessed
N0: No regional lymph node involvement
N1: Regional lymph node involvement (preauricular, cervical, submandibular)
N2: Distant lymph node involvement

Metastasis (M)
M0: No metastasis
M1: Systemic metastasis
 M1a: Single lesion to sites other than CNS
 M1b: Multiple lesions to sites other than CNS
 M1c: Prechiasmatic CNS lesion(s)
 M1d: Postchiasmatic CNS lesion(s)
 M1e: Leptomeningeal and/or CSF involvement

Pathologic classification (pTNM)
Primary tumor (pT)
pTX: Primary tumor cannot be assessed
pT0: No evidence of primary tumor
pT1: Tumor confined to eye with no optic nerve or choroidal invasion
pT2: Tumor with minimal optic nerve and/or choroidal invasion
 pT2a: Tumor superficially invades optic nerve head but does not extend past lamina cribrosa *or* tumor exhibits focal choroidal invasion
 pT2b: Tumor superficially invades optic nerve head, but does not extend past lamina cribrosa *and* exhibits focal choroidal invasion

continued

pT3: Tumor with significant optic nerve and/or choroidal invasion
- pT3a: Tumor invades optic nerve past lamina cribrosa, but not to surgical resection line *or* tumor exhibits massive choroidal invasion
- pT3b: Tumor invades optic nerve past lamina cribrosa, but not to surgical resection line *and* exhibits massive choroidal invasion

pT4: Tumor invades optic nerve to resection line or exhibits extraocular extension elsewhere
- pT4a: Tumor invades optic nerve to resection line, but no extraocular extension identified
- pT4b: Tumor invades optic nerve to resection line and extraocular extension identified

Regional lymph nodes (pN)

pNX: Regional lymph nodes cannot be assessed
pN0: No regional lymph node involvement
pN1: Regional lymph node involvement (preauricular, cervical)
N2: Distant lymph node involvement

Metastasis (pM)

cM0 No metastasis
pM1: Metastasis to sites other than CNS
- pM1a: Single lesion
- pM1b: Multiple lesions
- pM1c: CNS metastasis
- pM1d: Discrete mass(es) without leptomeningeal and/ or CSF involvement
- pM1e: Leptomeningeal and/or CSF involvement

Used with the permission from the American Joint Committee on Cancer (AJCC), Chicago, IL. The original source for this material is the AJCC Cancer Staging Manual, Seventh Edition (2010), published by Springer Science+Business Media.

TREATMENT RECOMMENDATIONS

Stage	Treatment recommendation
Unilateral intraocular	■ Laser therapy alone, or chemoreduction×6c → focal therapy. Chemo agents include vincristine, carboplatin, and etoposide. Focal therapy options include: ■ EBRT (35–46 Gy) for small tumors located within macula, diffuse vitreous seeding, or multifocal tumors ■ Cryotherapy is used in addition to EBRT or in place of photocoagulation for lesions <4 DD in the anterior retina ■ Photocoagulation is used for posteriorly located tumors <4 DD distinct from the optic nerve head and macula. It is occasionally used alone for small tumors, or in addition to EBRT ■ Episcleral plaque brachytherapy is used for either focal unilateral disease or recurrent disease following prior EBRT ■ Enucleation if the tumor is massive or if the eye is unlikely to have useful vision after treatment
Bilateral	■ Each eye is assessed individually. The worse eye is no longer routinely enucleated. If there is potential vision preservation in both eyes, bilateral chemoreduction ± EBRT with close follow-up for focal treatment may be used
Extraocular	■ Orbital EBRT + chemo for palliation. High-dose chemo with stem cell rescue may also be attempted in select cases. Intrathecal chemo may be given for patients with CNS or meningeal disease
Trilateral Retinoblastoma	■ Treat eyes as above. Neurosurgical resection, chemo, with cranial RT or CSI. MS is only 11 months, but as high as 24 months if caught early

RESULTS

- Five-year DFS: Intraocular >90%, extraocular (T4, N1, or M1) <10%.
- Eye preservations rates range among series from ~60 to 90% when using EBRT and depend on extent of disease. Group E patients have eye preservation rates of only 2%.
- Visual preservation rates range among series from ~65 to 100% for R-E Groups I–III but are lower for Groups IV–V.

XI

RADIATION TECHNIQUES

EBRT

- Indicated for small tumors involving macula, diffuse vitreous seeding, or multifocal tumors or those that failed prior chemo and local therapy.

- Pediatric anesthesia may be required.
- Simulate patient supine with thermoplastic head mask immobilization.
- 3DCRT is recommended (or IMRT if at an experienced center) using CT and/or MRI.
- Photons (4–6 MV) are used.
- For unilateral RB, four anterior oblique noncoplanar fields may be used (superior, inferior, medial, and lateral).
- For bilateral RB when both eyes require treatment, 3DCRT (or IMRT) is used with opposed lateral fields and anterior oblique fields.
- Depending on stage and anatomy, 0.5 cm bolus may be required
- At a minimum, the entire retina is treated including 5–8 mm of the optic nerve.
- Dose is 42–45 Gy in 1.8–2 Gy fractions.
- Critical structures to limit RT dose to include the opposite globe (including lens and retina), lacrimal glands, optic chiasm, pituitary gland, brainstem, posterior mandibular teeth, and upper C-spine.

EPISCLERAL PLAQUE BRACHYTHERAPY

- Refer to the chapter on orbital tumors (Chapter 3) for details of brachytherapy for orbital melanoma. Many of the techniques for RB are similar to treatment of melanoma.
- The treatment volume covers the tumor + radial (~2 mm) and deep (1–2 mm) margin.
- The dose to the tumor apex is 40 Gy (while the base receives 100–200 Gy).
- The dose rate is 0.7–1.0 Gy/h, and ~2–4 days of treatment are required.

COMPLICATIONS

- EBRT complications include dermatitis; depigmentation; telangiectasias; ectropion or entropion of the eyelid; loss of cilia of the scalp, eyebrow, or eyelid; facial/temporal bone hypoplasia; decreased tear production due to radiation damage to the lacrimal gland; direct corneal injury; cataracts; vitreous hemorrhage; retinopathy; hypopituitarism; and second tumors in radiation field.
- With plaque brachytherapy, the risk of orbital bone hypoplasia is low, but long-term retinopathy, cataract, maculopathy, paillopathy, and glaucoma are possible.

FOLLOW-UP

- H&P every 3 months for 1 year, every 4 months for second year, every 6 months for third and fourth years, then annually. Patients with bilateral or familial RB advised to have screening for CNS midline neuroblastic tumors with biannual CT or MRI of the brain until 5 years of age. In addition, they need screening of the contralateral eye every 2–4 months for up to 7 years.

REFERENCES

WILMS' TUMOR

D'Angio GJ, Breslow N, Beckwith JB, et al. Treatment of Wilms' tumor. Results of the Third National Wilms' Tumor Study. Cancer 1989;64:349-360.

D'Angio GJ, Evans A, Breslow N, et al. The treatment of Wilms' tumor: results of the Second National Wilms' Tumor Study. Cancer 1981;47:2302-2311.

D'Angio GJ, Evans AE, Breslow N, et al. The treatment of Wilms' tumor: Results of the national Wilms' tumor study. Cancer 1976;38:633-646.

Dome JS, Cotton CA, Perlman EJ, et al. Treatment of anaplastic histology Wilms' tumor: Results from the fifth National Wilms' Tumor Study. JCO 2006;24(15):2352-2358.

Green DM, Breslow NE, Beckwith JB, et al. Comparison between single-dose and divided-dose administration of dactinomycin and doxorubicin for patients with Wilms' tumor: a report from the National Wilms' Tumor Study Group. J Clin Oncol 1998;16:237-245.

Green DM, Breslow NE, Beckwith JB, et al. Treatment with nephrectomy only for small, stage I/favorable histology Wilms' tumor: a report from the National Wilms' Tumor Study Group. J Clin Oncol 2001;19:3719-3724.

Grundy PE, Breslow NE, Li S, et al. Loss of heterozygosity for chromosomes 1p and 16q is an adverse prognostic factor in favorable histology Wilms tumor: A report from the National Wilms Tumor Study Group. J Clin Oncol 2005;23:7312-7321.

Thomas PR, Tefft M, Compaan PJ, et al. Results of two radiation therapy randomizations in the third National Wilms' Tumor Study. Cancer 1991;68:1703-1707.

NEUROBLASTOMA

Castleberry RP, Kun LE, Shuster JJ, et al. Radiotherapy improves the outlook for patients older than 1 year with Pediatric Oncology Group stage C neuroblastoma. J Clin Oncol 1991;9:789-795.

Haas-Kogan DA, Swift PS, Selch M, et al. Impact of radiotherapy for high-risk neuroblastoma: a Children's Cancer Group study. Int J Radiat Oncol Biol Phys 2003;56:28-39.

Kun LE. Childhood Cancer. In: Cox JD, Ang KK, editors. Radiation oncology: rationale, technique, results. 8th ed. St. Louis: Mosby; 2003. pp. 913-938.

London WB, Castleberry RP, Matthay KK, et al. Evidence for an age cutoff greater than 365 days for Neuroblastoma risk group stratification in the Children's Oncology Group. J Clin Oncol 2005;23:6459-6465.

Mansur DB, Michaelski JM. Neuroblastoma, In: Halperin EC, Perez CA, Brady LW. Principes and practice of radiation oncology. 5th ed. Philadelphia: Lippincott, Williams, and Wilkins; 2008. pp. 1859-1871.

Matthay KK, Haas-Kogan D, Constine LS. Neuroblastoma. In: Halperin EC, Constine LS, Tarbell NJ, et al., editors. Pediatric radiation oncology. 4th ed. Philadelphia: Lippincott Williams & Wilkins; 2005. pp. 179-222.

Matthay KK, Reynolds CP, Seeger RC, et al. Long-term results for children with high-risk neuroblastoma treated on a randomized trial of myeloablative therapy followed by 13-*cis*-retinoid acid: A Children's Oncology Group Study. J Clin Oncol 2009;27:1007-1013.

Matthay KK, Villablanca JG, Seeger RC, et al. Treatment of high-risk neuroblastoma with intensive chemotherapy, radiotherapy, autologous bone marrow transplantation, and 13-cis-retinoic acid. Children's Cancer Group. N Engl J Med 1999;341:1165-1173.

Monclair T, Brodeur GM, Ambro PF, et al. The International Neuroblastoma Risk Group (INRG) staging system: An INRG Task Force Report. J Clin Oncol 2008;27:298-303.

Nitschke R, Smith EI, Shochat S, et al. Localized neuroblastoma treated by surgery: a Pediatric Oncology Group Study. J Clin Oncol 1988;6:1271-1279.

Perez CA, Matthay KK, Atkinson JB, et al. Biologic variables in the outcome of stages I and II neuroblastoma treated with surgery as primary therapy: a children's cancer group study. J Clin Oncol 2000;18:18-26.

Schmidt ML, Lal A, Seeger RC, et al. Favorable prognosis for patients 12 to 18 months of age with stage 4 nonamplified MYCN neuroblastoma: A Children's Cancer Group Study. J Clin Oncol 2005;23:6474-6480.

Spierer M, Tereffe W, Wolden S. Neuroblastoma and Wilms' Tumor. In: Leibel SA, Phillips TL, editors. Textbook of radiation oncology. 2nd ed. Philadelphia: Saunders; 2004. pp. 1273-1298.

Strother D, van Hoff J, Rao PV, et al. Event-free survival of children with biologically favourable neuroblastoma based on the degree of initial tumour resection: results from the Pediatric Oncology Group. Eur J Cancer 1997;33:2121-2125.

Wolden S. Neuroblastoma. In:Gunderson LL, Tepper JE, editors. Clinical radiation oncology, 2nd ed. Philadelphia: Churchill Livingston; 2007 pp. 1637-1643.

RHABDOMYOSARCOMA

Arndt CA, Stoner JA, Hawkins DS, et al. Vincristine, actinomycin, and cyclophosphamide compared with vincristine, actinomycin, and cyclophosphamide alternating with vincristine, topotecan, and cyclophosphamide for intermediate-risk rhabdomyosarcoma: children's oncology group study D9803. J Clin Oncol. 2009;27(31):5182-5188.

Bloch LE, Pappo AS. Pediatric soft tissue sarcomas. In: Gunderson LL, Tepper JE, editors. Clinical radiation oncology, 2nd ed. Philadelphia: Churchill Livingston; 2007. pp 1593-1603.

Breitfeld PP, Lyden E, Raney RB, et al. Ifosfamide and etoposide are superior to vincristine and melphalan for pediatric metastatic rhabdomyosarcoma when administered with irradiation and combination chemotherapy: a report from the Intergroup Rhabdomyosarcoma Study Group. J Pediatr Hematol Oncol 2001;23:225-233.

Breneman JC, Donaldson SS. Rhabdomyosarcoma. In: Halperin EC, Perez CA, Brady LW. Principes and practice of radiation oncology. 5th ed. Philadelphia: Lippincott Williams & Wilkins; 2008. pp. 1872-1885.

Crist W, Gehan EA, Ragab AH, et al. The Third Intergroup Rhabdomyosarcoma Study. J Clin Oncol 1995;13:610-630.

Crist WM, Anderson JR, Meza JL, et al. Intergroup rhabdomyosarcoma study-IV: results for patients with nonmetastatic disease. J Clin Oncol 2001;19:3091-3102.

Friedmann AM, Tarbell NJ, Constine LS. Rhabdomyosarcoma. In: Halperin EC, Constine LS, Tarbell NJ, et al., editors. Pediatric radiation oncology. 4th ed. Philadelphia: Lippincott Williams & Wilkins; 2005. pp. 319-346.

Kun LE. Childhood Cancer. In: Cox JD, Ang KK, editors. Radiation oncology: rationale, technique, results. 8th ed. St. Louis: Mosby; 2003. pp. 913-938.

Maurer HM, Beltangady M, Gehan EA, et al. The Intergroup Rhabdomyosarcoma Study-I. A final report. Cancer 1988;61:209-220.

Maurer HM, Gehan EA, Beltangady M, et al. The Intergroup Rhabdomyosarcoma Study-II. Cancer 1993;71:1904-1922.

Wharam Jr. MD. Pediatric Bone and Soft Tissue Tumors. In: Leibel SA, Phillips TL, editors. Textbook of radiation oncology. 2nd ed. Philadelphia: Saunders; 2004. pp. 1251-1272.

EWING'S SARCOMA

Donaldson SS, Torrey M, Link MP, et al. A multidisciplinary study investigating radiotherapy in Ewing's sarcoma: end results of POG no. 8346. Pediatric Oncology Group. Int J Radiat Oncol Biol Phys 1998;42:125-135.

Dunst J, Jurgens H, Sauer R, et al. Radiation therapy in Ewing's sarcoma: an update of the CESS 86 trial. Int J Radiat Oncol Biol Phys 1995;32:919-930.

Evans RG, Nesbit ME, Gehan EA, et al. Multimodal therapy for the management of localized Ewing's sarcoma of pelvic and sacral bones: a report from the second intergroup study. J Clin Oncol 1991;9:1173-1180.

Grier HE, Krailo MD, Tarbell NJ, et al. Addition of ifosfamide and etoposide to standard chemotherapy for Ewing's sarcoma and primitive neuroectodermal tumor of bone. N Engl J Med 2003;348:694-701.

Marcus KJ, Tarbell NJ. Ewing's Sarcoma. In: Halperin EC, Constine LS, Tarbell NJ, et al., editors. Pediatric radiation oncology. 4th ed. Philadelphia, PA: Lippincott Williams & Wilkins; 2005. pp. 271-290.

Marcus KJ, Marcus Jr RB. Ewing Tumor. In: Halperin EC, Perez CA, Brady LW. Principes and practice of radiation oncology. 5th ed. Philadelphia: Lippincott Williams & Wilkins; 2008. pp. 1886-1891.

Nesbit ME, Jr., Gehan EA, Burgert EO, Jr., et al. Multimodal therapy for the management of primary, nonmetastatic Ewing's sarcoma of bone: a long-term follow-up of the First Intergroup study. J Clin Oncol 1990;8:1664-1674.

Paulussen M, Ahrens S, Dunst J, et al. Localized Ewing tumor of bone: final results of the cooperative Ewing's Sarcoma Study CESS 86. J Clin Oncol 2001;19:1818-1829.

Paulussen M, Craft AW, Lewis I, et al. Results of the EICESS-92 Study: Two randomized trials of Ewing's Sarcoma treatment – Cyclophosphamide compared with ifosfamide in standard-risk patients and assessment of benefit of etoposide added to standard treatment in high-risk patients. J Clin Oncol 2008;27:4385-4393.

Schuck A, Ahrens S, Paulussen M, et al. Local therapy in localized Ewing tumors: results of 1058 patients treated in the CESS 81, CESS 86, and EICESS 92 trials. Int J Radiat Oncol Biol Phys 2003;55:168-177.

Schuck A. Pediatric sarcomas of bone. In: Gunderson LL, Tepper JE, editors. Clinical radiation oncology, 2nd ed. Philadelphia: Churchill Livingston; 2007. pp. 1605-1612.

Wharam Jr. MD. Pediatric Bone and Soft Tissue Tumors. In: Leibel SA, Phillips TL, editors. Textbook of radiation oncology. 2nd ed. Philadelphia: Saunders; 2004. pp. 1251-1272.

PEDIATRIC HODGKIN'S LYMPHOMA

Asselin B, Hudson M, Mandell LR, et al. Pediatric Leukemias and Lymphomas. In: Leibel SA, Phillips TL, editors. Textbook of radiation oncology. 2nd ed. Philadelphia: Saunders; 2004. pp. 1215-1251.

Donaldson SS, Link MP, Weinstein HJ, et al. Final results of a prospective clinical trial with VAMP and low-dose involved-field radiation for children with low-risk Hodgkins disease. J Clin Oncol 2007;25:332-337.

Greene FL, American Joint Committee on Cancer., American Cancer Society. AJCC cancer staging manual. 6th ed. New York: Springer-Verlag; 2002.

Hudson MM, Constine LS. Hodgkin's Disease. In: Halperin EC, Constine LS, Tarbell NJ, et al., editors. Pediatric radiation oncology. 4th ed. Philadelphia: Lippincott Williams & Wilkins; 2005. pp. 223-260.

Hudson MM, Krasin N, Link MP, et al. Risk-adapted, combined-modality therapy with VAMP/COPP and response-based, involved-field radiation for unfavorable pediatric Hodgkins disease. J Clin Oncol 2004;22:4541-4550.

Hudson MM, Asselin BL, Constine LS. Lymphomas in children. In: Halperin EC, Perez CA, Brady LW. Principes and practice of radiation oncology. 5th ed. Philadelphia: Lippincott Williams & Wilkins; 2008. pp. 1892-1912.

Hudson MM, Constine LS. Pediatric hodgkin's lymphomas. In: Gunderson LL, Tepper JE, editors. Clinical radiation oncology, 2nd ed. Philadelphia: Churchill Livingston; 2007. pp. 1657-1663.

Nachman JB, Sposto R, Herzog P, et al. Randomized comparison of low-dose involved-field radiotherapy and no radiotherapy for children with Hodgkin's disease who achieve a complete response to chemotherapy. J Clin Oncol 2002;20:3765-3771.

Ruhl U, Albrecht M, Dieckmann K, et al. Response-adapted radiotherapy in the treatment of pediatric Hodgkin's disease: an interim report at 5 years of the German GPOH-HD 95 trial. Int J Radiat Oncol Biol Phys 2001;51:1209-1218.

Ruhl U, Albrecht MR, Lueders H, et al. The German multinational GPOH-HD 95 trial: Treatment results and analysis of failures in pediatric Hodgkins disease using combination chemotherapy with and without radiation. Int J Radiat Oncol Biol Phys 2004;60:S131.

RETINOBLASTOMA

Abramson DA, McCormick B, Schefler AC. Retinoblastoma. In: Leibel SA, Phillips TL, editors. Textbook of radiation oncology. 2nd ed. Philadelphia: Saunders; 2004. pp. 1463-1482.

Freire JE, Kolton MM, Brady LW. Eye and Orbit. In: Halperin EC, Perez CA, Brady LW. Principes and practice of radiation oncology. 5th ed. Philadelphia: Lippincott Williams & Wilkins; 2008. pp. 778-799.

Halperin EC, Kirkpatrick JP. Retinoblastoma. In: Halperin EC, Constine LS, Tarbell NJ, et al., editors. Pediatric radiation oncology. 4th ed. Philadelphia, PA: Lippincott Williams & Wilkins; 2005. pp. 135-178.

Kun LE. Childhood Cancer. In: Cox JD, Ang KK, editors. Radiation oncology: rationale, technique, results. 8th ed. St. Louis: Mosby; 2003. pp. 913-938.

Lavey RS. Retinoblastoma. In: Gunderson LL, Tepper JE, editors. Clinical radiation oncology, 2nd ed. Philadelphia: Churchill Livingston; 2007. pp. 1625-1636.

Reese AB, Ellsworth RM. The evaluation and current concept of retinoblastoma therapy. Trans Am Acad Ophthalmol Otolaryngol 1963;67:164.

FURTHER READING

Bleyer WA. The U.S. pediatric cancer clinical trials programmes: international implications and the way forward. Eur J Cancer 1997;33:1439-1447.

Faria P, Beckwidth JB, Mishra K, et al. Focal versus diffuse anaplasia in Wilms Tumor: New definitions with prognostic significance. A Report from the National Wilms Tumor Study Group. Am J Surg Pathol 1996;20:909-920.

George RE, London WB, Cohn SL, et al. Hyperdiploidy plus nonamplified MYCN confers a favorable prognosis in children 12 to 18 months old with disseminated neuroblastoma: A Pediatric Oncology Group Study. J Clin Oncol 2005;23:6466-6473.

Halperin EC. Wilms' Tumor. In: Halperin EC, Constine LS, Tarbell NJ, et al., editors. Pediatric radiation oncology. 4th ed. Philadelphia, PA: Lippincott Williams & Wilkins; 2005. pp. 379-422.

Kalapurakal J, Thomas PRM. Wilms' Tumor. In: Perez CA, Brady LW, Halperin EC, et al., editors. Principles and practice of radiation oncology. 5th ed. Philadelphia: Lippincott Williams & Wilkins; 2008. pp. 1850-1858.

Kalapurakal J, Thomas PRM. Wilms' Tumor. In: Gunderson LL, Tepper JE, editors. Clinical radiation oncology, 2nd ed. Philadelphia: Churchill Livingston; 2007. pp 1613-1623.

Kun LE. Childhood Cancer. In: Cox JD, Ang KK, editors. Radiation oncology: rationale, technique, results. 8th ed. St. Louis: Mosby; 2003. pp. 913-938.

Spierer M, Tereffe W, Wolden S. Neuroblastoma and Wilms' Tumor. In: Leibel SA, Phillips TL, editors. Textbook of radiation oncology. 2nd ed. Philadelphia: Saunders; 2004. pp. 1273-1298.

PART XII
Palliation

Chapter 42
Palliation and Benign Conditions

Stuart Y. Tsuji and William M. Wara

INTRODUCTION

- This chapter will cover brain metastases, bone metastases, spinal cord compression, liver metastases, airway obstruction, superior vena cava obstruction, and gynecologic bleeding.

BRAIN METASTASES

PEARLS

- Most common type of intracranial tumor (incidence ~170,000/year in the US)
- Approximately 20–40% of all cancer patients develop brain metastases
- "Solitary" = one brain metastasis, only site of disease
- "Single" = one brain metastasis, other sites of disease
- Primary cancers most likely to metastasize to brain are lung, breast, and melanoma
- Hemorrhagic metastases: renal cell CA, choriocarcinoma, and melanoma

WORKUP

- H&P, MRI of brain with and without contrast
- If solitary lesion, obtain biopsy

PROGNOSTIC FACTORS

- RTOG Recursive Partitioning Analysis (Gaspar et al. 1997)

Class	Characteristics	Survival (months)
I	KPS 70–100, Primary controlled Age < 65 Mets to brain only	7.1
II	All Others	4.2
III	KPS < 70	2.3

- Graded Prognostic Index (Sperduto et al. 2008)

	Score			GPI score	Survival (months)
	0	0.5	1.0	3.5–4.0	11.0
Age	>60	50–59	<50	3	6.9
KPS	<70	70–80	90–100	1.5–2.5	3.8
Number of CNS metastases	>3	2–3	1	0–1	2.6
Extracranial metastases	Present	–	None		

TREATMENT RECOMMENDATIONS

STEROIDS

- Improve headache and neurologic function
- No impact on survival
- Start dexamethasone 4 mg q 6 h if patient has neurologic symptoms
- Taper as tolerated
- No role for steroids in asymptomatic patients

SURGERY, WHOLE-BRAIN RT (WBRT), STEREOTACTIC RADIOSURGERY (SRS)

Characteristics	Options
Single lesion RPA class I–II	■ Surgical resection + WBRT ■ WBRT + SRS ■ SRS alone (with SRS or WBRT for salvage prn) ■ WBRT alone
2–4 Lesions RPA class I–II	■ WBRT alone ■ WBRT + SRS ■ SRS alone (with SRS or WBRT for salvage prn) controversial

continued

>4 Lesions RPA class I–II	▪ WBRT alone ▪ WBRT + SRS controversial ▪ SRS alone (with SRS or WBRT for salvage prn) controversial
RPA class III	▪ WBRT alone

STUDIES

SURGERY

- Patchell et al. (1990): 54 patients with solitary brain lesion randomized to surgical removal of tumor plus WBRT (36 Gy in 12 fractions) vs. needle biopsy plus WBRT (same). Recurrence at original site, time to recurrence, MS, time to death from neurologic cause, and time with KPS ≥70 all significantly better in the surgery group. Six patients excluded when resection or biopsy did not demonstrate pathologic diagnosis of brain met.

POST-OP WBRT

- Patchell et al. (1998): 95 patients with solitary brain lesion treated with surgery randomized to WBRT (50.4 Gy in 28 fractions) vs. no further therapy. Post-op RT reduced recurrence at the original site and other sites in the brain. Patients in the RT group were less likely to die of neurologic causes. OS and duration of functional independence were not different.
- *EORTC 22952-26001* (Mueller et al. 2009): 345 patients with WHO PS 0–2, 1–3 brain mets treated with resection (GTR), or SRS (20 Gy) randomized to observation vs. WBRT (30 Gy in 10 fx). WBRT decreased 6, 24 months intracranial progression (15%, 31% vs. 40%, 54%) and neurologic death (25% vs. 43%), but no difference in OS or preservation of performance status.

WBRT ALONE OR WITH RADIOSENSITIZERS

- Suh et al. (2006): 515 RPA class I–II patients with ≥1 brain mets randomized to WBRT alone (30 Gy in 10 fractions) vs. WBRT (same) plus concurrent efaproxiral. Fifty percent of patients had ≥3 mets. Trend of MS benefit of efaproxiral (4.4 vs. 5.4 months). Largest improvement in breast cancer patients.
- Mehta et al. (2009): 554 patients with brain mets from NSCLC, KPS ≥70 randomized to WBRT alone (30 Gy in 10 fractions) vs. WBRT (same) plus concurrent motexafin gadolinium (MGd). Eighty percent of patients had >1 brain met. Trend of improved time to neurologic progression with MGd (10 vs. 15 months).

XII

Less salvage needed with MGd without change in MS (5.8 vs. 5.1 months).

SRS BOOST AFTER WBRT

- Andrews et al. (2004): 331 patients with 1–3 brain mets and KPS ≥70 randomized to WBRT (37.5 Gy in 15 fractions) plus SRS (15–24 Gy) vs. WBRT alone (same). Significant survival advantage with the addition of SRS in patients with single met (MS 6.5 vs. 4.9 months) and trends for advantage for RPA class I (11.6 vs. 9.6 months), lung histology (5.9 vs. 3.9 months), and tumor size >2 cm (6.5 vs. 5.3 months). Local control at 1 year and KPS at 6 months better with the addition of SRS.
- Kondziolka et al. (1999): 27 patients with 2–4 brain mets and KPS ≥70 randomized to WBRT alone (30 Gy in 12 fractions) vs. WBRT (same) plus SRS (16 Gy). Local failure 100% at 1 year after WBRT alone, 8% with the addition of RS. Nonsignificant OS benefit in the SRS group (MS 7.5 vs. 11 months).

SRS ALONE OR WITH WBRT

- *JROSG 99-1* (Aoyama et al. JAMA 2006): 132 patients with 1–4 mets and KPS ≥70 randomized to SRS (18–25 Gy) vs. WBRT (30 Gy in 10 fractions) → SRS (same). No difference in OS (8.0 vs. 7.5 months), neurologic or KPS preservation, or MMSE. WBRT reduced rate of new mets (63.7% vs. 41.5%), and improved 1-year LC (72.5% vs. 88.7%).
- Chang (Lancet Oncol. 2009): 58 patients with 1–3 mets and KPS ≥70 randomized to SRS (15–24 Gy) vs. SRS (same) → WBRT (30 Gy in 12 fractions). Worse neurocognitive decline at 4 months with WBRT (24% vs. 52%) by Hopkins Verbal Learning Test, despite better 1-year LC (67% vs. 100%) and 1-year distant brain tumor control (27% vs. 73%) with WBRT. Longer OS (15.2 vs. 5.7 months) for SRS alone. SRS alone patients received more salvage therapy, including repeat SRS (27/30 vs. 3/28).
- Sneed et al. (1999, 2002): Multiinstitutional and UCSF retrospective reviews of SRS vs. SRS + WBRT. No difference in OS by RPA class (I = 14–15 months, II = 7–8 months, III = 5 months). Brain FFP worse without WBRT, but brain FFP allowing for first salvage not different.

DOSE AND FRACTIONATION CONSIDERATIONS

- *RTOG fractionation papers* (Borgelt et al. 1980, 1981; Murrary et al. 1997): Multiple fractionation regimens evaluated. Most

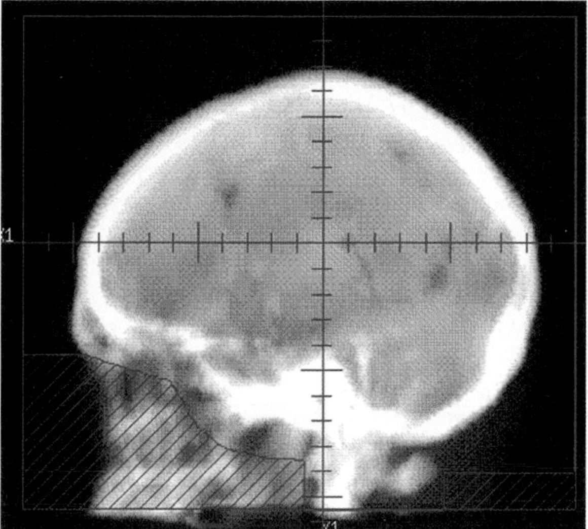

Fig. 42.1 Lateral DRR of a whole-brain radiation field

were similar for treatment response, duration of improvement, and OS. Worse outcomes with 10 Gy × 1 and 7.5 Gy × 2.

- Shaw et al. (2000): Maximum tolerated dose for single fraction radiosurgery: tumor diameter ≤20 mm, dose 24 Gy; diameter 21–30 mm, dose 18 Gy; diameter 31–40 mm, dose 15 Gy.

TECHNIQUES

WBRT

- Opposed laterals, flash anterior/posterior/superior (Fig. 42.1)
- Bottom of field at foramen magnum, inferior to C1, or inferior to C2
- Use eye block
- Acceptable fractionation schemes include 4 Gy × 5, 3 Gy × 10 (most common), 2.5 Gy × 15, and 2 Gy × 20
- Choose fractionation based on performance status and life expectancy

STEREOTACTIC RADIATION

- Consider increased dose gadolinium at the time of Gamma Knife SRS to improve the sensitivity of detection of brain metastases. Renal function must be assessed to avoid excess risk of gadolinium-associated nephrogenic systemic fibrosis.

- Gamma Knife SRS vs. FSRT recommended depending on number, size, location of mets.

COMPLICATIONS

- Neurocognitive deficits after WBRT in long-term survivors.
- Five percent rate of symptomatic brain necrosis after SRS, generally treated with steroids, sometimes requires surgery for intractable symptoms.

FOLLOW-UP

- Brain MRI scan with and without contrast every 3 months

BONE METASTASES

PEARLS

- Common cause of severe cancer pain
- Pain relief after RT can be expected in 60–90% of patients
- Good pain control may improve OS
- Sites of mets: spine (lumbar>thoracic) > pelvis > ribs > femur > skull
- Primary cancers most likely to metastasize to bone are breast, prostate, thyroid, kidney, and lung

WORKUP

- Bone scan is the primary imaging modality.
- Plain films should be used to look for fracture or impending fracture, but are not sensitive for diagnosis as cortical involvement occurs late.
- MRI is the procedure of choice when evaluating for spinal cord compression or nerve root compromise.
- Biopsy and/or PET scan are not routinely needed, but should be considered if radiographic studies are equivocal.

TREATMENT RECOMMENDATIONS

SURGERY

- Required for pathologic fracture or impending fracture.
- Mirels (1989): 12 point scoring system estimates risk of pathologic fracture based on the site of disease (upper extremity, lower extremity, peritrochanteric), amount of pain (mild, moderate,

functional), type of lesion (blastic, mixed, lytic), and size (<1/3, 1/3–2/3, >2/3 diameter of bone involved). Scores of 10–12 have 72–100% chance of fracture.

- Van der Linden et al. (2004): Data show that axial cortical involvement >30 mm and/or circumferential cortical involvement >50% predict for high rates of fracture.

EBRT

- Local field RT for discrete painful lesions
  - Avoid uninvolved sensitive tissues like perineum and joints when possible
  - Dose: 8 Gy × 1, 4 Gy × 5, or 3 Gy × 10
  - Wide-field ("hemibody") RT occasionally used for diffuse bone mets

RADIOPHARMACEUTICAL THERAPY

- Best for patients with multiple lesions that show uptake on bone scan.
- Should not be used for fractures, spinal cord compression, nerve root compression, or lesions with large extra osseous component.
- Patients must have adequate blood counts, no myelosuppressive chemotherapy for 4 weeks before and 6–8 weeks after treatment.
- Strontium-89 (β-emitter) response rates 40–95%, pain relief at 1–4 weeks, lasts up to 18 months. Improved response rate and duration with low-dose platinum.
- Samarium-153 (β- and γ-emitter) response rates 70–95%, pain relief at 1–2 weeks, lasts up to 4 months.

PHARMACOLOGIC THERAPIES AND SUPPORTIVE CARE

- Bisphosphonates are used in most patients with multiple bone mets
- Hormone therapy can be very effective in breast and prostate cancer
- Pain management is important (NSAIDs, narcotics, steroids, anticonvulsants, tricyclic antidepressants, electric stimulation, nerve blocks)
- Do not forget braces and walkers

STUDIES

EBRT DOSE

- Metaanalysis (Chow et al. 2007) of 16 randomized trials of single fraction vs. multiple fraction palliative RT regimens. No difference in response rates. Trend for increased risk of pathological fractures and spinal cord compression with single fraction RT. A 2.5× increased retreatment rate with single fraction RT.
- *Bone Pain Trial Working Party* (1999): 761 patients with painful bone mets randomized to 8 Gy in single fxn vs. 20 Gy in 5 fractions or 30 Gy in 10 fractions. No difference in time to pain relief, proportion achieving relief, duration of relief, or toxicity. Retreatment given more frequently after 8 Gy (23% vs. 10%).
- *RTOG 9714* (Hartsell, JNCI 2005, Howell et al. 2009): 898 patients with breast or prostate cancer and KPS ≥40 randomized to 8 Gy in 1 fxn vs. 30 Gy in 10 fractions. Higher acute toxicity with 30 Gy (17% vs. 10%). Pain CR/PR rates at 3 months were equivalent, 15%/50% for 8 Gy and 18%/48% for 30 Gy, but higher retreatment at 3 years for 8 Gy (18% vs. 9%). Same conclusions in subgroup of vertebral body mets.
- Tong et al. (1982): Various fractionation schemes evaluated. No differences seen in rates of pain relief.
- Blitzer (1985): Reanalysis of RTOG data with conclusion that more fractions with higher total dose were more effective for pain relief.
- See spinal cord compression for SBRT of spine bone metastases.

RADIONUCLIDE THERAPY

- Sartor et al. (2004): 152 patients with hormone-refractory prostate cancer randomized 2:1 to ^{153}Sm vs. nonradioactive ^{152}Sm. Better complete response (38% vs. 18%) with ^{153}Sm. No difference between arms in transient, mild marrow suppression.
- Oosterhof (Eur Urol 2003): 203 patients with hormone-refractory prostate cancer randomized to ^{89}Sr vs. EBRT. No difference in subjective response (~34%), response duration (4.5 months). MS 7.2 vs. 11 months for Sr vs. EBRT, despite similar toxicity.
- Sciuto et al. (2002): 70 patients with hormone-refractory prostate cancer randomized to ^{89}Sr±concurrent low-dose cisplatin. Better subjective response (91% vs. 63%), duration (120 vs. 60 days), survival without new painful mets (4 vs. 2 months), and less bone disease progression (27% vs. 64%) for cisplatin arm. No difference in toxicity.

- Porter et al. (1993): Randomized local field RT ± strontium 89 in patients with hormone-refractory prostate cancer. Patients in combined arm needed lesser analgesics, had fewer sites of new pain, had lower PSA and alk phos levels, and had better quality of life.

SPINAL CORD COMPRESSION

PEARLS

- Most important prognostic factor is ambulatory status
- Pain precedes neurologic dysfunction and is the most common presenting symptom

WORKUP

- MRI scan of entire spine to determine location and extent of disease and to rule out other sites of cord compression
- Biopsy required if metastatic disease has not been previously documented or if patient does not have proven cancer diagnosis

TREATMENT RECOMMENDATIONS

STEROIDS

- Start steroids immediately and then taper as tolerated
- Used for symptom relief (improved neurologic function, reduced pain)

SURGERY AND RT

- Maximum debulking surgery with appropriate spine stabilization followed by post-op RT is treatment of choice for patients with single region of cord compression and life expectancy >3 months.
- Laminectomy is not an alternative to maximal debulking and stabilization.
- If patient has multiple levels of compression or is not medically fit for surgery, then give immediate RT.

SBRT

- Delivers higher BED with greater conformality than EBRT
- Generally reserved for disease confined to 1–2 spinal segments, but not cases of cord compression

- Low-reported toxicity and risk of myelopathy, despite a range of dose and fractionation and its use in cases of reirradiation or postresection

TRIALS

- Patchell et al. (2005): Prospective randomized trial of surgery with post-op RT to 30 Gy vs. RT alone to 30 Gy. Surgery patients regained ability to walk more often (62% vs. 19%), retained ability to walk longer (122 vs. 13 days), and required less steroid and pain medication. Improved survival with surgery (126 vs. 100 days).
- Rades et al. (2005): Retrospective review of 204 patients with metastatic cord compression treated with EBRT of 8 Gy in 1 fxn or 30 Gy in 10 fractions. No difference in rate of motor function improvement, stability, or deterioration between treatments. Thiry-four percent of patients regained ability to walk.
- Rades et al. (2009): Prospective nonrandomized trial of 265 patients with metastatic spinal cord compression treated with short (1 or 5 fxn) vs. long (10, 15, or 20 fxn) course RT. Long-course RT achieved higher 1-year LC 61 vs. 81%. Motor function improvement (~35%) and OS (~25%) similar. Better OS with better KPS, no visceral mets, 1–3 vertebral mets, ability to ambulate, and use of bisphosphonates.
- Rades et al. (2008): Retrospective review of 124 patients reirradiated for in-field recurrence of metastatic cord compression. Motor function improved in 36%, stable in 50%. No radiation myelopathy at 11 months median follow-up with 24% of patients receiving cumulative BED < 100 Gy, including both courses of RT. [$BED = n*d*(1+d/\alpha\beta)$; n = # of fractions; d = dose per fraction; $\alpha\beta = 2$].

SBRT

- Gerzsten et al. (2007): Prospective single arm study of 393 patients (500 lesions) treated with SBRT (12.5–25 Gy in 1 fxn). Three hundred and forty-four lesions had received prior EBRT. Long-term improvement in 86% of patients treated for pain. For patient treated for imaging progression, LC was 90, 88% for primary and salvage SBRT. No episodes of radiation myelopathy.
- Sahgal et al. (2009): Retrospective review of 39 patients (60 mets) treated with SBRT (median 24 Gy in 3 fractions). Thirty-seven mets previously irradiated (median 36 Gy in 14 fractions) with 11

months interim. One- and two-year progression-free probability (per met) was 85 and 69%, respectively. No difference between primary and salvage. No radiation myelopathy or radiculopathy.

TECHNIQUES

- AP/PA gives more homogenous dose distribution and is the preferred technique
- With PA alone, one must decide between higher dose to the spinal cord or underdosing the tumor
  - Example: Lumbar spine met, cord depth (7.5 cm), anterior vertebral body depth (12 cm). With 6 MV dosed at 12 cm, cord would receive 128% of the prescription dose. If 18 MV is used, cord would receive 120% of the prescription dose. If the prescription is 3 Gy × ten fractions, total dose to the cord would be 36–38.4 Gy
- Dose schedules: 3 Gy × 10 (most common), 4 Gy × 5, 8 × 1, 2.5 Gy × 15

LIVER METASTASES

PEARLS

- MS 5–10 months without intervention
- Colo-rectal primary is most common with 50,000 cases of colorectal liver mets per year in the USA
- Liver has remarkable ability for regeneration and can grow back after 50% resection in just 3 weeks

WORKUP

- CT is primary imaging modality used for diagnosis and follow-up, special contrast protocols exist to maximize CT yield
- Ultrasound is particularly helpful intraoperatively
- MRI scan is good for distinguishing benign from malignant disease and can provide specific information about involvement of biliary tree

TREATMENT RECOMMENDATIONS

SURGERY

- Surgery with curative intent possible in ~10% of patients
- MS after complete resection is ~30 months with small number of patients surviving >10 year

- Contraindications for liver resection
  - Presence of extrahepatic disease (selected patients with limited pulmonary and liver mets are candidates for surgical resection of both sites of disease)
  - Complete resection not possible (unacceptable LF rates with + margins)
- Second resections can be performed for liver-only failures that meet criteria for surgery. Long-term survival after second resection is possible

CHEMOTHERAPY

- Systemic chemotherapy for unresectable mets is palliative
- Neoadjuvant chemotherapy can be used to shrink disease, increase resectability
- Adjuvant chemotherapy (including hepatic arterial chemotherapy) can be used to reduce LR rates and possibly improve survival

RADIOFREQUENCY ABLATION, CYROABLATION, ETHANOL INJECTION

- Alternative therapies for patients who are not surgical candidates
  - See Chap. 21 – Hepatobiliary

EBRT

- Whole Liver RT (3 Gy × 7) for symptomatic patients with multiple small lesions who are not candidates for other therapies.
- 3DCRT ± hepatic artery chemo is preferred over whole liver RT for patients with good KPS and limited metastatic disease.
- Stereotactic body irradiation and IMRT are promising, but remain investigational.

PAPERS

- McCarter and Fong (2000): Good review of surgical data.
- Rusthoven et al. (2009): Phase I/II trial of 47 patients (63 lesions) with 1–3 liver metastases, each <6 cm, treated with SBRT escalated from 36 to 60 Gy in 3 fractions. Two-year LC 92%. For 38 lesions treated to 60 Gy, LC 100% for ≤3 cm, 77% for >3 cm. OS 20.5 months. No radiation-induced liver disease, 2% incidence grade ≥3 toxicity.
- See Chap. 21 – Hepatobiliary for other studies.

RADIATION TECHNIQUES/TOLERANCE/COMPLICATIONS

- See Chap. 21 – Hepatobiliary

FOLLOW-UP

- Liver function tests 2–3 weeks after treatment
- Office visit every 3 months or as needed for symptoms
- CT scan every 3–6 months or sooner for recurrent symptoms

AIRWAY OBSTRUCTION

- Broncoscopy with stent placement
  - If successful, may result in immediate symptom relief
- Intraluminal brachytherapy
  - Use caution in previously treated areas near major vessels
- EBRT
  - Do not exceed spinal cord tolerance when using large fraction sizes
  - Accepted dose and fractionation schedules include: 10 Gy × 1, 8.5 Gy × 2 (1 week apart), 4 Gy × 5, 3 Gy × 10, 2.5 Gy × 15
  - If large fields will be necessary, use caution. Do not want to induce radiation pneumonitis in patients needing palliation for shortness of breath

SUPERIOR VENA CAVA SYNDROME

- Most frequently seen in lung cancer patients
- Biopsy required to evaluate for benign conditions and sensitive tumors
- Generally, symptoms improve because of collateral circulation
- Treatment includes supportive care, steroids, diuretics, and elevation of the head and torso
- Accepted external beam radiation therapy dose, and fractionation schedules include 3 Gy × 10, 4 Gy × 5, 2.5 Gy × 15

GYNECOLOGIC BLEEDING

- Treatment options
  - Vaginal packing

- EBRT: 3.7 Gy b.i.d. × 2 days, repeat every 2 weeks × 2 prn. Use CT scan to determine field borders
- Brachytherapy
- Electron cone

REFERENCES

Andrews DW, Scott CB, Sperduto PW, et al. Whole Brain Radiation Therapy with or without Stereotactic Radiosurgery Boost for Patients with One to Three Brain Metastases: Phase III Results of the RTOG 9508 Randomised Trial. Lancet 2004;363:1665-1672.

Aoyama H, Shirato H, Tago M, et al. Stereotactic Radiosurgery Plus Whole-Brain Radiation Therapy vs Stereotactic Radiosurgery Alone for Treatment of Brain Metastases: A Randomized Controlled Trial. JAMA 2006;295(21):2483-2491.

Blitzer PH. Reanalysis of the RTOG Study of the Palliation of Symptomatic Osseous Metastasis. Cancer 1985;55:1468-1472.

Bone Pain Trial Working Party. 8 Gy Single Fraction Radiotherapy for the treatment of Metastatic Skeletal Pain: Randomised Comparison with a Multifraction Schedule over 12 Months of Patient Follow-Up. Radiother Oncol 1999;52:111-121.

Borgelt B, Gelber R, Kramer S, et al. The Palliation of Brain Metastases: Final Results fo the First Two Studies by the Radiation Therapy Oncology Group. Int J Radiat Oncol Biol Phys 1980;6:1-9.

Borgelt B, Gelber R, Larson M, et al. Ultra-Rapid High Dose Irradiation Schedules for the Palliarion of Brain Metastases: Final Results of the First Two Studies by the Radiation Therapy Oncology Group. Int J Radiat Oncol Biol Phys 1981;7:1633-1638.

Chang EL, Wefel JS, Hess KR, et al. Neurocognition in patients with brain metastases treated with radiosurgery or radiosurgery plus whole-brain irradiation: a randomised controlled trial. Lancet Oncol 2009;10:1037-1044.

Chow E, Harris K, et al. Palliative Radiotherapy Trials for Bone Metastases: a Systematic Review. J Clin Oncol 2007;25:1423-1436.

Gaspar L, Scott C, Rotman M, et al. Recursive Partitioning Analysis (RPA) of Prognostic Factors in Three Radiation Therapy Oncology Group (RTOG) Brain Metastases Trials. Int J Radiat Oncol Biol Phys 1997;37:745-751.

Gerszten PC, Burton SA, Ozhasoglu C. Radiosurgery for Spinal Metastases: Clinical Experience in 500 Cases from a Single Institution. Spine 2007;32:193-199.

Hartsell WF, Scott CB, Bruner DW, et al. Randomized Trial of Short- Versus Long-Course Radiotherapy for Palliation of Painful Bone Metastases. J Natl Cancer Inst 2005;97:798-804.

Howell DD, James JL, Hartsell WF, et al. Randomized Trial of Short-Course Versus Long-Course Radiotherapy for Palliation of Painful Vertebral Bone Metastases: A Retrospective Analysis of RTOG 97-14. J Clin Oncol 2009;27:7s. ASCO 2009, abstract.

Kondziolka D, Patel A, Lunsford LD, et al. Stereotactic Radiosurgery Plus Whole Brain Radiotherapy Versus Radiotherapy Alone for Patients with Multiple Brain Metastases. Int J Radiat Oncol Biol Phys 1999;45:427-434.

McCarter MD, Fong Y. Metastatic Liver Tumors. Semin Surgl Oncol 2000; 19:177-188.

Mehta MP, Shapiro WR, Phan SC, et al. Motexafin Gadolinium Combined with Prompt Whole Brain Radiotherapy Prolongs Time to Neurologic Progression in Non-Small-Cell Lung Cancer Patients with Brain Metastases: Results of a Phase III Trial. Int J Radiat Oncol Biol Phys 2009;73:1069-1076.

Mirels H. Metastatic Disease in Long Bones. A Proposed Scoring System for Diagnosing Impending Pathologic Fractures. Clin Orthop Relat Res 1989; 249:256-264.

Mueller RP, Soffietti R, Abacioglu MU, et al. Adjuvant Whole-Brain Radiotherapy Versus Observation After Radiosurgery or Surgical Resection of 1-3 Cerebral Metastases: Results of the EORTC 22952-26001 Study. J Clin Oncol 2009;27:15s. ASCO 2009, abstract.

Murrary KJ, Scott C, Greenberg HM, et al. A Randomized Phase III Study of Accelerated Hyperfractionation Versus Standard in Patients with Unresected Brain Metastases: A Report of the Radiation Therapy Oncology Group (RTOG) 9104. Int J Radiat Oncol Biol Phys 1997;39:571-574.

Patchell RA, Tibbs PA, Regine WF, et al. Postoperative Radiotherapy in the Treatment of Single Metastases to the Brain. JAMA 1998;280:1485-1489.

Patchell RA, Tibbs PA, Regine WF, et al. Direct Decompressive Surgical Resection in the Treatment of Spinal Cord Compression Caused by Metastatic Cancer: A Randomised Trial. Lancet 2005;366:643-648.

Patchell RA, Tibbs PA, Walsh JW, et al. A Randomized Trial of Surgery in the Treatment of Single Metastases to the Brain. N Engl J Med 1990;322:494-500.

Porter AT, McEwan AJ, Powe JE, et al. Results of a Randomized Phase III Trial to Evaluate the Efficacy of Strontium-89 Adjuvant to Local Field External Beam Irradiation in the Management of Endocrine Resistant Metastatic Prostate Cancer. Int J Radiat Oncol Biol Phys 1993;25:805-813.

Rades D, Lange M, Veninga T, et al. Final Results of A Study Comparing Short-Course and Long-Course Radiotherapy (RT) for Local Control of Metastatic Spinal Cord Compression (MSCC). J Clin Oncol 2009;27:7s. ASCO 2009, abstract.

Rades D, Rudat V, Veninga T, et al. Prognostic Factors for Functional Outcome and Survival After Reirradiation for In-Field Recurrences of Metastatic Spinal Cord Compression. Cancer 2008;113:1090-1096.

Rades D, Stalpers LJA, Hulshof MC, et al. Comparison of 1 x 8 Gy and 10 x 3 Gy for Functional Outcome in Patients with Metastatic Spinal Cord Compression. Int J Radiat Oncol Biol Phys 2005;62:514-518.

Rusthoven KE, Kavanagh BD, Cardenes H, et al. Multi-Institutional Phase I/II Trial of Stereotactic Body Radiation Therapy for Liver Metastases. J Clin Oncol 2009;27(10):1572-1578.

Sahgal A, Ames C, Chou D, et al. Stereotactic Body Radiotherapy is Effective Salvage Therapy for Patients with Prior Radiation of Spinal Metastases. Int J Radiat Oncol Biol Phys 2009;74(3): 723-731.

Sartor O, Reid RH, Hoskin PJ, et al. Samarium-153-Lexidronam Complex for Treatment of Painful Bone Metastases in Hormone-Refractory Prostate Cancer. Urology 2004;63: 940-945.

Sciuto R, Festa A, Rea S, et al. Effects of Low-Dose Cisplatin on ^{89}Sr Therapy for Painful Bone Metastases from Prostate Cancer: A Randomized Clinical Trial. J Nucl Med 2002;43:79-86.

Shaw E, Scott C, Souhami L, et al. Single Dose Radiosurgical Treatment of Recurrent previously Irradiated Primary Brain Tumors and Brain Metastases: Final Report of RTOG Protocol 90-05. Int J Radiat Oncol Biol Phys 2000;47:291-298.

Sneed PK, Lamborn KR, Forstner JM, et al. Radiosurgery for Brain Metastases: Is Whole Brain Radiotherapy Necessary? Int J Radiat Oncol Biol Phys 1999;43:549-558.

Sneed PK, Suh JH, Goetsch SJ, et al. A multi-institutional review of radiosurgery alone vs. radiosurgery with whole brain radiotherapy as the initial management of brain metastases. Int J Radiat Oncol Biol Phys 2002;53:519-526.

Sperduto PW, Berkey B, Gaspar LE, et al. A New Prognostic Index and Comparison to Three Other Indices for Patients with Brain Metastases: An Analysis of 1,960 Patients in the RTOG Database. Int J Radiat Oncol Biol Phys 2008;70:510-514.

Suh JH, Stea B, Nabid A, et al. Phase III Study of Efaproxiral As an Adjunct to Whole-Brain Radiation Therapy for Brain Metastases. J Clin Oncol 2006;24:106-114.

Tong D, Gillick L, Hendrickson FR. The Palliation of Symptomatic Osseous Metastases: Final Results of the Study by the Radiation Therapy Oncology Group. Cancer 1982;50:893-899.

Van der Linden YM, Dijkstra PD, Kroon HM, et al. Comparative Analysis of Risk Factors for Pathological Fracture with Femoral Metastases. J Bone Joint Surg Br 2004;86:566-573.

FURTHER READING

Cowper SE. Nephrogenic Systemic Fibrosis: An Overview. J Am Coll Radiol 2008;5:23-28.

Dillehay GL, Ellerbroek NA, Balon H, et al. Practice Guideline for the Performance of Therapy with Unsealed Radiopharmaceutical Sources. Int J Radiat Oncol Biol Phys 2006;64: 1299-1307.

Finlay IG, Mason MD, Shelley M. Radioisotopes for the Palliation of Metastatic Bone Cancer: A Systematic Review. Lancet Oncol 2005;6:392-400.

Janjan NA, Delclos ME, Ballo MT, et al. Palliative Care. In: Cox JD, Ang KK, editors. Radiation Oncology: Rationale, Technique, Results. 8th ed. St. Louis: Mosby; 2003. pp. 954-986.

Johnson JD, Young B. Demographics of Brain Metastasis. Neurosurg Clin North Am 1996;7: 337-344.

Kagan RA. Palliation of Brain and Spinal Cord Metastases. In: Perez CA, Brady LW, Halperin EC, et al, editors. Principles and Practice of Radiation Oncology. 4th ed. Philadelphia: Lippincott Williams & Wilkins; 2004. pp. 2373-2384.

Leonard GD, Brenner B, Kemeny NE. Neoadjuvant chemotherapy before liver resection for patients with unresectable liver metastases from colorectal carcinoma. J Clin Oncol 2005;23:2038-2048.

Oosterhof G, Roberts JT, de Reijke TM, et al. Strontium^{89} Chloride Versus Palliative Local Field Radiotherapy in Patients with Hormonal Escaped Prostate Cancer: A Phase III Study of the

European Organisation for Research and Treatment of Cancer Genitourinary Group. Eur Urol 2003;44:519-526.

Perez CA, Grigsby PW, Thorstad W. Nonsealed Radionuclide Therapy. In: Perez CA, Brady LW, Halperin EC, et al, editors. Principles and Practice of Radiation Oncology. 4th ed. Philadelphia: Lippincott Williams & Wilkins; 2004. pp. 636-652.

Porter AT, Benda R, Ben-Josef E. Palliation of Metasteses: Bone and Spinal Cord. In: Gunderson LL, Tepper JE, editors. Clinical Radiation Oncology. 1st ed. Philadelphia: Churchill Livingstone; 2000. pp. 299-313.

Ratanatharathorn V, Powers WE, Temple HT. Palliation of Bone Metastases. In: Perez CA, Brady LW, Halperin EC, et al, editors. Principles and Practice of Radiation Oncology. 4th ed. Philadelphia: Lippincott Williams & Wilkins; 2004. pp. 2385-2404.

Sahgal A, Larson DA, Chang EL. Stereotactic Body Radiosurgery for Spinal Metastases: A Critical Review. Int J Radiat Oncol Biol Phys 2008;71:652-665.

Stevens, KR. The Liver and Biliary System. In: Cox JD, Ang KK, editors. Radiation Oncology: Rationale, Technique, Results. 8th ed. St. Louis: Mosby; 2003. pp. 493-496.

Chapter 43

Clinical Radiobiology and Physics

Gautam Prasad and Jean Pouliot

RADIOBIOLOGY PEARLS

The Four Rs of Radiobiology (rationale for fractionation of radiation)

- *Repair* – refers to DNA repair in response to sublethal or potentially lethal radiation damage. Fractionation of radiation allows normal tissues time to repair.
- *Reassortment* – refers to radioresistant cells that synchronize into a more radiosensitive phase of the cell cycle after a fraction of radiation. Over multiple fractions, more and more cells are redistributed into these radiosensitive phases.
- *Repopulation* – refers to tumor cell proliferation during the course of radiation therapy. This can be problematic with very low dose rates (VLDRs) or prolonged treatment durations.
- *Reoxygenation* – refers to the importance of oxygen in mediating the cytotoxic effects of radiation due to free radical production. As normoxic tumor cells are killed with each fraction, formerly hypoxic cells become oxygenated.

DNA DAMAGE AND IONIZING RADIATION

- Photons produce their effects through both direct action (one–third) and indirect action (two–thirds). Direct action refers to direct damage to DNA, whereas indirect action is mediated through free radicals produced through ionization of H_2O.
- DNA damage to the cell can come in several forms:
  - Base damage/single-strand breaks (SSBs) – repaired via base excision repair, not a major contributor to radiosensitivity.
  - Double-strand breaks (DSBs) – repaired via homologous recombination repair (in late S/G2, a DNA template is available) which is accurate, or nonhomologous end-joining which is error-prone. DSBs are a major contributor to radiosensitivity; ~40 DSBs are required to kill cell.

- Chromosome aberrations – result from unrepaired or misrepaired DSBs. Symmetric chromosome damage (e.g., translocations) tends to be nonlethal, whereas asymmetric damage (e.g., rings) tends to be lethal due to the loss of large amounts of DNA.
- *LET* (linear energy transfer) – refers to the average energy transferred to tissue per unit length of an ionizing particle (in keV/μm). Generally, heavy particles like protons and carbon ions have high LET, while photons have lower LET.
- *RBE* (relative biological effectiveness) – refers to the ratio of the dose of 250 keV X-rays (standard) required for a given effect compared to a different type of radiation. The greatest RBE for cell-killing occurs when LET reaches 100 keV/μm since this is the diameter of a DNA double helix.
- *OER* (oxygen enhancement ratio) – refers to the ratio of the dose necessary to provide an effect under anoxic conditions divided by the dose necessary to provide the same effect under aerobic conditions. At low LET (such as for X-rays or γ-rays), the OER is 2.5–3.0. This reflects that higher oxygen concentration leads to greater production of DNA-damaging free radicals by ionizing radiation. At high LET, OER approaches 1.0 since damage produced is mostly direct and oxygen-independent.

CELL SURVIVAL CURVES

- A cell survival curve graphs the relationship between dose and the surviving fraction of cells. Dose is plotted on a linear scale and surviving fraction on a logarithmic scale.
- The *linear-quadratic model (LQM)* refers to the fact that most radiation-induced aberrations are a linear-quadratic function of dose. At low doses, DSBs are likely to be caused by a single electron, and aberrations are directly proportional to dose (linear). At higher doses, DSBs are likely to be caused by separate electrons and are proportional to the dose squared (quadratic).
- According to the LQM, $S = e^{-\alpha(\text{alpha})D-\beta(\text{beta})D^2}$. Where *S* = surviving fraction, and α (alpha) and β (beta) represent the linear and quadratic components of cell-killing, respectively. The initial slope is determined by α (alpha), while the β (beta) causes the curve to bend.
- Most tumors and early-responding tissues (e.g., mucosa) have a high α (alpha)/β (beta) ratio (~10), whereas some tumors

(e.g., prostate) and late-responding tissues (e.g., spinal cord) have a low α/β ratio (~3).

- When treatments are fractionated, sublethal damage (SLD) can be repaired between treatments. This allows the "shoulder" of the survival curve to be repeated, thereby sparing late-responding tissues. This is the basis for hyperfractionation during which treatments are given twice per day or more to mitigate late effects.
- The *biological equivalent dose (BED)* refers to the effective total absorbed dose (in Gy) for a given fractionation scheme if it were given by standard fractionation (1.8–2.0 Gy/day).
  - BED = nd[1+d/(α(alpha)β(beta))], where n = number of fractions and d = the dose per fraction.

RADIATION AND THE CELL CYCLE AND DNA REPAIR

- The cell cycle for mammalian cells can be divided into G_1 (initial growth phase) → S (DNA replication phase) → G_2 (additional growth phase) → M (mitotic phase). In general, the G2/M phases are the most radiosensitive and late S phase is most radioresistant.
- Transition through the cell cycle is governed by cyclins and cyclin-dependent kinases (cdk). List of important checkpoints:
  - G1→S governed by p53, Rb, Cyclin D1/Cdk4/6, and Cyclin E/Cdk2
  - S governed by Cyclin A/Cdk2
  - G2→M governed by Cyclin B/A/Cdk1
- For a typical mammalian cell, a single fraction of radiation (1–2 Gy) results in >1,000 base damage, 1,000 SSB, and 40 DSBs. DSBs are the most relevant in terms of cell-killing.
- Base damage/SSB can be repaired by base excision repair (involves *XRCC1* gene) or nucleotide excision repair. DSBs can be repaired by less accurate nonhomologous end-joining (involves proteins Ku/XRCC4/Artemis/DNA ligase IV) or more accurate homologous recombination repair (involves proteins NBS/MRE11/Rad51/BRCA1/BRCA2).
- DNA damage can be categorized as:
  - Potentially lethal damage (PLD) – would ordinarily cause cell death, but can be modified by postirradiation environmental conditions; postulated that radiosensitive tumors repair PLD inefficiently, whereas radioresistant tumors have efficient mechanisms.

- Sublethal damage (SLD) – can be repaired in hours unless additional SLD is added; after a single fraction of radiation producing SLD, repair of DNA damage will occur; this is followed by reassortment of surviving cells into the more radiosensitive G2/M phase; if too much time elapses between fractions, cells will repopulate.
- Lethal damage – irreversible and leads to cell death by definition.

- Dose-rate effect refers to repair of SLD that occurs during long radiation exposure. Smaller doses per fraction lead to a repeat of the shoulder on the survival curve. Continuous low-date irradiation (such as I-125 seeds) would be considered an infinite number of infinitely small fractions leading to a survival curve with no shoulder and far shallower compared to acute exposures. The inverse-dose effect occurs when decreasing dose rate actually increases cell killing. This is because higher dose rates (HDRs) would cause arrest in radioresistant phases of the cell cycl
- Important hereditary syndromes that affect response to DNA damage:
  - Ataxia-telangiectasia (AT); autosomal recessive; *ATM* mutated; results in immune deficiency and high incidence of cancer.
  - Ataxia-telangiectasia-like disorder (ATLD); autosomal recessive; *MRE11* mutated.
  - Nijmegen breakage syndrome (NBS); autosomal recessive; *NBS1* mutated.
  - Fanconi anemia (FA); autosomal recessive; *FANCD2* mutated; enhanced radiosensitivity to tumors observed clinically.

EFFECT OF OXYGEN

- Oxygen "fixes" the free radical damage to DNA caused by X-rays. For this effect to be observed, oxygen must be present in the target at the time of irradiation or microseconds afterwards. Generally, at least 2% oxygen concentration results in maximum radiosensitization.
- In addition to rendering cells more radioresistant, both chronic and acute hypoxia also contribute to malignant and metastatic progression.
- In animal models, there is a wide range of percentage of hypoxic cells with an average of about 15%. After a fraction of radiation in which tumor cells in aerobic conditions are killed, the remaining hypoxic cells tend to become reoxygenated. In this way, fractionation of radiation can improve tumor cell kill.

- HIF-1, through its oxygen-sensitive HIF-1α subunit, is responsible for up-regulation of a number of hypoxia-induced genes. Under normoxic conditions, it is degraded by the von Hippel-Lindau (VHL) protein.

EFFECTS OF ACUTE TOTAL BODY IRRADIATION

- Clinical effects from acute radiation syndrome have been drawn from effects of survivors of atomic bombings of Hiroshima and Nagasaki, as well as various nuclear installation accidents.
- The LD50 (lethal dose in 50% of recipients) for humans who do not receive treatment for an acute dose is ~4 Gy; with antibiotics and careful nursing, the LD50 can be increased to 7–8 Gy; acute doses of ≥10 Gy are uniformly fatal; people receiving doses between 8 and 10 Gy may benefit from bone marrow transplantation.
- Temporally acute effects of radiation exposure can be divided into the following:
  - Prodromal radiation syndrome: (20+ Gy can be severe, <20 Gy variable) timing depends on dose, but can occur ~5 min – days; symptoms: fatigue, anorexia, nausea/vomiting; symptoms if supralethal doses received: fever, hypotension, immediate diarrhea.
  - Cerebrovascular syndrome (50–100 Gy): death occurs in 24–48 h; thought to primarily result from damage to intracranial blood vessels; symptoms: severe nausea/vomiting, ataxia, respiratory distress, coma, seizures.
  - Gastrointestinal syndrome (5–12 Gy): death occurs in 3–10 days; thought to result from death of intestinal crypt cells and/or apoptosis of vascular endothelial cells; symptoms: nausea/vomiting, prolonged diarrhea.
  - Hematopoietic syndrome (3–8 Gy): peak deaths at 30 days, continues for 60 days; results from death of hematologic stem cells resulting in eventual pancytopenia.

EFFECTS OF RADIATION ON EMBRYO/FETUS

- Preimplantation period (0–9 days): 0.05–0.15 Gy prenatal death.
- Organogenesis (10 days to 6 weeks): congenital malformations with increased risk for neonatal death, peak incidence of teratogenesis.
- Fetal period (6 weeks to birth): microcephaly (0–15 weeks), mental retardation (~40%/Sv at 8–15 weeks; 10%/Sv at 15–25 weeks), carcinogenesis (excess absolute risk ~6%/Gy).

COMMON EXPERIMENTAL TECHNIQUES USED IN RADIOBIOLOGY

- Western blot – identification/quantification of specific protein.
  - Cells of interest are lysed in the presence of protease inhibitor
  - Lysates are run through a polyacrlyamide gel by electrical current, which leads to separation based on size
  - The gel is transferred by electrical current to a membrane
  - The membrane is then probed with antibodies, which bind to the protein of interest
- Southern blot – identification/quantification of specific DNA sequence.
  - Cells of interest have their DNA extracted and digested by endonucleases
  - DNA is then run on a polyacrlyamide gel and transferred to a membrane (see Western blot)
  - Labeled probes complementary to the DNA sequence of interest are used to identify target sequence
- Northern blot – identification/quantification of a specific mRNA sequence; similar in principle to Southern blot.
- Polymerase chain reaction (PCR) – is used to greatly amplify a specific sequence of DNA which has many useful applications including diagnosis of disease and generation of hybridization probes for Southern/Northern blotting.
  - Purified DNA is denatured at high temperatures so that complementary strands separate
  - Temperature is lowered so that single-stranded DNA may anneal to specific primers to amplify sequences of interest
  - Temperature is increased so that *taq* polymerase amplifies sequences with primers
  - Each successive cycle doubles the DNA content
- Reverse-transcriptase (RT-PCR) – is similar to PCR except that it can be used to amplify specific mRNA sequences. During the first step, the mRNA of interest is converted to DNA using the reverse-transcriptase enzyme.
- Clonogenic assay – the gold standard to test cell survival (more precisely, reproductive cell death) after treatment with an agent(s). Cells are plated in plastic dishes, exposed to the agent(s) of interest and allowed to grow into colonies for several days to several weeks. Prior to experiment, untreated cells must be plated to determine the plating efficiency = (colonies counted/cells plated × 100%). To determine survival after exposure to an agent, use the formula colonies counted/cells plated × 100% × plating efficiency.

- RNA interference – gives the ability to "knock out" the expression of specific genes by the introduction of short-interfering RNAs (siRNAs), which can cleave and silence specific RNA sequences.
- Microarray (gene chip) analysis – allow simultaneous analysis of expression of many genes. Cells of interest have their RNA extracted and reverse-transcribed to DNA. These short sequences are then exposed to chips with preloaded labeled complementary DNA strands of target genes.

RADIATION SAFETY

Release criteria for patients treated with brachytherapy

Isotope	Activity at or below which patients may be released with instructions (mCi)	Dose rate at 1 m at or below which patients may be released with instructions	Activity at or below which patients may be released without instructions (mCi)	Dose rate at 1 m at or below which patients may be released without instructions
I-125	9	0.01 mSv/h (1 mrem/h)	2	0.002 mSv/h (0.2 mrem/h)
Pd-103	40	0.03 mSv/h (3 mrem/h)	8	0.007 mSv/h (0.7 mrem/h)
Ir-192	2	0.008 mSv/h (0.8 mrem/h)	0.3	0.002 mSv/h (0.2 mrem/h)
I-131	33	0.07 mSv/h (7 mrem/h)		

Release criteria can be based on either of these measures. For patients who exceed these levels, they can still be released with instructions if a calculation can be provided which proves no member of family or general public could receive more than 5 mSv (0.5 rem) as a result of exposure from the patient, or that lead shielding is provided (e.g., lead cap for brain patients) to reduce the dose rate level at 1 m.

ANNUAL OCCUPATIONAL DOSE LIMITS

Occupational effective dose equivalent (EDE) for whole body	50 mSv (5 rem)/year
Occupational EDE for declared pregnant workers (fetus)	0.5 mSv (0.05 rem)/month

continued

XII

General public EDE, frequent/ continuous exposure	1 mSv (0.1 rem)/year
General public EDE, infrequent exposure	5 mSv (0.5 rem)/year

Note: 1 rem = 0.01 Sv

Background radiation in the San Francisco Bay Area is in the range 2–2.5 mSv/year. Dose equivalent flying from San Francisco to New York round trip is <0.06 mSv. This is comparable to standing 24 h at one meter of a patient recently treated for prostate cancer with a permanent implant.

TUMOR MARKERS

Tumor marker	Primary tumor	Other tumors	Benign conditions
AFP	Hepatocellular carcinoma, nonseminomatous germ cell tumors (yolk sac tumors and embryonal cell carcinoma)	Gastric, biliary, and pancreatic	Cirrhosis, viral hepatitis, pregnancy
β-2 microglobulin	Multiple myeloma	Other B-cell neoplasms, lung, hepatoma, breast	Ankylosing spondylitis, Reiters syndrome
CA 125	Ovarian	Endometrial, fallopian tube, breast, lung, esophageal, gastric, hepatic, and pancreatic	Menstruation, pregnancy, fibroids, ovarian cysts, pelvic inflammation, cirrhosis, ascites, pleural and pericardial effusions, endometriosis
CA 15-3	Breast	Ovary, lung, prostate	Benign breast or ovarian disease, endometriosis, pelvic inflammatory disease, hepatitis, pregnancy, lactation

continued

CA 19-9	Pancreatic, biliary tract	Colon, esophageal, hepatic	Pancreatitis, biliary disease, cirrhosis
CA 27.29	Breast	Colon, gastric, hepatic, lung, pancreatic, ovarian, prostate	Breast, liver, and kidney disorders, ovarian cysts
Calcitonin	Medullary thyroid	Metastatic breast, lung, pancreas, hepatoma, renal cell, carcinoid	Zollinger-Ellison syndrome, pernicious anemia, chronic renal failure, cirrhosis, Paget's disease, pregnancy, benign breast, or ovarian disease
CEA	Colorectal	Breast, lung, gastric, pancreatic, bladder, medullary thyroid, head and neck, cervical, hepatic, lymphoma, melanoma	Cigarette smoking, peptic ulcer disease, inflammatory bowel disease, pancreatitis, hypothyroidism, cirrhosis, biliary obstruction
Gamma globulin	Multiple myeloma, macro-globulinemia	Leukemia	Chronic infections, hepatic disease, autoimmune diseases, collagen diseases
Neuron-specific enolase	Neuroblastoma, small cell lung cancer	Wilms' tumor, melanoma, thyroid, kidney, testicle, pancreas	
Prostatic acid phos-phatase	Prostate	Testicular, leukemia, non-Hodgkin's lymphoma	Paget's disease, osteoporsis, cirrhosis, pulmonary embolism, hyperpara-thyroidism

continued

PSA	Prostate	None	Prostatitis, BPH, prostate trauma, after ejaculation
Thyroglobulin	Differentiated thyroid cancer (not medullary)		Hyperthyroidism, Subacute thyroiditis, benign adenoma
β-HCG	Nonseminomatous germ cell tumors (embryonal cell carcinoma, choriocarcinoma), gestational trophoblastic disease	Rarely, gastrointestinal tumors, seminoma (occasional minimal)	Hypogonadal states, marijuana use

IMMUNOPHENOTYPING

- All lymphoid cells = CD45+
- B-cells = CD19+, CD20+, CD22+
- T-cells = CD2+, CD3+, CD5+, CD7+. CD4+ = helper cells, CD8+ = cytotoxic cells
- Natural-killer cells = CD16+, CD56+, CD57+
- Follicular cell lymphoma = CD 5−, CD10+, CD43−
- Mantle cell lymphoma = CD 5+, CD23−, CD43+
- MALT lymphoma = CD 5−, CD10−, CD23−
- Hodgkins' disease = CD15+, CD30+

CYTOGENETICS

- t(2:13) and t(1:13) = Alveolar rhabdomyosarcoma
- t(8:14) and t(8:22) = Burkitt's lymphoma and B-cell ALL (C-MYC gene)
- t(11:14) = Mantle cell lymphoma (BCL-1 gene, cyclin D1 overexpression)
- t(11:22) = Ewing's sarcoma and PPNET
- t(12:22) = Clear cell sarcoma
- t(14:18) = Follicular lymphoma and diffuse large B-cell lymphoma (BCL-2 gene)
- t(14:19) = Chronic lymphocytic leukemia (BCL-3 gene)
- t(X:18) = Synovial cell sarcoma

PHYSICS PEARLS

ATOMIC STRUCTURE AND NUCLEAR DECAY

- Atoms consist of a small central core or nucleus surrounded by a cloud of electrons in orbit; the vast majority of atomic mass lies in the nucleus.
- Elements and isotopes are denoted with the following abbreviation $^{X}_{Z}A$ where A is the element on the periodic table, X = mass number = neutrons + protons, Z = atomic number = protons = electrons.
- Gamma rays are produced intranuclearly (e.g., radioactive decay) and X-rays are produced extranuclearly (e.g., linear accelerator).
- Proton mass ~ Neutron mass ~1.01 atomic mass units (amu); mass-energy equivalence is described by Einstein's famous $E = mc^2$; therefore, 1 amu = 931.5 MeV (electron volt) defined as the kinetic energy acquired by passing an electron though a potential difference of 1 V.
- Arrangement of electrons is in orbits or shells denoted by K (innermost), L, M, N, O, etc. Maximum number of electrons per orbit is $2n^2$ (where n depends on shell, K = 1, L = 2, etc.).
- Four fundamental forces of nature in order of decreasing strength: strong nuclear, electromagnetic, weak nuclear, gravity.
- The binding energy of electrons refers to the magnitude of force (in Coulombs) between the electrons and nucleus; high Z atoms have greater binding energies because of greater nuclear charge; if inner orbital electrons are ejected from the atom, they will be filled by higher orbital electrons resulting in characteristic X-ray production.
- Nuclei are most stable at certain numbers of nucleons (neutrons + protons): 2, 8, 20, 82, 126. Also nuclei with odd numbers of protons and neutrons are less stable than those with even numbers of both.
- The rate of nuclear decay (or radioactivity) is described by $N = N_0 e^{-\lambda t}$, where N is activity at time (t) and N_0 is initial activity and λ is the rate decay constant; activity can be described in curies (Ci) where 1 Ci = 3.7×10^{10} dps (disintegrations/sec); 1 dps = 1 Becquerel (Bq) = 2.7×10^{-11} Ci.
- When $N = 0.5(N_0)$, the half-life ($T_{1/2}$) of a radioisotope has been reached; this can also be described as $T_{1/2} = 0.693/\lambda$; the mean life (T_{ave}) or average lifetime for decay of a radioactive nucleus can be described as $T_{ave} = 1/\lambda = 1.44 * T_{1/2}$.

XII

- *Radioactive equilibrium* refers to the ratio between the activity of the parent isotope and its daughter product.
  - In *transient equilibrium*, the $T_{1/2}$ of the parent is not too much greater than $T_{1/2}$ of the daughter.
  - In *secular equilibrium*, the half-life of the parent isotope is much longer than that of the daughter.

MODES OF RADIOACTIVE DECAY

Type	Formula	Notes
Alpha decay	${}^{A}_{Z}X \rightarrow {}^{A-4}_{Z-2}Y + {}^{4}_{2}He + Q$	Q = energy released
Positron decay (β plus decay)	${}^{A}_{Z}X \rightarrow {}^{A}_{Z-1}Y + {}^{0}_{+1}\beta + \nu + Q$	ν = neutrino; Q = energy released; produces positrons (useful in nuclear medicine)
Negatron decay (β minus decay)	${}^{A}_{Z}X \rightarrow {}^{A}_{Z+1}Y + {}^{0}_{-1}\beta + \tilde{\nu} + Q$	$\tilde{\nu}$ = antineutrino; Q = energy released; common in reactor-produced isotopes (e.g., ^{60}Co)
Electron capture	${}^{1}_{1}P + {}^{0}_{-1}\beta \rightarrow {}^{1}_{0}Y + \tilde{\nu} + Q$	An orbital electron (usually from K shell) is captured by nuclear proton which is converted to neutron; competitive with positron decay in nuclei with neutron deficiencies
Internal conversion	${}^{A}_{Z}X + {}^{0}_{0}\gamma \rightarrow {}^{A}_{Z}Y + {}^{0}_{-1}\beta$	A gamma ray is ejected from the nucleus, and in turn, ejects an orbital electron; the gamma ray is completely absorbed; the orbital vacancy is filled by an outer shell electron resulting in emission of a characteristic X-ray

PHOTONS AND THEIR INTERACTIONS

- The photon is a chargeless basic quantum particle that exhibits wave-particle duality.
- In linear accelerators (linacs), electrons are accelerated through an electric field and are rapidly decelerated in a target material such as tungsten. This results in the production of X-rays of varying energies. The basic unit of X-rays are photons.

- X-ray production can be achieved by two major mechanisms. In Bremmstrahlung radiation, an accelerated electron changes direction when it comes into the proximity of a positively charged nucleus, resulting in photon production. Characteristic X-rays are produced when an accelerated electron knocks an inner orbital electron out of its shell. This causes an outer shell electron to fill in the vacancy which subsequently results in photon production. The energy of this photon is the difference in binding energies of the two electrons.
- Photon beams are attenuated as they pass through matter and the degree of attenuation depends on both the thickness (x) and the linear attenuation coefficient (μ) of the material. This relationship can be described by $I(x) = I_0 e^{-\mu x}$. I_0 represents the intensity of the beam prior to attenuation, μ has units of (distance)$^{-1}$ and it represents the fraction of incoming photons that are removed from the beam per unit thickness of material.

COMMON PHOTON ENERGIES AND ATTENUATION PROPERTIES

Energy	~Tissue attenuation/cm (%)	~D_{max} (cm)
Co-60 (1.25 MV)	5	0.5
6 MV	3.5	1.5
18 MV	2.4	3.0

- The mass attenuation coefficient (μ_m) is equal to μ/ρ where ρ is the density of the material (in gm/cm^3). Unlike the linear attenuation coefficient, the mass attenuation coefficient does not vary much for different materials for photons in the therapeutic range.
- Derived from the above equation, the half-value layer [HVL] (e.g., the thickness of a given material required to attenuate the beam intensity to one-half) can be expressed as $\frac{I_0}{2} = I_0 e^{-\mu(HVL)}$. Solving for HVL yields, $HVL = \frac{0.693}{\mu}$.
- If all photons are of the same energy (monoenergetic), the first HVL is identical to subsequent HVLs. However, for polyenergetic photons, the first HVL is smaller than subsequent HVLs because of beam hardening. In other words, more material is required to remove the remaining higher energy photons.

SUMMARY OF MAJOR PHOTON INTERACTIONS

	Photoelectric effect	Compton scattering	Pair production
Brief description	Accelerated electron knocks inner orbital electron out of its shell; this leads to outer orbital electron filling in vacancy and production of characteristic X-ray	A photon hits an outer orbital electron causing it to be ejected from an atom; the photon is itself scattered	A photon hits the nucleus and produces an electron and positron
Prevalent at which energies in tissue?	$E < 30$ keV (diagnostic radiology)	30 keV $< E <$ 25 MeV (Linacs)	$E > 5$ MeV (present) $E > 25$ MeV (dominant)
Dependence of mass attenuation coefficient on atomic number	Z^3 (attenuation is variable based on Z of material; this results in good contrast between air, tissue, and bone)	Nearly independent of Z (proportional to electron density and provides poor contrast)	Z

BRACHYTHERAPY

- Brachytherapy is a form of radiation therapy where the radioactive source(s) are placed near or in the target to be treated.
- Brachytherapy can be categorized in different ways; by the source type, the anatomical site, the applicator type, the type of implants, or by the dose rate, HDR or LDR. None of these categories is complete by itself.
- There are three major types of brachytherapy implants: (1) Molds/plaques – used for superficial lesions where radioactive sources are placed over skin or orbital lesions, (2) Interstitial implants – radioactive sources are incased in wire or seeds and inserted in tumor (e.g., prostate), (3) Intracavitary implants – sealed radioactive sources are placed inside a body cavity (e.g., cervix). Temporary seed insertion and removal are now performed with computerized afterloaders.
- High-dose rate (HDR) implants use dose rates of >20 cGy/min. Lower than this is generally termed low dose rate (LDR).

MAJOR RADIONUCLEOTIDES USED IN BRACHYTHERAPY

Radionucleotide	Half-life	Photon energy (MeV)	HVL (mm Pb)	Clinical use
I-125	59.4 days	0.0028 avg	0.025	Permanent prostate implant
Pd-103	17.0 days	0.021 avg	0.008	Permanent prostate implant
Cs-131	9.7 days	0.029–0.034	0.030	Permanent prostate implant
Au-198	2.7 days	0.412	2.5	Permanent head and neck implant
Cs-137	30 years	0.662	5.5	Temporary intracavitary implants
Ir-192	73.8 days	0.38 avg	2.5	Temporary intracavitary or interstitial implants (HDR) for prostate, breast, cervix. Also used for skin
Co-60	5.26 years	1.25 avg	13.07	Older source for teletherapy
Ra-226	1,622 year	0.83 avg	12	Historical interest
Rn-222	3.83 days	0.83 avg	12	Temporary implant

- Note that the photon energies used in brachytherapy sources are far lower than for external beam. But more importantly, the sources are placed in or very close to the tumor. The inverse square law is of paramount importance in brachytherapy treatment planning. Briefly, this law states that the energy absorbed at a given distance from a point source is inversely proportional to the square of the distance of the source. This is denoted by $1/r^2$.
- There are three ways of quantifying radioactivity: (1) mCi (see above), (2) mg-Ra (milligram equivalent of radium) (obsolete), or (3) air-kerma strength (the current standard). Air-kerma strength is the dose rate in air at a specified distance in units of (Gy)(m^2)/h.
- Various systems exist for placing interstitial implants including:
  - Quimby system: radioactive sources are distributed uniformly over volume of tissue leading to nonuniform dose.
  - Manchester system: radioactive sources are distributed nonuniformly with the goal of ±10% dose uniformity.

XII

  - Paris system: developed for linear sources of iridium wire; sources are distributed uniformly for a planar implant, but follow a particular pattern for volume implants.
- All these systems have an important historical purpose, but have been replaced entirely by computerized dose planning. At UCSF, all HDR treatments are planned with inverse planning using IPSA, an image-based anatomy driven dose optimization tool. This is the equivalent of IMRT for brachytherapy.
- Modern implants are placed temporarily into a volume with the use of surgically placed catheters or intracavitary applicators. By positioning sources at a given position for variable periods of time (called dwell times), one can produce conformal dose distributions.

PHOTON DOSE DISTRIBUTIONS AND PLANNING FORMULAS

- In order to perform photon dose calculations, three key variables are important: (1) attenuation (see above) in tissue, (2) inverse square law (see above) or the distance from the radiation source, and (3) photon scattering due to the Compton effect (see above).
- Generally radiation doses are given in the unit Gray (Gy), which represents absorbed dose (specifically 1 J/kg of tissue). However, in clinical practice, this is difficult to measure, so we instead use monitor units (MUs). A MU represents a specific amount of charge collected in one of the beam monitoring ionization chambers.
- A *depth-dose curve* is a graphical illustration of photon attenuation as it passes through matter. Note that since photons exert their effects primarily through indirect action, the maximum dose is not at the surface. The fact that the maximum dose (D_{max}) is not at the skin gives photons their *skin sparing* effect. Note that the depth-dose curve for protons is notable for the *Bragg peak*. This refers to the dose of protons being distributed over a narrow range, unlike photons.
- Useful photon planning formulas:
  - *Equivalent square formula*: used to convert rectangular fields into square equivalents for ease of calculation; $E = 2XY/(X + Y)$, where E = equivalent square field size, and X and Y are the initial field dimensions.
  - *Wedge/hinge angle formula*: used to estimated necessary wedge angle when two beams are arranged at a particular hinge angle to each other in order to produce a more uniform dose distribution; *wedge angle = 90° – (hinge angle/2)*.

- *Skin gap formula for matching fields*: used to calculate the separation between two field edges (e.g., the gap) on the skin when they are matched at a given depth in tissue.
  - Skin gap = (L1/2)*(d/SSD1) + (L2/2)*(d/SSD2).
  - *L* = length of the field, *d* = depth of match, SSD = source to surface distance; for isocentric setups substitute SAD for SSD (Fig. 43.1).
- *Craniospinal radiation formulas*:
  - Collimator angle of cranial field to match the inferior border with the superior border of spine field = atan [(1/2 spine field length)/SSD] (Fig. 43.2).
  - Couch angle to make superior edge of spine field parallel to inferior border of cranial field = atan [(1/2 cranial field length)/SAD] (Fig. 43.3).

ELECTRON DOSE DISTRIBUTIONS

- Unlike photons, electrons deposit most of their dose at the surface. Also unlike photons, as the energy of electrons increases, the percentage of dose deposited at the surface increases.
- The 4:3:2 rule for electrons refers to the fact that the 90% isodose line for electrons is generally ≃MeV/4, the 80% isodose line is generally ≃MeV/3, and the effective range of electrons is ≃MeV/2.
- The amount of Pb shielding required for electrons may be estimated as MeV/2 (in mm).

ICRU DEFINITIONS

- Gross tumor volume (GTV): gross tumor by physical exam and/or imaging, including primary tumor, metastatic lymphadenopathy, or other metastases.

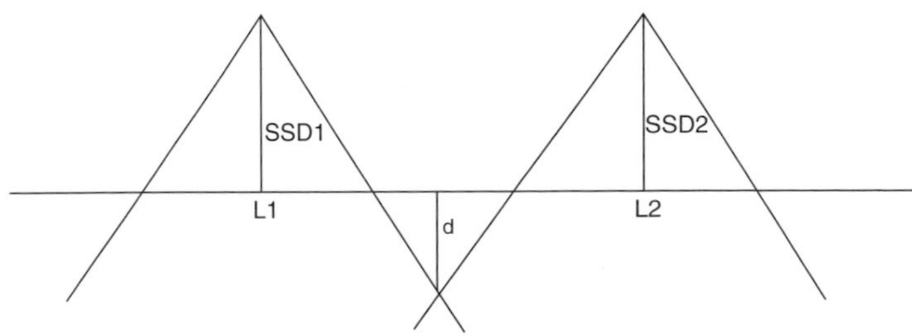

Fig. 43.1 Diagram for skin gap formula

XII

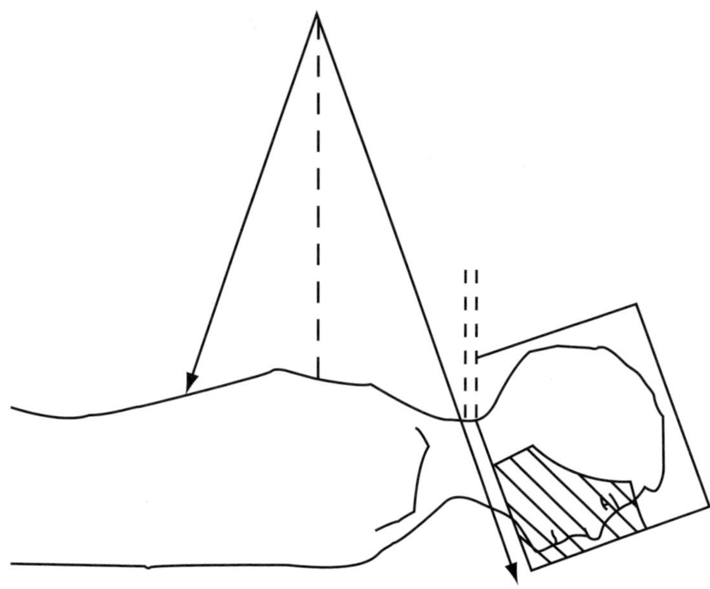

Fig. 43.2 Diagram of collimator angle of cranial field used to match divergence of spine field

- Clinical target volume (CTV): tissue volume that contains GTV and area at risk of subclinical microscopic disease.
- Internal margin (IM): may be added to CTV to compensate for internal physiological movement and variation in size, shape, or position of the CTV, such as related to filling of bladder or respiratory movement.
- Internal target volume (ITV): volume encompassing the CTV and IM (ITV = CTV + IM).
- Planning target volume (PTV): PTV = CTV + IM + setup margin (SM) for setup uncertainty. The penumbra of the beam(s) is not considered when delineating the PTV. However, when selecting beam sizes, the width of the penumbra has to be taken into account and the beam size adjusted accordingly.
- Organs at risk (OAR): normal tissues whose radiation sensitivity may significantly influence treatment planning and/or the prescribed dose.
- Planning organ at risk volume (PRV): analogous to PTV for OAR. PRV = OAR + IM + SM.

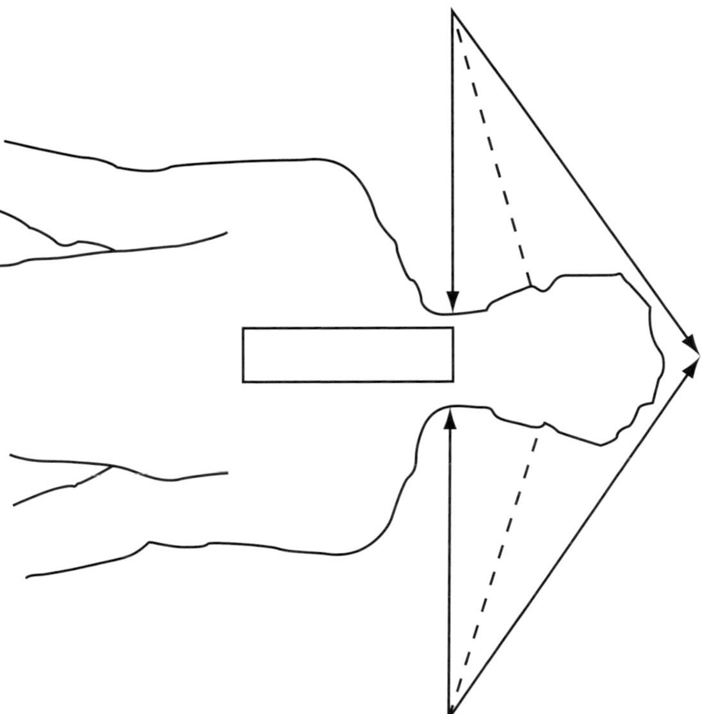

Fig. 43.3 Diagram of couch angle to make superior edge of spine field parallel to inferior border of cranial field

- Treated volume: volume enclosed by an isodose surface (e.g., 95% isodose), selected and specified by radiation oncologist as being appropriate to achieve the purpose of treatment. Ideally, treated volume would be identical to PTV, but may also be considerably larger than PTV.
- Irradiated volume: tissue volume receives a dose that is considered significant in relation to normal tissue tolerance. Dose should be expressed either in absolute values or relative to the specified dose to the PTV.

Acknowledgments Special thanks to Paula Petti and John Murnane for their Physics and Radiobiology teaching, which assisted in the preparation of this chapter.

FURTHER READING

Hall EJ, Amato JC. *Radiobiology for the Radiologist*. 6th ed. Philadelphia: Lippincott Williams & Wilkins, 2006.

ICRU. ICRU Report 50 – Prescribing, Recording and Reporting Photon Beam Therapy. *Med Phys* 21(6):833-4, 1994.

ICRU. *Prescribing, Recording and Reporting Photon Beam Therapy (Supplement to ICRU Report 50), ICRU Report 62*. Bethesda: ICRU, 1999.

ICRU. *Prescribing, Recording and Reporting Photon Beam Therapy (Supplement to ICRU Report 50), ICRU Report 62*. Bethesda: ICRU, 1999.

Kahn, FM. *The Physics of Radiation Therapy*. 3rd ed. Philadelphia: Lippincott Williams & Wilkins, 2003.

Appendices

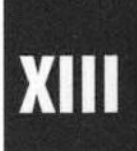

APPENDIX A: PERFORMANCE STATUS SCALES

KARNOFSKY PERFORMANCE STATUS

100	Normal; no complaints; no evidence of disease
90	Able to carry on normal activity; minor signs or symptoms of disease
80	Normal activity with effort; some signs or symptoms of disease
70	Cares for self; unable to carry on normal activity or to do active work
60	Requires occasional assistance, but is able to care for most of his/her personal needs
50	Requires considerable assistance and frequent medical care
40	Disabled; requires special care and assistance
30	Severely disabled; hospital admission is indicated although death not imminent
20	Very sick; hospital admission necessary; active support treatment necessary
10	Moribund; fatal processes progressing rapidly
0	Dead

From Karnofsky D, Abelman W, Craver L, Burchenal J. The use of nitrogen mustards in the palliative treatment of carcinoma. Cancer 1948;1:634-656, with permission.

ECOG PERFORMANCE STATUS

0	Fully active, able to carry on all pre-disease performance without restriction
1	Restricted in physically strenuous activity but ambulatory and able to carry out work of a light or sedentary nature (e.g., light house work, office work)
2	Ambulatory and capable of all self-care but unable to carry out any work activities. Up and about more than 50% of waking hours

3	Capable of only limited self-care, confined to bed or chair more than 50% of waking hours
4	Completely disabled. Cannot carry on any self-care. Totally confined to bed or chair
5	Dead

From Oken MM, Creech RH, Tormey DC, et al. Toxicity and Response Criteria of The Eastern Cooperative Oncology Group. Am J Clin Oncol 1982;5:649-655, with permission

APPENDIX B: COMMONLY PRESCRIBED DRUGS

SKIN

Name	Use	Dose	Comments
Aquaphor (OTC)	Dry desquamation	Apply b.i.d.–t.i.d.	Original ointment (14 oz jar) or healing ointment (1.75 oz tube or 3.5 oz jar)
Eucerin (OTC)	Dry desquamation	Apply prn	Lotion 4–16 oz, Cream 2–16 oz
Hydrocortisone (OTC)	Dry desquamation	Apply q.i.d.	0.5–1%
Dermoplast (OTC) topical anesthetic	Dry desquamation	Apply t.i.d.	Spray (2 and 2.75 oz) or lotion (3 oz)
Desonide (tridesilon)	Dry-moist desquamation	Apply b.i.d.–t.i.d.	0.05% cream
Domeboro soaks (OTC)	Moist desquamation	Moist soak 20 min t.i.d.–q.i.d.	Dissolve one tablet or packet in 1 pint water
Aquaphor/xylocaine 5% ointment	Moist desquamation	Apply t.i.d.	Pharmacist mix 1:1
Neosporin (neomycin, polymixin B, bacitracin; OTC)	Moist desquamation	Apply b.i.d.–q.i.d.	Cream (7.5 g)
Bacitracin	Moist desquamation	Apply b.i.d.–t.i.d.	Ointment (30 g)
Silvadene creme 1%	Moist desquamation	Apply t.i.d.	Tube (20 or 85 g) or jar (50, 400, and 1,000 g)
Telfa (OTC nonadhesive pads)	Moist desquamation	Apply prn	
Hydrogel wound dressings (e.g., Vigilon, Radicare, Geliperm)	Moist desquamation	Apply prn	

Pentoxifylline (trental)	Ulceration	400 mg po t.i.d.	Avoid if recent cerebral bleed or retinal hemorrhage. If GI or CNS side effects, decrease to 400 mg b.i.d.; if they persist, discontinue
Clotrimazole topical 1%	Yeast infection	Apply b.i.d.	12, 24 g tubes
Fluconazole	Yeast infection	200 mg po ×1, then 100 mg po qd ×14 days	
Acyclovir	Herpes	200 mg po 5×/day × 10 days for herpes infections. For zoster, 800 mg po 5×/day × 7–10 days	
Valacyclovir	Herpes	500 mg po b.i.d. × 3 days (recurrent)	
Diphenhydramine (benadryl; OTC)	Pruritis	25–50 mg po q6h	
Hydroxyzine (vistaril)	Pruritis	25 mg po t.i.d.–q.i.d.	

Drug selection, method and duration of administration, and dosage should be verified by the reader with the most current product information provided by the manufacturer.

HEAD AND NECK

Name	Use	Dose	Comments
Cortisporin ophthalmic	Conjunctivitis or keratitis	Apply ointment or 1–2 gtts suspension q3–4h	Contraindicated for viral infections or ulcerative keratitis and after foreign body removal. Do not use for more than 5–10 days. Caution if glaucoma
Lacrilube (OTC)	Dry eye	Apply qhs	
Saline solutions (OTC)	Dry eye	Apply prn	
Proparacaine hydrochloride 5%	Topical anesthetic for conjunctiva	2 gtts	Use care when manipulating eye because abrasions will not be felt
Auralgan (benzocaine/antipyrine otic)	Otic analgesic	2–4 gtt OTIC q.i.d. prn	Contraindicated if perforated tympanic membrane
Cortisporin otic suspension	External otitis	4 gtts OTIC q6h × 7–10 days	
Diphenhydramine (benadryl; OTC)	Antihistamine, sedating	25–50 mg po q4–6h	
Loratadine (OTC; claritin)	Antihistamine, nonsedating	10 mg po qd	
Pseudoephedrine (OTC)	Decongestant	30–60 mg po q4–6h prn	Max. 240 mg/day
Dextromethorphan/guaifenesin	Antitussive/expectorant	1–2 tablets po b.i.d. or 10 mL po q4h	Tablets 30/600 or solution 10/100/5 mL. Max. 4 tablets/day or 60 mL/day
Ibuprofen (OTC)	Parotitis	600 mg po t.i.d.	Should resolve rapidly after first several treatments
Ulcerease (OTC)	Apthous ulcers, mucositis	Rinse or gargle prn. Do not swallow	6 oz bottle

"Triple mix," "Magic mouthwash," "BLM mouthwash" (benadryl elixir, viscous lidocaine 2%, maalox)	Mucositis	2 tsp po 10 min ac and qhs. Swish and spit prn	Pharmacist mix 1:1:1 in a 600 mL bottle. Swallow no more than 8 tsp/day
Sucralfate	Mucositis	2 tsp swish and swallow q.i.d.	Suspension 1 g/10mL. Do not use within 30 min of lidocaine (interferes with binding)
Fluconazole	Candidiasis	200 mg po ×1, then 100 mg po qd × 14 days	
Nystatin suspension	Candidiasis	5 mL swish and swallow q.i.d.	Continue 2 days postsymptom resolution
Amifostine (ethylol)	Xerostomia	200 mg/m² IV qd over 3 min, 15–30 min before RT	Monitor BP
Artificial saliva (OTC)	Xerostomia	Apply prn	e.g., Salivart, xerolube, saliva substitute
Baking soda mouthwash (OTC)	Xerostomia	1–3 tsp swish and spit prn	Mix 1 tsp baking soda, 1 tsp salt, 1 quart water
Fluoride carriers	Xerostomia		Arrange via dental consultation
Pilocarpine (salagen)	Xerostomia	5–10 mg po t.i.d.	Requires some salivary function. Max. 30 mg/day. Caution if asthma, glaucoma, liver dysfunction, cardiovascular disease, COPD
Cevimeline (evoxac)	Xerostomia	30 mg po t.i.d.	Max. 90 mg/day. Similar cautions as pilocarpine

Drug selection, method and duration of administration, and dosage should be verified by the reader with the most current product information provided by the manufacturer .

LUNG

Name	Use	Dose	Comments
Albuterol	Asthma	2 puffs q4h prn	
Dextromethorphan/guaifenesin (OTC)	Antitussive/ expectorant	1–2 tablets po b.i.d. or 10 mL po q4h	Tablets 30/600 or solution 10/100/5 mL. Max. 4 tablets/ day or 60 mL/day
Benzonatate (tessalon Perles)	Cough	100–200 mg po t.i.d.	Max. 600 mg/day
Tylenol with codeine (300/30)	Cough	1–2 tablets po q4h prn	Max. 12 tablets/day
Ibuprofen (OTC)	Mild radiation pneumonitis	600–800 mg po q6–8h	
Prednisone	Radiation pneumonitis	1 mg/kg at diagnosis with slow taper over weeks	
Beclomethasone	Radiation pneumonitis	2 puffs q.i.d. or 4 puffs b.i.d.	May help reduce systemic steroid dose
Methylprednisolone (solu-medrol)	Status asthmaticus	0.5–1 mg/kg IV q6h	Start 2 mg/kg

Drug selection, method and duration of administration, and dosage should be verified by the reader with the most current product information provided by the manufacturer.

BREAST

Name	Use	Dose	Comments
Tamoxifen (nolvadex)	Breast cancer	10 mg po b.i.d. or 20 mg qd	Binds to estrogen receptors, producing estrogenic and antiestrogenic effects
Raloxifene (evista)	Breast cancer	60 mg po qd	Selective estrogen receptor modulator
Anastrozole (arimidex)	Breast cancer, postmenopausal	1 mg po qd	Aromatase inhibitor, nonsteroidal
Letrozole (femara)	Breast cancer, postmenopausal	2.5 mg po qd	Aromatase inhibitor, nonsteroidal
Exemestane (aromasin)	Breast cancer, postmenopausal	25 mg po qd	Aromatase inhibitor, steroidal
Fulvestrant (faslodex)	Breast cancer, metastatic	250 mg IM q month	Binds to estrogen receptors (ER), downregulates ER protein, producing antiestrogenic effects
Megestrol (megace)	Breast cancer, palliative	40 mg po q.i.d.	Progestin
Clonidine	Hot flashes	0.1 mg po b.i.d.	Antihypertensive, watch for rebound hypertension
Venlafaxine (effexor)	Hot flashes	50–75 mg po qhs	
Paroxetine (paxil)	Hot flashes	20 mg po qd	

Drug selection, method and duration of administration, and dosage should be verified by the reader with the most current product information provided by the manufacturer.

GASTROINTESTINAL

Name	Use	Dose	Comments
Triple mix (benadryl elixir, maalox, viscous lidocaine 2%)	Esophagitis	2 tsp po 10 min ac and qhs. Swish and spit prn	Pharmacist mix 1:1:1 in a 600 mL bottle. Swallow no more than 8 tsp/day
Miracle mouthwash	Esophagitis	Mix 60 mL tetracycline oral suspension (125 mg/5 mL), 30 mL mycostatin oral suspension (100,000 U/mL), 30 mL hydrocortisone oral suspension (10 mg/5 mL), and 240 mL benadryl solution (12.5 mg/5 mL)	
Sucralfate	Esophagitis	2 tsp swish and swallow q.i.d.	Suspension 1 g/10 mL. Do not use within 30 min of lidocaine (interferes with binding)
Fluconazole	Candidiasis	200 mg po × 1, then 100 mg po qd ×14 days	
Mylanta (aluminum, magnesium, and simethicone; OTC)	Dyspepsia, flatulence	15–30 mL po q.i.d. prn	200/200/20 per 5 mL susp (1 bottle = 355 or 710 mL)
Famotidine (pepcid; OTC)	GERD	20 mg po b.i.d.	
Omeprazole (prilosec; OTC)	GERD	20–40 mg po qd	
Megestrol (megace) suspension	Appetite stimulant	400–800 mg po qd	
Dronabinol (marinol)	Appetite stimulant	2.5 mg po b.i.d.	
Chlorpromazine (thorazine)	Hiccups	25–50 mg po t.i.d.–q.i.d.	
Metoclopramide (reglan)	Gastroparesis N/V	10 mg po qac, qhs 5–10 mg po/IV q6–8h prn	Give 30 min before meals
Prochlorperazine (compazine)	N/V	5–10 mg po q6–8h	
Promethazine (phenergan)	N/V	12.5–25 mg po/pr/IV q4–6h	
Ondansetron (zofran)	N/V	8 mg po t.i.d.	First dose 1–2 h before RT

Granisetron (kytril)	N/V	2 mg po ×1 or 1 mg po q12h	
Palonosetron (aloxi)	N/V	0.5 mg po ×1	
Dolasetron (anzemet)	N/V	100 mg po × 1	
Lorazepam (ativan)	N/V	Anticipitory: 1–2 mg po 45 min before treatment. Adjunct: 0.5–1 mg po t.i.d.	
Simethicone	Flatulence	80–120 mg po qac and qhs	Max. 480 mg/day. Chew tablets before swallowing
Loperamide (imodium; OTC)	Diarrhea	4 mg ×1, then 2 mg po after each unformed stool	Max. 16 mg/day
Atropine/diphenoxylate (lomotil)	Diarrhea	1–2 tablets po t.i.d.–q.i.d. prn	Max. 8 tablets/day
Bismuth subsalicylate (pepto-bismol; OTC)	Diarrhea	2 tablets po q1h prn	Max. 4,200 mg/day
Metamucil	Constipation	1–3 tsp in juice qd with meals	Bulking agent
Colace	Constipation	100 mg po b.i.d.	Stool softener
Bisacodyl (dulcolax)	Constipation	10 mg po or pr	Laxative
Senna	Constipation	2–4 tablets po qd – b.i.d.	Stool softener and laxative
Fleet enema	Constipation	1–2 as directed pr prn	
Anusol HC (hydrocortisone)	Perianal pain Proctitis	1–2.5%, apply q.i.d.25 mg supp pr b.i.d.–t.i.d.	
Hydrocortisone enema	Proctitis	1 pr qhs, retain for 1 h	
Proctofoam HC 2.5%	Proctitis	Apply pr t.i.d.–q.i.d.	

Drug selection, method and duration of administration, and dosage should be verified by the reader with the most current product information provided by the manufacturer.

GENITOURINARY

Name	Use	Dose	Comments
Phenazopyridine (pyridium)	Dysuria	200 mg po t.i.d.–q.i.d.	Urine turns orange
Tolterodine (detrol)	Bladder spasm	2 mg po b.i.d.	Anticholinergic
Flavoxate (urispas)	Bladder spasm	100–200 mg po t.i.d.–q.i.d.	Anticholinergic
Oxybutynin (ditropan)	Bladder spasm	5 mg po b.i.d.–t.i.d.	Anticholinergic
Finasteride (Proscar)	BPH	5 mg po qd	Type-2 alpha reductase inhibitor
Dutasteride (avodart)	BPH	0.5 mg po qd	Type-1 and -2 alpha reductase inhibitor
Doxazosin (cardura)	Bladder outlet obstruction	1–8 mg po qd (start 1)	Alpha-1 blocker
Terazosin (hytrin)	Bladder outlet obstruction	1–10 mg po qhs (start 1)	Alpha-1 blocker
Tamsulosin (flomax)	Bladder outlet obstruction	0.4–0.8 mg po qd	Selective alpha-1a blocker
Alfuzosin (uroxatral)	Bladder outlet obstruction	10 mg po qd	Selective alpha-1a blocker
Trimethoprim/ sulfamethoxazole	Urinary tract infection	1 DS tablet po b.i.d. × 5–7 days	
Ciprofloxacin	Urinary tract infection	250 mg po b.i.d. × 3–7 days	
Sildenafil (viagra)	Erectile dysfunction	25–50 mg po × 1	Max. 100 mg. Contraindicated with nitrates. Caution if HTN, cardiovascular disease

Tadalafil (cialis)	Erectile dysfunction	10 mg po ×1	Lasts up to 36 h, max. 20 mg. Contraindicated with nitrates, alpha-blockers. Caution if HTN, cardiovascular disease
Vardenafil (levitra)	Erectile dysfunction	5–10 mg po × 1	Max. 20 mg. Contraindicated with nitrates, alpha-blockers. Caution if HTN, cardiovascular disease
Bicalutamide (casodex)	Prostate cancer	50 mg po qd	Antiandrogen. Monitor LFTs at baseline, every month × 4
Flutamide (eulixen)	Prostate cancer	250 mg po q8h	Antiandrogen. Monitor LFTs every month × 4
Leuprolide (lupron)	Prostate cancer	Depot (1 month = 7.5 mg, 3 months = 22.5 mg, 4 months = 30 mg)	Gonadotropin-releasing hormone analog, inhibits gonadotropin release
Goserelin (zoladex)	Prostate cancer	Depot (1 month = 3.6 mg, 3 months = 10.8 mg)	Gonadotropin-releasing hormone analog, inhibits gonadotropin release
Pentoxifylline (trental)	Chronic hematuria or radiation cystitis	400 mg po t.i.d.	Avoid if recent cerebral bleed or retinal hemorrhage. If GI or CNS side effects, decrease to 400 mg b.i.d.; if they persist, discontinue
Vitamin E (tocopherol)	Chronic hematuria or radiation cystitis	1,000 IU po qd	

Drug selection, method and duration of administration, and dosage should be verified by the reader with the most current product information provided by the manufacturer.

GYNECOLOGIC

Name	Use	Dose	Comments
Replens vaginal moisturizer (OTC)	Vaginitis	One applicator full q2–3 days prn	
Premarin vaginal cream	Atrophic vaginitis	1/2–2 g PV 1–3×/weeks	Conjugated estrogens
Metronidazole	Bacterial vaginitis	500 mg po b.i.d. × 7 days	
Fluconazole	Candidiasis	150 mg po ×1; if refractory, 100 mg po qd ×14 days	
Miconazole	Candidiasis	1 supp qhs ×3 or cream qhs × 7 days	

Drug selection, method and duration of administration, and dosage should be verified by the reader with the most current product information provided by the manufacturer.

NERVOUS SYSTEM

Name	Use	Dose	Comments
Dexamethasone (decadron)	Brain or tumor edema	RT induced: 2–6 mg po q6–8h; tumor induced: 10–25 mg IV ×1, then 4–10 mg po/IV q6 h; impending herniation: as high as 100 mg IV ×1, then 25 mg IV q6h	
Meclizine	Vertigo	25–50 mg po qd	
Scopolamine patch	Vertigo	Apply behind ear, 1 patch q3 days	
Phenytoin (dilantin)	Seizure	300–400 mg po div qd – t.i.d.	Monitor therapeutic levels
Carbamazepine (tegretol)	Seizure Trigeminal neuralgia	800–1,200 mg po div b.i.d.–q.i.d. Start 200 mg b.i.d.200–400 mg po b.i.d.	Monitor therapeutic levels
Phenobarbital	Seizure	60 mg po b.i.d–t.i.d.	Monitor therapeutic levels
Levetiracetam (keppra)	Seizure	500–1,500 mg po q12h, start at 500 mg q12h, max. 3,000 mg/day, taper gradually to discontinue	
Gabapentin (neurontin)	Seizure, neuropathic pain	300–1,200 mg po t.i.d.	

Drug selection, method and duration of administration, and dosage should be verified by the reader with the most current product information provided by the manufacturer.

PSYCHIATRIC

Name	Use	Dose	Comments
Lorazepam (ativan)	Anxiety	0.5–2 mg po/IV q6–8h prn	
Haldol (haloperidol)	Agitation, psychosis	0.5–5 mg po/IM q1–4h	
Temazepam (restoril)	Insomnia	7.5–30 mg po qhs	Short-term treatment
Ambien (zolpidem)	Insomnia	5–10 mg po qhs	Short-term treatment
Trazodone	Insomnia	25–50 mg po qhs	

Drug selection, method and duration of administration, and dosage should be verified by the reader with the most current product information provided by the manufacturer.

Name	Use	Dose	Comments
Acetominophen (OTC)	Mild–moderate	325–1,000 mg po q4–6h prn	Max. 1 g/dose, 4 g/day
Aspirin (OTC)	Mild–moderate	325–650 mg po q4h prn	Max. 4 g/day
Ibuprofen (motrin; OTC)	Mild–moderate	200–800 mg po q4–6h prn	Max. 3,200 mg/day
Naproxen (naprosyn)	Mild–moderate	250–500 mg po b.i.d.	Max. 1,500 mg/day
Celecoxib (celebrex)	Mild–moderate	200 mg po qd	
Codeine	Mild–moderate	15–60 mg po qd	Max. 60 mg/dose, 360 mg/day
Acetaminophen/codeine (Tylenol #2, #3, #4)	Mild–moderate	1–2 tablets po q4–6h prn	300 mg/15, 30, or 60 mg
Hydrocodone/ acetaminophen (vicodin, lortab elixir)	Moderate–severe	1–2 tablets po q4–6h prn 5–15 mL po q4–6h prn	5/500 mg or ES 7.5/750 mg 7.5/500 mg per 15 mL
Oxycodone	Moderate–severe	5–30 mg po q4h prn	5, 15, 30 mg tablets
Oxycodone/acetaminophen (percocet)	Moderate–severe	1–2 tablets po q4–6h prn	2.5/325, 5/325, 7.5/325, 10/325, 7.5/500, or 10/650 mg
Oxycontin	Moderate–severe	10–160 mg po b.i.d. prn	10, 20, 40, 80 mg tablets. Start 10 mg b.i.d.
Morphine	Moderate–severe	10–30 mg po q3–4h prn 2.5–10 mg IV q2–6h prn	10, 15, 30 mg tablets
MS Contin	Moderate–severe	15–30 mg po q8–12h prn	15, 30, 60, 100, 200 mg tablets
Morphine elixir (roxanol)	Moderate–severe	10–30 mg po q4h	20 mg/mL solution
Fentanyl transdermal (duragesic)	Moderate–severe	25–100 μg/h patch q72h	For opiate tolerant patients. Start 25 μg
Fentanyl oral transmucosal (actiq)	Moderate–severe	1 unit po prn	For opiate tolerant patients. Start 200 μg, titrate up to 1,600 μg. Dissolve in mouth, do not chew or swallow

continued

Name	Use	Dose	Comments
Cyclobenzaprine (flexeril)	Muscle spasm	5–10 mg po tid	Therapy should be limited to 3 weeks maximum
Pamidronate (aredia)	Bone mets	90 mg IV q 3–4 weeks	Monitor renal function. Dental exam prior to treatment
Zoledronic acid (zometa)	Bone mets	4 mg IV q 3–4 weeks	Monitor renal function. Dental exam prior to treatment

Drug selection, method and duration of administration, and dosage should be verified by the reader with the most current product information provided by the manufacturer.

MISCELLANEOUS

Name	Use	Dose	Comments
Epinephrine	Anaphylaxis	0.1–0.5 mg SC (1:1,000) q10–15 min or 0.1–0.25 mg IV (1:10,000) over 5–10 min	For urticaria, give benadryl 25–50 mg. For hypotension, add IV fluids, elevate legs, and add O_2. May need atropine 0.6 mg IV push (repeat up to 3 mg total)
Diphenhydramine (benadryl)	Anaphylaxis	25–50 mg PO/IV q6–8h	Max. 100 mg/dose, 400 mg/day

Drug selection, method and duration of administration, and dosage should be verified by the reader with the most current product information provided by the manufacturer.

APPENDIX C: INTRAVASCULAR CONTRAST SAFETY

IDENTIFY PATIENTS AT INCREASED RISK FOR WHOM LOW-OSMOLALITY CONTRAST MEDIA IS PREFERRED

- History of prior contrast reaction.
- Asthma.
- Prior severe allergic reactions to other materials.
- Patients with congestive heart failure, dysrhythmia, unstable angina, recent myocardial infarction, pulmonary HTN.
- Renal insufficiency (particularly with diabetes).
- Diabetes melitus.
- Metformin – must be discontinued at the time of exam and not re-started until renal function re-evaluated 48 h exam.
- Multiple myeloma (due to paraprotein renal insufficiency).
- Sickle cell.
- Pheochromocytoma.
- Myasthenia gravis.

PREMEDICATION REGIMEN FOR AT-RISK PATIENTS WHO REQUIRE IV CONTRAST ADMINISTRATION

- Encourage good oral or IV hydration for at least 12 h before and after injection.
- Prednisone 50 mg po at 13 h, 7 h, and 1 h before contrast medium injection.
- Benadryl 50 mg po or IV 1 h before contrast medium injection.
- Use nonionic low osmolatity contrast medium.

MANAGEMENT OF ACUTE REACTIONS IN ADULTS

- *Urticaria*: Stop the injection. Give diphenhydramine PO/IM/IV 25–50 mg. If severe urticaria, give epinephrine SC (1:1,000) 0.1–0.3 mL (=0.1–0.3 mg) if no cardiac contraindications.
- *Facial or laryngeal edema*: Assess patient. Give oxygen via mask. Start at 6–10 L/min. Give epinephrine SC or IM (1:1,000)

0.1–0.3 mL (=0.1–0.3 mg). If hypotension present, give epinephrine (1:10,000) slowly IV 1–3 mL (=0.1–0.3 mg). Repeat up to 1 mg as needed. If not responsive, call for assistance (e.g., cardiopulmonary arrest code team).

- *Bronchospasm*: Assess patient. Give oxygen via mask. Start at 6–10 L/min. Monitor vital signs. Give bronchodilator (e.g., Albuterol 2–3 puffs). If unresponsive to inhaler, use epinephrine as above. If not responsive or oxygen saturation persists <88%, call for assistance (e.g., code team).
- *Hypotension*: Assess patient. Elevate legs or Trendeleburg position. Give oxygen via mask at 6–10 L/min. Monitor vital signs, pulse oximetry, ECG. Secure IV access and administer IV fluids (normal saline or Ringer's lactate). If persistent bradycardia, administer atropine 0.6–1 mg IV slowly. If poorly responsive, call for assistance (e.g., code team). Ensure complete resolution of hypotension prior to discharge.
- *Hypertension*: Assess patient. Give oxygen via mask at 6–10 L/min. Monitor vital signs, pulse oximetry, ECG. Give sublingual nitroglycerine 0.4 mg (may repeat ×3). If no response, consider labetalol 20 mg IV. If poorly responsive, call for assistance (e.g., code team) or transfer to Emergency Department.
- *Seizures or convulsions*: Assess patient. Give oxygen via mask at 6–10 L/min. Monitor vital signs, pulse oximetry. Consider diazepam 5 mg IV or midazolam 0.5–1 mg IV. If poorly responsive, call for assistance (e.g., code team) or transfer to Emergency Department.
- *Pulmonary edema*: Assess patient. Elevate torso. Give oxygen via mask at 6–10 L/min. Monitor vital signs, pulse oximetry. Consider furosemide 20–40 mg IV slowly, morphine 1–3 mg. Call for assistance (e.g., code team) or transfer to Emergency Department.

Abbreviations

3D	3-dimensional
3DCRT	3-dimensional conformal radiotherapy
5-FU	5-flourouracil
AA	Anaplastic astrocytoma
ABMT	Autologous bone marrow transplant
abstr.	Abstract
ACS	American Cancer Society
ACTH	Adrenocorticotropic hormone
ADR	Doxorubicin
AFP	Alpha fetoprotein
AIDS	Acquired immune deficiency syndrome
AMD	Dactinomycin
AML	Acute myeloid leukemia
AP	Anterior-posterior
APR	Abdominoperineal resection
ASCO	American Society of Clinical Oncology
ASTRO	American Society for Therapeutic Radiology and Oncology
BCC	Basal cell carcinoma
BCG	Bacillus Calmette-Guerin
bPFS	Biochemical progression-free survival
BUN	Blood urea nitrogen
c	Cycles (e.g., =for two cycles)
ca	Cancer
CALGB	Cancer and Leukemia Group B
CBC	Complete blood count
cCR	Clinical complete response
CESS	German Cooperative Ewing's Sarcoma Study
cGy	CentiGray
Chemo	Chemotherapy
Chemo-RT	Chemo-radiotherapy
CHOP	Cyclophosphamide, doxorubicine, vincristine, & prednisone

CIS	Carcinoma in situ
CN	Cranial nerve (e.g., CN X)
COG	Children's Oncology Group
CR	Complete response
Cr	Creatinine
CR	Complete response
CSF	Cerebrospinal fluid
CSI	Craniospinal irradiation
CSS	Cause-specific survival
CT	Computed tomography
CTV1	Clinical target volume 1
CTV2	Clinical target volume 2
Cu	Copper
CXR	Chest X-ray
CY	Cyclophosphamide
D&C	Dilation and curettage
DCIS	Ductal carcinoma in situ
DES	Diethylstibestrol
DFS	Disease-free survival
DLBCL	Diffuse large B cell lymphoma
DLCO	Diffusing capacity
DM	Distant metastases
Dmax	Maximum dose
DRE	Digital rectal exam
DRR	Digitally-reconstructed radiograph
DSS	Disease specific survival
DVH	Dose-volume histogram
EBCTCG	Early Breast Cancer Trialists' Collaborative Group
EBRT	External beam radiation therapy
EBV	Epstein–Barr virus
ECE	Extracapsular extension
ECOG	Eastern Cooperative Oncology Group
EFS	Event-free survival
EFRT	Extended field radiotherapy
EGD	Esophogastroduodenoscopy
EORTC	European Organisation for Research and Treatment of Cancer
EPID	Electronic portal imaging device
ERCP	Endoscopic retrograde cholangiopancreatography
ESR	Erythrocyte sedimentation rate
ETE	Extra-thyroid extension
EtOH	Alcohol
EUA	Exam under anesthesia

EUS	Endoscopic ultrasound
FEV1	Forced expiratory volume in 1 second
FFF	Freedom from failure
FFP	Freedom from progression
FFS	Failure-free survival
FH	Family history
FOBT	Fecal occult blood test
fx	Fraction(s)
GBM	Glioblastoma multiforme
GERD	Gastroesophageal reflux disease
GHSG	German Hodgkin's Study Group
GS	Gleason score
GTR	Gross total resection
GTV	Gross tumor volume
GU	Genitourinary
Gy	Gray
H&N	Head and neck
H&P	History and physical exam
hCG	Human chorionic gonadotropin
HCV	Hepatitis C virus
HDR	High dose rate
HIV	Human immunodeficiency virus
HNPCC	Hereditary non-polyposis colon cancer
HPV	Human papilloma virus
HTN	Hypertension
HVL	Half-value layer
Hx	History
IC	Intracavitary
IDL	Isodose line
IESS	Intergroup Ewing's Sarcoma Study
IE	Ifosfamide and etoposide (VP-16)
IFN	Interferon
IFRT	Involved-field radiation therapy
IGRT	Image-guided radiotherapy
IJROBP	*International Journal of Radiation Oncology Biology Physics*
IMRT	Intensity modulated radiotherapy
INSS	International Neuroblastoma Staging System
Int	Intergroup
IORT	Intraoperative radiation therapy
IS	Interstitial
IVC	Inferior vena cava
IVP	Intravenous pyelogram

JCO	*Journal of Clinical Oncology*
JPA	Juvenile pilocytic astrocytoma
LAR	Low anterior resection
LC	Local control
LCSG	Lung Cancer Study Group
LDH	Lactate dehydrogenase
LDR	Low dose rate
LF	Local failure
LFTs	Liver function tests
LN	Lymph node(s)
LND	Lymph node dissection
LR	Local recurrence/relapse
LRC	Local-regional control
LRF	Local-regional failure
LVEF	Left ventricular ejection fraction
LVSI	Lymphovascular space invasion
MALT	Mucosa associated lymphoid tissue
MFH	Malignant fibrous histiosarcoma
mm	millimeter
MRC	Medical Research Council
MRI	Magnetic resonance imaging
MRSI	Magnetic resonance spectroscopy imaging
MS	Median survival
MUGA	Multiple gated acquisition scan
N0	Node negative
N+	Node positive
NCCN	National Comprehensive Cancer Network (www.nccn.org)
NCI	National Cancer Institute
NCIC	National Cancer Institute of Canada
NED	No evidence of disease
NEJM	New England Journal of Medicine
NHL	Non-Hodgkin's Lymphoma
NPV	Negative predictive value
NPX	Nasopharynx
NSABP	National Surgical Adjuvant Breast and Bowel Project
NSCLC	Non-small cell lung cancer
NSGCT	Non-seminomatous germ cell tumor
NWTS	National Wilms' Tumor Study
OPX	Oropharynx
OS	Overall survival
PA	Posterior-anterior
Pb	Lead

pCR	Pathologic complete response
PET	Positron emission tomography
PLAP	Placental alkaline phosphatase
PNET	Primitive neuroectodermal tumor
PNI	Perineural invasion
Post-op	Post-operative
PPV	Positive predictive value
PR	Partial response
Pre-op	Pre-operative
PS	Performance status
PSA	Prostate specific antigen
PTV	Planning target volume
PUVA	Psoralen and ultraviolet light A
QOL	Quality of life
RAI	Radioactive iodine
RBE	Relative biological effectiveness
RCC	Renal cell carcinoma
RFS	Relapse-free survival
RP	Radical prostatectomy
RT	Radiation therapy
RTOG	Radiation Therapy Oncology Group
S/P	Status post
SCC	Squamous cell carcinoma
SCID	Severe combined immunodeficiency
SCLC	Small cell lung cancer
SCV	Supraclavicular
SI	Sacroiliac
SIADH	Syndrome of inappropriate antidiuretic hormone
SPEP	Serum protein electrophoreses
SRS	Stereotactic radiosurgery
STD	Sexually transmitted disease
STLI	Subtotal lymphoid irradiation
STR	Subtotal resection
SWOG	Southwest Oncology Group
T&O	Tandem & Ovoid
TAH/BSO	Total abdominal hysterectomy / bilateral salpingo-oophorectomy
TBI	Total body irradiation
TCC	Transitional cell carcinoma
TMP/SMX	Trimethoprim/sulfamethoxazole
TNM	Tumor Node Metastasis
TRUS	Transrectal ultrasound
TSH	Thyroid stimulating hormone

TURBT	Transurethral resection of bladder tumor
UA	Urinalysis
UCSF	University of California, San Francisco
UPEP	Urine protein electrophoreses
US	United States of America
US	Ultrasound
USO	Unilateral salpingo-oophorectomy
UVB	Ultraviolet light B
VAC	Vincristine, actinomycin-D, and cyclophosphamide
VDC	Vincristine, doxorubicin, cyclophosphamide
VDCA	Vincristine, doxorubicin, cyclophosphamide, and actinomycin-D
VCR	Vincristine
VP-16	Etoposide
VM	Vincristine and melphalan
WHO	World Health Organization
WLE	Wide local excision

Index

O

S

T